A Comprehensive Guide to **Rehabilitation** of the Older Patient

A Comprehensive Guide to Rehabilitation of the Older Patient

FOURTH EDITION

Edited by

Shane O'Hanlon, MB BCh, BAO, LLB, MSc, MRCPI
Consultant Geriatrician
Department of Geriatric Medicine
St Vincent's University Hospital

Associate Clinical Professor
Department of Medicine
University College Dublin
Dublin
Ireland

Marie Smith, BSc, MSc
Nursing Quality Manager
The Royal Hospital Donnybrook

Honorary Lecturer
RCSI School of Nursing and Midwifery
Dublin
Ireland

Foreword writer

Timothy L. Kauffman, PT, PhD, FAPTA, FGSA
Consultant
Lancaster
Pennsylvania
United States of America

ELSEVIER

First edition 1999
Second edition 2007
Third edition 2014
Fourth edition 2021

Notices

Practitioners and researchers must always rely on their own experience and knowledge in evaluating and using any information, methods, compounds or experiments described herein. Because of rapid advances in the medical sciences, in particular, independent verification of diagnoses and drug dosages should be made. To the fullest extent of the law, no responsibility is assumed by Elsevier, authors, editors or contributors for any injury and/or damage to persons or property as a matter of products liability, negligence or otherwise, or from any use or operation of any methods, products, instructions, or ideas contained in the material herein.

ISBN: 978-0-7020-8016-6

Content Strategist: Poppy Garraway Smith
Content Development Specialist: Fiona Conn/Veronika Watkins
Project Manager: Srividhya Vidhyashankar
Design: Bridget Hoette
Illustration Manager: Narayanan Ramakrishnan
Marketing Manager: Ed Major

With thanks to the British Geriatrics Society for use of the cover image

Printed in Poland
Last digit is the print number: 9 8 7 6 5 4 3 2 1

Working together
to grow libraries in
developing countries

www.elsevier.com • www.bookaid.org

Emily Ainger, BSc, MBBS
Elderly Medicine
Leeds Teaching Hospitals Trust
Leeds
United Kingdom

Sujo Anathhanam, MB BCh, MRCP
Centre for Health of Older People
Leeds Teaching Hospitals NHS Trust
Leeds
United Kingdom

Suzanne Arkill, BMBS, MPhys
Department of Health Sciences
University of Leicester
Leicester
United Kingdom

Simon Conroy, MB BCh, PhD, FRCP
Department of Health Sciences
University of Leicester
Leicester
United Kingdom

Amit Arora, MSc, MD, FRCP
Consultant Geriatrician
Department of Geriatric Medicine
University Hospitals of North Midlands
Newcastle under Lyme
London, United Kingdom

**Terry Aspray, MBBS, MD,
FRCP, FRCP(E)**
Consultant Physician
The Bone Clinic
Freeman Hospital
Newcastle upon Tyne
United Kingdom

Hon Clinical Senior Lecturer
The Medical School
Newcastle University, Newcastle upon Tyne
United Kingdom

**Taranjit Badh, BDS, LLM, MFDS
RCPS (Glasg), Dip Clin Ed**
Senior Community Dentist
Midlands Partnership Foundation NHS Trust
Staffordshire
United Kingdom

Rita Bakhru, MD, MS
Assistant Professor of Medicine
Department of Internal Medicine
Section on Pulmonary, Critical Care,
    Allergy and Immunology
Wake Forest University School of Medicine
Winston-Salem
United States of America

**Anna Bargent, BSc (Biological Sciences),
BSc (Occupational Therapy)**
Frailty Practitioner
Advanced Specialist Occupational Therapist
Royal Berkshire NHS Foundation Trust,
Reading, Berkshire, United Kingdom

Jenny Basran, BSc, MD
Associate Professor of Medicine
Head of the Division of Geriatric Medicine
Saskatchewan Health Authority
University of Saskatchewan
Saskatoon
Canada

Naomi Bates, BSc (Hons)
Advanced Diploma in Dietetic Practice
    (BDA)
Nutrition and Dietetics
St Vincent's University Hospital
Dublin, Ireland

Kate Bennett, BSc, MSc, PGCert
Clinical Lead Physiotherapist
NHS Solent Trust
Southampton, Hampshire
United Kingdom

Robbie Bourke, MB BCh, BAO, MRCPI
Mercer's Institute for Successful Ageing
St James's Hospital
Dublin
Ireland

Giulia Rivasi, MD
Department of Geriatrics and Intensive
    Care Unit
University of Florence and Azienda
    Ospedaliero Universitaria Careggi
Florence
Italy

Rose Anne Kenny, MD
Mercer's Institute for Successful Ageing
St Jame's Hospital
Department of Medical Gerontology
Trinity College Dublin
Dublin
Ireland

Lisa Jane Brighton, BSc (Hons), MSc
Research Assistant
Cicely Saunders Institute of Palliative Care,
    Policy and Rehabilitation
King's College London
London
United Kingdom

Thomas Nathaniel Bryce, MD
Professor
Rehabilitation and Human Performance
Icahn School of Medicine at Mount Sinai,
    New York
New York
United States of America

Elinor Burn, MB BCh, MRCP
Department of Medicine for the Elderly
University Hospitals of Derby and Burton
Derby
United Kingdom

Eileen Burns, MB BCh, MD, FRCP
Centre for the Health of Older People
Leeds Teaching Hospitals
Leeds
United Kingdom

**Elissa Burton, BSc (Hons), MBus,
GradDip (Hlth Econs), PhD**
Senior Research Fellow
School of Physiotherapy and Exercise
    Science
Curtin University
Perth
Australia

Kit Byatt, MBBS, FRCP
Former Consultant
Department of Geriatric Medicine
The County Hospital
Hereford, United Kingdom

Aine Carroll, DPhil, MB BCh, BAO, MD
Professor
Department of Healthcare Integration and
    Improvement

Consultant
Rehabilitation Medicine
University College Dublin
National Rehabilitation Hospital

Professor
School of Medicine
University College Dublin
Dublin
Ireland

**Paul Carroll, MSc, H Dip Musculoskel
Med, H Dip Pall Care, MB BCh,
BAO, MRCP (UK), MRCPI**
Consultant in Rehabilitation Medicine
National Rehabilitation Hospital
The Royal Hospital Donnybrook
St. Vincent's University Hospital
Dublin
Ireland

Lisa Cogan, MSc, MB BCh, MRCPI
Consultant Physician in Geriatric
    Medicine
The Royal Hospital Donnybrook
St. Vincent's University Hospital
Dublin
Ireland

Marie Condon, BSc, MSc
Senior Physiotherapist
Department of Physiotherapy
Cork University Hospital
Cork
Ireland

Deirdre Connolly, PhD, MSc,
PG Dip Stats, Dip COT
Associate Professor in Occupational
    Therapy
Discipline of Occupational Therapy
Trinity College Dublin
Dublin, Ireland

Simon Conroy, MB BCh, PhD
Geriatric Medicine
University Hospitals of Leicester
Leicester
United Kingdom

Lesley Corcoran, BSc (Hons)
Clinical Specialist Physiotherapist in
    Acquired Brain Injury
Department of Physiotherapy
National Rehabilitation Hospital
Dublin
Ireland

Catherine Cornell, BSc (Hons)
Physiotherapy Clinical Specialist (ABI)
Department of Physiotherapy
National Rehabilitation Hospital
Dublin
Ireland

Fiona Craven, BSc
Senior Speech and Language Therapist
Speech & Language Therapy Dept.
HSE, Ireland East Hospital Group
Dublin
Ireland

Morgan Crowe, BAgrSc, PhD,
DSc, MRIA, Dipl ACAP
Consultant Physician in Geriatric
    Medicine
University College of Dublin
Clinical Associate Professor
University College of Dublin
School of Medicine
St Vincent's University and Royal Hospital,
Dublin, Ireland

Consultant Physician in Geriatric Medicine
Medicine for the Elderly
St.Vincents University Hospital
Royal Hospital
Dublin
Ireland

Consultant Physician in Geriatric Medicine
Medicine for the Elderly
St Vincents University Hospital, Dublin.4
Ireland

Consultant Physician in Geriatric Medicine
Department of Medicine for the Elderly
Royal Hospital,
Dublin
Ireland

Clinical Associate Professor
 School of Medicine
University College Dublin
Dublin
Ireland

Vanda Cummins, BSc (Hons), TCD
Senior Physiotherapist
Primary Care Services
HSE
Dublin
Ireland

Clinical Researcher
School of Physiotherapy
Royal College of Surgeons
Dublin
Ireland

Audrey Daisley, BSc, MSc Clin
Psych, DClin Psych C Psychol
Consultant Clinical Neuropsychologist
Lead for Oxford Centre for Enablement
    Clinical Neuropsychology
Psychological Medicine at the Oxford
    Centre for Enablement
Oxford University Hospitals
NHS Foundation Trust
Oxford, United Kingdom

Mary Danoudis, MPhysio,
Applied Science (Physio)
Research physiotherapist
Clinical Research Centre for Movement
    Disorders and Gait
Parkinson's Foundation Centre of
    Excellence
Monash Health, Kingston Centre
Victoria
Australia

Carol de Wilde, BSocSc,
MSocSc (Social Work)
Principal Social Worker
Department of Social Work
St Columcille's Hospital
Loughlinstown, Dublin, Ireland

Brian Dolan, OBE, MSc(Oxon),
MSc(Nurs), RMN, RGN
Professor
Health Service 360
Consultancy, Stratford upon Avon
Warwickshire, United Kingdom

Claire Dow, B.Med.Sci, MBBS, FRCP
Consultant Geriatrician
Older People's Services
Barts Health NHS Trust
London, United Kingdom

Rachael Doyle, BAO, DME, DCE,
DCH, D Obs, MB BCh, MD, FRCPI
Consultant Physician in Geriatric Medicine
Associate Clinical Professor
UCD School of Medicine

Department of Geriatric Medicine
St. Vincent's University Hospital
St Columcille's Hospital
Dublin
Ireland

Sarah Duggan, MSc
Senior Speech and Language Therapist
Department of Speech and Language
    Therapy
Mater Misericordiae University Hospital
Dublin, Ireland

Eoin Fahy, MB BCh, BAO,
BMedSc, MRCPI
Interventional Cardiologist
Cardiology Department
Beaumont Hospital
Dublin
Ireland

Emma Finch, BSc (Hons)
Senior Speech and Language Therapist
Clinical Speech and Language Studies
Department of Speech and Language
    Therapy
Mater Misericordiae University Hospital
Dublin, Ireland

Paul Finucane, MSc, FRCPI, FRACP
Senior Staff Specialist Geriatrician
Conjoint Professor
University of New South Wales
Adjunct Professor
University of Notre Dame
Australia
Professor Emeritus
University of Limerick
Limerick, Ireland

Professor
Aged Care
Murrumbidgee Local Health District
New South Wales
Australia

Donal Fitzpatrick, MB BCh, BAO
Geriatrics
Cork University Hospital
Cork
Ireland

**Matthew Fuller, BSc, BSc
(Hons), PgCert, SRP, MCSP**
Clinical Specialist Physiotherapist
Guys and St. Thomas' NHS Foundation
    Trust
Department of Physiotherapy
St Thomas Hospital
London
United Kingdom

**Marissa C. Galicia-Castillo, MD,
MSEd, CMD, FACP, AGSF, FAAHPM**
Professor
Internal Medicine/Geriatrics/Palliative
    Medicine
Eastern Virginia Medical School

Medical Director
Palliative Medicine
Sentara Norfolk General Hospital
Norfolk
United States of America

Hannah Gallagher, MBBS, MA
Geriatrics Registrar
Aintree Hospital
Liverpool
United Kingdom

**Paul Gallagher, MB BCh,
BAO, PhD, FRCPI**
Department of Geriatric Medicine
Cork University Hospital
Cork
Ireland

Rose Galvin, BSc, PhD
Senior Lecturer in Physiotherapy
School of Allied Health
Ageing Research Centre
Health Research Institute
Limerick, Ireland

John F. Garvey, MB BCh, BAO, PhD
Consultant Respiratory Physician
Respiratory Medicine
St. Vincent's University Hospital
Dublin
Ireland

Gillian Gibson, BSc (Hons)
Podiatry
Private Practice
Langport
United Kingdom

William Gibson, MB BCh, MRCP, PhD
Division of Geriatric Medicine
University of Alberta
Alberta
Canada

Rebecca Golder, BSc (Hons)
Senior Occupational Therapist
Guys and St Thomas' NHS Foundation
    Trust
London
United Kingdom

Virginia Golightly, MS, PT, DPT
Acute Physical Therapist
Department of Acute Physical Therapy and
    Occupational Therapy
Wake Forest Baptist Health
Winston-Salem
United States of America

**Adam Lee Gordon, MB BCh,
MMedSci (Clin Ed), PhD**
Professor of Care of Older People
Division of Medical Sciences and Graduate
    Entry Medicine
University of Nottingham
Derby
United Kingdom

Margot Gosney, MD, FRCP
Elderly Care Medicine
Royal Berkshire NHS Foundation Trust
Reading
United Kingdom

Frances Horgan, PhD
Associate Professor of Physiotherapy
School of Physiotherapy
Royal College of Surgeons in Ireland
Dublin, Ireland

**Robert Iansek, BMedSc,
MBBS, PhD, FRACP**
Professor
Clinical Research Centre for Movement
    Disorders and Gait
Kingston Centre

School of Clinical Sciences,
Monash University
Monash Medical Centre
Victoria
Australia

Thomas Jackson, BSc, MBBS, PhD
Clinician Scientist in Geriatric Medicine
Institute of Inflammation and Ageing
University of Birmingham, Birmingham
West Midlands
United Kingdom

Jo Jethwa, BSc (Hons)
Highly Specialised Neuro-Oncology
    Physiotherapist
Richard Wells Rehabilitation Unit
The Royal Marsden Hospital
London
United Kingdom

**Timothy L. Kauffman, PT,
PhD, FAPTA, FGSA**
Consultant
Lancaster
Pennsylvania
United States of America

Yi-Yen Karen Kee, MSc, MBBS, FRCP
Department of Stroke and Elderly Care
    Medicine
Croydon University Hospital
Croydon
United Kingdom

Vaughan Keeley, PhD, FRCP
Consultant Physician in Lymphoedema
Department of Lymphoedema
Royal Derby Hospital

Honorary Professor
Medical School
University of Nottingham
Nottingham
United Kingdom

Cliff Kilgore, BSc (Hons), MA
Consultant Nurse Older People
Advanced Nurse Practitioner
Visiting Fellow, Healthcare
Bournemouth University
Bournemouth, United Kingdom

Consultant Nurse
Intermediate Care and Older People
Dorset Healthcare University Foundation
    NHS Trust, Bournemouth
Dorset
United Kingdom

Rosalind Kings, MB BCh, MRCP
Consultant Geriatrician and Lead for
    Frailty
Care of the Elderly
West Hertfordshire Hospitals NHS Trust
Watford
United Kingdom

Neva Kirk-Sanchez, PT, PhD
Associate Professor
Department of Physical Therapy
University of Miami
Miller School of Medicine
Florida
United States of America

Kimberley Kok, MBBS, MA, MRCP (UK) (Geriatric Medicine)
Specialty Registrar in Geriatric and General
   Internal Medicine
Department of Elderly Care
University Hospital Lewisham
London
United Kingdom

Ny-Ying Lam, MD
Assistant Professor
Department of Rehabilitation Medicine
University of Washington
Washington
United States of America

Talia Lea, BA (Hons), MSc
Advanced Nurse Practitioner
Vascular Surgery
Guys and St Thomas' NHS Foundation
   Trust, London
United Kingdom

Hannah Leach, BSc (Hons)
Highly Specialist Oncology and Palliative
   Care Physiotherapist
Department of Physiotherapy
The Royal Marsden Hospital
London
United Kingdom

Rebecca Lee, MB BCh, MRCP (UK)
Division of Geriatric Medicine
University of Alberta Alberta
Canada

Anna Lewis, MB BCh, MRCP
Geriatric Medicine
Nottingham University Hospitals
Nottingham
United Kingdom

Matthias Linke, DO
SCIM Fellow
Icahn School of Medicine at Mount Sinai
New York
United States of America

Belinda Longhurst, BSc (Hons), Dip HE
Podiatry Assistant
Lecturer
SMAE Institute in collaboration with
   Queen Margaret University
Edinburgh
United Kingdom

Howard Luks, MD
Chief
Sports Medicine
Orthopedic Surgery
Westchester Medical Center
New York
United States of America

Helen Mackie, MBBS, FARM (RACP), DipMSM, Cert TM, CertCLINED
Medical Director
Lymphoedema Service
Mt Wilga Hospital

Clinical Lead
ALERT
Macquarie University Hospital
Macquarie University
New South Wales
Australia

Matthew Maddocks, PhD
Senior Lecturer
Cicely Saunders Institute of Palliative Care
   Policy and Rehabilitation
King's College London
London
United Kingdom

Gill Main, BSc (Hons)
SLT Service Manager and Clinical
   Lead
Speech and Language Therapy
South Ayrshire HSCP
NHS Ayrshire and Arran
Scotland
United Kingdom

Laura Masterson, BSc, Pg Dip, MSc
Department of Nutrition and Dietetics
Health Service Executive (HSE)
Dublin, Ireland

Tahir Masud, MBBS, MA, MSc, FRCP
Professor of Geriatric Medicine
Geriatric Medicine
University Hospitals NHS Trust
Nottingham
United Kingdom

Jacinta McElligott, MB BCh, BAO
Rehabilitation Medicine
National Rehabilitation Hospital
Dublin
Ireland

Senior clinical lecturer
Rehabilitation Medicine
Trinity College Dublin, Dublin
Dublin
Ireland

Paul McElwaine, MB
Consultant Geriatrician
Clinical Senior Lecturer
Department of Medical Gerontology
Tallaght University Hospital
Dublin, Ireland

Kate McGoldrick, BSc
Independent Occupational Therapist
NHS (Greater Glasgow & Clyde) Specialist
   Occupational Therapist
Glasgow
United Kingdom

Ellen McGough, PT, PhD
Associate Professor
Department of Rehabilitation
   Medicine
University of Washington
Washington
United States of America

Dara Meldrum, BSc, MSc, PhD
Senior Research Fellow
Academic Unit of Neurology
School of Medicine
Trinity College Dublin
Dublin
Ireland

Hannah Moorey, BSc, MB BCh
Institute of Inflammation and
   Ageing
University of Birmingham
Birmingham
United Kingdom

Fiona Murphy, BSc (Hons)
Senior Occupational Therapist
Department of Occupational
   Therapy
Guys and St Thomas' NHS Foundation
   Trust
London
United Kingdom

Deirdre Murray, BSc (Physiotherapy), PhD
Research Fellow
Academic Unit of Neurology
Trinity College Dublin
Dublin
Ireland

Meenakshi Nayar, BMBS, BMedSci, MRCP
Clinical lead
Neurological Rehabilitation
London
United Kingdom

Mary Ni Lochlainn, MB BCh, BAO
Academic Specialist Registrar
Older Persons Unit
Guy's and St Thomas' Hospital
London
United Kingdom

Sean Ninan, MB BCh, MRCP
Consultant Geriatrician
Department for Elderly Medicine
Leeds Teaching Hospitals NHS Trust
Leeds
United Kingdom

Marissa O'Callaghan, MB BCh, BAO, MRCPI
Respiratory Department
St Vincent's University Hospital
Dublin
Ireland

Rónán O'Caoimh, MB, MRCPI, MSc, MPH, PhD
Consultant Physician
Geriatric Medicine
Mercy University Hospital

IRL Senior Lecturer in Geriatric Medicine
Clinical Sciences Institute
National University of Ireland Galway
Galway
Ireland

Shane O'Hanlon, MB BCh, BAO, LLB, MSc, MRCPI
Consultant Geriatrician
Department of Geriatric Medicine
St Vincent's University Hospital

Associate Clinical Professor
Department of Medicine
University College Dublin
Dublin
Ireland

Desmond O'Neill, MD, FRCPI
Professor
Medical Gerontology
Trinity College Dublin
Dublin
Ireland

Fiona O'Reilly, MSc, BSc, MCSP, MISCP
Specialist Neurorehabilitation Service
The Royal Hospital Donnybrook
Dublin, Ireland

Daniel Oh, MD, MS
Resident Physician
Physical Medicine and Rehabilitation
New York Presbyterian - Columbia and Cornell
New York
United States of America

George Peck, MBBS, BSC, MRCP
Consultant Physician and Geriatrician
St Mary's Hospital
London
United Kingdom

Ciara Preston, BSc (Hons), DClin Psych
Consultant Clinical Psychologist
Department of Clinical Neuropsychology
Oxford Psychological Medicine Centre
Oxford Centre for Enablement
Nufflield Orthopaedic Centre
Oxford University Hospitals
NHS Foundation Trust
Oxford, United Kingdom

Joanna Preston, MBBS, MSc, MRCP(UK, Geriatric Med)
Senior Health
St. George's NHS University Hospitals
Foundation Trust
London
United Kingdom

Angeline Price, MSc (Advanced Clinical Practice), RN
Ageing and Complex Medicine
Salford Royal NHS Trust
Salford
United Kingdom

Rachel Prusynski, DPT, NCS
Physical Therapist
Research Associate
Department of Rehabilitation Medicine
University of Washington
Washington
United States of America

Roisin Purcell, MB BCh, BAO, MRCPI
Geriatric Medicine
OLH&CS Harold's Cross
St James' Hospital
Dublin, Ireland

Kenneth Rockwood, MD
Division of Geriatric Medicine
Dalhousie University
Halifax
Canada

Lorna Roe, PhD
Research Assistant Professor
Centre for Health Policy and
Management
School of Medicine
Trinity College Dublin
Dublin, Ireland

Roman Romero Ortuno, Lic Med, MSc, MRCP(UK), PhD
Associate Professor
Discipline of Medical Gerontology
Global Brain Health Institute
Trinity College Dublin
Dublin, Ireland

Ibrahim Roushdi, BSc, MBBS, FRCS(Orth), DipHandSurg
(Hand and Upper Limb Unit)
Robert Jones and Agnes Hunt Orthopaedic
Hospital
Shropshire
United Kingdom

Sheila Ryan, BSc, Master of Applied Physiotherapy (Manual Therapy)
Senior Physiotherapist
Rheumatic and Musculoskeletal Disease Unit
Our Lady's Hospice and Care Services
Dublin, Ireland

Andrew Scott, MB BCh, BAO, MRCPI
Respiratory Specialist Registrar
Respiratory Department
St. Vincent's University Hospital
Dublin
Ireland

Cliona Small, MB BCh, BAO
Department of Orthogeriatrics
St. Vincent's University Hospital
Dublin
Ireland

Marie Smith, BSc, MSc
Nursing Quality Manager
The Royal Hospital Donnybrook

Honorary Lecturer
RCSI School of Nursing and Midwifery
Dublin
Ireland

Gavin Snelson, BSc, MSc
Team Lead Physiotherapist Older Peoples
Medicine
Department of Physiotherapy
Newcastle NHS Foundation Trust
Newcastle
United Kingdom

Tadhg Stapleton, BSc, MSc, PhD
Assistant Professor in Occupational
Therapy
Discipline of Occupational Therapy
Trinity College Dublin
Dublin, Ireland

Louise Statham, MPharm
Senior Lecturer in Clinical Pharmacy
Faculty of Health Sciences and Wellbeing
University of Sunderland
Sunderland
United Kingdom

Honorary Lead Clinical Pharmacist
Osteoporosis
Bone Clinic
Newcastle upon Tyne Hospitals NHS
Foundation Trust, Newcastle upon Tyne
United Kingdom

Joel Stein, MD
Simon Baruch Professor and Chair
Rehabilitation and Regenerative Medicine
Columbia University
Vagelos College of Physicians and Surgeons

Professor and Chair
Rehabilitation Medicine
Weill Cornell Medical College

Physiatrist-in-Chief
Rehabilitation Medicine
NewYork-Presbyterian Hospital
New York
United States of America

Jennifer Stewart, PhD, RN
Assistant Professor
Department of Community-Public Health
Johns Hopkins University School of
    Nursing
Baltimore, Maryland

Jacqueline Stow, MB BCh, MRCPCH
Consultant in Rehabilitation Medicine
Prosthetic Department
National Rehabilitation Hospital
Dublin
Ireland

Emily Stowe, BSc, MSc
Clinical Specialist Physiotherapist
Farleigh Hospice
Essex
United Kingdom

**Rachel Tams, DClin Psych,
PGDip, CPsychol**
Consultant Clinical Neuropsychologist
Department of Clinical Neuropsychology
Oxford Centre for Enablement
Oxford University Hospitals
NHS Foundation Trust
Oxford, United Kingdom

**Arturo Vilches-Moraga,
LMS, DGM, MSc, FRCP**
Consultant Geriatrician and Physician
Ageing and Complex Medicine
Salford Royal NHS Foundation Trust

Honorary Senior Lecturer
Faculty of Medical and Human Sciences
University of Manchester
Salford
United Kingdom

Adrian Vyse, BSc (Hons), MSc
Clinical Specialist Physiotherapist for Older
    People
In-Patient Therapies
West Hertfordshire Hospitals NHS Trust
Watford
United Kingdom

**Adrian Wagg, MB, FRCP (Lond),
FRCP (Edin), FHEA**
AHS Professor
Department of Medicine
University of Alberta
Alberta
Canada

Iain Wilkinson, MBBS, MA, FRCP
Consultant Orthogeriatrician
Medicine for the Elderly
Surrey and Sussex Healthcare
NHS Trust, Redhill
Surrey
United Kingdom

Honorary Senior Lecturer
Brighton and Sussex Medical School
Brighton
United Kingdom

Wilby Williamson, BMBS, DPHIL
Assistant Professor
Department of Physiology
School of Medicine
Trinity College Dublin
Dublin, Ireland

Richard Wong, MB BChir, MD, FRCP
Consultant Geriatrician
Geriatric Medicine
University Hospitals of Leicester NHS Trust
Leicester
United Kingdom

FOREWORD

"Old people, on the whole, have fewer complaints than young; but those chronic diseases which do befall them generally never leave them"

Hippocrates
Aphorisms, Section II

The goal of rehabilitation is to help people recover from illness or regain/maintain function at the highest quality of life despite those diseases, chronic and acute. At the time that Hippocrates wrote that aphorism, rehabilitation of older people was not comprehensive or multidisciplinary and most likely did not exist other than water, sun, and proper nutrition.

This compilation of 75 chapters defines rehabilitation of older people like no other text and breathes life into this underutilized and underrecognized, albeit essential and coveted area of care for older persons. Building on the earlier editions, the editors set out to expand its use to all disciplines as well as to center on patients and their families. The inclusion of learning objectives, case studies, summary points and multiple-choice questions make this text invaluable for students and practitioners in the field of rehabilitation. This 4th Edition is loaded with great tables, figures and concise boxes which accentuate the information for experts, students, and non-medical readers. The mass of international contributors with an expanse of degrees and disciplines potentiates the value of this book.

Over 30 years ago I was asked to write a book about geriatric rehabilitation. Recognizing the idiosyncrasies as well as the breadth and depth of ageing, I conceptualized the Geriatric Rehabilitation Manual 1st and 2nd Editions which grew into the 3rd Edition of A Comprehensive Guide to Geriatric Rehabilitation.

I was the lead editor for all three editions.

Those who study from or use this 4th Edition will understand that the contributors and the editors recognize that "Ageing...the passage of time...brings with it an abundance of experiences within the psychosocial, economic and medical milieu..." It is diverse, complex, and challenging. The study of ageing is the study of life and, "Above all else, ageing is to be venerated" (Geriatric Rehabilitation Manual, Preface, 1st and 2nd Editions).

With great honor and pleasure, I pass the torch into the very capable hands of these two co-editors, Shane O'Hanlon and Marie Smith.

Timothy L. Kauffman, PT, M.S, PhD,
Fellow American Physical Therapy Association,
Fellow Gerontological Society of America
Lancaster, Pennsylvania, United States of America

"The hope of the world lies in the rehabilitation of the living human being, not just the body but also the soul."

Vaclav Havel

It has been an absolute pleasure for us to be invited to work on this project that we hope will benefit all readers, whether health professional, caregiver, or a person going through rehabilitation. One of our strong beliefs is that this book should be accessible to a wide readership. We hope that it is found not only in medical libraries, but also in many different clinical settings, and in public libraries too. We support the democratisation of health information - ultimately we want this book to help as many people as possible! If that means it is just as useful to the daughter of someone undergoing stroke rehabilitation in a specialised unit as it is to the physiotherapy student on the renal ward then we will be delighted.

We spent a lot of time choosing the right chapters, and the right authors. We thank the hundreds of people who helped us to crowdsource the list of subjects that we should cover, and the many others who provided advice and feedback. The result is a book that has had a huge amount of input from a varied team of people, and covers topics never seen before in similar books. We particularly thank the authors for bringing their experience in complex areas and doing a superb job of condensing it into readable chapters. You can start the book from the beginning for a logical tour through all aspects of rehabilitation, or go directly to areas where you need specific information. Throughout the book, the emphasis is on holistic management of rehabilitation with the older person at the centre.

We wish to thank our families for their patience with us and our deadlines. We are indebted to the previous editors for guiding the book to this point, where we humbly accept the responsibility for further nurture. We thank the lay reviewers - members of the public who kindly gave their time to provide feedback, which was invaluable. We also thank all the team at Elsevier, who were with us every step of the way.

Rehabilitation is about maximising quality of life and independence – something that benefits not just the individual, but society as a whole. How much support is provided for this process also reflects on society. We hope that this book encourages readers to help raise the profile of rehabilitation of older people, and we are proud to play our small part by compiling this text.

Shane O'Hanlon, Consultant Geriatrician
Marie Smith, Nursing Quality Manager
Dublin, Ireland

CONTENTS

UNIT 6 Planning for Discharge

INTRODUCTION

This book remains faithful to its title. It really is a ***comprehensive*** guide to rehabilitation of the older patient and provides a practical framework for anyone involved in the rehabilitation process. The book comprises 75 chapters written by a multidisciplinary group of authors and is structured into six units. Unit 1 introduces the reader conceptually to the rehabilitation process applied specifically to older people and describes the importance of person-centred care and comprehensive holistic assessment. Shared decision making, respecting patients' values and beliefs, understanding their concerns, and facilitating their participation in the rehabilitation plan are all stressed as being vital in achieving successful outcomes. The quality of interpersonal skills including a caring and sympathetic approach, an appropriate environment and understanding the important roles of families and carers are also discussed.

Units 2 and 3 describe in detail how the rehabilitation process works and how it can be supported. Chapters on how to assess rehabilitation potential and on setting goals are well composed, and there is an excellent overview of different types of equipment available to the novice as well as the experienced clinician. This section also focuses on how the expertise of different allied healthcare professionals including physiotherapists, occupational therapists, nurses, speech therapists, psychologists and social care workers are employed in the rehabilitation process. The importance of mental health and capacity, nutritional requirements, avoiding deconditioning, keeping people engaged in the process as well as measuring progress are discussed in detail and in my opinion are important components of the book. The next unit focuses on the common issues that often exist or arise in individual patients during rehabilitation, how these pose a challenge and how to overcome them. These issues include pain, psychological factors including depression and impaired cognition, visual and hearing loss, skin fragility, continence, and foot problems.

The next specialised rehabilitation section of the book is composed of chapters that outline specific issues arising in a wide range of different conditions including stroke, movement disorders and progressive neurological conditions, vestibular disorders, cardiac and pulmonary disorders, cancer and many more. Practical advice on how to individualise rehabilitation and overcome barriers will help to achieve successful outcomes. There are also excellent chapters on rehabilitation following surgery, intensive care admission, spinal injury, trauma, and amputation. Community geriatric medicine and rehabilitation is now rapidly developing in many countries and an extremely helpful chapter is devoted to this theme.

The final section is an innovative one which is dedicated to the discharge planning process and therefore provides useful chapters on the home environment assessment, home care support, advance care planning, driving, health promotion, and previously under-recognised issues such as loneliness, which can impact on quality of life. The holistic approach, which takes into account physiological, psycho-social, spiritual, and cultural factors, is a real strength of the book. Another helpful aspect is the many case studies that are used to illustrate important principles. The MCQs after every chapter also allow the reader to test their knowledge. I thoroughly recommend this book to health and social care professionals who are new to the subject as well as experienced rehabilitation professionals who want to improve their understanding and skills to enable them to provide better outcomes for patients. It will also be useful for patients and carers seeking guidance through the rehabilitation process.

Professor Tahir Masud, Consultant Geriatrician,
President of the British Geriatrics Society (2018-2020)
Nottingham, UK

Introduction to Rehabilitation for Older People

Person-Centred Care

Marie Smith

LEARNING OBJECTIVES

- Explain the concept of person-centred care
- Describe person-centred care in healthcare practice
- Discuss the elements of a person-centred practice framework

---

CASE

Alex is a 72-year-old gentleman who likes to spend time reading books. He used to work as a clerical officer in the firm close to his home. Alex is married to Tess and together they like to read, watch sport on television and go for walks with their dog Frankie. One day on his way back from the shop, Alex collapsed on the road and was brought to a local hospital for examination. He was diagnosed with a haemorrhagic stroke. He was seen by a specialist team and was prescribed medication. He needed the assistance of two people with walking and transferring from his bed to a chair. Alex was assessed and treated immediately by the stroke rehabilitation team, and was recommended to attend a further rehabilitation programme in a nearby hospital once medically stable. He agreed to attend; however, he told his wife that he was feeling anxious about it, and he was also worried that he may have another stroke.

CONCEPT OF PERSON-CENTRED CARE

In recent years, person-centredness has been discussed within health and social care at a global level. The importance of providing person-centred care is highlighted in international and national guidelines and standards of conduct (Department of Health, 2001; Nursing & Midwifery Council, 2008; WHO, 2015). According to the guidelines, person-centred care is a standard of care where the person/patient is at the centre of the delivery.

There have been numerous debates about the concepts underpinning person-centredness. Generally, person-centredness has been recognised as a multidimensional concept; however, what is fundamental to this concept is an understanding about being a person. For example, how the person thinks about values, how the person expresses their beliefs, how he/she engages emotionally in a relationship or how the person wants to live are core attributes of being a person.

Person-centredness is concerned with a meaningful relationship that is built on trust, respect and recognition of 'me as a person'. As McCormack and McCance (2017) point out,

there are four concepts at the heart of person-centredness – being in a relationship, being in a social world, being in a place and being with self. Being in a relationship emphasizes practice that helps to develop therapeutic relationships. Being in the social world means that the person is creating and recreating the meaning of life through connection with others. Knowing myself, knowing my own values and making sense of what is happening to me captures the idea of being with self. Finally, being in a place encourages the person to recognise what is happening around them and to notice the impact of care on their experience (Price, 2019).

In a healthcare environment the concept of person-centred care is related to all who are involved in caring for others. It applies to patients, families, carers, nurses, doctors and other healthcare professionals of a multidisciplinary team.

Commonly, the idea of person-centred care is understood at a basic level; however, healthcare professionals often find it challenging to recognise the concept and to deliver it in practice. The challenge is in the delivery of care that is relationship focused, collaborative and holistic in comparison to care that is fragmented and medically/disease orientated. There have been several frameworks developed to help and support the delivery of person-centred care and to merge the real and the theoretical (Kelly et al., 2019; Santana et al., 2018). For example, a Person-centred Practice Framework developed from research by McCormack and McCance (2017) focuses on person-centred practice with older people. The Person-centred Framework consists of four domains as presented in Fig. 1.1. This framework will be briefly discussed in the next few paragraphs.

ELEMENTS OF THE PERSON-CENTRED PRACTICE FRAMEWORK

The Prerequisites

The first domain of the framework is the prerequisites and they are considered as key elements in the delivery of person-centred care. They focus on the healthcare professional's ability and professional competence.

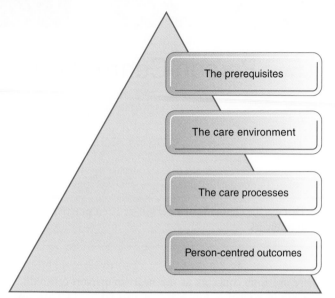

FIG. 1.1   Elements of person-centred practice framework.

- A professional who is professionally competent, who is constantly learning and developing new skills and using these skills in practice can contribute significantly to the delivery of person-centred care. However, if learning and education is focused only on technical skills, then there could be a challenge that the healthcare professional will not see a patient as a person.
- Person-centred care is dependent on the quality of interpersonal skills that the healthcare professional has. Effective verbal and non-verbal communications coupled with good listening skills are beneficial to the process, but they are not enough. If the healthcare professional wants to build a trusting relationship and to engage in important conversation, then the development of advanced communication skills is a necessity.
- The healthcare practitioner can become person-centred through reflection in action (while doing something) or on action (after things were done). Furthermore, receiving feedback and working with that feedback can help the professional to increase self-awareness.
- Values and beliefs of the healthcare professional have an impact on the delivery of person-centred care. To facilitate the process, values (what people think should be carried out) and beliefs (what is true or not) need to come together. For example, the concept of person-centeredness is shared by all involved in care and lived in everyday practice.
- To be committed to the job is another fundamental part of the framework but it does not necessarily mean that the person is kind or going the extra mile. Commitment to the job could be explained by taking mindful action (based on the research evidence) towards another person.

The Care Environment

The true potential of a healthcare professional cannot be fully realised if the delivery of a person-centred care environment does not support a person-centred way of working. Box 1.1 presents an overview of seven features of a care environment that facilitates person-centred care as described in the framework.

Person-Centred Care Processes

This part of the framework focuses specifically on the patient and care delivery through various actions such as working with a patient's beliefs and values, sharing decision-making, engaging with the patient authentically, being sympathetically present and providing holistic care.

One of the elements of person-centred care as described in the framework is for healthcare professionals to **know a patient's values and beliefs** and how the patient makes sense of what is happening to him/her. Being aware of a patient's values helps the practitioner to see and appreciate the person as a unique human being. However, very often the first contact that the healthcare professional has with a patient is driven by gathering information for assessment and goal planning. In this respect it is important to obtain the objective; however, it should not be to the detriment of getting to know the patient as a person.

One of the roles of a healthcare professional in delivering person-centred care is **to facilitate the participation of a patient in decision-making** by providing a patient with information and integrating patient values into the relevant practice. Furthermore, the role involves being with the patient while empowering them to actively participate in the decision of care. In shared decision-making the patient and the practitioner are actively involved and each of them brings knowledge and experience to the presenting situation. At the centre of decision making is a therapeutic relationship where there is respect and trust of each other's values, equally their knowledge and experience. Through negotiation, the patient and practitioner learn from each other and together they discover new ways forward.

Healthcare professionals have an opportunity to engage with the patient while delivering care. Furthermore, **the engagement can be authentic** if the focus is on the interaction with that particular patient and at that particular time. However, full engagement is also dependent on the healthcare professional's ability to connect, and is influenced by the care environment. Full engagement means that there is an equal connection and collaborative decision-making between both parties where values and beliefs are taken into account.

Being sympathetically present describes the way of being present with the patient, with his/her uniqueness and values. Showing acceptance and understanding of the patient's losses and limitations as well as considering a person's needs and life perspectives is central to building a therapeutic relationship and thus providing person-centred care. Simply being with the person, being available in that moment without the need to be doing something to the person; this is essential to person-centred care.

Person-centered care involves **taking care of the whole person**, paying attention to the physiological, psychological, developmental, spiritual, cultural and the sociological needs of the patient.

Person-Centred Outcomes

Person-centred outcomes are essential elements of the framework, and they represent the results of the delivery of person-centred care. The results are expressed by patients as a good care experience, a feeling of involvement in care, a feeling of well-being and being valued and the presence of a healthy (therapeutic) culture. The next paragraph will present 'a narrative' of a patient experience of person-centred care.

"My name is Alex and for the last year I was a patient in the rehabilitation hospital. I would like to share some thoughts on my experience. I was very happy with the care that I received. At first, I was a bit apprehensive of the rehabilitation team. The first day, everybody was very nice and welcoming but they all asked too many technical questions such as do you have pain, do you have allergies, how often you go to the toilet…and I wanted to tell them about my worries and my dog, but they were all very busy. I was afraid that if I started my exercises, I could have another stroke. But I was more worried as to how I was going to be able to manage at home, would I be able to bring my dog Frankie for a walk? And what about my wife, would she be able to manage?

As the days passed, I got to know the staff and they showed a real interest in me as a person. They learned about my fears, my wife and my dog. I felt that some of the staff members were really listening to me and they were interested in what I had to say about myself, they were just there present with me. They made my stay in hospital more pleasant. They took time to explain things, and they talked to me not down to me.

They also asked my opinion about the care that they were giving me. Not only that, they also included my suggestions into the care situation. I felt like I was part of the team. The staff knew what they were doing, they came across as professional and competent; I also noticed that they were nice to each other.

A couple of weeks later I was discharged from the hospital. I was not only able to walk on my own with a stick but I felt that the interactions and discussions made my stay in hospital more meaningful and prepared me for my life at home."

SUMMARY POINTS

- Person-centred care is concerned with a meaningful relationship that is built on trust, respect and recognition of who the person is

- To understand about being a person is fundamental to the concept of person-centred care
- The elements of a Person-centred Practice Framework can help and support delivery of person-centred care

MCQs

Q.1 Which of the following does not define person-centred care?
  a. Therapeutic relationship
  b. Including older person views and preferences in healthcare delivery
  c. Focusing only on person-reported outcomes
  d. Encouraging the person to be involved in providing care
  e. Supporting the person to be responsible for their own health

Q.2 How can the healthcare professional support the delivery of person-centred care?
  a. Designing new research, reflecting on the care provided
  b. Empowering the person to take responsibility for their own life
  c. Listening to the person's stories
  d. Identifying clinical risks and discussing patients worries, wishes and requests
  e. All the above

REFERENCES

Department of Health. (2001). *National service framework for older people.* London.

Kelly, F., Reidy, M., Denieffe, S., & Madden, C. (2019). Older adults' views on their person-centred care needs in a long-term care setting in Ireland. *Journal of Nursing, 28*(9), 552–557.

McCormack, B., & McCance, T. (2017). *Person-centred practice in nursing and healthcare, theory and practice.* West Sussex, UK: Wiley Blackwell.

Nursing and Midwifery Council. (2008). *The code: standards of conduct, performance and ethics for nurses and midwives.* London.

Price, B. (2019). *Delivering person-centred care in nursing.* London, UK: Sage Publications.

Santana, M., Manalili, K., Jolley, R., Zelinsky, S., Quan, H., & Lu, M. (2018). How to practice person-centered care: a conceptual framework. *Health Expectations, 21*, 429–440.

World Health Organization. *WHO global strategy on people-centered and integrated health services.* Retrieved from https://apps.who.int/iris/bitstream/handle/10665/155002/WHO_HIS_SDS_2015.6_eng.pdf;jsessionid=D2EF16E30A3B2E761F84F72B5D7EB640?sequence=1.

FURTHER READING

McCance, T., McCormack, B., & Dewing, J. (2011). An exploration of person-centredness in practice. *Journal of Issues of Nursing, 16*(2), 1–11.

McCrae, N. (2013). Person-centred care: rhetoric and reality in public healthcare system. *Journal of Nursing, 22*(19), 1125–1128.

Moore, L., Britten, N., Lydahl, D., Naldemirci, O., Elam, M., & Wolf, A. (2016). Barriers and facilitators to the implementation of person-centred care in different healthcare contexts. *Scandinavian Journal of Caring Science, 31*, 662–673.

Oxelmark, L., Ulin, K., Chaboyer, W., Bucknall, T., & Ringdal, M. (2017). Registered nurses' experiences of patient participation in hospital care: supporting and hindering factors patient participation in care. *Journal of Caring Science, 32*, 612–621.

Pope, T. (2012). How person-centred care can improve nurses' attitudes to hospitalised older persons. *Nursing Older People, 24*(1), 32–36.

Riding, S., Glendening, N., & Heaslip, V. (2017). Real world challenges in delivering person-centred care: a community-based case study. *Journal of Community Nursing, 22*(8), 391–394.

Sjögren, K., Lindkvist, M., Sandman, P. -O., Zingmark, K., & Edvardsson, D. (2017). Organizational and environmental characteristics of residential aged care units providing highly person-centred care: a cross sectional study. *BMC Nursing, 16*, 44.

2

Comprehensive Assessment of Older People

Suzanne Arkill & Simon Conroy

LEARNING OBJECTIVES

- Describe the importance of a holistic (biopsychosocial approach) approach to the care of older people
- Identify the components of Comprehensive Geriatric Assessment (CGA), as one specific, well-evidenced approach for older people with acute care needs
- Describe the International Classification of Function framework
- Explain how CGA can be applied in a rehabilitation setting

FRAILTY AND COMPREHENSIVE ASSESSMENT

The global population is steadily ageing and more patients are being admitted to hospital year on year. Many are 'frail' (see Chapter 4 Frailty) or vulnerable to catastrophic functional decline in the face of even apparently innocuous illnesses; this often manifests as a frailty syndrome (Box 2.1).

Frailty syndromes are complex to unpick, so a clear, comprehensive and structured approach is vital. Comprehensive Geriatric Assessment (CGA) is one such approach that has been studied in hospitalised older people (Ellis et al., 2017). There is growing consensus that CGA is most effective when applied to moderately to severely frail older people in urgent care settings, identified using the Clinical Frailty Scale (Fig. 2.1) (Rockwood et al., 2005).

The Clinical Frailty Scale (CFS) is a quick and simple tool describing degrees of frailty based on symptoms and functional status:

- Patients scoring 1–3 are very fit, active and independent, with a risk of death of 2% during hospital admission.

BOX 2.1 Frailty Syndromes

Cognitive impairment – delirium and/or dementia
Incontinence/constipation
Malnutrition
Falls
Gait disorders
Pressure ulcers
Sleep disorders
Sensory disorders
Fatigue
Polypharmacy
End of life scenarios

- Patients scoring 4–6 are vulnerable but with a mortality risk of less than 6%.
- Patients scoring 7 are severely frail and completely dependent, with a risk of death of 11% during hospital admission.
- Patients scoring 8 are very severely frail and completely dependent, with a risk of death of 24% during hospital admission.
- Patients scoring 9 are terminally ill with a life expectancy of less than six months (Wallis et al., 2015).

COMPREHENSIVE GERIATRIC ASSESSMENT

Patients receiving CGA are more likely to be alive and at home, and have an improved quality of life compared to patients who have received standard care.

What is comprehensive geriatric assessment?

Comprehensive Geriatric Assessment is defined as a multi-dimensional, multidisciplinary diagnostic and therapeutic process conducted to determine the medical, mental and functional problems of older people with frailty so that a co-ordinated and integrated plan for treatment and follow-up can be developed (Fig. 2.2) (Rubenstein et al., 1991).

The aim of CGA is to use the skills and expertise of the multidisciplinary team (MDT) in order to provide a person-centred approach to improve an older person's quality of life. Typical team members come from geriatric medicine, nursing, physiotherapy, pharmacy, occupational therapy and social worker. Other team members might come from psychiatry, podiatry, dietetics, audiology or optometry – it will depend upon the individual patient's identified needs. The specific areas usually assessed during CGA are listed in Box 2.2.

A range of tools can be used to quantify problems within each of these domains (see for example https://www.bgs.org.uk/resources/how-cga-chapter-2-self-assessment).

Clinical Frailty Scale*

 1   Very Fit – People who are robust, active, energetic, and motivated. These people commonly exercise regularly. They are among the fittest for their age.

 2   Well – People who have **no active disease symptoms** but are less fit than category I. Often, they exercise or are very **active occasionally**, e.g. seasonally.

 3   Managing Well – People whose **medical problems are well controlled,** but are **not regularly active** beyond routine walking.

 4   Vulnerable – While **not dependent** on others for daily help, often **symptoms limit activities.** A common complaint is being "slowed up", and/or being tired during the day

 5   Mildly Frail – These people often have **more evident slowing,** and need help in **high order IADLs** (finances, transportation, heavy housework, medications). Typically, mild frailty progressively impairs shopping and walking outside alone, meal preparation, and housework.

 6   Moderately Frail – People need help with **all outside activities** and with **keeping house.** Inside, they often have problems with stairs and need **help with bathing** and might need minimal assistance (cuing, standby) with dressing.

 7   Severely Frail – Completely dependent for personal care, from whatever cause (physical or cognitive). Even so, they seem stable and not at high risk of dying (within ~ 6 months).

 8   Very Severely Frail – Completely dependent, approaching the end of life. Typically, they could not recover even from a minor illness.

9   Terminally Ill – Approaching the end of life. This category applies to people with **a life expectancy <6 months,** who are **not otherwise evidently frail.**

Scoring frailty in people with demantia

The degree of frailty corresponds to the degree of dementia. Common **symptoms in mild dementia** include forgetting the details of a recent event, though still remembering the event itself, repeating the same question/story, and social withdrawal.

In **moderate dementia,** recent memory is very impaired, even though they seemingly can remember their past life events well. They can do personal care with prompting.

In **severe dementia,** they cannot do personal care without help.

FIG. 2.1   Clinical Frailty Scale (Rockwood et al., 2005).

Specific CGA elements
Cognition

Assessment of a patient's ability to think, understand and perceive the world around them is crucial. Recognising and differentiating between delirium (new or worsening confusional state caused by an acute precipitating factor) and dementia (a long-term confusional state) is of paramount importance (see Chapter 30 Cognitive Problems). Where cognition appears to be impaired, baseline cognition is best obtained from careful questioning of the patient's relatives and carers. The use of a validated screening tool such as the 4-AT (MacLullich, Ryan, & Cash, 2014) on admission is especially useful. If delirium is present, then causes should be identified (e.g. infection, metabolic disturbance, medication, pain, constipation, urinary retention, etc.) and consideration given

FIG. 2.2 Comprehensive Geriatric Assessment (CGA): domains of assessment.

BOX 2.2   Components of Comprehensive Geriatric Assessment

CGA domains
Cognition
Continence
Mobility and falls risk
Mood
Nutrition
Pain
Activities of daily living and functional status
Social support
Medication and polypharmacy
End of life care, legal and ethical issues
Vision or hearing difficulties
Goals of care

to looking for underlying dementia. These issues will have a significant impact upon rehabilitation plans.

Continence

Bowel and bladder control impact on a patient's physical health (skin problems, falls, urine infections), dependence and self-esteem. It is important to establish a patient's baseline continence and investigate if there have been any changes and over what timescale. Consider the likely causes (e.g. overactive bladder, blocked urine outflow, weak pelvic floor or functional incontinence for example related to immobility). Bladder scanning with a handheld ultrasound machine can be done with very little training, and shows how much urine is left in the bladder. Bladder scanning and bladder diaries can be useful in differentiating between causes in the first instance. See Chapter 35 Bladder and Bowel Problems for further advice.

Mobility and Falls Risk

Falls can cause significant distress, pain, serious complications, loss of confidence and independence, and can have a huge effect on a patient's quality of life. A patient's baseline mobility needs to be established and if this has changed, establish over what period and why? Physiotherapists and occupational therapists are invaluable and may use tools, such as a Timed Up and Go (TUG) test (Eagles et al., 2017), to test how quickly a person can get out of a chair, walk 3 m and return to sit in the chair. Longer times are associated with functional decline, falls and dying.

Falls in older people are usually multifactorial; try to identify at least five contributing factors. Examples might include poor vision, lighting, loose carpets, frequent toilet trips in the dark, sensory impairment, muscle weakness, ill-fitting footwear, sedating medication or alcohol. Identifying multiple factors is critical to outline the rehabilitation interventions that will be necessary to reduce falls risk – there is very rarely just one cause in this population. See Chapter 28 Falls, Dizziness and Funny Turns.

Mood

Depression and/or anxiety (e.g. related to fear of falling) are common and may often be missed. MDT members who spend considerable time with the patient, such as nurses and therapists, are well placed to recognise signs of low mood and anxiety. A patient's baseline mood should be assessed, ideally using validated scales such as the Geriatric Depression Score (GDS) or Hospital Anxiety and Depression Scale (HADS). Where problems are identified, input from the old age psychiatry team should be considered. See Chapter 29 Anxiety and Depression for more details.

Nutrition

Older patients are at increased risk of malnutrition. Patients should be asked about their usual diet, how food is obtained and cooked, and whether they require assistance to eat. The Malnutrition Universal Screening Tool (MUST) is a useful screen for malnutrition risk. Examine oral health (see Chapter 33 Oral Health) and swallowing problems, especially in at-risk groups, such as people with stroke. Consider simple nutritional supplementation and review acceptability. If the patient has complex nutritional needs and simple measures are not working, then consider dietician input (see Chapter 17 Nutrition and Hydration).

Pain

Older patients may have difficulty communicating that they are in pain, for example due to reduced verbal communication. Carers, relatives, nursing staff, other members of the MDT and the patient through non-verbal cues may help understand the patient's pain level. Pain reassessment following treatment should continue on a regular basis. Chapter 25 Pain provides practical advice.

Functional Status and Activities of Daily Living (ADLs)

Establish how much personal care the patient is able to undertake themselves, i.e. washing, cleaning, shopping, cooking and transferring around the home. What do they struggle with and why? Is additional support or formal assessment required? Additional consideration should be given to driving and the use of technology. Chapter 13 Occupational Therapy: Function and Cognition explains the role of assessments of ADLs.

Social Support

What existing home support does the patient have from friends and family, and how frequently does this occur? Are they lonely and/or isolated? Are there any especially vulnerable times? Does the patient require additional support?

Medication

Many older patients have a complex medical background and may be on several medications, some of which may no longer be appropriate. Older patients may be particularly susceptible to the effects of 'polypharmacy' (see Chapter 37 Optimising Pharmacotherapy), and careful review of their medications is essential. Several tools are available, such as the STOPP-START tool (for evidence-based medication reviews) and the Anticholinergic Burden Scale (for anticholinergic side effects such as confusion and constipation). Drug side effects commonly affect rehabilitation (e.g. urinary retention leading to catheterisation).

Vision or Hearing Difficulties

This is an often-neglected area where real improvements in the patient's quality of life can be made. Establish if the patient requires glasses or a hearing aid and when their last vision and hearing tests took place. Chapter 39 Vision and Hearing explains how to assess further.

End of Life Care, Legal and Ethical Issues

It is important to consider the likely outcomes; the CFS provides some idea about prognosis. This might lead to a discussion about preferred priorities for care and 'what matters to the patient' which may be more important to address than 'what is the matter with the patient'. Is there an advance care plan in place and if not, would the patient benefit from one? For people with cognitive or sensory impairment that impacts upon communication, consider if there is an existing legal instrument (e.g. power of attorney for health and/or finance)?

Goals of Care

The main aims of treatment and overall care should be patient-centred with patient wishes, functionality and physiological fitness taken into account. Well-defined and realistic rehabilitation goals should be jointly determined between the patient and the MDT, and re-evaluated at regular intervals (see Chapter 10 Setting Rehabilitation Goals). These goals should be made clear to the patient, family and MDT. Rehabilitation teams often use SMART goals: Specific, Measurable, Achievable, Realistic and Time sensitive. For example, the treatment aim might be to walk 5 m with a wheeled Zimmer frame in 1 week in order to allow the patient to mobilise to their toilet unaided at home. Most important is that the goal has meaning to the patient; it is all too easy to set goals that satisfy or assure the clinical team, but that have little meaning to the patient themselves!

THE INTERNATIONAL CLASSIFICATION OF FUNCTIONING, DISABILITY AND HEALTH

Another way to approach complexity is through the International Classification of Function, Disability and Health (ICF, Fig. 2.3), which was developed by the World Health Organization (WHO). Instead of considering a patient in terms of their disease, the ICF model places the emphasis on the health needs of the patient by considering bodily function, structure and activity.

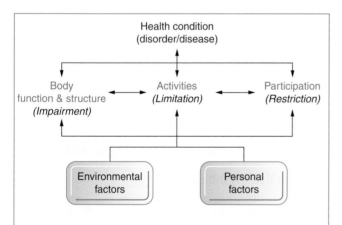

- Body functions are defined in terms of physiological function.
- Body structures are defined anatomically in terms of organs, limbs and related components.
- Activities are defined in a similar way to activities of daily living and refer to actions the patient takes such as walking, driving, engaging in a conversation.
- Participation in society is in relation to a patient's wishes and the role they want to adopt. If a patient wishes to engage in an activity but is unable to or in a reduced capacity, then the patient has participation restriction.
- Environmental factors are physical or societal mechanisms that influence a patient's participation in activities.
- Personal factors refer to a patient's personal preference with regards to performing activities.

FIG. 2.3 The International Classification of Function and Health.

As Fig. 2.3 demonstrates, the patient's health condition, body structure and function, activity, participation, environmental and social factors are all interrelated.

For example, two men who are unable to walk (activity), in wheelchairs (environmental factor), who have lost a limb (body structure) and watch a football match (participation). One has previously been a professional footballer and would still like to play (personal factors) and is now restricted to a non-playing role, whereas the other man attends the match to watch as a spectator. The activity and participation level is the same, but the achievement of personal goals is very different for both men. Both CGA and the ICF can be used to guide an approach to improving outcomes for older people with rehabilitation needs in urgent care settings. They are both underpinned by a holistic, biopsychosocial approach to care, in contrast to the more typical, medically dominant model of care sometimes seen in acute hospital settings.

CASE

Eric is an 83-year-old man who is admitted to the emergency department with confusion and a fall. He lives alone and was found by his neighbors. He is diabetic and has cardiovascular disease, and had recently had a below-the-knee amputation of his left leg. He takes many different medications and has carers once a day.

Collateral history: Eric's neighbours were worried that they hadn't seen him for a couple of days and noticed that unusually the curtains were open at night. They saw Eric on the floor and called an ambulance. Eric normally has one carer a day to help him bathe and dress but he had been coping at home with most of his ADLs following the leg amputation 4 months ago. His neighbours go shopping for him sometimes, and he has been leaving the house less frequently and looks like he has lost weight recently. His neighbours report that he has become more forgetful. The house was dirty with unwashed dishes and dirty clothes lying around.

Background history: Eric uses a wheelchair and has a mobility scooter for outside. He lives in a bungalow. He is normally continent of urine and bowels; however, there was a strong smell of urine when paramedics found him. His wife died 2 years ago. He smokes but does not drink alcohol.

Past medical history: diabetes, cardiovascular disease – peripheral vascular disease and 2 x TIAs (transient ischaemic attacks), hypertension.

Medication: Codeine 30 mg four times a day, metformin 1 g twice a day and the following medications once a day: gliclazide 80 mg, amlodipine 5 mg, atorvastatin 40 mg, aspirin 75 mg, ramipril 2.5 mg.

On examination: Eric is clinically dehydrated with a dry mouth. His blood pressure is 107/65 mmHg (normally 134/83). He is confused and not orientated to time, place or person. AMTS (Abbreviated Mental Test Score) = 0/4, but he is responsive to commands and voice. His chest is clear and abdomen is soft with mild discomfort in the lower abdomen on palpation. A rectal exam reveals a loaded rectum. The left knee is clean and the amputation wound has healed. There are grade 3 sacral pressure sores present. Eric is tachycardic, has a temperature of 38 degrees Celsius and a heart rate of 110. Eric also complains of pain in his limb that has been amputated.

Investigations: Bladder scan 80 ml (normal), estimated glomerular filtration rate (eGFR) 32 (baseline 68), urea 14 (high), creatinine (Cr) 158 (high), white blood cell count (WCC) 12.8 (high), C-reactive protein (CRP) 150 (high), creatine kinase (CK) = 1400 (high), Mg = 0.67 (low) and phosphate = 0.85 (normal). Blood glucose = 3.2 (low). Other bloods were normal. A CT head scan showed moderate small vessel disease with no acute findings.

1) Outcome without CGA

Eric was treated on the traditional care pathway. Sepsis was identified and he was treated with antibiotics, IV fluids and laxatives. Some medication was held but recommenced once the sepsis had resolved. Eric was declared 'medically fit' for discharge; however, he subsequently required his social circumstances to be assessed which delayed his discharge. Whilst awaiting a social assessment, Eric developed a hospital-acquired pneumonia and delirium that further prolonged his stay in hospital.

2) Outcome with CGA

Eric had a CFS of 7; CGA was undertaken for him and the following problem list was generated:
1) Sepsis likely to sacral pressure sore
2) Acute kidney injury secondary to sepsis, long lie, dehydration and medication
3) Dehydration
4) Hypoglycaemia

5) Hypotension
6) Constipation secondary to reduced oral intake and opiates
7) Polypharmacy
8) Poor nutrition
9) Hyperactive delirium secondary to above
10) Increased care needs
11) Ongoing limb pain, possibly due to phantom limb pain

The acute medical issues were dealt with immediately, and a medication review reduced his blood pressure medication, stopped opiates and commenced neuropathic analgesia (nerve pain medication, gabapentin) for ongoing limb pain. Laxatives and nutritional supplements were started. His antidiabetic medication gliclazide was stopped due to the risk of hypoglycaemic episodes – Eric's lifestyle had changed recently with reduced oral intake.

Multidisciplinary assessment early in the admission found a reduction in Eric's function and difficulty in carrying out ADLs. Pressure sore reducing equipment was ordered, and an additional social care package was requested to help support his return home. Eric had a significant decline in physical strength resulting in poor transfers. Rehabilitation was started from day 1 of his admission to try and build up his strength in order for him to be able to transfer better. Recognising that rehabilitation might take longer than his recovery from the acute illness, a rehabilitation placement was secured for him and he was transferred as soon as he was sufficiently functionally stable. Clear patient goals were identified that the rehabilitation team used as a basis for their assessment and treatment.

SUMMARY POINTS

- Comprehensive Geriatric Assessment (CGA) is a process that looks at many different aspects of a patient's background and current situation and involves the expertise of many different teams to identify problems and optimise management
- CGA helps identify and manage complex problems that an older frail adult may be facing including medical, mental and functional problems so that a coordinated and integrated plan for treatment and follow-up can be developed

- Anyone in the MDT can initiate CGA, as long as the team together are able to deliver the relevant competencies
- CGA can help identify problems in older people with complexity, especially those who present with frailty syndromes
- An ICF approach to evaluation of a patient is an internationally recognised and validated method, and especially useful in a rehabilitation setting

MCQs

Q.1 Which of the following statements regarding CGA is correct?
   a. CGA can only be implemented by a doctor
   b. All older patients admitted to hospital should undergo CGA
   c. CGA has been shown to improve outcomes for older patients in acute hospital settings
   d. CGA is carried out at one specific time
   e. There is a standard template for CGA
Q.2 Which of the following components are part of CGA?
   a. Cognition
   b. Continence

   c. Medication
   d. Social support
   e. All of the above
Q.3 Which one of the following components is not part of the International Classification of Functioning, Disability and Health?
   a. Body functions
   b. Personal factors
   c. Activities
   d. Medications
   e. Body structures

REFERENCES

Eagles, D., Sirois, M. J., Perry, J. J., Lang, E., Daoust, R., Lee, J., Griffith, L., Wilding, L., Neveu, X., & Emond, M. (2017). Timed Up and Go predicts functional decline in older patients presenting to the emergency department following minor trauma. *Age Ageing, 46*(2), 214–218.

Ellis, G., Gardner, M., Tsiachristas, A., Langhorne, P., Burke, O., Harwood, R. H., Conroy, S. P., Kircher, T., Somme, D., Saltvedt, I., Wald, H., O'Neill, D., Robinson, D., & Shepperd, S. (2017). Comprehensive geriatric assessment for older adults admitted to hospital. *Cochrane Database of Systematic Reviews*(9), CD006211.

MacLullich, A., Ryan, T, & Cash, H. (2014). 4AT-Rapid assessment test for delirium. Retrieved from: www.the4at.com (Accessed October 2014).

Rockwood, K., Song, X., MacKnight, C., Bergman, H., Hogan, D. B., McDowell, I., & Mitnitski, A. (2005). A global clinical measure of fitness and frailty in elderly people. [see comment]. *CMAJ Canadian Medical Association Journal, 173*(5), 489–495.

Rubenstein, L. Z., Stuck, A. E., Siu, A. L., & Wieland, D. (1991). Impacts of geriatric evaluation and management programs on defined outcomes: overview of the evidence. *Journal of the American Geriatrics Society, 39*(9 pt 2), 8S–16S discussion 17S-18S.

Wallis, S. J., Wall, J., Biram, R. W., & Romero-Ortuno, R. (2015). Association of the clinical frailty scale with hospital outcomes. *QJM: An International Journal of Medicine, 108*(12), 943–949. doi: 10.1093/qjmed/hcv066.

3

Effects of Ageing

Paul Finucane & Jennifer Stewart

LEARNING OBJECTIVES

- Describe the changes seen in the body's organ systems with ageing

- Explain how these changes affect the rehabilitation of older people

INTRODUCTION

Healthcare has evolved in recent decades such that there is now an ever-increasing focus on older people, even nonagenarians and centenarians. While the breakdown of health in older age is always related to the onset and/or progression of disease, coincidental physiological decline and an associated lack of physiological 'reserve' present an increasingly important backdrop against which disease occurs. Physiological reserve is the capacity of a tissue, organ or body system to maintain its function when it comes under stress. This implies that a lack of reserve is not always apparent when an organ or body system is at rest but becomes evident when exposed to a physiological or pathological stress. Take for example, resting heart rate which remains constant throughout life. However, when exposed to a stress such as exercise, heart rate in the older person takes longer to increase than in the young, fails to achieve a similar maximal rate and takes appreciably longer to regain the resting state once the stress is removed.

A reduction in physiological reserve with increasing age (part of the concept of frailty – see Chapter 4) greatly increases susceptibility to the onset and progression of disease. When older people become unwell, this tends to trigger a cascade of secondary problems in body systems that are not initially compromised. An example is the older person in whom the onset of a respiratory tract infection triggers the added problems of atrial fibrillation and heart failure. These in turn can lead to a sharp functional decline which results in a fall and a fracture. A lack of physiological reserve means that recovery from illness is less assured, generally takes longer to achieve and may be partial rather than total.

DEFINITIONS OF AGEING

A chronologically based definition is that ageing begins at birth or even at conception. An alternative perspective is that ageing equates to vulnerability or susceptibility to death. Actuarial data indicate that humans are least susceptible to death at around the age of 10 years. The likelihood of death increases very gradually thereafter until around the age of 40 in males (slightly older in females); thereafter, the probability of death escalates exponentially year on year. Depending on the organ or body system involved, functional decline can be observed from as early as late teens to as late as early 30s. A good rule of thumb is that various physiological functions decline at a rate of about 10% per decade from the age of 30 years. Thus, the average healthy 90-year-old needs to contend with something in the region of a 60% decline in a wide range of functional parameters.

Age-related changes in organs and body systems can usefully be classified as:
- Structural changes
- Functional changes
- Changes to protective and reparative/restorative processes.

The major body systems that impact on the body's ability to recover from illness are the cardiovascular, respiratory, musculoskeletal, nervous systems and special senses. Changes seen in these systems with age are summarised in basic terms in Table 3.1, and in visual form in Fig. 3.1. The detailed physiological changes are discussed in depth below.

THE CARDIOVASCULAR SYSTEM IN OLDER PEOPLE

Structure of the Heart and Blood Vessels

The major age-related structural changes in the heart and blood vessels are listed in Table 3.2.

When not affected by disease, total heart size remains unchanged in females and decreases in males. However, the atria and intraventricular septum show an age-related increase in size relative to other parts and this impacts on cardiac contractility. At a cellular level, gross anatomical changes are accompanied by an asymmetrical increase in the size of cardiac myocytes. Within the conducting system, there is apoptosis of pacemaker cells together with the build-up of fat, elastic and collagen.

With regard to blood vessels, it is difficult to separate age-related structural changes from those that result from pathological stimuli (e.g. hypertension) and lifestyle factors (e.g. poor diet, smoking, lack of exercise). However, it is clear that large arteries dilate and stiffen with age (Fleg & Strait, 2012).

TABLE 3.1 Summary of changes in organ systems with age.	
ORGAN SYSTEM	**CHANGES SEEN WITH AGE**
Cardiovascular	In older people, heart function is generally preserved when at rest. However, during exercise or other stress, the heart's ability to pump blood becomes less effective with age. Maximal heart rate reduces and rhythm abnormalities are also more common. Blood pressure generally increases with ageing due to stiffening of blood vessels. This also increases the pressure against which the heart must work to eject blood. Finally, the ability of the heart to repair its cells declines with age.
Respiratory	As we age, the overall size of our chest cavity decreases, leaving the lungs with less space to expand. Muscle strength decreases and leads to a weaker cough. The cells that 'clean' the airways become less effective and the lung has less ability to repair damage.
Musculoskeletal	Muscle mass reduces with age leading to decreased strength. Bone density reduces (particularly in females), and cartilage becomes thinner and weaker. The discs in our spine become more susceptible to injury. The ability of the system to repair itself lessens.
Nervous	Brain volume reduces, reactions slow and planning/problem-solving abilities decrease. Memory can become less effective. The autonomic nervous system, which controls bodily functions such as temperature regulation, bladder and bowel function as well as sexual function, can deteriorate.
Special senses	Vision gets worse, usually causing long-sightedness but also affecting depth perception and visual fields narrow. The ability to hear deteriorates over time and balance becomes more unstable. All of these can profoundly affect rehabilitation and the ability to function independently.

Intimal walls thicken due to the migration of vascular smooth muscle cells from the media to the intima where they subsequently proliferate. Within the media, reduced elastin and increased collagen deposition further reduce vascular compliance.

Function of the Heart and Blood Vessels

The major age-related functional changes in the heart and blood vessels are also listed in Table 3.2. At rest, systolic function is preserved in the normal ageing heart (Kyriazis & Saridi, 2010). However, when subjected to a physiological stress such as exercise, cardiac output falls due in part to a reduction in cardiac stroke volume but to a greater extent to a reduction in maximal heart rate. In diastole, early diastolic filling is reduced due to impaired cardiac relaxation. As a consequence, diastolic filling becomes more dependent on the late 'active' phase that coincides with atrial contraction. As with systolic function, the impact of impaired relaxation during diastole is most evident when the heart is stressed. The structural changes in the conducting or electrical pathway outlined earlier predispose to sinus bradycardia, heart block, sick sinus syndrome and cardiac dysrhythmias. The β-adrenergic modulated response to exercise which includes an increase in heart rate, greater cardiac contractility and enhanced cardiac relaxation is reduced with ageing.

Both systolic and diastolic blood pressures increase with ageing. Increasing stiffness of the vessel wall in large arteries results in a particular increase in systolic blood pressure and

thus increases afterload on the heart – the pressure against which the heart must work to eject blood during systole. Through nitrous oxide (NO) production and otherwise, the endothelium plays a crucial role in modulating vascular tone, vascular permeability and responses to inflammation. Age-related endothelial dysfunction results in decreased bioavailability of NO which couples with an age-related increase in oxidative stress. These and other complex biochemical processes impair vasodilatation and predispose to inflammation and atherosclerosis. The net result is to further increase cardiac afterload.

Cardioprotection and Repair Processes

These become increasingly defective with age and lead to disordered remodelling and organ dysfunction. Cardiac cells die and are replaced throughout life with new cells which are mainly derived from precursor cells in bone marrow and adipose tissue. However, cardiac cell turnover declines from a peak of about 1% per year in youth to something far less in old age. Furthermore, newly generated cardiac cells are relatively short-lived so new cell formation fails to keep pace with cell death. At the chromosomal level, each time a cell divides the telomeres shorten and this reduces telomerase activity which predisposes to cellular dysfunction and cell death. Reduced NO bioavailability, increased oxidative stress and other biochemical factors also interfere with the ability of ageing blood vessels to repair and remodel.

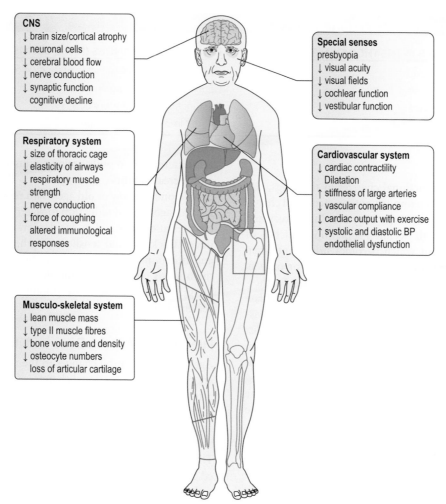

FIG. 3.1   Summary of the principal age-related changes in the human body that impact on rehabilitation.

TABLE 3.2 **Cardiovascular system.**	
STRUCTURAL CHANGES IN THE HEART AND BLOOD VESSELS	**FUNCTIONAL CHANGES IN THE HEART AND BLOOD VESSELS**
Increased thickness of intraventricular septum	Reduced stress-induced cardiac contractility
Atrial enlargement	Reduced stress-induced rise in heart rate
Increased size of cardiac myocytes	Reduced ventricular relaxation in diastole
Apoptosis of cells in conducting system	Dysregulation of cellular calcium exchange
	Decreased adrenergic responsiveness in the heart and blood vessels
Dilatation, increased thickness and reduced compliance in large arteries	Endothelial dysfunction

THE RESPIRATORY SYSTEM IN OLDER PEOPLE

Structure of the Thorax and Lungs

The major age-related structural changes in the thorax and lungs are listed in Table 3.3.

Factors such as spinal kyphosis, narrowing of the intercostal spaces and atrophy of intercostal muscles cause an age-related reduction in the dimensions of the thoracic cage, and this impairs the efficiency of breathing. Within the lung, there is loss of airway elasticity and enlargement of alveolar sacs without alveolar wall destruction. However, these changes seldom compromise gas exchange (Occhipinti et al., 2017).

TABLE 3.3   Respiratory system.

STRUCTURAL CHANGES IN THE THORAX AND LUNGS	FUNCTIONAL CHANGES IN THE LUNGS
Reduced size of thoracic cage	Reduced strength of muscles of respiration
Reduced elasticity of airways	Reduced force of coughing
Enlargement of alveolar sacs	Dysfunction of respiratory cilia
	Altered immunological responses

Function of the Lungs

The major age-related functional changes in the lungs, also listed in Table 3.3, are more important than structural changes and become apparent from the early 20s. Inspiratory and expiratory muscle strength declines, something which is of little relevance at rest but which becomes important when exercise or illness increases metabolic demands for oxygen. Older people cough less forcefully than the young. Furthermore, the ciliated cells which remove inhaled particulate matter from the upper and lower airways become increasingly dysfunctional, further reducing lung 'hygiene'. Complex age-related changes in immunity result in increased levels of proinflammatory cytokines, and these both attenuate and prolong immune responses within the lung, predisposing to chronic inflammation. The same processes impact on the ability of the damaged lung to repair itself and to minimise the onset of long-term structural damage and fibrosis.

THE MUSCULOSKELETAL SYSTEM IN OLDER PEOPLE

Structure of Muscle, Bone and Joints

The major age-related structural changes in the musculoskeletal system are listed in Table 3.4 (Roberts et al., 2016).

An age-related reduction in muscle mass becomes apparent in one's 30s, accelerates with advancing years and has clear implications for rehabilitation of the older patient. At a cellular level, the loss of fast-twitch type II muscle fibres (that produce more strength but that easily fatigue) exceeds the rate of loss of slow-twitch type I fibres (that produce less strength but are fatigue-resistant). Regarding bone, throughout life the maintenance of its integrity depends on physiological resorption being offset by new bone formation – i.e. balanced osteoclastic and osteoblastic activity. A shift in stem cell differentiation with ageing results in reduced osteoblast and increased adipocyte formation – this contributes to the 'fatty' bone marrow of old age. With regard to articular cartilage, an age-related reduction in water content and structural changes at cellular and molecular levels result in tissue of reduced thickness and tensile strength. Age-related structural and functional changes in the cellular components of both the nucleus pulposus and annulus fibrosus result in a loss of integrity and increased susceptibility to injury of the intervertebral discs.

Function of Muscle, Bone and Joints

Age-related structural changes in the musculoskeletal system are paralleled by functional changes as also listed in Table 3.4. Muscle strength declines in parallel with muscle mass, due in part to the disproportionate loss of type II muscle fibres. With regards to bone, functional changes in osteoclast and osteoblast activity have the net effect of reducing bone density. These cellular changes in bone are compounded by age-related endocrine dysfunction (particularly reduced sex hormone activity) such that osteoclasts in particular are released from the inhibitory effects of oestrogen. This largely explains the female propensity to post-menopausal osteopenia and osteoporosis. The 40 billion osteocytes in adult human bone act as mechanoreceptors and help to maintain the integrity of bone and cartilage; an age-related reduction in osteocyte number and function further contribute to bone and cartilage loss. Chondrocytes also show a multifactorial functional decline, in part related to oxidative stress.

Repair Processes of the Musculoskeletal System

The ability of the tissues of the musculoskeletal system to maintain turnover and to repair themselves lessens with advancing years.

TABLE 3.4   Musculoskeletal system.

STRUCTURAL CHANGES IN MUSCULOSKELETAL SYSTEM	FUNCTIONAL CHANGES IN MUSCULOSKELETAL SYSTEM
Reduced lean muscle mass with disproportionate loss of type II muscle fibres	Reduced muscle strength
Reduced bone volume and density	Increased bone turnover with impaired remodelling
Relative reduction in osteoblast and increase in osteoclast numbers	Relative reduction in osteoblast and increase in osteoclast activity
Reduced osteocyte number	
Reduced thickness of articular cartilage	Reduced tensile strength of articular cartilage
Loss of integrity of intervertebral discs	Reduced chondrocyte activity

TABLE 3.5 Nervous system.

STRUCTURAL CHANGES IN THE BRAIN AND NERVES	FUNCTIONAL CHANGES IN THE BRAIN AND NERVES
Reduced brain size with cortical atrophy and ventricular dilatation	Cognitive decline
Loss of neuronal cells	Reduced integrity of blood–brain barrier
Deterioration of myelin sheath	Slowing of nerve conduction
Dendritic loss	Reduced synaptic function
Reduced cerebral blood flow	

THE NERVOUS SYSTEM IN OLDER PEOPLE

Structure of the Brain and Nerves

While it is particularly challenging to disentangle pathological changes in the ageing brain and nerves from those that are purely physiological, the major age-related structural changes are listed in Table 3.5.

On average, the brain loses 5% of its volume per decade from the age of 40 years, accelerating with increasing age and associated with decreased neuronal cell size and with cell death (Peters, 2006).

Function of the Brain and Nerves

Table 3.5 also lists the major age-related functional changes in the brain and nerves. While such things as slowed reaction times and decreased executive function are clearly age-related phenomena, these are not readily explained by observed structural changes in the brain and nerves. There is uncertainty around the relationship between age-related cognitive decline on the one hand and the pathologies that cause dementia on the other. Even more mysterious is the response of the ageing brain to the physiological stress of acute illness and how this results in the altered level of consciousness, disorganised thinking and inattention that we recognise as delirium (see Chapter 30 Cognitive Problems). Finally, age-related dysfunction of the autonomic nervous system can contribute to the often-challenging problem of orthostatic hypotension and also to impaired temperature regulation, obstructive uropathy, constipation and sexual dysfunction.

Repair Processes in the Brain and Nerves

Ageing brains and nerves maintain some ability to offset structural and functional losses. For example, as compensatory mechanisms, the non-dominant cerebral hemisphere becomes more activated with ageing and dendritic sprouting can increase the number of neuronal synapses. A range of strategies that aim to promote so called 'neuroplasticity' in the ageing brain continue to be developed and investigated.

THE SPECIAL SENSES IN OLDER PEOPLE

Structure and Function of the Eye

Every part of the eye from the lid to the retina is impacted both structurally and functionally by the ageing process (Salvi, Akhtar, & Currie, 2006). Yet, the visual problems that require rehabilitation or that impact the rehabilitation of the older person are almost always disease rather than age-related. Nevertheless, sclerosis of the lens and loss of elasticity in its capsule cause presbyopia (long-sightedness) and age-related structural changes in the retina at a cellular level result in reduced visual acuity, reduced visual fields, decreased contrast sensitivity and with the latter, the ability to perceive depth. As these age-related changes can be modified (e.g. with spectacles or with modification of the environment) they are worthy of consideration.

Structure and Function of the Ear and Vestibular System

Age-related oxidative stress results in apoptosis of cochlear cells and in reduced hearing, a process that accelerates in response to environmental stimuli such as cumulative noise exposure. Hearing loss can profoundly influence disability and often makes the rehabilitation of the older person all the more challenging. Ageing also affects the vestibular system, with vestibular hair cells and vestibular neurones both decreasing in number, a phenomenon attributed to genetic factors and to oxidative stress. Function in the semicircular canals, utricle and saccule has all been shown to decline with age and this predisposes to postural instability, particularly in the context of coexisting reduced vision, compromised proprioception and muscle weakness. Once established, these structural and functional changes persist because vestibular hair cells and vestibular neurons lack the capacity to regenerate. See Chapter 39 Vision and Hearing for more information.

THE IMPORTANCE OF PHYSIOLOGICAL DECLINE IN THE REHABILITATION SETTING

Physiological decline with age is seen in practically all tissues, organs and body systems. The challenges in rehabilitating older people differ fundamentally from those in younger people. With older people, the major body systems (cardiovascular, respiratory, musculoskeletal, neurological) may be compromised by structural and functional decline, have diminished physiological reserve and can be highly susceptible to the stress of disease and/or rehabilitation. Rehabilitation strategies need to be tailored accordingly. One major consideration is that older people will require more time to optimise their functional status. Short-term and long-term rehabilitation goals will therefore need to be modified.

Despite all of this, the great majority of older people and even very old people retain the ability to benefit from a rehabilitation programme following health breakdown. Indeed the benefits of rehabilitation are often greatest in this age group where seemingly small functional gains can translate into major improvements in the quality of remaining life.

SUMMARY POINTS

- As a 'rule of thumb', various physiological functions decline in most body systems at a rate of about 10% per decade from the age of 30 years
- Physiological decline and a lack of physiological reserve are seldom apparent while the body is at rest but become increasingly important as the body is stressed, particularly by the onset of disease
- A lack of physiological reserve means that recovery from illness is less assured in older people, generally takes longer to achieve and may be partial rather than total
- Rehabilitation programmes need to be tailored to the individual and allow for reduced physiological reserve
- Even in extreme old age, people not only have the ability to benefit from rehabilitation but often have a disproportionately high gain in terms of improved quality of life

MCQs

Q1. Which one of the following is true?
   a. A reduction in physiological reserve is also known as acopia
   b. Physiological reserve can be estimated at the end of the bed
   c. Lack of reserve is caused by anxiety
   d. When older people become unwell they tend to have just one problem
   e. Physiological reserve is the capacity of a tissue, organ, or body system to maintain its function when it comes under stress

Q2. Which one of the following is true?
   a. Maximal heart rate increases with age
   b. The overall size of our chest increases with age
   c. Bone density drops more in men than women
   d. Subtle memory loss can be explained by the ageing process
   e. Visual fields become wider as we age

REFERENCES

Fleg, J. L., & Strait, J. (2012). Age-associated changes in cardiovascular structure and function: a fertile milieu for future disease. *Heart Failure Reviews, 17*, 545–554.

Kyriazis, I., & Saridi, M. (2010). Senescence of the cardiovascular system due to aging and the resulting increase in cardiovascular risk. *Health Science Journal, 4*, 68–76.

Occhipinti, M., Larici, A. R., Lorenzo, B., & Incalzi, R. A. (2017). Aging airways: between normal and disease. A multidimensional diagnostic approach by combining clinical, functional and imaging data. *Aging Disease, 8*, 471–485.

Peters, R. (2006). Ageing and the brain. *Postgraduate Medical Journal, 82*, 84–88.

Roberts, S., Colombier, P., Sowman, A., Mennan, C., Rölfing, J. H. D., Guicheux, J., & Edwards, J. R. (2016). Ageing in the musculoskeletal system: cellular function and dysfunction throughout life. *Acta Orthopaedica, 87*, 15–25.

Salvi, S. M., Akhtar, S., & Currie, Z. (2006). Ageing changes in the eye. *Postgraduate Medical Journal, 82*, 581–587.

FURTHER READING

Smith, G. S. (2013). Aging and neuroplasticity. *Dialogues in Clinical Neuroscience, 15*, 3–5.

Strait, J. B., & Lakatta, E. G. (2012). Aging-associated cardiovascular changes and their relation to heart failure. *Heart Failure Clinics, 8*(1), 143–164.

4

Frailty

Lorna Roe, Wilby Williamson & Roman Romero-Ortuno

LEARNING OBJECTIVES

- Explain the concept of frailty in older adults
- List tools that can be used to identify older adults living with frailty
- Describe the positive and potentially negative aspects of the biomedical narrative of frailty

- Describe common management strategies for frailty
- Outline the evidence for rehabilitation potential of older adults living with frailty

INTRODUCTION

The World Health Organization defines healthy ageing as the process of developing and maintaining the functional ability that enables well-being in older age; and 'functional ability' as the interaction between a person's physical, mental, and psychological capacities and the environment they inhabit (World Health Organization, 2015). Being able to think, move, feel and react to the external environment is essential to participate in society, form relationships and express ourselves. Before we think about maintaining or restoring physical, mental or psychological function, it is good to think about how these functions work prior to decline.

In reality, the performance of a simple task relies on all of the physiological systems running simultaneously and efficiently. For example, in navigating an uneven path, our brains (nervous system) interpret sensory information, our legs (musculoskeletal system) perform the movement and our heart (cardiovascular system) pumps blood around the body distributing oxygen and glucose, fuelling the brain and muscles.

Homeostasis – Maintaining Order in Our Body

Homeostasis is an overall governing mechanism that takes care of each physiological system by repairing damaged cells and generating new ones, much like a car mechanic might repair or buy new parts while servicing your car. Homeostasis is a 24/7 job as there are always issues that need to be resolved. For example, your body temperature might be too high, which triggers a negative feedback loop to reduce the temperature to the normal range (through nerves, the temperature-regulatory control centre in your brain, sweat glands and blood flow). As homeostasis depends on negative feedback loops, anything that interferes with the latter can disrupt homeostasis and lead to disease.

For example, diabetes is a disease caused by a broken feedback loop involving the hormone insulin. When we eat a big meal our glucose levels rise, triggering the secretion of insulin. Diabetes occurs when a person cannot make enough insulin, or when cells in the body stop responding to insulin, or both. Under these conditions, blood sugar levels remain high for a long period after a meal leading to short-term and longer-term damage. Breakdowns in feedback loops can compromise the function of the entire body, because all of the physiological systems are linked and depend on each other in crucial ways.

Frailty – a State of 'Disorder'

As all of our physiological systems depend on each other to perform, the more problems there are, the more likely we are to break down under stress. 'Frailty' is a term that describes a situation when an older adult is vulnerable to breakdown, as the body has accumulated too many problems. Frailty increases the risk of adverse outcomes such as falls, delirium, sarcopenia, cognitive impairment, disability, hospitalisation and death (Campbell and Buchner, 1997; Theou and Rockwood, 2012).). Much can be done for older adults living with frailty to manage and in some cases, reverse the condition.

WHAT DOES 'FRAILTY' MEAN?

The condition 'frailty' has three core characteristics: (1) vulnerability, (2) deficit accumulation, and (3) gradient.

Vulnerability

Frailty is synonymous with 'vulnerability'. Older adults living with frailty are at increased risk of adverse outcomes due to their reduced ability to 'bounce back' after a stressor event (Clegg et al., 2013) such as a new drug, minor infection, or minor surgery. For example, a healthy older adult might be hospitalised with a urinary tract infection, but will recover quickly following treatment. However, an older adult living with frailty will typically take longer to recover, may experience complications in hospitals such as confusion, disorientation, agitation, delirium, lose muscle tone and weight, and may also experience issues once leaving the hospital, such as reduced functional ability and increased care needs (Clegg et al., 2013) (Fig. 4.1).

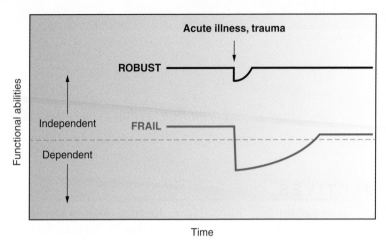

FIG. 4.1 Frail older adults' risk of change in health status after an acute illness (Modified from Clegg et al., 2013. Reproduced with permission).

In acute hospital settings, frailty adds to the severity of the acute illness in predicting inpatient mortality (Romero-Ortuno et al., 2016) and is associated with adverse functional trajectories during acute hospitalisation (Lyons et al., 2019), longer lengths of stay in hospital (Roe, 2016; Roe et al., 2017) and increased risk of future hospitalisations and nursing home admission (Hastings et al., 2008).

Deficit Accumulation

While it is a normal part of ageing to experience a gradual decline in the working of physiological systems, for older adults with frailty this decline is accelerated and numerous problems accumulate (Fulop et al., 2010). Frailty develops as a consequence of age-related decline across many physiological systems, which collectively results in vulnerability to sudden health status changes triggered by minor stressors (Clegg et al., 2013). While frailty is associated with disease, it can occur in the absence of disease, and problems can arise from a poorly functioning immune system (e.g. inflammageing), nervous system (e.g. neuroendocrine dysregulation) and digestive system (e.g. nutritional and metabolic alterations) which are also thought to determine frailty. Social factors also determine frailty, such as gender, education and neighbourhood deprivation. This link between social/environmental exposures and the development of later life health problems reinforces the need for a lifecourse approach to healthy ageing which addresses early/mid-life social determinants of health such as poverty (e.g. income or food poverty), discrimination (e.g. ethnicity or sexual orientation) and social conditions (e.g. poor housing or education) (Marmot, 2018).

Gradient

Frailty is commonly thought to be a one-way process involving grades: healthy or 'robust'; moving to those on the cusp of frailty: 'pre-frail'; and finally those who are 'frail'. In reality, the process is not linear, and there can be movement between stages (Gill et al., 2006, De Vries et al., 2011, Fallah et al., 2011,

Etman et al., 2012). For example, researchers examining frailty transitions in a study of non-disabled community-dwelling adults aged 70 years or older found that the experience of frailty can include recovery for many individuals (Gill et al., 2006).

Additionally, needs and experiences vary within each stage. For example, some older adults with frailty would need home care, while others might need palliative care which is well described, for example in the nine stages of the Clinical Frailty Scale (Rockwood, 2005).

How Can We Identify and Measure Frailty in Older Adults?

Although frailty is often clinically recognisable, operational criteria vary. There are over 20 different validated measures of frailty (Sternberg et al., 2011), but no agreed 'gold standard' measure. However, a consensus paper on frailty measurement concluded that measures ought to evaluate frailty across multiple dimensions including physical performance, gait speed, mobility, nutritional status, mental health, and cognition (Rodriguez-Manas et al., 2013).

While comprehensive geriatric assessment (CGA) holistically examines an older adult (Pilotto et al., 2017), in practice each frailty measure explores certain CGA components or domains. For example, some measures have a stronger focus on the presence of chronic illnesses, some on objective physical performance measures, while others are more multidimensional and include chronic illness, physical factors, disability, cognition and psychosocial aspects. In addition, some frailty measures were designed for use in a clinical setting, some for use in population setting, and others for use in both clinical and population settings (Dent et al., 2016). Two very commonly used measures of frailty are the frailty phenotype and the frailty index.

Frailty Phenotype

Fried et al. (2001) developed the frailty phenotype measure of frailty. The phenotype approach considers frailty as a clinical

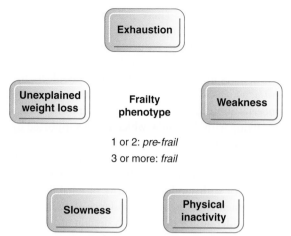

FIG. 4.2 Components of the frailty phenotype (Based on Fried et al., 2001).

syndrome, comprising five specific indicators: unintentional weight loss, self-reported exhaustion, low physical activity, slow gait speed and weak grip strength (see Fig. 4.2).

Those with three or more of the five factors were judged to be frail, those with one or two factors as pre-frail and those with no factors as not frail or robust. According to this model, multimorbidity gives rise to frailty, and frailty is a pre-disability state (Fried et al., 2004).

Frailty Index

Rockwood and colleagues (Rockwood et al., 2005) developed a frailty index measure of frailty. This approach considers frailty as an accumulation of health problems where "the number of things that are wrong with you" is more important than "what is wrong with you" in determining if you are frail. The original index containing over 90 possible deficits was later revised to a much more manageable minimum of 30 deficits (Searle et al., 2008). Deficits must satisfy basic criteria such as being associated to poor biological outcomes, accumulate with age and not saturate too early (i.e. develop too high a prevalence at younger ages). The frailty index is a simple calculation: divide the number of deficits present in the person by the total number of deficits considered (Fig. 4.3). This gives a score ranging from 0 (none of the deficits present) to 1 (all deficits present) (e.g., 20 deficits present of a possible 92 gives a frailty index of 20/92 = 0.22). A value

Frailty index:

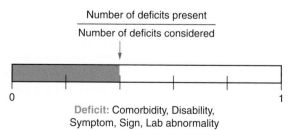

FIG. 4.3 Summary of the frailty index approach (Based on Searle et al., 2008).

of around 0.7 appears to be a threshold beyond which death is very likely.

While the frailty index is a continuous measure of frailty, cut-points have been established which allow people to categorise older adults as frail (score of 0.25 or more) (Searle et al., 2008).

Comparison of Frailty Measures

Depending on how you measure frailty, the prevalence of frailty in community-dwelling adults aged 65 years and older ranges between 5% and 60% (Collard et al., 2012, Sternberg et al., 2011). In Ireland, researchers using data from The Irish Longitudinal Study on Ageing (TILDA) estimated the prevalence of frailty among community-dwelling adults aged 65 years and older at 8% (Fried Phenotype) and 24% (Frailty Index) (Roe et al., 2017).

All frailty assessment tools identify people who are vulnerable to adverse outcomes (Theou et al., 2014), but each measure will identify a different group of older adults (De Vries et al., 2011), with partial overlap. Because measures have been developed from different theoretical constructs, they are capturing slightly different mechanisms and trajectories and hence do not identify the same older adults as frail. This is because different frailty tools address different domains of health. In choosing a measure it is important to remember that some were designed to be screening instruments and others were designed to be more comprehensive outcome, or prognostic indices (Martin and Brighton, 2008).

How Can We Best Manage Frailty?

The British Geriatrics Society (BGS) 'Fit for Frailty' guidelines caution that we may put older adults with frailty at risk of significant harm if healthcare interventions are planned for them without recognising their frailty (Turner, 2015). For example, older adults with frailty are at risk of potentially inappropriate prescribing where clinical guidelines fail to present modifications for frailty (Boyd et al., 2005), creating the need for medication reviews. Frailty assessment is becoming a feature of mainstream services outside of specialist geriatric hospital care. For example, in England in 2017, frailty identification became a contractual requirement for GPs (Travers et al., 2019).

Comprehensive Geriatric Assessment

Frailty tools are only measures of risk and need to be followed up with a more comprehensive assessment to fully understand what is going on. CGA is a process of care with a multidimensional holistic assessment of an older person's health and well-being, care planning, service activation and ongoing monitoring (Pilotto et al., 2017) (see Chapter 2 Comprehensive Assessment of Older People).

CGA in the hospital setting has been found to improve survival rates and the chances of independent living 6–12 months following a hospital admission for older adults classified as frail (Ellis et al., 2017). In the community, CGA may also offer health benefits (Garrard et al., 2019).

Care Needed in Using 'Labels'

While frailty identification is important, care is needed in using the label 'frail' with older adults and their families (De Witte et al., 2013). Frailty can be interpreted as a label denoting losses and diminished function. In a clinical encounter, frailty can be the sole objective for care, when for some older adults their frailty is not the source of their difficulty. Some frailty measures consist of objective measures of health and well-being, and overlook the social and emotional experiences of the individual and their individual strengths and capacities. Finally, by examining frailty from the perspective of the individual, we fail to address the social and environmental determinants of health. For example, 'risk of falling' can be driven by poor muscle strength but also by poor street design.

It is important that every older adult living with frailty is treated in clinical settings as a unique individual with different expectations, hopes, fears, strengths and abilities, as well as different types and levels of need and support (Turner, 2015). The starting point of care should be what is important to the individual with frailty, their family and carers ('nothing about me without me'). These may not be centred on the management of a specific disease or the achievement of disease-based outcomes (such as keeping blood sugar levels at a specific level) but instead focus on the priorities of the older adult. Sometimes the goals will contradict medical goals; for example, patients with high blood pressure may want to forego treatments which make them hypotensive at times and thus liable to fall or feel dizzy (Turner, 2015). Understanding an individual's goals and planning treatment and support strategies to achieve those goals involves the process of personalised care planning. The role that frailty plays is being able to *identify* those older adults who are on the cusp of decline and to apply clinical evidence that helps to remove or minimise stressors. This involves addressing the rehabilitation needs of older adults with frailty.

What is the Rehabilitation Potential of an Older Adult Living With Frailty?

Older adults have the right to be able to attain and maintain maximum independence, with the assistance of comprehensive rehabilitation services, through article 26.1 of the UN *Convention on the Rights of Persons with Disabilities*. However, older adults can experience barriers to rehabilitation services.

Firstly, adults with 'hidden' disabilities such as dementia may experience barriers to care when rehabilitation is viewed in terms of physical rehabilitation following injury (Clare, 2017). Cognitive rehabilitation (CR) applies basic rehabilitation principles to enable people with dementia and other long-term progressive neurodegenerative conditions to maintain or optimise functioning (Clare, 2017). The aim of CR is not to improve cognition, but to facilitate improved management of functional disability. Potential targets include everyday functioning, activities of daily living, self-care, language and communication, social interaction and the effects of dementia-related physical disability (Clare, 2017). There is a small but growing evidence base demonstrating that CR is effective in supporting everyday functioning, reducing disability and delaying institutionalisation (Clare, 2017). There is also evidence that physical activity may be beneficial in older people living with dementia, which is important as at times there are unfounded concerns about the safety risks of promoting exercise in persons living with dementia, which is not supported by evidence (Zieschang et al., 2017).

Secondly, it is important to challenge the viewpoint that older adults with frailty always have 'poor rehab potential', or they cannot withstand the intensity of rehabilitation programmes, when there is ample evidence showing the contrary. Even older adults in the ninth decade of life can show increases in muscle strength from resistance exercise training, despite the age-related changes in muscle strength (Travers et al., 2019). Rehabilitation in this context can include physical activity, health education, nutrition supplementation, home visits and counselling. A review of interventions in primary care settings which address frailty found muscle strength training and protein supplementation were placed highest for effectiveness and ease of implementation (Travers et al., 2019).

Additionally, a consortium in the UK, 'Moving Medicine', produced a number of evidence reviews on physical exercise across a range of conditions. In the context of physical exercise and 'Falls and Frailty', they found that physical activity benefits the oldest-old, including those living in long-term care facilities (Moving Medicine, 2019). Moving Medicine found no evidence to suggest exercise is harmful in frail populations. The Moving Medicine consortium found good evidence that physical exercise decreases both the risk and rate of falls, improves the ability to perform activities of daily living, reduces the risk of falls-related fractures, improves functional ability, leads to improvements in walking speed, balance and muscle strength, and can reduce the severity and progression of frailty. Based on their evidence review, they recommended that older adults should aim to:

1. Be active daily, in bouts of at least 10 minutes and in total at least 150 minutes per week.
2. Do muscle strengthening and balance activities on at least 2 days per week.

It needs to be acknowledged that rehabilitation in the context of frailty is not straightforward. For example, an older woman living with frailty and osteoporosis with recurrent fractures on weight-bearing activities might be encouraged by healthcare staff to limit her physical activity to reduce the risk of future fractures. However, an alternative approach might try to break the cycle of fractures by discussing with her alternative ways she can exercise safely, such as using a home exercise bike instead of walking. This solution isn't risk free, but can improve her musculoskeletal health and her physical and mental well-being. By creating a rapport with the woman, it's possible to discuss what goals are important to her, what the risks are with achieving these goals and then tailoring a care plan to manage risks and maximise outcomes.

Finally, truly transformative power comes from approaching rehabilitation not as a prescribed treatment but as a way of life. In many cultures 'care and respect' for older adults is demonstrated by doing activities for them, when in reality older adults would benefit from the time, encouragement and support to stay engaged in activities, even if they can't do them as quickly, or as effectively, as before. This requires changes in attitudes; policies to ensure the built environment support people of all abilities to function; and the opportunities for older adults to participate in activity, for example, the National Physical Activity Programme for Older People 'Go for Life' provided by Age and Opportunity (Citizens Information, 2019).

CONCLUSION

Frailty measures are tools to identify older adults with complex needs who are at risk of adverse outcomes. With evidence from the research identifying the benefits of rehabilitation programmes even for the oldest-old, therapists can confidently intervene and expect positive outcomes. The key will be to identify those adults with frailty, to holistically assess their needs and capacities at baseline and to work with the older adult and their families to determine what is important and how rehabilitation can support them to maintain the functions which provide meaning as they continue into their older-old years.

SUMMARY POINTS

- The clinical concept of frailty refers to a syndrome or a state of vulnerability to stressors
- Frailty is not a diagnosis; the identification of frailty needs to be followed by a diagnostic process of multidisciplinary comprehensive geriatric assessment (CGA)
- Frailty is also an indication for rehabilitation. There is evidence that physical activity and nutrition can delay or reverse frailty in populations
- Frailty is not (and should not be accepted as) a marker of 'poor rehabilitation potential'
- Medical professionals need to be aware of the potential negative consequences that a 'frailty label' may have for patients
- It is important that medical professionals educate patients that frailty is dynamic and potentially remediable, and focus on their lived experience as well as the purely medical aspects

MCQs

1. Which one of the following is not a component of the clinical definition of frailty?
   a. Multiple physiological systems dysregulation
   b. Vulnerability to stressors
   c. Higher risk of adverse outcomes
   d. Progression to dementia
   e. Reduced physiological reserve
2. Which one of the following is not defining the frailty phenotype?
   a. Low physical activity
   b. Exhaustion
   c. Unexplained weight loss
   d. Weakness
   e. Falls
3. Which two of the following have good evidence for delaying and/or reversing frailty?
   a. Advanced care planning
   b. Medication listing
   c. Exercise interventions
   d. Activation of a summary care record
   e. Nutritional optimisation

REFERENCES

Boyd, C. M., Darer, J., Boult, C., Fried, L. P., Boult, L., & Wu, A. W. (2005). Clinical practice guidelines and quality of care for older adults with multiple comorbid diseases. *Journal of American Medical Informatics Association, 294*, 716–724.

Campbell, A. J., & Buchner, D. M. (1997). Unstable disability and the fluctuations of frailty. *Age Ageing, 26*, 315–318.

Citizens information. (2019). Go for Life programme [Online]. Retrieved from www.citizensinformation.ie (Accessed 12 September, 2019).

Clare, L. (2017). Rehabilitation for people living with dementia: a practical framework of positive support. *PLOS Medicine, 14*, e1002245.

Clegg, A., Young, J., Iliffe, S., Olde Rikkert, M., & Rockwood, K. (2013). Frailty in elderly people. *The Lancet, 381*, 752–762.

Collard, R. M., Boter, H., Schoevers, R. A., & Oude Voshaar, R. C. (2012). Prevalence of frailty in community-dwelling older persons: a systematic review. *Journal of the American Geriatrics Society, 60*, 1487–1492.

Dent, E., Kowal, P., & Hoogendijk, E. O. (2016). Frailty measurement in research and clinical practice: a review. *European Journal of Internal Medicine, 31*, 3–10.

de Vries, N. M., Staal, J. B., van Ravensberg, C. D., Hobbelen, J. S. M., Olde Rikkert, M. G. M., & Nijhuis-van der Sanden, M. W. G. (2011). Outcome instruments to measure frailty: a systematic review. *Ageing Research Reviews, 10*, 104–114.

De Witte, N., De Donder, L., Dury, S., Buffel, T., Verté, D., & Schols, J. (2013). A theoretical perspective on the conceptualisation and usefulness of frailty and vulnerability measurements in community dwelling older persons. *APORIA, 5*, 13–21.

Ellis, G., Gardner, M., Tsiachristas, A., Langhorne, P., Burke, O., Harwood, R. H., Conroy, S. P., Kircher, T., Somme, D., Saltvedt, I., Wald, H., O'Neill, D., Robinson, D., & Shepperd, S. (2017). Comprehensive geriatric assessment for older adults admitted to hospital. *Cochrane Database of Systematic Reviews, 9*, CD006211.

Etman, A., Burdorf, A., Van der Cammen, T. J., Mackenbach, J. P., & Van Lenthe, F. J. (2012). Socio-demographic determinants of worsening in frailty among community-dwelling older people in 11 European countries. *Journal of Epidemiology and Community Health, 66*, 1116–1121.

Fallah, N., Mitnitski, A., Searle, S. D., Gahbauer, E. A., Gill, T. M., & Rockwood, K. (2011). Transitions in frailty status in older adults in relation to mobility: a multistate modeling approach employing a deficit count. *Journal of American Geriatrics Society, 59*, 524–549.

Fried, L. P., Ferrucci, L., Darer, J., Williamson, J. D., & Anderson, G. (2004). Untangling the concepts of disability, frailty, and comorbidity: implications for improved targeting and care. *Journal of Gerontology A Biological Sciences and Medical Sciences, 59*, 255–263.

Fried, L. P., Tangen, C. M., Walston, J., Newman, A. B., Hirsch, C., Gottdiener, J., Seeman, T., Tracy, R., Kop, W. J., Burke, G., & McBurnie, M. A. (2001). Frailty in older adults: evidence for a phenotype. *Journal of Gerontology A Biological Sciences and Medical Sciences, 56*, M146–M156.

Fulop, T., Larbi, A., Witkowski, J. M., McElhaney, J., Loeb, M., Mitnitski, A., & Pawelec, G. (2010). Aging, frailty and age-related diseases. *Biogerontology Journal, 11*, 547–563.

Garrard, J. W., Cox, N. J., Dodds, R. M., Roberts, H. C., & Sayer, A. A. (2019). Comprehensive geriatric assessment in primary care: a systematic review. *Aging Clinical and Experimental Research, 32*, 197–205.

Gill, T. M., Gahbauer, E. A., Allore, H. G., & Han, L. (2006). Transitions between frailty states among community-living older persons. *Archives of Internal Medicine, 166*, 418–423.

Hastings, S. N., Purser, J. L., Johnson, K. S., Sloane, R. J., & Whitson, H. E. (2008). Frailty predicts some but not all adverse outcomes in older adults discharged from the emergency department. *Journal of the American Geriatrics Society, 56*, 1651–1657.

Lyons, A., Romero-Ortuno, R., & Hartley, P. (2019). Functional mobility trajectories of hospitalized older adults admitted to acute geriatric wards: a retrospective observational study in an English university hospital. *Geriatrics & Gerontology International, 19*, 305–310.

Marmot, M. (2018). Just societies, health equity, and dignified lives: the PAHO Equity Commission. *The Lancet, 392*, 2247–2250.

Martin, F. C., & Brighton, P. (2008). Frailty: different tools for different purposes? *Age Ageing, 37*, 129–131.

Mitnitski, A. B., Mogilner, A. J., & Rockwood, K. (2001). Accumulation of deficits as a proxy measure of aging. *ScientificWorld Journal, 1*, 323–336.

Moving Medicine. (2019). Prescribing movement for falls and frailty [Online]. Retrieved from: http://movingmedicine.ac.uk/disease/fallsandfrailty/ (Accessed 17 July 2019).

Pilotto, A., Cella, A., Pilotto, A., Daragjati, J., Veronese, N., Musacchio, C., Mello, A. M., Logroscino, G., Padovani, A., Prete, C., & Panza, F. (2017). Three decades of comprehensive geriatric assessment: evidence coming from different healthcare settings and specific clinical conditions. *Journal of the American Medical Directors Association, 18*, 192e1–192e11.

Rockwood, K. (2005). A global clinical measure of fitness and frailty in elderly people. *Canadian Medical Association Journal, 173*, 489–495.

Rockwood, K., Andrew, M., & Mitnitski, A. (2007). A comparison of two approaches to measuring frailty in elderly people. *The Journal of Gerontology: Series A, 62*, 738–743.

Rodriguez-Manas, L., Feart, C., Mann, G., Vina, J., Chatterji, S., Chodzko-Zajko, W., Gonzalez-Colaco Harmand, M., Bergman, H., Carcaillon, L., Nicholson, C., Scuteri, A., Sinclair, A., Pelaez, M., Van Der Cammen, T., Béland, F., Bickenbach, J., Delamarche, P., Ferrucci, L., Fried, L. P., Gutierrez-Robledo, L. M., Rockwood, K., Rodriguez Artalejo, F., Serviddio, G., & Vega, E. (2013). Searching for an operational definition of frailty: a Delphi method based consensus statement: the frailty operative definition-consensus conference project. *Journal of Gerontology B Psychological Sciences & Social Sciences, 68*, 62–67.

Roe, L. (2016). An exploration of frailty and resource use in the Irish older population and the implications for the policy and practice of integrated care: a mixed methods study PhD thesis. Trinity College Dublin, Dublin.

Roe, L., Normand, C., Wren, M., Browne, J., & O'Halloran, A. (2017). The impact of frailty on healthcare utilisation in Ireland: evidence from the Irish longitudinal study on ageing. *BioMed Central Geriatrics, 17*, 203.

Romero-Ortuno, R., Wallis, S., Biram, R., & Keevil, V. (2016). Clinical frailty adds to acute illness severity in predicting mortality in hospitalized older adults: an observational study. *European Journal of Internal Medicine, 35*, 24–34.

Searle, S. D., Mitnitski, A., Gahbauer, E. A., Gill, T. M., & Rockwood, K. (2008). A standard procedure for creating a frailty index. *BioMed Central Geriatrics, 8*, 24.

Sternberg, S. A., Schwartz, M. A., Karunananthan, S., Bergman, H., & Clarfield, M. (2011). The identification of frailty: a systematic literature review. *Journal of the American Geriatrics Society, 59*, 2129–2138.

Theou, O., Brothers, T. D., Pena, F. G., Mitnitski, A., & Rockwood, K. (2014). Identifying common characteristics of frailty across seven scales. *Journal of the American Geriatrics Society, 62*, 901–906.

Theou, O., & Rockwood, K. (2012). Should frailty status always be considered when treating the elderly patient? *Aging Health, 8*, 261–271.

Travers, J., Romero-Ortuno, R., Bailey, J., & Cooney, M. T. (2019). Delaying and reversing frailty: a systematic review of primary care interventions. *British Journal of General Practice, 69*, e61–e69.

Turner, G. (2015). Fit for frailty II: developing, commissioning, and managing services for people living with frailty in community settings: guidance for GPs, geriatricians, health service managers, social service managers and commissioners of services. *A Report by the British Geriatrics Society and the Royal College of General Practitioners and AGE UK London.*

World Health Organization (2015). *World Report on Ageing.* Geneva: World Health Organization.

Zieschang, T., Schwenk, M., Becker, C., Uhlmann, L., Oster, P., & Hauer, K. (2017). Falls and physical activity in persons with mild to moderate dementia participating in an intensive motor training: randomized controlled trial. *Alzheimer Disease & Associated Disorders, 31*, 307–314.

5

Rehabilitation for Older People

Morgan Crowe, Kate Bennett & Shane O'Hanlon

LEARNING OBJECTIVES

- Explain the concept of rehabilitation
- Describe how rehabilitation can help older people to restore or maximise their functional ability
- Describe the settings for rehabilitation
- Explain how prehabilitation may help before surgery or cancer treatment

IMPAIRMENT, DISABILITY, FRAILTY

Older people represent the fastest growing sector of the population with dramatic increases predicted in the very old. In the UK, the proportion aged 85 years and over is expected to double over the next 25 years. Despite negative stereotyping, most older people are active, living at home and are engaged in society. They are however at risk of several disease processes such as stroke, arthritis or falls/fractures, which may have adverse physical and psychological effects. Following a stroke for example, a patient may be left with arm and leg weakness, depression or dementia. Such deficits are classified as impairments and may result in disability or limitation in performing functions such as basic activities of daily living (ADLs) or instrumental ADLs (see Table 5.1). The concept of disability or inability to perform these functions is very relevant in rehabilitation as hospital-based medicine tends to focus on the disease process and the ensuing impairments and does not always address disability which is a major concern for the patient.

Whilst disability is common in old age, it is important to keep in mind that most community dwelling older people are not disabled. In the Irish Longitudinal study of Aging (TILDA) which is a prospective study of a representative sample of the community living population in Ireland, only 15.5% of the 65- to 75-year-old age group were disabled in performing basic or instrumental ADLs. Whilst this figure increases to 34.6% in the 80+ group, the majority (65.4%) were completely independent. Disability therefore even in very older persons should prompt a search for the underlying cause or causes.

Alternatively some older people may suffer a dramatic decline in physical and mental well-being following minor issues such as an infection or treatment with a new medication. This may reflect the condition of frailty or increased vulnerability due to a decline in the older person's physiological and psychological reserves (see Chapter 4 Frailty). Between 25% and 50% of people aged over 85 years are considered to be frail indicating that most very old patients are not frail. Frailty therefore should not be considered an inevitable part of ageing, but it is more common in the very old and is associated with a higher risk of adverse outcomes and disability. The consequence of such disability may be very serious and, particularly if complicated by social isolation or unsuitable home circumstances, may result in loss of independence, and need for hospitalisation or nursing home care.

EVOLUTION OF REHABILITATION

Although dramatic advances have been made in the medical and surgical treatment of many diseases in recent years, patients are still often left with substantial disability after an illness. However, it is often possible through nursing care and allied health professional input in collaboration with the patient and family/carers to improve function and help the patient to regain independence. Someone with poor mobility following a stroke may be supported through rehabilitation to walk and perform usual daily activities with the help of aids if needed. Basic adaptions of the home following assessment by the occupational therapist such as provision of rails or moving the bed downstairs may allow the patient to move around safely and facilitate return home. Alternatively patients subject to prolonged bed rest following an acute illness may rapidly become deconditioned and dependent. Encouragement and support to mobilise, dress and self-care will often enable discharge home. The process of facilitating older people to function at the highest possible level and regain personal autonomy despite disabling diseases or acute insults is the essence of rehabilitation.

> *"Rehabilitation is a process that aims to restore or maximise functional ability"*

In the UK, the benefits of rehabilitation for older people were first identified by Dr Marjory Warren (1897–1960) who in 1935 was given responsibility for 714 chronically ill, mostly older patients in West Middlesex Hospital in London (Matthews, 1984). Most of these had multiple medical conditions, poor functional status and adverse social circumstances. They were regarded as incurable and referred to as inmates. She immediately moved to raise the standard of

TABLE 5.1	**Activities of daily living and instrumental activities of daily living**
Activities of daily living	Bathing and showering
	Personal hygiene and grooming
	Dressing
	Toileting
	Mobility
	Self-feeding
Instrumental activities of daily living	Cleaning and managing the house
	Managing money
	Moving within the community
	Preparing meals
	Shopping
	Taking medications
	Using the telephone

care adopting a very active multidisciplinary assessment and rehabilitation approach. Every patient was examined and medical treatment was administered where appropriate. She constantly stressed the dangers of immobility including incontinence, pressure sores, muscle atrophy and contractures. Vacated wards were used as gyms, and exercise programmes were introduced in which patients were encouraged to participate. Proper footwear and mobility aids were provided where necessary. Certain structural alterations were undertaken to promote mobility including removing obstructions, widening doors and installing handrails. Patients were encouraged to dress in their day clothes and to take responsibility for their personal care including washing and dressing: 'Nothing that a patient can do for himself should be done for him'. Meals were taken together to facilitate socialising and appropriate diets were provided, considering many patients were edentulous. Additional linen was obtained where incontinence was a problem although many patients regained continence as their mobility improved.

As a result of her work, the number of long-stay beds was reduced from 714 to 240 with many patients being discharged home or to residential care. The turnover of the unit was trebled. As there were 70,000 hospital beds in England with similar chronic sick patients, her work attracted the attention of the health planners in the newly established National Health Service. She constantly argued for special units in general hospitals for older people to establish correct diagnosis and institute treatment and rehabilitation pointing out that much disability could be avoided and many patients discharged home rather than to long-term hospital care. This eventually led to the development of acute assessment and rehabilitation units in newly created departments of geriatric medicine in acute hospitals. Over the past 20 years statistical analysis of the many randomised controlled trials on older patients admitted acutely to hospital have conclusively shown the benefits of multidisciplinary care and rehabilitation compared to usual care in reducing mortality and increasing the number of patients being discharged home (Bachmann et al., 2010). Interestingly, the research suggests that the patients who benefit most from this approach are those managed in designated wards as advocated by Dr Warren many years ago.

REHABILITATION IN OLDER PEOPLE

Rehabilitation in older people differs in many respects to younger patients. Multiple disease processes are more common in the older population and they are often on multiple medications which may affect ability to rehabilitate successfully. Thus a patient with a hip fracture may also have dementia resulting in 'poor carry over' of physiotherapy training or the same patient may have chronic kidney disease requiring regular haemodialysis which may make full participation in rehab extremely challenging. Older patients are often coming from a baseline of pre-existing disability which may necessitate adaptation of rehab goals.

Bed rest and immobility are tolerated very poorly in older people with frailty. Even short periods result in rapid decline in muscle strength and aerobic capacity due to pre-existing sarcopenia (muscle wasting). This predisposes older people to such complications as constipation, urinary and faecal incontinence, delirium (sudden onset of confusion), pressure sores and contractures. Finally patients may have been living in unsuitable accommodation or have limited home support. In some cases the older person may have been caring for a disabled spouse or partner.

The rehabilitation process must therefore include a number of important elements. Assessment must be comprehensive, taking into consideration all the patient's underlying medical conditions, both current and in the past, and accompanying medications. Appropriate treatment of all medical and surgical issues must be ensured underlining the importance of access to the facilities and expertise of the general hospital. The patient's baseline function, cognition and frailty status should be estimated. Objective assessment of the patient's current functional and cognitive status should be performed using simple validated tools, such as Barthel Index of ADLs, Timed Up and Go test, Abbreviated Mental Test Score (AMTS) or Montreal Cognitive Assessment (MOCA). Weight should be noted. These measurements serve as comparisons with previous or subsequent values and help in assessing progress. Rehabilitation focused services/settings should be organised around principles of enabling people to function optimally in the context of both their intrinsic capacity and current health state (Clare, 2017).

COMPONENTS OF REHABILITATION

Rehab is not a single intervention and involves a team, including doctors, nurses, physiotherapists, occupational therapists (OTs), and medical social worker with appropriate input from speech and language therapists, dieticians and clinical psychologists. Effective communication is essential and is facilitated by multidisciplinary team (MDT) meetings which should take place at least weekly. Here a practical management plan including goals can be discussed taking into consideration the patient's and family wishes and expectations. This must be flexible depending on the patient's progress or complications. Discharge planning will explore the need for home modifications or additional carer support to allow the patient to manage at home.

Given the risks of immobilisation in older people, rehab should commence as soon as possible following hospital admission rather than waiting until after illness has resolved (Fig. 5.1). Patients who commence the rehabilitation process early tend to do better functionally, and have a reduced length of stay (Kunik et al., 2006). Such an approach is often frustrated in the acute hospital by competing pressures on limited staff to prioritise management of patients with acute medical problems. This is compounded by the perception that patients must await transfer to a dedicated rehab ward or hospital resulting in delays of days or weeks during which time the patient is labelled as 'awaiting rehab' – something that should never happen. There is evidence that higher intensity of therapy can result in greater gains in functional independence and a shorter length of stay as an inpatient (Jette et al., 2005); therefore, patients should be seen regularly by all appropriate professionals to optimise their recovery.

It is not always feasible for someone following an emergency procedure (such as abdominal surgery), or an acute illness such as pneumonia, to start rehabilitation immediately. In these cases there may be medical factors to take into account before effective rehabilitation can begin. Early rehabilitation is promoted as soon as reasonably possible; there is benefit however to completing an initial assessment with the individual and/or their family to provide background history, explore previous levels of function and determine rehabilitation goals. Getting patients out of bed and into their day clothes is a simple intervention that can be instituted by nursing staff and helps to promote recovery. The End PJ Paralysis movement has helped to empower staff, patients and families to do just that.

SETTINGS FOR REHABILITATION

Rehabilitation may be provided in a number of locations. For inpatients these range from general medical wards or designated rehab wards in the general hospital to stand-alone rehab units/hospitals. Patients managed in designated wards with a coordinated MDT particularly benefit compared to patients managed on general wards even with advice from a specialist MDT. For example, for patients admitted with acute stroke, access to a specialist stroke rehab unit is recommended by the Royal College of Physicians based on robust evidence about their efficacy.

Stand-alone rehab facilities in a unit separate to the general hospital promote multidisciplinary care in a less frantic and pressurised atmosphere compared to a busy acute hospital and is very conducive to successful rehabilitation for certain patients. However, transferring patients to such units may have some disadvantages including risk of medication errors or delays, or breaks in continuity of rehab, particularly if acute medical problems necessitate transfer back to the acute hospital. Many older patients with cognitive impairment tolerate transfer to a different hospital with unfamiliar staff poorly, particularly if they have already had multiple moves in the initial admitting hospital which increases the risks of complications such as delirium. Despite these disadvantages, stand-alone rehab units may be particularly useful for older patients who are medically stable and doing well with rehab but deemed to require a longer period of inpatient rehab with a view to discharge home. This environment also allows for complex discharge planning while appropriate care and equipment is sourced. Arrangements for follow-up to assess progress at home by the hospital team or the patient's GP should be put in place. Further rehab at the day hospital, day centre or at home may be required to maintain function and prevent hospital readmission.

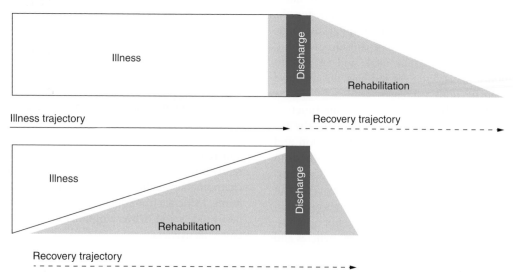

FIG. 5.1 The top panel shows the 'traditional' rehabilitation mindset, where illness was treated first. The bottom panel shows the integrative model, where rehabilitation begins on admission and gradually increases as recovery proceeds.

REHABILITATION IN THE COMMUNITY

Community rehabilitation is usually less intensive than rehabilitation in any inpatient setting. It can be provided in the person's usual place of residence or other settings such as day hospitals or community rehabilitation units (see Chapter 63 Rehabilitation in the Community). The aim is to achieve any outstanding goals and ensure the return to baseline function is complete.

The first purpose built day hospital was developed by Dr Lionel Cosin in Cowley Road Hospital, Oxford in 1957. He recognised the need to get older people back to their home or avoid inpatient hospital admission. The day hospital is staffed by medical and nursing personnel with variable input from physiotherapists, OTs and other allied health professionals and facilitates medical assessment, nursing care and rehabilitation without need for hospital admission. It is usually located on an acute hospital or rehabilitation hospital campus where it has access to existing medical or rehabilitation expertise and facilities. As the patient attends on a day basis from their own home, transport is an essential component of any effective service. Where rehabilitation is the main indication, patients may attend for any time from 6–12 weeks depending on progress in meeting their goals. At this time they should be discharged with advice from the physiotherapist to continue an appropriate exercise program at home or in a day centre. The day hospitals may also offer subspecialty services such as heart failure, bone protection, falls or stroke secondary prevention clinics. Whilst these may also be provided in the outpatient department, availability of more time and meals in a multidisciplinary environment makes the day hospital particularly suitable for many frail older people.

Other developments to expedite discharge to home or provide rehab at home include an Early Supported Discharge Service. In some cases earlier discharge may be possible if the patient's rehab can be continued at home, e.g. using a 'Discharge to Assess' model. This may include a coordinated MDT of therapists, nurses and doctors who work together to continue rehab at home following hospital discharge. Early supported discharge should also be considered for hip fracture patients who are medically stable and are able to transfer and mobilise short distances and have the cognitive ability to participate in continued rehab.

If goals are unable to be achieved or baseline function is not attained, the community team will ensure the individual has achieved their optimal level of function and that appropriate equipment and input to enable them to remain safely in their own home are provided. Community rehabilitation teams are multidisciplinary and can provide input for a finite period of time. Patients are often referred when discharged from inpatient care but a significant number of referrals come from GPs, care agencies and other community-based services. These referrals will be for people who don't require hospital admission but have some impairment of function. Whilst they remain able to stay in their usual place of residence, they require therapy input in order to regain their usual level of function or ascertain appropriate support and equipment in order to remain safely in their own home.

REHABILITATION IN RESIDENTIAL SETTINGS

Provision of ongoing community rehabilitation in residential settings (e.g. a care home) can be widely variable. If the service is unable to be provided, this can cause disappointment for both the individual and their immediate family who may have been reliant on this intervention.

In residential settings the level of staff involvement with rehabilitation programmes or interventions can also vary hugely. Staff undertaking exercise programmes or other interventions need to know exactly what is expected of them, how to perform any interventions appropriately and effectively and also who to contact with any issues/queries about the intervention in the immediate weeks following input. There should also be a pathway in place for the staff to re-refer to the community rehabilitation team should the needs of the person change and a review of their functional ability be required.

PREHABILITATION

As noted above many older persons have frailty which increases their risk of serious adverse outcomes following events that stress their system. Complications following surgery occur in up to 50% of patients, many of whom are older people with frailty. Prehabilitation refers to pre-operative or pre-cancer treatment programmes including exercise, psychological and nutritional interventions aimed at improving physiological reserve and reducing incidence of post-operative complications. Evidence from systemic reviews of prehabilitation has revealed improved outcomes in exercise capacity and cardiorespiratory fitness following surgery for lung cancer although results in patients undergoing colorectal surgery have been less conclusive. Many research studies are currently taking place examining various ways to conduct prehabilitation. Exercise interventions have shown promising results in patients undergoing treatment for breast, prostate, gynaecological and haematological cancers in terms of improving quality of life and reducing fatigue. Prehabilitation programmes are currently offered at many institutions prior to surgery or cancer chemotherapy. Patients may participate in the hospital or at home. Evidence from ongoing trials may help to identify the best models and delivery options to optimise outcome and cost-effectiveness.

SUMMARY POINTS

- Rehabilitation is the process of facilitating people to function at the highest possible level
- There is evidence from trials that rehabilitation reduces mortality and increases the chance of returning home
- Rehabilitation can occur in many settings such as an acute hospital, a stand-alone rehabilitation unit or in a person's own home
- Newer models are examining prehabilitation, with the aim of avoiding or reducing the deconditioning associated with illness or its treatment

MCQs

Q.1 Which of the following is true about rehabilitation?
  a. It only occurs in rehabilitation units
  b. Rehabilitation should only begin once acute illness has resolved
  c. There is little evidence for benefit
  d. Rehabilitation can occur in many settings including acute hospitals, the community and nursing homes
  e. Rehabilitation is only performed by a physiotherapist

Q.2 Which of the following is true about transfer to stand alone rehabilitation units?
  a. It is always necessary after an illness or operation
  b. Some people may become more confused due to the transfer
  c. There are no risks involved in the transfer of care
  d. They are suitable for medically unstable patients
  e. They are not suitable for complex discharge planning

REFERENCES

Bachmann, S., Finger, C., Huss, A., Egger, M., Stuck, A. E., & Clough-Gorr, K. (2010). Inpatient rehabilitation specifically designed for geriatric patients: systematic review and meta-analysis of randomised controlled trials. *British Medical Journal, 340,* c1718.

Clare, L. (2017). Rehabilitation for people living with dementia: a practical framework of positive support. *PLoS Medicine, 14*(3), e1002245.

Jette, D. U., Warren, R. L., & Wirtalla, C. (2005). The relation between therapy intensity and outcomes of rehabilitation in skilled nursing facilities. *Archives of Physical Medicine and Rehabilitation, 86*(3), 373–379.

Kunik, C. L., Flowers, L., & Kazanjian, T. (2006). Time to rehabilitation admission and associated outcomes for patients with traumatic brain injury. *Archives of Physical Medicine and Rehabilitation, 87*(12), 1590–1596.

Matthews, D. (1984). Dr. Marjory Warren and the origin of British geriatrics. *Journal of the American Geriatrics Society, 32*(4), 253–258.

6

The Rehabilitation Team

Claire Dow

LEARNING OBJECTIVES

- Introduce the different multidisciplinary team members involved in rehabilitation
- Briefly describe the roles of team members
- Explain how team members work together to achieve the patient's goals

This chapter provides a brief introduction to the members of the multidisciplinary rehabilitation team (MDT) and how it works together to provide high-quality care for older people undergoing rehabilitation.

CASE

George is admitted to the emergency department (ED) following a fall at home. This is the third time he has fallen in the last few weeks and his wife and children are becoming increasingly concerned about him.

He had a stroke 3 years ago from which he recovered well. He was left with a slight limp on his left leg and some word finding difficulties, especially when he is anxious. His wife Anne reports that he has been slightly more forgetful over the last 12–18 months and he has become more worried about leaving the house as he has felt more unsteady on his feet over the last few months. He needs some help with getting washed in the morning (struggling to get in and out of the bath) and Anne has to help with putting his socks and shoes on as he struggles to bend over now. They live together in a three-bedroom house with the toilet and bathroom upstairs. Their son lives 15 miles away and their daughter 10 miles away. Both visit weekly to help with the heavy shopping and they all go out for a weekend meal together (which George and Anne look forward to).

In the ED George is assessed by the **nursing** and **medical** teams. He has bad bruising to his left-hand side where he fell, but fortunately has not broken any bones. He also has a skin tear on his left arm and is noted to have non-blanching redness over his sacrum (lower back). He has had a bad cough recently and is found to have a chest infection and blood pressure at the lower end of the normal range (110/65 mmHg).

He is assessed by the **physiotherapist** and **occupational therapist** in the ED who find he is too frightened to stand up and walk due to the pain on the left side and fear of falling again. He finds it difficult to express how he is feeling and can appear quite upset at times. A decision is made to admit him to the hospital for further assessment and treatment.

He is admitted to the older adults ward where his care is discussed in the **board round** the following morning at which the medical team, nursing team, physiotherapist, occupational therapist and **social worker** are present. Due to his communication difficulties a referral to the **speech and language therapist** is made.

He continues to be quite anxious about getting out of bed, and Anne admits his memory has been worse than she had previously admitted to her children. A cognitive assessment is undertaken and referral to the **clinical psychologist** is also made to see what strategies could be helpful in managing his anxiety and to arrange cognitive rehabilitation. A medication review is undertaken by the medical team and **pharmacist,** and his chest infection is improving.

In the board round the following day, goals that have been identified by the team are discussed and plans set to meet these. A key worker (the occupational therapist) coordinates his rehabilitation with the team and keeps George and Anne (and their family) up to date with the goals which they have jointly agreed and planned.

George recovers over the next 3 days, and plans are made for him to go home with the appropriate equipment to help with bathing, and a reablement package of care is set up to help whilst he continues to recover. The **community therapy team** will continue to work with George to improve his confidence on the stairs and outside. The **district nursing team** will monitor his skin tear and his **GP** is asked to review his blood pressure (as some of his medications have been stopped on admission). A referral to the local **memory service** is also made for review regarding his memory once he has recovered from his hospital admission. He is discharged home after 5 days in hospital.

MEMBERS OF THE REHABILITATION TEAM

Team members vary depending on the setting, the person's needs and local resources. This section briefly describes the role of each team member, and there are chapters dedicated to many of these where more detail can be found later in the book. Fig. 6.1 shows one possible configuration of the rehabilitation team.

Patient and Their Family

The patient undergoing rehabilitation is the key member of the team, and it is essential to ensure that they are included in plans around their rehabilitation (especially if the person has issues with cognition or communication, to ensure that they know what is happening). Family members are also an important part of the team, and may provide most of the support when the person is ready to go home to continue their rehabilitation there.

Medical Team

In a hospital setting this will comprise of a specialist doctor (for example in the UK they would most commonly be a consultant geriatrician, but there are also consultants in Rehabilitation Medicine and Stroke Medicine who take a lead in this area), and the trainees in their team. They will undertake the assessment of medical conditions and treatments given and often will be a key person on the rehabilitation team (and may take a lead in meetings). In a community setting this may be the general practitioner or community geriatrician who will be involved.

Nursing Team

The nursing team not only comprises of the registered nursing team but also the invaluable work of the healthcare support worker (may also be called nursing assistant or healthcare assistant). Nurses are often the main contact for families and the main advocate for the people that they care for. The nursing assessments are a key part of the multidisciplinary assessment around an older person as they will give important information for example about continence, nutrition, hydration, worries and fears of the person. The healthcare support worker will often be privy to information that the person 'doesn't want to bother the nurse/doctor with' but may be the key piece of information about the person that leads to them meeting their rehabilitation goals.

In many rehabilitation teams there will also be clinical nurse specialists (CNS) who have extended skills in the care of adults undergoing rehabilitation. They will have undertaken additional qualifications in areas such as prescribing (and stopping) medications, advanced assessment skills and leadership of teams. The CNS leads the rehabilitation team in some units and can lead to enhanced outcome for patients and their families (Royal College of Nursing Policy Briefing, 2009).

Physiotherapist

The physiotherapist will undertake assessments of the older person taking into account not only their ability to walk and transfer, but also how their other conditions, treatments and other interventions can impact upon them. They will then formulate a treatment plan with the person to meet their goals (for example being able to walk up the stairs, go outside into the garden) how they can support this. They work in a variety of settings such as the ED, acute medical units, rehabilitation units and in the community to do this and will often undertake preventative work as well as rehabilitative work. They may be supported by a therapy support worker who can assist the person to meet their goals (Chartered Society of Physiotherapists, 2019).

Occupational Therapist

The occupational therapist will consider the physical, psychological, social and environmental needs of the person that they are working with (Royal College of Occupational Therapists, 2019). This will include hearing from the person and their family about what concerns they have about being at home after rehabilitation, how their underlying health conditions may impact upon this and how to help the person adapt to this as well as looking at interventions including assistive technology, equipment, links with social care and the voluntary sector to support the person when they return home. They too work across all the care settings.

Social Worker

Social workers will be able to undertake an assessment of the needs of an older person both in the hospital and at home. This will look at their needs, strengths and wishes working with individuals and families directly to help them make changes and solve problems, organising support, making recommendations or referrals to other services and agencies (British Association of Social Workers, 2019).

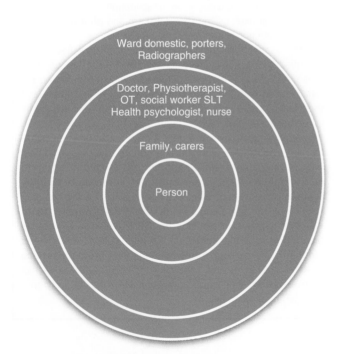

FIG. 6.1 Members of the rehabilitation team.

BOX 6.1   All Team Members Help Patients with Rehabilitation

The Importance of the Porter by Yusuf Yousuf (Pictured in Fig. 6.2)

The portering colleagues will bring valuable holistic input to the care of the patient that paints a bigger picture outside the clinical diagnosis they have presented with. For instance, when transporting patients from different settings around the hospital, porters (as non-clinical staff) are more likely to engage with patients about their hobbies, fear and what they most look forward to once they are home. This will bring them respite from the constantly buzzing ward, where they are likely to have conversations (which can also be repetitive) that predominantly revolve around their illness.

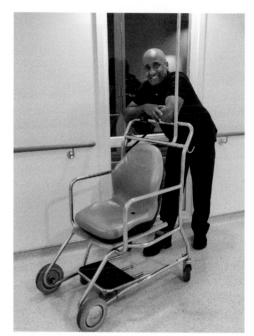

FIG. 6.2   The porter.

Speech and Language Therapist

Speech and language therapists undertake assessment and treat people who are having problems with talking and communicating their needs as well as assessing people who have swallowing and eating problems. They work closely with the person, their family and the wider MDT to provide tailored support for the person (Royal College of Speech and Language Therapists, 2019).

Clinical Psychologist

The clinical psychologist in the team can use their skills to promote rehabilitation and well-being. In a rehabilitation setting they may investigate why a person is behaving in a certain way that can impact on their rehabilitation and help them to regain control of the situation. They may also see how the event that now requires rehabilitation impacts on the individual, families and carers (Health Education England, 2019).

Other Team Members

The above shows the core members of the MDT involved in rehabilitation of an older adult but there are many other members of the team who will be involved ranging from pharmacists, radiographers and theatre staff to the ward domestic staff, volunteers and portering staff (see Box 6.1).

HOW DO WE COORDINATE THE REHABILITATION OF AN OLDER ADULT?

Working in a MDT and coordinating the rehabilitation of an older adult requires good communication between the team members. Regular MDT meetings are key in this and can range from the daily 'board round', where every person on the ward is briefly discussed with the goals for the day set and issues raised the previous day are discussed, to the weekly MDT meeting where a more in-depth discussion may take place. Many acute hospital units have moved towards the daily board round and use of tools such as the SAFER patient flow bundle (NHS Improvement, 2019) to ensure that the older person requiring rehabilitation does not get 'stranded' in hospital longer than they need to be there (see Fig. 6.3).

Ensuring all members of the team can contribute is key to these meetings and how this is done will vary according to the team. Ellis and Sevdalis (2019) give a good overview of how team working can be improved. Lessons can be learnt from work in behavioural science and how teams work in other areas. They suggest that team training in the MDT should occur to enhance how the team works once it is set up (including simulation training and patient feedback into the training) and use established leadership frameworks to identify who the best person in the team is to lead the MDT, along with other points regarding skills and competencies to improve how we deliver care to our patients and their carers.

SUMMARY POINTS

- The rehabilitation team will vary and flex according to the needs of the older person undergoing rehabilitation
- All team members bring their unique skills to the care of the person
- Rehabilitation may take place in many different settings and can start as soon as the person arrives into hospital or before this
- Ensuring that the team communicates with the person, their family and each other is a key part of successful rehabilitation

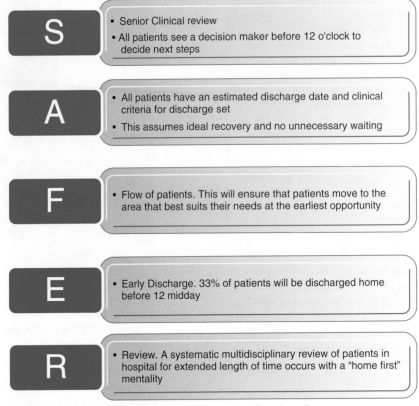

FIG. 6.3 The SAFER patient flow bundle.

MCQs

1. Rehabilitation is best undertaken at which of the following times?
   a. After the acute illness has resolved
   b. When the person has returned home
   c. As soon as the person is admitted to the acute hospital
   d. When the person is ready to move to an inpatient rehabilitation unit
   e. In a nursing home
2. The person best placed to coordinate the care of the older adult is:
   a. The doctor
   b. The nurse
   c. The physiotherapist
   d. The person whose skills meet the needs of the patient best
   e. The occupational therapist
3. Communication between team members best takes place:
   a. Weekly
   b. Monthly
   c. Daily
   d. Only if necessary
   e. In formal meetings

REFERENCES

British Association of Social Workers. (2019). What do social workers do? Retrieved from https://www.basw.co.uk/resources/become-social-worker/what-do-social-workers-do/ (Accessed September 1 2019).

Chartered Society of Physiotherapy. (2019), What is physiotherapy? Retrieved from https://www.csp.org.uk/careers-jobs/what-physiotherapy (Accessed September 1 2019).

Ellis, G., & Sevdalis, N. (2019). Understanding and improving multidisciplinary team working in geriatric medicine. *Age and Ageing, 48*, 498–505.

Health Education England. (2019). Health careers. https://www.healthcareers.nhs.uk/explore-roles/psychological-therapies/roles/health-psychologist (Accessed September 1 2019).

NHS Improvement. (2019). The SAFER patient flow bundle. https://improvement.nhs.uk/resources/safer-patient-flow-bundle-implement/ (Accessed September 1 2019).

Royal College of Nursing Policy Unit. (2009). Policy Briefing 14/2009. Specialist nurses make a difference. Retrieved from https://www.rcn.org.uk/about-us/policy-briefings/pol-1409#tab1 (Accessed September 1 2019).

Royal College of Occupational Therapy. (2019). What is occupational therapy? Retrieved from https://www.rcot.co.uk/about-occupational-therapy/what-is-occupational-therapy (Accessed September 1 2019).

Royal College of Speech and Language Therapists. (2019). What is speech and language therapy. Retrieved from https://www.rcslt.org/speech-and-language-therapy#section-1 (Accessed September 1 2019).

7

What Can Patients and Families Do to Help with Rehabilitation?

Rachel Tams

LEARNING OBJECTIVES

- Describe the key challenges people may face when entering into rehabilitation
- Identify a number of practical ways that patients and families can engage in rehabilitation to help the process to gain the best results
- Explain why self-care is important when engaging in rehabilitation

INTRODUCTION

Coming into a rehabilitation ward or unit can present a patient and their families with many challenges. For many older people, rehabilitation will follow a sudden, unexpected (and often traumatic) event such as a stroke, heart attack or fall, or a significant deterioration in an existing health condition. While the rehabilitation process may start early in the acute hospital setting (as soon as the individual is well enough to actively engage in rehabilitation), it often involves transfer from the acute setting to a ward/unit that has rehabilitation as its primary focus. For many patients and families, this will be their first experience of rehabilitation and there may be uncertainty about what to expect and what is expected of them (what the 'rules' are). It is important to note at the start of this chapter that rehabilitation settings for older adults can be incredibly diverse, with services ranging from highly structured specialist neurorehabilitation services to smaller, fragmented general services. While rehabilitation units/wards vary considerably, they generally involve:

- a longer stay than acute hospital settings
- multiple interventions with many different therapists
- more active patient/family involvement.

During rehabilitation, families may also be faced with difficult decisions (e.g. around future care). To add to the complexity, this may be happening within the context of new or worsening cognitive or communication difficulties, and significant mood issues as all involved struggle to adjust to the new situation. This chapter is written both for individuals undergoing rehabilitation and their family members, and focuses on how they can actively support the rehabilitation process by:

- being well-prepared practically
- becoming well-informed
- making sure the rehabilitation team know the patient's personal story

- following key recommendations of the rehabilitation team
- actively contributing to/engaging in the rehabilitation plan
- maintaining ongoing and effective communication with the team.
- attending to emotional self-care.

This chapter concludes with some advice on how to deal with difficult issues that might arise during the rehabilitation journey. See also the Resources section for a summary of practical ways to support rehabilitation and get the best results.

Being Well-Prepared Practically

To be able to engage fully in rehabilitation, it is important that you/your relative have any existing sensory difficulties corrected. Glasses or hearing aids should be brought in from home to ensure effective communication. Suitable comfortable clothing and footwear is required, as rehabilitation will involve being active in the gym or on the ward. Other items from home that might be helpful to bring in include those that help people stay in touch with significant others, activities to occupy free time, items that bring comfort or help as an aid to memory. See Box 7.1 for examples of useful items.

BOX 7.1   Useful Items to Bring to Rehabilitation

Glasses/hearing aids
Comfortable clothing/footwear
Phone/list of important phone numbers
Radio
Books/audiobooks/favourite magazines
Games – e.g. cards, crossword puzzles
Knitting/craft activities
Family photos/albums
Special blanket/pillow/cushion
Notebook and pen
Diary

Becoming Well-Informed

We know that being well-informed is important in helping everyone cope and adjust to longer-term changes. Gathering information and becoming better informed can help to address concerns, increase motivation and help manage expectations. The information provided routinely to patients and families may vary across settings. It can therefore be helpful for you to be proactive in seeking information if not automatically offered. This might involve completing some independent research (looking at websites, reading available literature), contacting local/national organisations, in addition to communicating with the rehabilitation team. It can be useful to gather the following:

Information About the Rehabilitation Setting Itself

As a start, it is helpful to know about the particular rehabilitation setting you (or your relative) have been referred to. Some background research may be helpful when transfer to rehabilitation is first mentioned (e.g. looking at website/leaflets) about the unit; asking questions about why a referral is being made. It may in some situations be possible to visit the onward rehabilitation setting before transfer. It is particularly important to know what to expect in the first few days after admission, as the rehabilitation unit/ward may be run in a very different way to more familiar hospital settings. It is expected that a team member would orientate you/your relative to the ward and provide relevant information. If this doesn't happen, however, families can play an important role in asking some key questions (outlined in Box 7.2).

Information About Current Areas of Difficulty and the Rehabilitation Plan

After their initial assessments the rehabilitation team will be able to give information about your/your relative's particular pattern of strengths and difficulties. This information will help everyone understand what they are experiencing/observing and the rationale behind rehabilitation tasks. The rehabilitation setting may have a particular structure in place for feeding back to patients and families (e.g. regular review meetings). However, if this is not the case, requesting time to talk through the assessments and rehabilitation plan with the professionals involved in care is important. You might find asking for written summaries, or to meet again after you have had time to absorb information, helpful.

Making Sure the Rehabilitation Team Know Your/Your Relative's Personal Story

The patient's story should be at the centre of rehabilitation to ensure that the rehabilitation plan is meaningful to them.

It is therefore essential that the team supporting you/your relative know something of your personal story. This includes personal history, likes/dislikes, values and motivators, who is important to you, previous experiences of illness, cultural issues and wishes regarding future care. Rehabilitation units may have a structured way of gaining this information and using it in rehabilitation. The Rivermead system of goal planning (Davis et al., 1992), for example, which has been widely adopted in neurorehabilitation, places the patient at the heart of the process by using a life goals questionnaire to guide initial goal planning. This semi-structured interview collects information from patients and families on important life goals, wishes and expectations, and sets up a collaborative system of goal setting.

For some patients, because of cognitive/communication difficulties, it may not be possible to provide this information themselves. In this case the family can play an important role in increasing the team's understanding. Bringing in photos from home, providing background history and other key information can all help the team better identify and engage with the patient. For people with dementia it is helpful to fill in and share the "This is me" leaflet; this useful tool can be downloaded from the Alzheimer's Society UK website. Alzheimer's Disease International (which provides a directory of worldwide Alzheimer's Disease Associations) may also be a useful starting place for sourcing similar resources. Website links are provided at the end of this chapter. Tools like "This is me" may be particularly important if the service is more fragmented and there are frequent changes in staff. Such information can ensure that assumptions about what the patient wants to achieve are avoided. It can also help the team understand decisions and preferences that may differ from theirs or seem unwise to others. For more information, see Chapter 19 The Patient Story.

Following Key Recommendations of the Rehabilitation Team

In order to help manage areas of difficulty and reduce risks, it is important to follow (or support your relative to follow) key advice provided by the team. Advice will be individualised, depending on initial assessment and will cover several areas. Some examples are provided in Box 7.3.

> **BOX 7.2   Example Questions**
>
> Can I visit at any time during the day?
> Can I attend therapy sessions? – this is usually encouraged but it is important to check
> What will my/my relative's daily timetable consist of?
> Who are the different professionals in the team?
> When/how do we all meet and discuss progress?

> **BOX 7.3   Examples of Advice from the Rehabilitation Team**
>
> - Communication difficulties – using pictures and gesture to support understanding of spoken language
> - Memory difficulties – writing down key information such as planned family visits on an easily visible white board in the bedroom
> - Reduced mobility – advice on the safest ways to get out of bed; the level of supervision or equipment needed to walk safely; use of powered wheelchair
> - Swallow difficulties – advice on what food is safe to eat
> - Timing and length of visits – e.g. shortened visits, restricted number of visitors if tiring or overwhelming

There may be times such recommendations are frustrating and you/your relative may not fully understand or agree with them. It is important for you to raise concerns with the team, so they can talk to you about the reasons behind recommendations and the plan going forward. Learning as much as you can about ongoing difficulties (and the best ways to reduce their impact) will stand you in good stead in the longer term.

Actively Contributing to/Engaging in the Rehabilitation Plan

Engaging fully in rehabilitation sessions, and working on the tasks set between sessions, is important to maximise progress. While this sounds obvious, there are many reasons why someone may struggle to engage in rehabilitation. Reluctance to engage may reflect many factors, including low mood, feeling frightened, not being fully aware of difficulties or changes in thinking skills and communication. Being as involved as possible in guiding the programme (through contributing to goals set), being well-informed by asking questions and raising concerns will all help with engagement. See Chapter 23 Keeping People Engaged in Rehabilitation for more detailed discussion on this important area. As family members you can play an important role in contributing/supporting this process by helping your relative understand what they are working on and why (as well as providing encouragement and emotional support). While it is good practice for family members to be actively included in rehabilitation, this may require you adopting a more proactive stance with the rehabilitation team in some settings (e.g. asking how you can support the process, what goals to work on during visits, whether you can attend therapy sessions) particularly when services are more fragmented.

Visits out of the rehabilitation unit (e.g. short trips or days out with family) can also be immensely useful both in terms of you/your relative's emotional well-being (having family time away from the rehabilitation setting) and as an opportunity to practice skills they are working on in the 'real world'. This could even be to an outside area of the rehabilitation centre, just to get some fresh air (see Fig. 7.1). If you would like some time away from the unit (whether it's to attend a

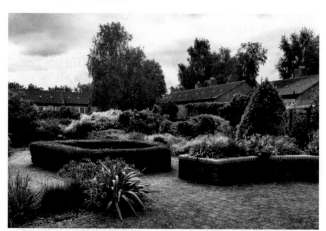

FIG. 7.1 An example of an outside area in a rehabilitation centre that is accessible to patients and families.

special family event or to just get away together for a coffee and a change of scene), then do talk this through with the team. They will advise on any particular issues that are relevant to your specific situation.

Maintaining Ongoing/Effective Communication with the Team

Honest and open communication with the team will help you/your relative throughout the rehabilitation journey. It is likely that you will be faced with hearing difficult information, and making difficult decisions at times. It is important for the team to be aware of your wishes and views (both patient and family members), even if it can feel difficult or uncomfortable to express these. It may be helpful for families to identify one person within the team to serve as their key contact (many units will operate a keyworker system or equivalent). Families can help by letting teams know how they prefer to communicate, e.g. face to face, phone, emails or setting up a communication book (if visiting at times when team members are not around).

Meetings with the team provide a good opportunity for you to meet with all involved in the rehabilitation programme, ask questions, hear about progress and be involved in discharge planning. These meetings may have different names in different settings (e.g. Care Planning Meetings, Multidisciplinary Team Meetings, Goal Planning Meetings, Discharge Meetings, Review Meetings). If you are not sure what the meeting is about, it is important to ask the team. It is recognised that such meetings can be overwhelming to some people (e.g. due to the large number of team members who may attend, or because of the nature of the discussion) and if you would prefer to have smaller meeting, have someone attend to support you, or receive feedback separately, it is helpful to say so. If relatives are unable or choose not to attend, it can be helpful to think of other ways to feed into the process (for example, making a list of questions beforehand or requesting written feedback afterwards).

Attending to Emotional Self-Care

Rehabilitation is almost always associated with significant changes (e.g. to health, independence, family roles), and thus can be an extremely emotional journey. Coping with these is complex, affecting individuals and families in different ways. In addition, rehabilitation may place particular stresses on family (e.g. if the rehabilitation setting is at a distance from the family home, balancing supporting your relative with other work/family commitments). As the person undergoing rehabilitation, emotional support may be offered (depending on the setting). If you/family members are concerned about mood, feed this back to the team and ask if an assessment by a psychologist or doctor can be conducted.

Family members are often the most important source of emotional support and encouragement for the patient. However, we know that relatives are likely to be experiencing high levels of distress themselves (anxiety and depression are common). In order to best support a patient, it is important that you also consider your own self-care needs. This may involve not visiting quite as regularly. Family members often feel pressure to visit every day, which can place a huge strain on them. While family visits are usually actively encouraged (and may be of great importance to your relative), visiting less frequently may help you engage in activities that are good for your emotional well-being (e.g. taking time for yourself, seeing friends, drawing on support groups/online resources), and thus will benefit your relative in the long run.

If you feel you are really struggling to cope, seeking more formal support may be necessary. Ask about counselling support (the rehabilitation unit may provide some family support) or see your General Practitioner to discuss further.

Dealing with Difficult Issues

Communication between the patient, family and team is particularly important when difficult issues arise. You may not agree with the views of the team, for example or you may not wish to follow the rehabilitation programme or the advice of others. This may escalate into you/your relative wishing to leave against advice. Talking to the team (a recurring theme throughout this chapter!) in order to express your wishes while gaining clear information about their recommendations is an essential starting point. If your/your relative's reluctance to engage reflects cognitive difficulties, for example, this may be addressed through using aids to help understanding (e.g. an information folder providing a clear summary of rehabilitation goals and progress). As a family member you can use such resources to support your relative. If reluctance to engage reflects a clear difference in opinion, then further discussion and attempting to work collaboratively are important. It may be helpful to clarify what the alternatives to the rehabilitation setting are. You may be able to continue with rehabilitation as an outpatient in a day hospital or other setting, for example, or to access community rehabilitation in your own home. While this usually involves less intensive therapy and thus may not achieve optimal results, it may have advantages in some cases. Clarifying the specific advantages/disadvantages of different options may help you when weighing up the alternatives and making a decision.

Differences in opinion around discharge options may also arise. You may disagree with the views of the team or your relative/other family members. Return home may involve adaptations, equipment, or a formal care package (which may involve financial assessments) to be deemed safe, or may not be viewed as an option at all. All of the above can be unfamiliar and anxiety-provoking. Again it is essential to have clear two-way communication: you will need information from the team about the level of required support they anticipate on discharge, and to communicate your own views and wishes to the team (e.g. if an option is unacceptable to you). This can be hard, but it is essential that the views of all are taken into consideration.

It is important when such challenging situations arise that issues of risk and mental capacity are considered. In most countries, if an individual has capacity to make a particular decision (i.e. fully understands the decision, the advantages/disadvantages of options faced and risks associated), they are supported in law to make that decision. This is the case even if the decision expressed (for example, around discharge destination) seems "risky" and unwise to others. In general, no one can be kept in rehabilitation against their will, unless they are deemed to lack capacity to make that decision. If someone doesn't have the capacity to make a particular decision, family members can often play an important role in what happens next by contributing to discussions about what is in their relative's best interests. Check your local laws to see what applies in your country and how this might affect you.

SUMMARY POINTS

- Both the individual engaged in rehabilitation and their family members have an active part to play in ensuring rehabilitation is successful and meets all needs
- As a patient or relative you are required to take on this active role while faced with many challenges and uncertainty
- The role of families in supporting and advocating for their relative is even more important when services are fragmented
- The recommendations in this chapter provide some ideas to take forward, in order to help navigate this journey and prepare for the future

REFERENCES

Alzheimer's Society (UK). This is me. Retrieved from https://www.alzheimers.org.uk/get-support/publications-factsheets/this-is-me.

Davis, A., Davis, S., Moss, N., Marks, J., McGrath, J., Hovard, L., Axon, J., & Wade, D. (1992). First steps towards an interdisciplinary approach to rehabilitation. *Clinical Rehabilitation, 6,* 237–244.

FURTHER READING

UK based: Age UK (www.ageuk.org.uk)
Headway – the brain injury association (www.headway.org.uk)

The Stroke Association (www.stroke.org.uk)
International: Alzheimer's Disease International (www.alz.co.uk)

8

What Can We Do to Help Patients and Families?

Audrey Daisley

LEARNING OBJECTIVES

- Describe the family impact of illness and the importance of providing rehabilitation services that are 'family-minded'
- Describe key information and support needs of families during a relative's rehabilitation
- Explain the ways in which families may be helped during the rehabilitation process

CASE

Jack is in his 80s and recently had a fall; the cause isn't known yet and so he has been admitted to the hospital for further tests. This is the first time Jack has been in hospital and away from his wife Sarah. Jack and Sarah have two children, Bobby and Clare, who live away and are busy with their own families. Jack is missing Sarah as she hasn't been able to visit too often; she's recovering from cancer and does not drive. Clare has been staying with Sarah but has just gone home to her own family as she is helping to look after her mother-in-law who has dementia. When Clare came to see Jack on the ward, she often became upset and angry with the staff, sometimes shouting at them and was frequently abrupt and offhand with them. She made a formal complaint about the care her father has received and has a meeting planned with the ward manager next week to discuss this. The team looking after Jack had been expecting this as they had heard from the admitting team that Clare had been shouting and angry with them too. Jack has been apologising to staff for his daughter's behaviour and seems very upset by the whole situation. Jack's son has visited once or twice and is always polite and calm with the staff.

As you read this chapter, consider what the key family issues are and what the healthcare team could do to help. In particular, reflect on how it might feel to be looking after Jack.

INTRODUCTION

The previous chapter entitled 'What can patients and families do to help rehabilitation?' drew attention to the key issues and concerns that illness, hospitalisation and participating in rehabilitation can give rise to. The journey through illness can be difficult for patients and families to navigate; the effects of ill-health typically 'ripple out' and reverberate around the family system affecting everyone (Utz, Berg, & Butner, 2017). In turn, the resulting family distress can impact on the older adult's recovery and adjustment, highlighting the important, but often overlooked, reciprocal influence that family members can have on each other (Martire et al., 2008). This points to the importance of rehabilitation teams being able to rise to the challenge of knowing how best to help patients *and* their families in order to maximise outcomes for all.

The research in this area offers some guidance with studies consistently showing that patients and their families benefit from:

- A welcoming supportive 'family-minded' rehabilitation environment
- Positive relationships with the professionals
- Clear and honest information (e.g. about their diagnosis and prognosis)
- Meaningful and supported involvement in making decisions about treatment and rehabilitation options
- Psychological support and
- Advice with practical issues.

However, providing such a myriad of support to patients and their families, particularly at times of significant distress and uncertainty, is not a simple undertaking. Whilst some rehabilitation teams have considerable expertise in offering this type of support and are able to tailor it to each patient and family, others may be less resourced or lack the training, supervision or commitment to deliver family-focused support, leaving both staff teams and families feeling as if needs are not being met.

In this chapter we address the question 'what can we do to help patients and their families?' by providing a brief overview of some ways in which staff, from all disciplines and at all levels of experience, can respond to the information and support needs of their older patients' families. As is a key theme in this book, the patient story – the older person's life narrative of who they are, their preferences, their individuality and expectations and the relationships that are important to them – should underpin and inform any supportive interventions and approaches that we undertake.

1) Fostering a family-focused environment

Whilst patients typically describe the process of rehabilitation as being more relaxed, meaningful and less formal than other hospital interactions, the high expectation of active and sustained family involvement can place greater demands on their relatives. It is essential that healthcare teams create environments that encourage, facilitate and invite this crucial input from families. This ethos of 'family mindedness' should be reflected in how the facility operates and in its physical layout. See the Resources section for practical advice on how this can be achieved and a checklist for creating a family-friendly environment.

2) Supporting patient and family understanding of the illness/diagnosis and the process of rehabilitation by making information readily available and understandable

Whilst families have extensive information needs when an older person is hospitalised, research has shown that obtaining clear details about a relative's diagnosis and treatment can be problematic for many (Higgins et al., 2007). Information or access to rehabilitation professionals may not always be readily forthcoming, and some family members find themselves apologising to staff for being a 'nuisance'. Some withdraw from the process and can (mistakenly) be seen by staff as disinterested or indifferent. Others may have a more assertive approach to communicating with staff which can result in them being incorrectly labelled as 'difficult' or 'demanding'. In particular, older patients and families report that obtaining the 'truth' about their situation can be challenging (Marzanski, 2000). As a result, families may end up feeling distressed, ignored, disliked, uninformed, unclear as to how to help their relative or how to support the rehabilitation efforts and unable to plan ahead. This is likely to impact on the older person's progress.

Healthcare teams can take steps to ameliorate this by developing clear family-focused information-sharing protocols or pathways, based on clinical and research evidence regarding the typical information needs of families of older people (e.g. Steiner, Pierce, & Salvador, 2016). Some helpful strategies for effective sharing of information include the following.

- Having a proactive and positive approach to providing families with information; this conveys, from the outset, that family needs are recognised, valued, understood and will be met. This is likely to foster more meaningful, collaborative and effective working relationships between the staff team and the older person's relatives.
- A commitment to truth-telling and the honest and supportive sharing of diagnostic and prognostic information including 'bad news'.
- Assigning a key information contact person to each patient and their family, so it is clear who families should direct their questions to.

- Encouraging family members to similarly assign a key information recipient who can serve as a 'hub' for the rest of the family; this can avoid unnecessary duplication and can clarify issues around who information can (and cannot) be shared with in line with local policies on confidentiality. This is particularly important when an older person's capacity to consent to information sharing may be compromised due to illness.
- Ensuring that information-giving is an ongoing process rather than a single event. It can be particularly helpful to provide families with additional, updated information at key times in the rehabilitation journey such as admission to the new ward, at times of significant progress or set-back and as discharge approaches.
- Providing families with written summaries or audio recordings of important and complex discussions can be helpful to aid their understanding and ability to process and reach a decision and compensate for information likely to be forgotten as a result of anxiety during the consultation. Further adapting these to accommodate the needs of the older relatives (e.g. in large print) is essential.
- Involving patients and families in decision-making. The process of 'shared decision-making' is part of patient and family centred care, along with collaborative conversations, decision support and decision aids (see Fig. 8.1).
- Support factual information exchange with experiential learning for families; e.g. including them actively in their relative's therapy sessions to assist 'learning through doing'. The presence of family in therapy sessions can also serve as a motivator or source of reassurance for the more fearful or confused older adult, leading to increased and more meaningful engagement in rehabilitation (Lawler, Taylor, & Shields, 2015).

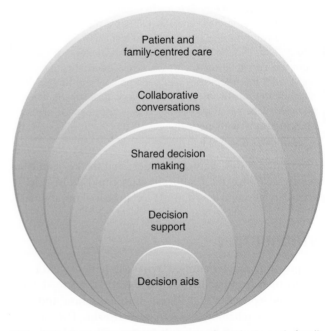

FIG. 8.1 Decision-making is part of patient and family centred care.

3) Caring for the carers – providing emotional support to family members

The impact of illness on family members is well documented with much of the research pointing to the negative consequences for relatives such as anxiety, depression and, depending on the type of illness, the experience of 'burden'. Frameworks have been offered to guide professional understanding of family reactions; a popular idea is that relatives pass through predictable stages, each characterised by different emotional reactions, such as shock, anger and acceptance. Whilst it is true that these emotions are common, not every relative will experience them and not in a straightforward linear fashion; it is more helpful for professionals to hold in mind a flexible and personalised perspective on how the older person and their family might experience their illness and how distress might be communicated. Family reactions to illness are thus highly individual, can range from mild to severe in nature (with only a small number requiring referral to psychological support services) and can be influenced positively when families feel as though their needs are being met.

Healthcare teams can help in the following ways:

- Having an open and proactive approach to providing emotional support that normalises asking for help.
- Remembering that most families do not require formal psychological support and benefit from being listened to.
- Taking time to reflect and be curious about why a family is distressed or angry, asking 'what is the person trying to communicate to me?' and 'what problem are they trying to solve?'; more overt, and sometimes challenging, behaviours such as anger, aggression, shouting and swearing at staff usually mask deeper levels of distress, sadness and fear.
- Being familiar with the family issues that can give rise to distress when an older person is unwell. These include anticipatory grief arising from the fear that the person might die, worry about a diagnosis, prognostic uncertainty (e.g. in cancer treatment), anxiety about having to assume a carer role (this can be a significant issue for the spouse of an older person who may not be in good health themselves) and fears that the older person might not be well enough to return home. A particular issue facing the families of older people with neurological illness (such as stroke or Parkinson's disease) is adjusting to the changes in thinking or personality that often accompany such conditions. This is referred to as 'ambiguous loss' – an incomplete and highly distressing loss of someone as they were, without them dying. Work in this area has been usefully applied in the care of older people with conditions such as Alzheimer's disease and acquired brain injuries (Boss, 2011).
- Validate and normalise family concerns: the family member may feel a range of conflicting and confusing emotions which can cause further distress (e.g. a relative may find themselves feeling both anger and guilt towards their relative at the same time). It is helpful to listen and reassure.
- Signpost relatives towards educational materials and self-help resources.
- Know what support services are available to refer family members on to. Many hospitals have access to clinical psychology or counselling services.
- Remember that most families cope well when they are offered good information about their relative's situation and when they feel that their concerns have been heard and understood.

4) Providing practical support

The provision of practical support and guidance is another way that rehabilitation staff can help families. Family members typically require help and signposting with issues relating to applying for state benefits and accessing funding for carer support, navigating the legal system (e.g. what to do if their relative loses mental capacity to make important decisions) and knowing how to access equipment, aids and adaptations to their house. Helping families access social workers, care managers and third sector organisations can be helpful.

If we return to Jack and his family, whom we met at the beginning of this chapter, we can see that a number of issues come into play when thinking about their situation.

- Illness can have a huge emotional impact on family members. Not all family members will react in the same way and their response will be affected by many factors, including their pre-illness relationship with the person who is unwell, their own health and circumstances, the amount of support they have and how much they understand about their relative's condition and treatment.
- How family members express distress is individual to them; some relatives show emotions in ways that are expected and understandable to us (e.g. sadness seen through crying) but others may communicate their distress and worry in other ways – such as asking frequent questions, becoming easily frustrated and angry with staff. It is important to hold this in mind when trying to support relatives. It can be tempting to want to support the person who is less challenging to us. This will likely leave other relatives feeling more isolated and increasingly distressed, creating a vicious cycle of emotionally distressing communication between family and staff. Jack's daughter, Clare, is likely to be in need of emotional support and reassurance; yet it will probably be difficult for the team to approach her. Her reputation for being 'difficult' that was passed on from the staff in the previous hospital won't have helped, and it is a reminder that we should try to be careful about how our assumptions and expectations might impact negatively on how family members perceive us.
- Family distress can affect the patient's mood and ability to focus on their treatment/rehabilitation. This can lead to less positive outcomes for all. Supporting families is, therefore, a good additional way of supporting your patient. This will be important for Jack's recovery as he seems to be very worried about how his daughter is feeling and behaving.
- Family members will likely have other caring responsibilities, and it is important for healthcare teams to be aware of this when planning the patient's discharge. Jack's children have probably been very worried about their mother who is recovering from an illness and now they are faced with their

father being unwell. In addition, Clare's mother-in-law is also requiring her support. It is helpful to understand what other life events family members are dealing with.

- Family members who are infirm, unwell or unable to travel may feel isolated from and left out of the discussions about their relative's care and treatment. It is important to try to include, with the patient's consent, these family members in plans for discharge to avoid things breaking down in the future. This might require the healthcare team to make an extra effort to contact and stay in touch with these family members. Jack's wife is not able to visit him often; she may need some regular telephone updates from staff looking after Jack; this means she can ask questions or raise concerns about issues that she might not want her children to know about.

- Information about the relative's illness, treatment and prognosis (where consented to), along with a listening ear, and signposting towards further help when needed, should be offered to all family members. There is some uncertainty about the cause of Jack's fall and the family are likely to be fearing the worst. Letting families know that we understand how worried they are can be very supportive, even if we do not yet have definite information for them.

- Supporting families can be a very emotional undertaking, and healthcare teams need support to talk about the personal impact of this work and develop strategies for knowing how to support even the most distressed relatives. Ward staff are likely to dread talking to Clare and worry that she will make a complaint about them. They might benefit from discussing this with close colleagues.

SUMMARY POINTS

- Healthcare professionals are well placed to offer support to both patients and their families that focuses on enhancing knowledge of the illness, the processing of difficult emotions, families feeling heard and understood and supported with practical problems

- There can be barriers to providing family support such as lack of time, confidence, training or support
- A culture of family mindedness in health settings is the starting point for developing services that will enhance outcomes for all and, importantly, instil hope

MCQs

Q.1 Which one of the following is true about sharing information?
  a. Written information and audio recordings should be avoided
  b. Individual family members should be encouraged to come separately, to reinforce information
  c. Relatives should not be encouraged to join the patient's therapy sessions
  d. A key information contact person should be assigned to each patient and their family

Q.2 Which one of the following is true about how healthcare teams can help to care for the carers?
  a. Advise them to ask for help in another location in the first instance
  b. Teams should validate and normalise family concerns
  c. Encourage them to find information by themselves
  d. Avoid talking to carers when they are angry

REFERENCES

Boss, P. (2011). *Loving someone who has dementia: how to find hope when coping with stress and grief.* San Francisco, CA: Jossey-Bass.

Higgins, I., Joyce, T., Parker, V., Fitzgerald, M., & McMillan, M. (2007). The immediate needs of relatives during the hospitalisation of acutely ill older relatives. *Contemporary Nurse, 26*(2), 208–220.

Lawler, K., Taylor, N. F., & Shields, N. (2015). Involving family members in physiotherapy for older people transitioning from hospital to the community: a qualitative analysis. *Disability and Rehabilitation, 37*(22), 2061–2069.

Martire, L. M., Schultz, R., Reynolds, C. F., Morse, J. Q., Butters, M. A., & Hinrichsen, G. A. (2008). Impact of close family members on older adults' response to depression treatment. *Psychology and Aging, 23*(2), 447–452.

Marzanski, M. (2000). On telling the truth to patients with dementia. *Western Journal Of Medicine, 173*(5), 318–323.

Steiner, V., Pierce, L. L., & Salvador, D. (2016). Information needs of family caregivers of people with dementia. *Rehabilitation Nursing, 41*(3), 162–169.

Utz, R. L., Berg, C., & Butner, J. (2016). It's a family affair: reflections about ageing and health within a family context. *The Gerontologist, 57*(1), 129–135.

Rehabilitation: How it Works

9

Rehabilitation Potential and Selection for Rehabilitation

Kate Bennett

LEARNING OBJECTIVES

- Describe the concept of rehabilitation potential
- Identify indicators of rehabilitation potential and where rehabilitation is unlikely to be successful

- Identify practical considerations prior to undertaking rehabilitation

CASE

Queenie is a 92-year-old lady currently living in a nursing home where full care is provided. She recently had a stroke, leaving her with a dense left-sided hemiplegia (paralysis) in hospital. Prior to her stroke, Queenie used a wheeled walking frame to move from her bed to her chair with the assistance of the staff at the nursing home. On her return from hospital, Queenie needed to move from her bed to her chair with a hoist. She had been provided with a specialist seating system in the form of a reclining chair that was able to be moved around the home. She was referred to the community rehabilitation team on discharge from hospital for a review, to see if she had regained any function and to decide if she had any rehabilitation potential. The main goal was for Queenie to be able to sit out in her chair and be wheeled to the communal areas, and she expressed that she wanted to do this and would like to be able to complete the transfer in standing rather than being hoisted.

WHAT IS REHABILITATION POTENTIAL?

Rehabilitation potential is a process which involves complex clinical judgement and prognostication on the projected benefits of undertaking a targeted programme of rehabilitation. The assessment of rehabilitation potential should take into account physical and psychological factors identified during multidisciplinary assessments along with individual patient needs and wants and the availability of family support. It involves developing an understanding of who will participate with rehabilitation, in and outside the therapy setting, who can support this and who is likely to benefit.

Cowley (2020).

Successful rehabilitation includes the maintenance of self-care activities at a higher level than that maintained by an 'untreated' population.

Muller, Tobis, & Kelman (1963).

Rehabilitation potential is a term used by clinicians to describe the ability of a person to return to a previous level of function following a period of illness or injury. This return to function follows a period of input carried out by various professions, including physiotherapists, occupational therapists and speech and language therapists amongst others. The resultant level of function may not be the same as the person's previous, or baseline, level of function. For example, someone previously completely independent who has a stroke may not return to complete independence in activities of daily self-care but may be able to complete some aspects independently and others with assistance. More accurately, rehabilitation potential describes the ability of a person to progress on from their current state brought about by illness or injury to a level of functional ability.

INDICATORS OF REHABILITATION POTENTIAL

Every person who has deviated from their baseline level of function should be given the opportunity to undertake a period of rehabilitation with the aim of returning back to their baseline level of function. However people can recover from illness or injury at varying speeds and progress at different rates to attain different levels of function.

The UN Convention on the Rights of Persons with Disabilities states that people with disabilities (which include physical and cognitive disabilities) have the right to attain and maintain maximum independence (United Nations Convention, 2006) through comprehensive rehabilitation services and programmes. Therefore every person considered to have a disability who has suffered an impairment of their normal level of independence should be given the opportunity to undertake a period of multidisciplinary rehabilitation in order to regain their independence.

There is no definitive assessment or measure for rehabilitation potential. Determination of rehabilitation potential is largely experiential and will depend on a number of factors. These include clinician experience (both of other individuals with the same condition and their general experience as a practising clinician), case studies, best practice and evidence from research trials, and intrinsic factors relating to the individual, such as motivation, cognition, physical ability and other factors. External factors, such as the illness or injury, environment, equipment, availability of therapy staff and time, should also be considered.

The best way to determine if someone has the potential to regain function is to undertake a period of functional rehabilitation and assess if there has been any progress made following this period. This should take place after a thorough assessment of physical function to ascertain current ability, which will give the clinician a baseline measure that can be used to compare progress with and also assist in the setting of goals for rehabilitation. The next chapter will discuss goals and goal setting in more detail. See also Chapter 22 Measuring Progress with Rehabilitation. The rehabilitation process requires continual assessment to evaluate if outcomes from decisions regarding input are favourable or non-favourable and whether further input is likely to result in further progress in a recalibration cycle (Fig. 9.1).

For the case at the beginning of this chapter, an assessment of sitting balance was undertaken to check Queenie's ability to sit independently. Once the ability to sit independently was determined, the ability to stand was assessed. Once the ability to stand with an appropriate aid was determined, the next stage was to attempt a step. It was very quickly apparent that Queenie was not able to step so the input then went back to

focusing on the ability to stand and the amount of assistance/support required to achieve this. Progress within rehabilitation may sometimes appear to be more of a sideways step rather than moving directly forwards. As long as progress is being made, then continuing with the rehabilitation process is appropriate.

Whilst there are some incidences where it is apparent that a person is not demonstrating potential to completely regain function, there is no definitive method of determining this. However, if a patient has made no significant progress in several consecutive sessions, or appears to be regressing, further input is unlikely to result in progress. This may be due to the disease process, cognitive decline or a further significant illness or injury that has again reduced functional ability. Any sudden changes should prompt early discussion with the medical team, to rule out infection, dehydration or other medical issues that may affect rehabilitation. There is evidence that depression and cognitive impairment are predictors of poor rehabilitation outcomes, but that this could potentially be mitigated by engagement in the rehabilitation process (Lenze et al., 2004). It is therefore important to address these issues where possible to optimise engagement before ceasing input.

PRACTICAL CONSIDERATIONS FOR UNDERTAKING REHABILITATION

When undertaking a period of rehabilitation, it is important to consider what is a realistic level of function that is achievable and sustainable. For example, if an individual can only perform a standing transfer with three people, but only two carers are provided during care visits, it is worth considering if a standing transfer is the most appropriate method of transfer in this setting. Other considerations need to be taken into account when individuals move between settings. If they need daily input to assist with mobility practice in an inpatient setting, it is not realistic to expect that a community team will be able to provide this level of input long term.

Motivation and ambition to progress and achieve goals also need to be considered; if someone isn't willing to carry out their home exercise programme or mobility practice between therapy sessions, they are not going to progress as quickly and resources may be better used for other individuals. In this case, the use of a measure such as the Patient Activation Measure to assess levels of engagement and motivation may be appropriate (Development of the Patient Activation Measure (PAM), 2004).

USE OF THE TERM 'NO REHABILITATION POTENTIAL'

The use of the phrase 'no rehabilitation potential' is not now considered appropriate. No one is should be labelled as having no potential, but their potential may be limited due to factors such as cognitive state, lack of motivation and physical disability. These individuals should still be offered the chance

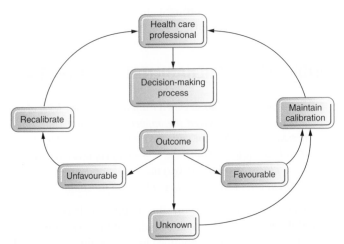

FIG. 9.1 The cycle of determining if further input is likely to be beneficial. (Adapted with permission from The feedback sanction. P. Croskerry. Academic Emergency Medicine 7(11):1232–1238, 2000).

to rehabilitate, and this only should be ceased when it is clear there is no progress to be made.

It is also important to recognise that while the therapist may have ideas about how far a patient can progress, it is up to the individual to determine what is important for them and what they want to achieve. This could be very basic things such as:

- Receiving visitors in a chair rather than in the bed
- Being able to access a shower rather than having to have strip washes or bed baths
- Being able to access a toilet rather than using a commode
- Being able to sit out in the garden.

These simple things can make a huge difference to someone's quality of life and go a long way to preserving their sense of dignity.

Patients also have the right to decline input if they have the capacity to make that decision. If a patient lacks capacity, then the appropriateness of input would be discussed with family/friends or an official advocate and the rest of the multidisciplinary team, and a decision whether or not to proceed would be made.

CASE CONCLUSION

On assessing Queenie, she was able to sit on the edge of the bed and maintain her own balance without needing support and was able to complete a standing transfer from the bed into her specialised chair using a specific piece of equipment.

This needed practice to ensure the safety of both staff and Queenie. Queenie undertook a period of rehabilitation lasting 3 weeks where she was seen 2–3 times a week in her nursing home by the community team to practice the transfers. In between visits the staff were asked to hoist Queenie to her chair daily so she got used to being out in her chair after staying in bed for long periods of time.

A progress review was completed after the first 3 weeks. At the review, the staff reported that Queenie was declining to sit in her chair, preferring to stay in bed all of the time because she didn't enjoy being out of her bed and in an upright position in the chair. Queenie was reviewed by her GP, and the case was discussed with the staff, therapists and Queenie herself. Although Queenie stated she enjoyed the therapy sessions, she felt this was due to the fact she was seeing different people and 'having visitors' rather than the actual standing practice and being sat in her chair. Queenie was judged to be able to make the decision around sitting in her chair for herself and it was decided at this point to stop rehabilitation input. Queenie was therefore discharged from the service but the staff at her nursing home were given the option to re-refer her if Queenie changed her mind and wanted to sit out in her chair regularly.

This case illustrates how someone with rehabilitation potential was given the opportunity and input to enable to progress to a higher level of function, and also how it was the person's choice to not pursue this further, despite having the ability both physically and cognitively to engage in the rehabilitation process.

SUMMARY POINTS

- There is no definitive indicator or measure for rehabilitation potential
- Rehabilitation can be very effective in improving quality of life and physical function even if individuals aren't able to return to their previous level of function
- Everybody should be given the choice and opportunity to realise their potential before rehabilitation is deemed to be inappropriate
- Rehabilitation goals can be simple things that have a huge impact on a person's quality of life

MCQs

Q.1 In which of these settings can effective rehabilitation take place?
   a. The acute setting
   b. Intermediate/ step down inpatient care setting
   c. Usual place of residence
   d. All of the above
   e. None of the above

Q.2 When should rehabilitation commence for people in an inpatient setting?
   a. A few days after admission
   b. When the person is medically stable
   c. When the person is able to walk with their usual aid
   d. When the person is ready for discharge
   e. When they are ready to transfer to a rehab facility

REFERENCES

Cowley, A. Assessment of Rehabilitation Potential in Frail Older people in the Acute Healthcare Setting: A Mixed Methods Study. 2020. E-thesis, University of Nottingham.

Development of the Patient Activation Measure (PAM): conceptualizing and measuring activation in patients and consumers." Hibbard J H, Stockard J, Mahoney E R, Tusler M. Health Services Research. 2004 Aug;39(4 Pt 1): 1005-26.

Lenze, E. J., Munin, M. C., Dew, M. A., Rogers, J. C., Seligman, K., Mulsant, B. H., & Reynolds, C. F., III (2004). Adverse effects of depression and cognitive impairment on rehabilitation participation and recovery from hip fracture. *International Journal of Geriatric Psychiatry, 19*(5), 472–478.

Muller, J. N., Tobis, J. S., & Kelman, H. R. (1963). The rehabilitation potential of nursing home residents. *American Journal of Public Health and the Nation's Health, 53*(2), 243–247.

United Nations. (2006). Convention on the Rights of Persons with Disabilities. Section 26 (1). 2006 [cited 2019 Aug 14].

10

Setting Rehabilitation Goals

Kate Bennett

LEARNING OBJECTIVES

- Describe the theory behind setting rehabilitation goals
- List factors for consideration when setting rehabilitation goals

- Explain how to set appropriate long-term and short-term goals

CASE

Robbie was an 82-year-old man admitted to hospital following a urinary tract infection (UTI). Robbie lived in a ground floor flat with his wife who was also his main carer. His flat had seven external concrete steps up to the entrance doors but within the flat all rooms were on the same level. Robbie had a stroke in the past which left him with limited function in his right hand and a right-sided foot drop. Prior to admission, he was able to walk around his flat with a tripod stick in his left hand and was able to access both his toilet and his level access shower. He had been housebound for several years due to his inability to complete the steps outside the main doors. When Robbie was discharged home he had to use a wheelchair initially, but was able to transfer from his wheelchair to his recliner chair with assistance of one person and a walking frame. Despite the limitations in his hand, he had enough function to use it for transferring, but wasn't able to control a walking frame with it. Robbie had been assessed by the inpatient therapy team in the hospital and had been set goals of progressing his mobility and transfers with a view to completing stairs. Robbie's ultimate goal was to walk out of his flat and be able to walk outside.

INTRODUCTION TO GOAL SETTING

'Rehabilitation involves working with people to achieve the goals that are important to them' (Clare, 2017)

Goal setting is a key part of the rehabilitation process that is considered to be an effective behaviour change technique (Epton, Currie, & Armitage, 2017) and results in improved health for older people with chronic conditions (Vermunt et al., 2017). There are many benefits of setting clear and concise goals; without goals the rehabilitation process can lack purpose, resulting in decreased motivation from both staff and the individual involved. A lack of support from family and friends can also be an issue as they do not appreciate the purpose and potential outcome of the intervention. Goal setting should always be person-centred and meaningful to the person involved.

Patient participation is known to ensure personally relevant goals are set, and results in greater satisfaction with the rehabilitation experience (Rice et al., 2017). It can also help people achieve a higher quality of life and an increased sense of self-efficacy. There is also some evidence to suggest that for patients with impairments who are unable to fully take part in the goal setting process, suggested goals at the level of impairment by the therapists involved can act as a route to patient-centred goals at their level of activity and participation (Leach et al., 2009).

If the person is not able to return to their baseline level of function, goals need to be set that reflect what level of function is needed to enable the individual to return to their usual place of residence. If the individual is not returning to their usual place of residence but an alternative is being considered (for example, a care home), it is important to understand what is needed for the individual to be able to move into that setting successfully.

FACTORS TO CONSIDER WHEN SETTING REHABILITATION GOALS

Goals should always be set using the SMART guidelines (see Table 10.1).

An example of goal setting using these guidelines is provided below and considered under each of the headings:

'I want to be able to complete the stairs using a bannister on the left-hand side going up with no help by the end of next week.'

Specificity

This goal clearly states exactly what the person wants to achieve. It has a definite end point and a definite purpose. It also gives a very clear description of what achievement of this goal looks like for this person.

Measurable

The goal is measurable – the number of steps the person needs to be able to complete at home can be counted. The goal could also be measured in time if preferred.

TABLE 10.1 **Description of SMART goals.**	
Specific	• What exactly do you wish to achieve? • Where do you want to be at the end of the intervention? • Where do you want to achieve this? • Is there anyone else you want to involve in this goal?
Measurable	• How will you know when the goal is achieved? • What evidence is there to prove the goal has been achieved? • How will progress be measured?
Achievable	• Do you have a good chance of achieving your goal? • Do you have access to the resources needed to achieve the goal?
Realistic/ relevant	• Is the goal in line with priorities/ objectives?
Time-bound	• When will the goal be achieved by?

Achievable

The goal needs to be achievable both physically and within the specified time frame. If the person is currently being hoisted from bed to chair, it is likely that they won't achieve this goal in this time frame.

Realistic/Relevant

Goals need to be relevant to the person they are relating to. So completing stairs for someone who lives in a level access bungalow isn't a relevant goal. Equally, if someone hasn't climbed the stairs for 20 years, then it is not realistic that it will be achievable.

Time-bound

The above goal is clearly time-bound. There is potential for both therapists and individuals to keep plugging away trying to achieve a simple goal when in reality no progress is being made. Time-bound goals prevent this by providing the opportunity to review progress at certain points. Time-bound goals can also be motivating; the individual may work harder in therapy sessions than they otherwise would and may also complete exercises/mobility practice in their own time in order to ensure they achieve the goal in the specified time period.

GOAL SETTING AND BASELINE FUNCTION

The purpose of goal setting is to assist the person to return to their baseline level of function where possible. If a return to the previous level of function isn't feasible due to the nature of the illness/injury suffered, then it should focus on returning to the highest possible level of function achievable for that person. This should be determined through discussions with them, all members of the multidisciplinary team involved in their care and any carers/family members whom the person wishes to be involved. If the person is unable to partake fully in goal setting, consideration should be given to involving a patient advocate. Goals should always be documented (Fig. 10.1).

The return to baseline function is often a slow process. Therefore, the progress towards this should consist of both long-term and short-term goals. Long-term goals should focus on the end point of rehabilitation; once these have been achieved

the rehabilitation process can be considered to be complete. Short-term goals are the stepping-stones to this achievement.

> Short term goals are goals that can be achieved in the near future.
> Example: walking 5 metres with a walking frame and supervision.
>
> Long term goals are goals that are more far reaching and take longer to achieve.
> Example: walking 500m to the shop independently with a walking stick.

GOAL SETTING FOR DIFFERENT ENVIRONMENTS

Using SMART goals allows for goal setting in differing environments. For example, a goal of walking 5 m could translate into a goal of being able to walk to the toilet in an acute or intermediate care setting; or in someone's home, being able to walk to the front door to answer it. Goals are usually set after the initial assessment has been completed; this could be on the acute hospital ward or in the person's own home, depending on when they receive rehabilitation input. The attainment of goals set in hospital should follow patients through to any other inpatient settings and, if outstanding, into the community setting. They should be regularly reviewed to check for appropriateness and relevance, e.g. a goal of walking to the toilet could mean walking 5 m on one ward, 20 m on a different ward or up a flight of stairs at home. This is why SMART goal setting principles should be used, so that every person involved in the patient's care knows exactly what they are trying to achieve.

GOAL SETTING IN RESIDENTIAL CARE

It is easy to overlook goal setting for those in residential care, but some care homes require a certain level of mobility to enable residents to be able to live there. The rehabilitation process should not stop however when the person has reached the minimum level of mobility required but should carry on until they have reached their full potential.

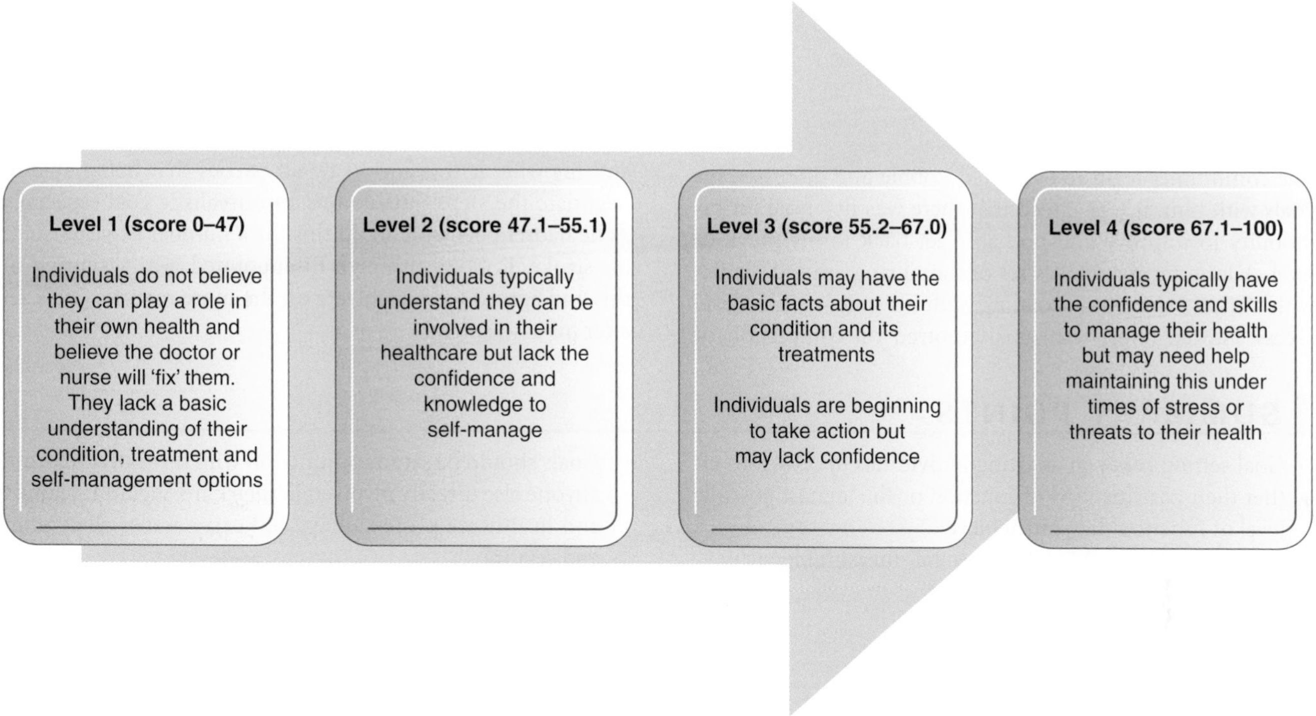

Level 1 (score 0–47)

Individuals do not believe they can play a role in their own health and believe the doctor or nurse will 'fix' them. They lack a basic understanding of their condition, treatment and self-management options

Level 2 (score 47.1–55.1)

Individuals typically understand they can be involved in their healthcare but lack the confidence and knowledge to self-manage

Level 3 (score 55.2–67.0)

Individuals may have the basic facts about their condition and its treatments

Individuals are beginning to take action but may lack confidence

Level 4 (score 67.1–100)

Individuals typically have the confidence and skills to manage their health but may need help maintaining this under times of stress or threats to their health

FIG. 10.1 Description of Hibbard's four stages of the Patient Activation Framework (Adapted with permission from Roberts NJ, Kidd L, Dougall N, et al. Measuring patient activation: the utility of the Patient Activation Measure within a UK context–Results from four exemplar studies and potential future applications. *Patient Educ Couns.* 2016;99(10):1739-46).

CONSIDERATIONS FOR UNDERTAKING REHABILITATION GOAL SETTING

The needs of the person should be balanced with what a realistic outcome is given their injury/illness. Goal setting also takes into account the environment(s) in which rehabilitation input will be taking place and any limitations this creates. Goals should always be clearly documented and handed over to the next team involved in the person's care for continuity.

The potential input of family, friends and carers also needs to be considered. If a person needs assistance with an exercise programme, it needs to be clear who is able to provide that assistance on an ongoing basis. It is imperative not to assume that family/friends or carers/care staff will be able to provide this assistance regularly long term. Likewise with individuals in residential care, an agreement must be reached and documented in the care plan regarding how much input the care staff should be undertaking.

ENGAGEMENT IN THE REHABILITATION PROCESS

The Patient Activation Measure (PAM) is a validated, commercially licenced tool which helps to measure the spectrum of skills, knowledge and confidence in patients and captures the extent to which people feel engaged and confident in taking care of their condition. (NHS, 2019).

A key component to success in rehabilitation is patient engagement. If a person is not engaged with the process, the chances of success are slim. A person's level of engagement can be gauged by using a validated measure such as the Patient Activation Measure (Hibbard et al., 2004) (see Fig. 10.1). The Patient Activation Measure (PAM) can be used to design and evaluate appropriate interventions. It may be that if a person is not engaged in the process, therapy input at this stage is futile but may be appropriate at a later stage.

UNREALISTIC GOALS

Goals need to be realistic. If not, rehabilitation is set up to fail before it has started. At times individuals want to pursue unrealistic goals. In these instances, it is wise to discuss the goal with the individual and their thoughts around how achievable it may be, and how they see themselves achieving it. This may be tricky depending on if the person has any cognitive impairment and in these cases involving the advocate for the person is vital so the plan is clear. For example, people with dementia may lack insight into their abilities or their potential for improvement. A stepwise approach to goal setting can be beneficial because there may be aspects of the goal the individual can achieve and by progressing through the steps they may come to their own realisation that the main goal is un-achievable.

CONCLUSION OF CASE

The community team re-evaluated Robbie and discussed his goals with him. It was agreed that there was potential for his mobility to improve and probably get back to his previous level. A long-term goal was set of mobilising around his flat with a tripod stick and accessing both his toilet and his level access shower. Short-term goals centred on completion of a daily exercise programme to improve his muscle strength with his wife assisting at weekends, working on transfers with his tripod stick instead of his frame and mobilising short distances initially with his wheelchair behind him for when he needed to sit. After long discussions with both Robbie and his wife, it was agreed by all parties that being able to negotiate the steps outside was an unrealistic goal especially as he hadn't been able to do this for a number of years since his stroke. Robbie, although disappointed, was accepting of this and agreed to concentrate on the more realistic goals set after his assessment.

SUMMARY POINTS

- Goal setting is key in assisting individuals to return to either their baseline level of function or the highest possible level of function they can achieve
- Goals should be SMART – specific, measurable, achievable, realistic/relevant, time-bound
- Goals should be set in conjunction with the individual and anyone else directly involved in their care, including family and healthcare professionals, and carry across all settings and sectors

MCQs

Q.1 Which of the following is true about goal setting?
   a. People with dementia should not be involved in the process
   b. For people being discharged to a care home, goals should only be to reach the minimum necessary level of function
   c. Unrealistic goals should be included, in case unexpected improvements occur
   d. Goals should be set as soon as the initial rehabilitation assessment has been completed
   e. The purpose of goal setting is to keep patient expectations low

Q.2 Which of the following is true about rehabilitation goals?
   a. Patients don't need to be involved in choosing goals they want to achieve
   b. Without goals the rehabilitation process can lack purpose
   c. Goals should not be shared with the patient or family
   d. Goals should reflect a level of function needed to keep the patient in hospital
   e. If patients lack insight into their abilities, no goals should be set

REFERENCES

Clare, L. (2017). Rehabilitation for people living with dementia: a practical framework of positive support. *PLoS Medicine, 14*(3), e1002245.

Epton, T., Currie, S., & Armitage, C. J. (2017). Unique effects of setting goals on behavior change: systematic review and meta-analysis. *Journal of Consulting and Clinical Psychology, 85*(12), 1182–1198.

Hibbard, J. H., Stockard, J., Mahoney, E. R., & Tusler, M. (2004). Development of the Patient Activation Measure (PAM): conceptualizing and measuring activation in patients and consumers. *Health Services Research, 39*(4), 1005–1026.

Leach, E., Cornwell, P., Fleming, J., & Haines, T. (2009). Patient centred goal-setting in a subacute rehabilitation setting. *Disability and Rehabilitation, 32*(2), 159–172.

NHS. (2019). https://www.england.nhs.uk/ourwork/patient-participation/self-care/patient-activation/pa-faqs/.

Rice, D. B., McIntyre, A., Mirkowski, M., Janzen, S., Viana, R., Britt, E., & Teasell, R. W. (2017). Patient-centered goal setting in a hospital-based outpatient stroke rehabilitation center. *American Academy of Physical Medicine and Rehabilitation, 9*(9), 856–865.

Vermunt, N. P. C. A., Harmsen, M., Westert, G. P., Olde Rikkert, M. G. M., & Faber, M. J. (2017). Collaborative goal setting with elderly patients with chronic disease or multi-morbidity: a systematic review. *BMC Geriatrics, 17*, 167.

11

Rehabilitation Equipment

Frances Horgan, Rose Galvin, Deirdre Connolly & Tadhg Stapleton

LEARNING OBJECTIVES

- Describe the range of equipment available for rehabilitation of activities of daily living and mobility of older adults
- Identify common safety concerns associated with mobility equipment
- Explain the impact of different case complexities on the availability of rehabilitation aids for older adults

CASE

Hamish is an 84-year-old retired farmer admitted to hospital with a wrist fracture and bruising of his arm after a fall in a slippery yard. Hamish is referred for rehabilitation and complains of deep aching pain and stiffness in both of his knees. He notes that this pain was initially felt when lifting heavy materials, but more recently he had experienced pain in the absence of any physical activity or exertion. He is no longer able to walk his dog due to the severity of his pain. The physiotherapist and the occupational therapist have reported a brief summary of their assessment findings as follows:
- Independent in most areas of self-care.
- Mobilising without any aids although tends to hold on to furniture or the wall as walking; there are concerns about his balance.

INTRODUCTION

This chapter outlines the broad range of equipment that is available in the rehabilitation of older adults to support their needs around activities of daily living, mobility and function. It focuses particularly on activities including eating, dressing, personal hygiene, bed mobility and mobility aids, including wheelchair use. It is recommended that a thorough assessment should be completed by the occupational therapist or the physiotherapist to assess a person's ability and requirements for rehabilitation equipment. This comprehensive assessment will ensure that any equipment that is provided is tailored to the older adult's needs and reduces the risk of non-use of such equipment.

EATING

Before providing any specific eating equipment for older adults, it is important to ensure the person is in an optimal upright position to facilitate safe and independent eating and that the swallowing status of the individual has been assessed with respect to food consistency. Other considerations include the person's upper limb ability such as no use, partial or full use of one or both upper limbs.

Suitable cutlery, tableware and provision of additional equipment such as non-slip table mats are typical rehabilitation equipment that can facilitate safe and independent eating. The type of cutlery will depend on the person's level of ability but can include padded cutlery to facilitate a stronger grip or combined cutlery such as a combined knife and fork which facilitates eating with one hand only. Lightweight cutlery is used for older adults with reduced upper limb strength. Options available for drinking include double handled mugs, insulated mugs, mugs with lids or mugs with a nose cut-out. A fixed or clip-on straw can also be useful for older adults with decreased upper limb strength or dexterity; however, a swallowing assessment is required to ensure this is a safe option. Plates with raised sides can help a person to gather up their food if they can only use one hand for eating.

DRESSING

It is important that older adults are facilitated to wear their own clothes as soon as possible on admission to hospital. Different types of clothing facilitate easier dressing such as garments with the minimal number of fasteners like buttons and zips. Examples include loose t-shirts, sweatpants and shoes with Velcro fastenings. Equipment to minimise effort required by people with decreased mobility or reduced manual dexterity incudes long-handled reachers, dressing sticks, stocking or tights aid, long shoehorn, elasticated or spiral laces, button hook or a pull ring for zippers. Some individuals will have to adhere to specific precautions for dressing. For example, older adults admitted to hospital for a total hip replacement will have to follow specific post-surgery precautions while dressing to avoid dislocation of the hip or excessive pain. Common precautions include putting trousers on the operated leg first and using devices such as long-handled reachers to avoid excessive bending of the hip. Fig. 11.1 shows some examples of adaptive aids.

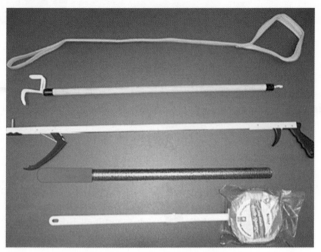

FIG. 11.1 Adaptive aids. Top to bottom: leg lifter, dressing stick, reacher, long shoehorn, long-handled sponge. (From Niederhuber JE, Armitage JO, Kastan MB, Doroshow JH, Tepper JE. *Abeloff's Clinical Oncology*, 6th edn. Elsevier Inc., 2020, with permission.)

PERSONAL HYGIENE: BATHING, WASHING, SHOWERING AND TOILETING

There is a wide range of equipment available to assist with personal care and hygiene. Equipment ranges from fixed equipment in the bathroom environment such as wall-mounted grab bars located beside the toilet, in a shower cubicle and beside a bathtub. Wall-mounted, or free-standing, shower seats are helpful for individuals with reduced balance and mobility.

Mobile equipment is available to enable staff to safely provide assistance to those who cannot walk from their bedroom to the bathroom. Examples of mobile equipment include a commode, shower chair (see Fig. 11.2) and hoist. For physically dependent or bed-bound older adults, a shower trolley

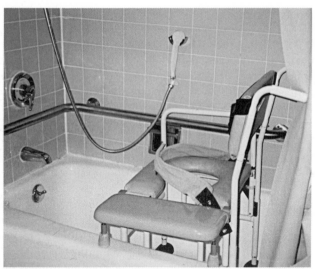

FIG. 11.2 Bathroom setup with shower or commode chair and hand-held shower head. (From Umphred DA, Burton GU, Lazaro RT, Roller ML. *Umphred's Neurological Rehabilitation*, 6th edn. Elsevier, 2013, with permission.)

facilitates safe and regular showering and good hygiene routine. Shower trolleys allow older adults to be showered while lying down on a comfortable and soft mattress. They are height-adjustable and of sufficient width to turn the individual easily. It is important to have equipment available on the ward that matches that which an individual may use when discharged home.

There is a wide range of options to facilitate safe and independent toileting. Typical equipment includes non-slip floor mats, raised toilet seats or toilet surrounds which provide support when getting on/off the toilet. For more dependent patients, a shower chair with a commode seat is a useful option as it facilitates both toileting and showering.

BED MOBILITY

There is a range of equipment available to assist older adults to move from lying to sitting and to get in/out of bed safely and independently. Hoists provide a mechanical means by which dependent older adults can be moved or transferred from one place or position to another. An over-bed trapeze bar, a bed-rope ladder (also known as bed pull-up) and side bed lever are used to assist movement from lying to sitting. Side bed levers are also used to push up from sitting to standing when getting in and out of bed. For those with difficulty lifting their legs into bed when getting into bed, a leg lifter can be used if the person has adequate upper limb strength and sitting balance. A leg lifter consists of a strap with a foot loop and hand loop (see Fig. 11.1). The foot is placed in the foot loop and the hand loop is used to elevate the leg onto the bed. A floor mat sensor pad may be appropriate for patients with cognitive impairment and reduced mobility. This alerts staff if a person who is at a high risk of falling attempts to get out of bed unsupervised.

MOBILITY EQUIPMENT

A mobility aid can assist when an older adult feels insecure when walking, experiences weakness or pain, or has had a fall. To ensure that the appropriate device is selected, the older person's needs, lifestyle and home environment should be assessed. Common equipment in a rehabilitation gym that supports improvements in mobility include parallel bars, pedal exercisers, stationary bikes, treadmills and stairs. Walking/mobility equipment may perform a number of functions:
- Offers greater stability and balance by providing a wider support base.
- Facilitates the walking pattern in terms of speed and evenness of stride. The equipment may also help maintain an upright body posture.
- Increasing the confidence of the older person in his/her walking ability.
- Weight redistribution – some of the weight carried through the legs when walking is transferred through the arms of the frame or stick as it is leant on for support. This may help reduce pain in the joints, muscles and ligaments in the lower limbs.

Types of Mobility Equipment

Wheelchairs and Seating

It is vital, when medically able to do so, that older adults are facilitated to mobilise as much as possible. It is important to have a range of wheelchairs and seating options to provide the appropriate level of support and mobility to accommodate individuals with varying functional abilities. Both manual (Fig. 11.3) and powered (Fig. 11.4) wheelchairs are available to facilitate safe and independent mobility. Wheelchairs have many adjustable features to ensure optimal seating position. A range of pressure-relieving and supportive cushions to prevent skin damage and optimise seating endurance such as gel, air and moulded foam cushions are commercially available. Options for customised cushions, backrest/trunk supports and other seating supports are available but require the input of a specialised seating therapist. Suitable armchairs should be available for older adults who can transfer in/out of bed and sit out for periods of time during the day. Options for suitable armchairs include adjustable arm rests, back heights and chair legs. Riser/recliner chairs can be useful to assist standing up from sitting but also need to be assessed for safety. A riser/recliner chair is an electric powered armchair allowing the user to adjust it to lift them into a standing position, or safely lower them into a seated, or lying, position.

Walking Frames and Rollator Frames

The rehabilitation process is a gradual progression towards independent and unassisted walking and may commence with the use of a walking frame to give the user confidence

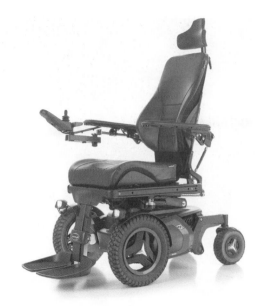

FIG. 11.4 Powered wheelchair. (From Chui K, Jorge M, Sheng-Che Y, Lusardi M. *Orthotics and Prosthetics in Rehabilitation*, 4th edn. Elsevier, 2020, with permission.)

before progressing to another walking aid. It is very important to have the frame at the correct height for use. Most walking frame models are available with adjustable telescopic legs so that their height can be altered (Fig. 11.5). A folding frame can easily be stored within the home if it does not need to be used all the time. Other modifications to walking frames include bags or baskets to store personal belongings, tray

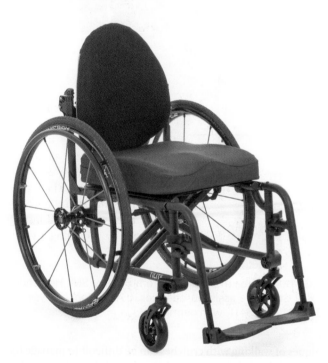

FIG. 11.3 Manual wheelchair (with a precontoured seat and back). (From Chui K, Jorge M, Sheng-Che Y, Lusardi M. *Orthotics and Prosthetics in Rehabilitation*, 4th edn. Elsevier, 2020, with permission.)

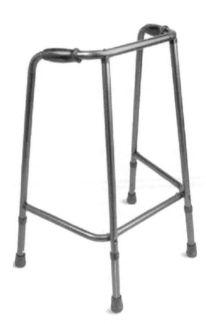

FIG. 11.5 Walking frame. The height of the legs is adjustable. (From Cetin E, Muzembo J, Pardessus V, Puisieux F, Thevenon A. Impact of different types of walking aids on the physiological energy cost during gait for elderly individuals with several pathologies and dependent on a technical aid for walking. *Ann Phys Rehabil Med.* 2010;53(6-7):399–405, with permission.)

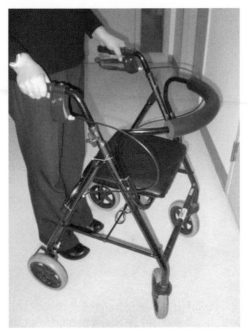

FIG. 11.6 Wheeled walking frame. The crossbar can be used as an aid to standing up from a chair without armrests. (From Elsevier Interactive Patient Education © 2019 Elsevier Inc., with permission.)

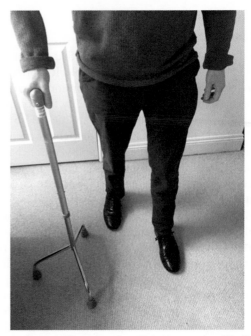

FIG. 11.7 Tripod. (From Bradley SM, Hernandez CR. Geriatric assistive devices. *Am Fam Physician.* 2011;84(4):405–11, with permission.)

attachments and seats to allow individuals to rest. Wheeled frames are useful for people who find it difficult to use a traditional walking frame as they make a more continuous walking pattern possible, and do not need to be lifted clear off the ground to move forwards (Fig. 11.6). Walking frames and rollator frames are often not practical for long-term use because they are difficult to manoeuvre in tight spaces and cannot be used on a flight of stairs. It is important to liaise with community physiotherapy colleagues to be aware of the home situation so that an appropriately sized walking frame is available.

Tripod/Quadripod

A tripod/quadripod (Fig. 11.7) is often prescribed as a progression from a Zimmer frame or rollator frame as it facilitates increased independence in mobility for the older person. A tripod/quadripod has a walking stick style shaft and a three- or four-point base. It is free standing and is more stable than a standard walking stick. It is very important to have the tripod or quadripod at the correct height for use. All tripods and quadripods are made of metal, usually aluminium or steel, and have a telescopic mechanism for adjusting.

Crutches

Crutches (Fig. 11.8) provide a higher level of mobility – they allow for a quicker walking pattern and can be used safely on stairs with the correct technique. As the person increases in confidence and is allowed to put more weight through their weaker leg, they will progress onto one or two sticks. The tech-

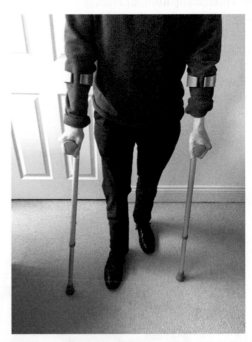

FIG. 11.8 Forearm crutches. (From Bradley SM, Hernandez CR. Geriatric assistive devices. *Am Fam Physician.* 2011;84(4):405–11, with permission.)

niques of walking with crutches can be difficult to manage for older adults. It is important that safe mobility with crutches is taught when they are prescribed and also that safe transfer techniques are considered. Crutches may not always be

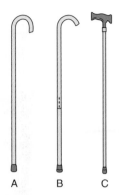

FIG. 11.9 (A) C-handle or crook-top stick. (B) Adjustable aluminium stick. (C) Functional grip stick. (From Webster J, Murray D. *Atlas of Orthoses and Assistive Devices,* 5th edn. Elsevier © 2019, with permission.)

the appropriate choice of mobility aid for the older person, and prescription will depend on lots of factors including the personal and environmental factors.

Walking Sticks (Canes)

Walking sticks (Fig. 11.9) are routinely prescribed for older adults who present with slight balance problems. Similar to other mobility aids, it is important that a walking stick is prescribed by a healthcare professional, usually a physiotherapist or an occupational therapist. It is not uncommon for older adults to use a walking stick that has not been prescribed for them. This is not recommended due to safety risks around incorrect height or wear and tear of rubber ferrules at the base of the stick. If the height is incorrect, then the support will not be adequate. Some walking sticks are made of wood, which must be measured and cut to the correct height. Metal sticks are available in a variety of fixed heights and the nearest suitable height should be chosen.

Safety

All mobility equipment should be checked regularly for signs of wear and tear. Particularly vulnerable parts include the rubber ferrules, which must be replaced if the slip-resistant rings become worn down, or if the rubber shows signs of cracking. Equipment that is height-adjustable can show signs of stress at the height setting after prolonged use. Handgrips can also become worn.

Rehabilitation Robotics

Rehabilitation robotics is an area of rehabilitation focused on facilitating rehabilitation through the use of robotic devices. Rehabilitation robotics includes devices that are designed to assist in improving function in the arm or hand or in the leg or foot. Other robotic devices are designed to improve mobility but are often only available in specialist rehabilitation centres. For example, exoskeleton devices have been shown to improve arm function and walking ability in people with stroke. However, the amount of time spent using these devices is an important determinant of improvements in arm function and walking ability. Rehabilitation using robotics is generally reported to be well tolerated and enjoyed by older adults.

CASE CONCLUSION

Following a detailed assessment and intervention by the occupational therapist and physiotherapist in hospital, Hamish was provided with the following rehabilitation aids:

- A non-slip table mat to support eating with one hand.
- A raised toilet seat and non-slip floor mat in the bathroom to support personal hygiene; he was supplied with a shower sleeve to wear over the wrist cast when showering. Initially he was provided with a free-standing shower seat so he could shower from a seated position to reduce slip or fall risk while showering. He was advised to hold the wall-mounted grab bars for safety when entering and exiting the shower.
- His family were advised to bring in 'easy-to-don' clothing (clothing with minimal fasteners/buttons) to enable Hamish to dress himself more independently. For upper body dressing Hamish was advised to don clothing over the fractured upper limb first.
- A walking stick for outdoor mobility.

As Hamish's fractured wrist would be considered a temporary disability and recovery would be expected some of the equipment used in the early stage of his rehabilitation may only be needed on a temporary basis. However, given his age and other functional issues such as pain and decreased mobility he may need to use some of the equipment such as the free-standing shower seat and walking stick in the longer term after discharge to reduce his fall risk.

SUMMARY POINTS

- Rehabilitation equipment should be assessed and provided on an individualised basis, depending on the unique needs of the person
- Common types of equipment are those that assist with activities of daily living such as eating, dressing, hygiene and mobility
- As needs change, equipment may no longer be needed as people recover
- Equipment should be checked regularly for wear and tear

MCQs

Q.1 Older adults are prescribed lightweight cutlery because of:

   a) Reduced muscle strength

   b) Increased muscle strength

   c) Improved coordination

   d) All of the above

Q.2 Which of the following provides the most support for older adults when mobilising?

   a) Walking stick

   b) Crutch

   c) Tripod

   d) Zimmer frame

Q.3 Walking sticks should be:

   a) Prescribed by a healthcare professional

   b) Tailored to the individual's height

   c) Safety checked regularly

   d) All of the above

12

Physiotherapy: How It Works

Fiona O'Reilly

LEARNING OBJECTIVES

- Describe in basic terms how physiotherapy works
- Explain the role of physiotherapy in assessment and management of falls
- Explain the value of movement as an essential element of what it means to be healthy

CASE

Sarah is a 78-year-old retired postwoman who lives alone in a two-story house. She fell at home, fracturing the left hip. Following hospitalisation for a left hemiarthroplasty (partial hip replacement), Sarah was referred to a multidisciplinary day hospital service to continue her physiotherapy rehabilitation programme.

"Walking is man's best medicine" (Hippocrates, c 400 BC)

Functional movement is an essential element of health and well-being, it is purposeful and is influenced by internal and external factors.

WHAT IS PHYSIOTHERAPY?

The goal of physiotherapy is to 'develop, maintain and restore maximum movement and functional ability throughout the lifespan. It is provided in circumstances where movement and function are threatened by ageing, injury, pain, diseases, disorders, conditions or environmental factors and with the understanding that functional movement is central to what it means to be healthy' (WCPT, 2019).

The provision of skilled physiotherapy integrates clinical experience, research-based knowledge and patient values to maximise quality of life and movement potential for individuals of all ages. Physiotherapists work with patients with wide-ranging conditions in hospital and community-based settings and play an important role within the interdisciplinary rehabilitation team.

PHYSIOTHERAPY: HOW IT WORKS

Physiotherapists are movement specialists. Physiotherapy practice is rooted in movement physiology research; brain cells and nerves, muscle and load-bearing bone are all subject to the same basic 'use it or lose it' principle. These cells, when 'stressed' by movement (exercise) or weight bearing (standing, stepping, walking), are responsive and adaptable, and in the right conditions result in increased output or remodelling. This process is referred to as 'plasticity' (Rea, 2017).

The physiotherapist's role is to assess the nervous, muscle and skeletal (bone) systems for condition-specific impairments. Based on assessment findings, the physiotherapist designs a person-centred programme involving movement and exercise that places sufficient demands on the body to challenge nerves and increase activation of muscles. This increased muscle activity can serve to maintain or improve muscle strength, flexibility and a patient's ability to regain meaningful physical movement and function.

Even in situations of very limited movement, e.g. in the case of a patient with brain injury who has severe global weakness, physiotherapy intervention could involve providing an adequate stable posture to allow small controlled movement of the head by setting up a seating system or providing physical support. In a person who has just had surgery following a fractured ankle, it may be to provide specific advice about when they can commence more challenging tasks, putting full weight on the limb, and prescribing a specific strengthening exercise programme that they can carry out for themselves (Fig. 12.1).

As a holistic practitioner, the physiotherapist places great value on the need for creating 'trust' and a 'rapport' with the patient to instil motivation, encourage self-efficacy or 'self-belief' and a willingness to explore their limits of ability.

ASSESSMENT OF MOVEMENT AND BALANCE

In addition to examining the integrity of muscles and joint movement, the physiotherapist will look for impairments related to:
- ability to maintain a stable posture when sitting or standing
- ability to respond to balance displacement in changing postures such as moving from lying to sitting or standing up
- dynamic standing balance such as reaching while standing or navigating an obstacle while walking.

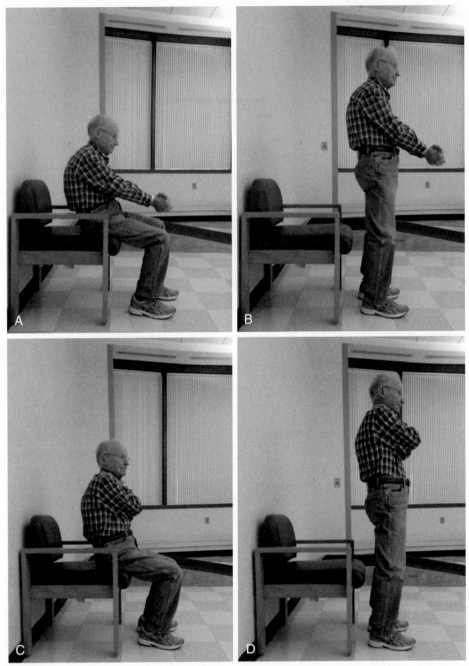

FIG. 12.1 Functional strengthening progression example. (With permission from Pastva AM, Duncan PW, Reeves GR. Strategies for supporting intervention fidelity in the rehabilitation therapy in older acute heart failure patients (REHAB-HF) trial. *Contemp Clin Trials.* 2018;64: 118—127.)

Balance Assessment Tools

Physiotherapists use assessment tools to rate performance across various tasks requiring balance control to identify functional limitations or the capacity to perform various tasks, and also to re-evaluate the outcome of interventions. Introducing complexity such as environmental change or dual tasking, such as walking and talking, can further test the real-life attentional demands of a task.

The Berg Balance Scale (BBS) (Berg et al., 1989) and Timed Up and Go (TUG) (Shumway-Cook, Brauer, & Woollacott,

2000) are commonly used by physiotherapists to measure functional ability. The BBS includes 14 items assessing both static and dynamic aspects of balance in order of advancing difficulty. A cut-off score of 46/56 has been identified as useful to predict falls. Muir et al. (2008) also suggest that a cut-off score of 40/56 is particularly useful to predict those who will have multiple falls and injurious falls. The TUG is a gait-based functional mobility test that is easy to administer, reliable and has high sensitivity (87%) for predicting falls (Shumway-Cook et al., 2000). This test involves the functional task of standing

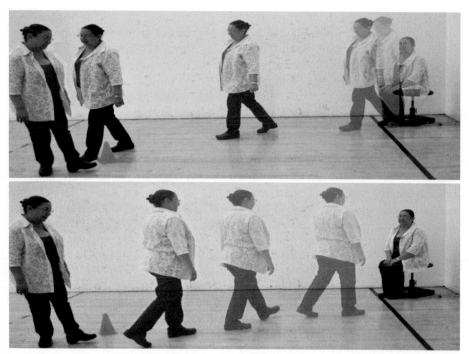

FIG. 12.2 The Timed Up and Go test. (From Lee S-P, Dufek J, Hickman R, Schuerman S. Influence of procedural factors on the reliability and performance of the timed up-and-go test in older adults. *Int J Gerontol.* 2016;10(1):37—42, with permission.)

up from a chair, walking 3 m, returning to the chair to sit down, and is timed (see Fig. 12.2). Importantly, this test allows the patient to utilise a walking aid, and requires limited endurance to complete. Patients taking ≥14 seconds to perform the test are generally classified as at high risk of falls.

In busy clinical practice, de Villiers and Kalula (2015) suggest a combination of elements of various functional balance assessments would include the TUG, Romberg's test (which assesses sensory pathways by removing visual compensation), assessing for postural sway with eyes open and closed (identifying slowed postural reflexes), the sternal nudge (assessing postural response to external displacement) and the functional reach test (testing limits of stability).

Gait Assessment

The physiotherapist will also assess the quality of movement and walking patterns (gait) to tease out those factors that have potential to improve with intervention. Age-related gait impairments such as increased variability of step length or shorter single support time (time on one foot) during dual task gait (walking while talking for example) have been identified as risk factors for falls in older adults (Bauer et al., 2015).

Assessment of gait speed is particularly important, as a reduction in speed is an indicator of 'fear of falls', a risk factor for falls and disability, and is used to screen people for frailty. A walking speed of less than 0.8 m/s and not being able to walk more than 350 m in 6 minutes are suggestive of frailty (Vieira, Palmer, & Chaves, 2016). Falls among older people with frailty are particularly concerning because the low reserve across multiple physiological systems

that characterises frailty may increase complications with recovery (Fried et al., 2004).

CASE CONTINUED

Patient History

Further relevant information to the physiotherapist's assessment includes the fact that Sarah has had a number of falls in the past 6 months; she has a recent diagnosis of osteoporosis following a DEXA scan with a T-score of −2.8; and has hypertension (high blood pressure) and coronary heart disease. Her current medications include furosemide and metoprolol for hypertension, ibuprofen (an anti-inflammatory drug) for long-term arthritis pain and she was commenced on alendronic acid for osteoporosis during hospitalisation.

Examination

Physical examination revealed: a mild thoracic kyphosis (stooping posture); independent gait with a walking frame, weight bearing as tolerated, limited due to pain; rated by Sarah as 3/10 on a Numeric Rating Scale (NRS).

Manual muscle strength testing revealed: left hip strength of 3/5; knee and ankle strength 4/5 and some tightness at end of range in both knee joints and ankles. She also had difficulty with activities of daily living (ADLs); decreased balance with a Berg Balance score of 38/56, and limited endurance as she was only able to mobilise 24 m in 2 minutes before requiring a rest period. Rating of perceived exertion (RPE) at rest was reported as 1/10, and after gait was rated as 8/10. Sarah had not been on a regular exercise programme.

The physiotherapist sought to establish whether the cause of falls could be intrinsic in nature, possibly due to orthostatic hypotension (dropping of blood pressure on standing) caused by taking antihypertensive (blood pressure lowering) medication. Sarah has experienced multiple falls in the past, and her Berg Balance score indicates she is at risk for further falls. Based on this, the physiotherapist establishes if 'fear of falling' has produced activity-limiting behaviours for Sarah, such as restricting her mobility outside the home, potentially contributing to reduced exercise capacity. Physiotherapists will be sensitive to the risk of increasing isolation and consider the need for referral to the social worker. The therapist determined if the patient has managed to get up following previous falls, if she is able to summon help in case of an emergency and if she will require a pendant alarm system.

Goal Setting

Following assessment, the physiotherapist helps guide the patient to set functional goals in the commonly used SMART format: specific, measurable, achievable, realistic/relevant and time-bound (see Chapter 10 Setting Rehabilitation Goals). In Sarah's case, the long-term goal is to return to being an independently functioning, community-dwelling individual with a predicted achievement date of 3 months after surgery. To achieve this long-term goal, several short-term impairment and activity-based goals are set. These included:

1. Safe and independent gait with full weight bearing on the left leg with progression to use of a walking stick.
2. Independent stair climbing.
3. Increase hip strength to 4/5 to enable progression to walking stick.
4. Increase Berg score to 46/56 to decrease risk of falls and demonstrate detectable change.
5. To be able to walk outdoors safely to her local shops using a stick only.

The therapist continues to monitor and evaluate the patient's progress and if necessary, adjusts goals or intervention accordingly.

Physiotherapy Interventions

The physiotherapist may utilise a number of approaches when addressing balance instability and risk of falls including restorative, compensatory or accommodating strategies. Therapeutic exercise is a primary restorative approach (Moreland et al., 2003). Prescribing foot orthotics may be considered a compensatory approach and provision of walking aid an accommodating approach.

Physiotherapy-led group exercise programmes have been shown to reduce falls by 29% and the risk of falling by 15% and individual exercise programmes by 32% and 22%, respectively (Gillespie et al., 2012).

Recommendations for fall prevention practice include (Sherrington et al., 2017):

1. Balance training that is highly challenging, individualised and progressive. It should incorporate:

a) reducing the base of support (e.g. standing with two legs close together, standing with one foot directly in front of the other, standing on one leg)
b) moving the centre of gravity and controlling body position while standing (e.g. reaching, transferring body weight from one leg to another, stepping up onto a higher surface) and
c) standing without using the arms for support, or if this is not possible then aiming to reduce reliance on the upper limbs (e.g. holding onto a surface with one hand rather than two, or one finger instead of the whole hand).

2. At least 3 hours of exercise each week.
3. Ongoing participation in exercise is necessary or benefits will be lost.
4. Walking training may be included in addition to balance training, but high-risk individuals should not be prescribed brisk walking programmes.
5. Strength training may be included in addition to balance training.
6. Exercise providers should make referrals for other risk factors to be addressed.

Sarah's proposed rehabilitation programme is described in the Resources section. It includes progressive hip strengthening exercises targeting weaker hip abduction, gluteal, hamstring and quadriceps muscles. Once full weight bearing on the affected leg is achieved, task-specific training for independent walking with a stick and stair climbing is progressed, in addition to progressive balance training (see Fig. 12.3). Since Sarah is taking a beta-blocker, which dampens the cardiac response to exercise, the traditional target heart rate using the Karvonen formula (ACSM, 2009) to calculate the intensity of exercise cannot be effectively utilised. The RPE is

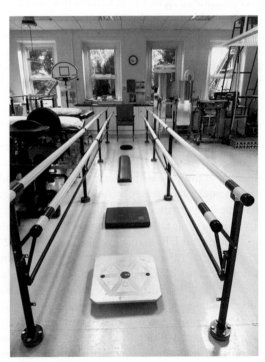

FIG. 12.3 Balance training.

used to monitor physical stress in lieu of heart rate and blood pressure. Sarah is taught how to perform a safe technique for getting off the floor, and she is educated around how to reduce potential hazards for falls in her home.

Finally, onward referral to a community-based falls prevention exercise programme in addition to advice about increasing levels of physical activity completes this episode of physiotherapy rehabilitation.

SUMMARY POINTS

- The goal of physiotherapy is to develop, maintain and restore maximum movement and functional ability
- Physiotherapists are movement specialists and design person-centred rehabilitation programmes

- Physiotherapists, as healthcare providers, are also health educators and health promoters and serve people throughout the life span
- Common physiotherapy interventions include balance training, walking training and strength training; these help to reduce the risk of falls in older people

MCQs

Q.1 Which of the following is the commonly known physiological principle that physiotherapists often use to underpin their interventions?
  a. Only use it if you can
  b. Don't use it if it's too much effort
  c. Use it or lose it
  d. Use it and lose it anyway
  e. Don't use it because you're going to lose it

Q.2 Which of the following are evidence-based restorative components of physiotherapy intervention to reduce falls risk?
  a. Advice about home hazards
  b. Strengthening and balance exercises that are individualised, challenging and progressive

  c. Backward chaining technique for getting off the floor
  d. Provision of a foot orthosis
  e. Provision of a walking stick

Q.3 According to Sherrington et al. (2017) what amount of exercise is required for effective falls prevention?
  a. 30 minutes per week for 6 months
  b. 2.5 hours per week and ongoing participation
  c. 3 hours per week and ongoing participation
  d. 3 hours per week for 6 months
  e. 5 hours per week

REFERENCES

American College of Sports Medicine (ACSM). (2009). *ACSM's guidelines for exercise testing and prescription* (8th edn.). Baltimore, MD: Lippincott Williams & Wilkins.

Bauer, C. M., Gröger, I., Rupprecht, R., Marcar, V. L., & Gaßmann, K. G. (2015). Prediction of future falls in a community dwelling older adult population using instrumented balance and gait analysis. *Zeitschrift für Gerontologie and Geriatrie, 49*(3), 232–236.

Berg, K. O., Wood-Dauphinee, S. L., Williams, J. T., & Gayton, D. G (1989). Measuring balance in the elderly: preliminary development of an instrument. *Physiotherapy Canada, 41,* 304–311.

de Villiers, L., & Kalula, S. Z. (2015). An approach to balance problems and falls in elderly persons. *SAMJ: South African Medical Journal, 105*(8), 695.

Fried, L. P., Ferrucci, L., Darer, J., Williamson, J. D., & Anderson, G. (2004). Untangling the concepts of disability, frailty, and comorbidity: implications for improved targeting and care. Review. *The Journals of Gerontology: Series A: Biological Sciences and Medical Sciences, 59*(3), 255–263.

Gillespie, L. D., Robertson, M. C., Gillespie, W. J., Sherrington, C., Gates, S., Clemson, L. M., & Lamb, S. E. (2012). Interventions for preventing falls in older people living in the community. *Cochrane Database of Systematic Reviews, 9,* CD007146.

http://onlinelibrary.wiley.com/doi/10.1002/14651858. CD007146.pub3/abstract.

Moreland, J., Richardson, J., Chan, D., O'Neill, J., Bellissimo, A., Grum, R., & Shanks, L. (2003). Evidence-based guidelines for the secondary prevention of falls in older adults. *Gerontology, 49*(2), 93–116.

Muir, S. W., Berg, K., Chesworth, B., & Speechley, M. (2008). Use of the Berg Balance Scale for predicting multiple falls in community-dwelling elderly people: a prospective study. *Physical Therapy, 88*(4), 449–459.

Rea, I. M. (2017). Towards ageing well: use it or lose it: exercise, epigenetics and cognition. *Biogerontology, 18*(4), 679–691.

Sherrington, C., Michaleff, Z., Fairhall, N., Paul, S., Tiedemann, A., Whitney, J., Cumming, R., Herbert, R., Close, J., & Lord, S. (2017). Exercise to prevent falls in older adults: an updated systematic review and meta-analysis. *British Journal of Sports Medicine, 51,* 1750–1758.

Shumway-Cook, A., Brauer, S., & Woollacott, M. (2000). Predicting the probability of falls in community-dwelling older adults using the Timed Get Up & Go test. *Physical Therapy, 80,* 896–903.

Vieira, E. R., Palmer, R. C., & Chaves, P. H. (2016). Prevention of falls in older people living in the community. *BMJ, 353*:i1419.

WCPT.org. (2019). Policy statement: description of physical therapy | World Confederation for Physical Therapy. Retrieved from: https://www.wcpt.org/policy/ps-descriptionPT (Accessed 4 March 2019).

13

Occupational Therapy: Function and Cognition

Anna Bargent

LEARNING OBJECTIVES

- Explain how occupational therapy helps people to overcome the effects of disability
- Describe the role of the occupational therapist
- Identify different types of occupational therapy assessments
- Describe interventions offered by occupational therapists

CASE

Mira is an 83-year-old woman. She lives on her own in a house with stairs. Her bathroom is upstairs and she does not have a downstairs toilet. She showers daily.

Mira usually walks around her home without the use of a walking aid. She uses a stick when walking outdoors. She is a keen gardener and enjoys cooking her own meals at home.

Mira has macular degeneration, and needs large print in order to read. She takes multiple medications on a daily basis. Her family live locally but work full time. She does not usually require daily support from others.

Mira fell in her garden, and fractured her T12 vertebra (one of the bones that form the spine). This was managed conservatively without any surgery, and Mira was prescribed pain medication and exercise. She is transferred to a rehabilitation ward and is keen to get home as soon as possible.

WHAT IS OCCUPATIONAL THERAPY?

Occupation refers to practical, purposeful and meaningful activities that allow people to live independently and have a sense of identity. Occupations may be essential day-to-day tasks, such as self-care, work or leisure.

What makes occupational therapists (OTs) unique is that they therapeutically use occupations to help people of all ages overcome the effects of disability caused by illness, ageing or accident. This may include practising self-care activities, providing specialist equipment to enable a person to manage an activity independently or teaching someone how to complete a task in a different way. OTs work holistically, considering the whole person and their needs, whether these be physical, environmental, psychological or social. They are practical problem-solvers, with a focus on facilitating independence.

OTs work with people of all ages with a wide range of conditions, most commonly those who have difficulties due to a mental illness, physical or learning disabilities. They work in a variety of settings including hospitals, community-based health services and social care services. They also work in housing, prisons, education and voluntary organisations. They work as independent practitioners (RCOT, 2019).

OCCUPATIONAL THERAPY AND REHABILITATION

OTs use meaningful activities to help people gain or regain skills; strength and confidence to carry out the occupations they wish to do. They address *occupational performance* – how a person carries out an occupation, including what the desired outcomes are for that person. They are specialists in how people function.

Using task analysis, OTs identify the components required to carry out an activity. They consider the requirements of the task itself and the person completing it, including physical and cognitive requirements. This includes the person's ability to 'sequence' a task – to carry it out in an order that makes sense. OTs use this information to understand why a person may find it difficult to carry out or finish a task, and make recommendations to enable a person to do so more independently. The American Occupational Therapy Association Occupational Therapy Practice Framework helps to guide task analysis (AOTA, 2002).

In the context of rehabilitation, OTs consider:

What can you do now? (assessment)

What do you want/need to do? (goals)

How are we going to help you to do this? (intervention)

Interventions may include practising an activity, or parts of an activity, to increase confidence. They may include modifying an activity to facilitate independence, for example by using equipment or teaching someone how to carry out an activity in a different way. They may also include developing skills and abilities that are common across several occupations.

OTs may use activities that appear unrelated, to build up strength, balance or other skills, to enable a person to be more independent across a range of occupations. For example, the action of standing up from a sitting position, and sitting from standing position, is transferrable across a range of functional activities. This action is performed when transferring on or off a bed, chair and toilet.

Within a rehabilitation service, OTs may assess, prescribe a rehabilitation programme and review progress. The rehab programme itself may be delivered by therapy assistants, overseen by a qualified OT. Rehabilitation may start in a hospital or rehabilitation unit, and then continue in someone's own home.

ASSESSMENT OF COGNITION

Assessment of cognition forms part of the assessment by an OT. Other members of the multidisciplinary team may also assess cognition. Some of the cognitive assessments used are brief, for example, the Mental Status Questionnaire (MSQ) or Abbreviated Mental Test Score (AMTS) have 10 questions. Others are more comprehensive assessments, for example the Mini Mental State Examination (MMSE) or Montreal Cognitive Assessment (MoCA), which are scored out of 30.

Assessment of cognition can include memory, attention and concentration, processing of information, language, object recognition and recall. The way a person processes information, and the speed at which they make sense of information, affects the way a person understands the world and interacts with it. It is important for OTs and the wider multidisciplinary team to be aware of any cognitive difficulties an older person may be experiencing, in order for rehabilitation to address or factor in any deficits.

Identification of impairments in cognition can help to predict changes in occupational performance – for example, impairments with short-term memory and recall may indicate a person will find it more difficult to remember new information, and may require additional strategies to support them in this.

ASSESSMENT OF FUNCTION

For assessment of function, OTs may use a range of assessment tools and measures to assess and review a person's occupational performance of given tasks. These may include standardised subjective assessments such as the Canadian Occupational Performance Measure (COPM) or objective assessments such as the Barthel Index (see Table 13.1). These measures can be used at the start of the rehabilitation process to look at occupational performance prior to interventions, and can also be used as outcome measures to review a person's performance during or following rehabilitation interventions.

A person's usual routine and way of carrying out an activity will be discussed prior to any functional assessment to confirm previous level of occupational performance and to help plan rehabilitative interventions. The areas of self-care, including washing, dressing and toileting, are often assessed. Assessing self-care is important for many reasons, including hygiene, skin integrity and dignity.

Kitchen tasks are commonly used for both assessment and interventions. A kitchen assessment is not 'just making a cup of tea'; it is a multifaceted assessment, completed by carrying out a usual daily task (see Fig. 13.1). Performance components assessed during a kitchen assessment include orientation to the environment and the task itself; sequencing; safety; risk assessment and management; physical abilities; short-term memory; attention and concentration, to name but a few.

Assessing a person's ability to transfer from one surface to another is important when considering their ability to function within an environment, especially during activities of daily living. Key transfers include between bed, chair and toilet. The environment and furniture itself is considered, alongside the person's physical and cognitive abilities, to transfer and reposition themselves. For example, using the toilet includes the transfer itself, alongside clothing management and personal hygiene tasks. The location of the toilet within the person's own environment is also a factor. Fear of falling can play a role in a person's ability to transfer. Consideration should be made of appropriate furniture, mobility aids, equipment and number of people required to assist with the transfer during assessment.

EQUIPMENT

Equipment can be used to modify tasks and facilitate independence. It can be used to compensate for loss of function in the short term, and to enable people to carry on living independent lives in the long term. Commonly issued equipment in a rehabilitation setting includes walking aids; toileting equipment such as commodes, toilet frames or toilet seats; dressing aids including long-handled shoehorns and dressing sticks ('grabbers') – see Chapter 11 Rehabilitation Equipment for more information.

CASE: MIRA – ASSESSMENT

Cognitive assessment indicated that Mira had some short-term memory difficulties.

Mira lacked confidence in her ability to walk, following her fall. She was fearful of falling again. It was painful and effortful for her to turn in bed and transfer from bed initially. She required assistance of two people to transfer from bed and to take a few steps with a frame, to sit on a chair located next to her bed.

As she was unable to stand without assistance, Mira needed help to wash and dress. She was unable to bend down to reach her feet.

Mira was not keen to practice any kitchen activities until such time as she was able to stand by herself.

CASE: MIRA – INTERVENTIONS

Mira practised bed transfers at least twice daily, at logical times in her usual routine – morning and evening. These practices were carried out with the therapists, therapy assistants and

TABLE 13.1   The Barthel Index.

Parameter	Status	Score
Eating	Totally independent	10
	Needs help to cut meat, bread, etc.	5
	Dependent	0
Washing	Independent: enters and leaves the bathroom alone	5
	Dependent	0
Dressing	Independent: can put on and take off clothes, button clothes and tie shoelaces	10
	Needs help	5
	Dependent	0
Personal hygiene	Independent for washing face, hands, brushing hair, shaving, putting on makeup, etc.	5
	Dependent	0
Stools	Normal continence	10
	Occasional episodes of incontinence, or needs help to administer suppositories or laxatives	5
	Incontinence	0
Micturition	Normal continence or able to take care of catheter if inserted	10
	Maximum one daily episode of incontinence, or needs help to take care of catheter if inserted	5
	Incontinence	0
Use of toilet	Independent to go to the toilet, take off and put on clothing	10
	Needs help to go to the toilet, but can clean self	5
	Dependent	0
Movement	Independent to go from chair to bed	15
	Minimal physical help or supervision needed	10
	Needs great degree of help, but is capable of staying seated alone	5
	Dependent	0
Walking	Independent, walks 50 m alone	15
	Needs physical help or supervision to walk 50 m	10
	Independent in wheelchair without help	5
	Dependent	0
Stairs	Independent to go up and down stairs	10
	Needs physical help or supervision	5
	Dependent	0

From Niitsu M, Ichinose D, Hirooka T, et al. Effects of combination of whey protein intake and rehabilitation on muscle strength and daily movements in patients with hip fracture in the early postoperative period. *Clin Nutr.* 2016;35(4):943–9.

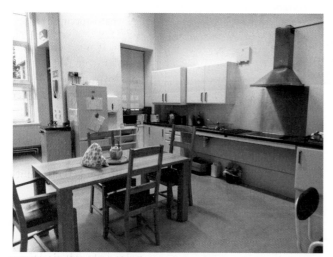

FIG. 13.1   The therapy kitchen. This area on the rehabilitation ward can be used to assess everyday tasks such as cooking and cleaning.

also with the nursing staff, as part of the multidisciplinary rehabilitation team. When Mira needed to go to the toilet during the day, she practised transferring to/from a chair and a toilet, and also practised walking to/from the toilet. At mealtimes, she was encouraged to join others in social dining on the ward. This encouraged good, balanced nutrition during her recovery and also involved walking practice to and from the dining area. In this way, mobility and transfer practice was woven into her daily routine. Mira's confidence and ability to carry out transfers increased with practice and encouragement. Her mobility also improved.

With practice, Mira was able to stand up from a chair by herself, but found sitting onto and standing up from the toilet was difficult, as the toilet was low. A raised toilet seat was provided for use both on the ward and at home. Mira was able to stand independently from this higher surface. She required support and encouragement to be able to consistently transfer out of bed by herself.

Mira was keen to be able to wash and dress herself without support – she was a proud lady and found it embarrassing that she initially required support to have a strip-wash. Through the use of dressing aids, Mira found she was able to dress herself slowly, using the new techniques taught to her.

Mira was unable to remember some of the recommended dressing techniques to allow her to dress herself independently. She was given a large print information sheet to remind her, due to her visual impairment. Leaflets were also provided on managing activities of daily living following a fracture and exercise sheets provided, to help reinforce advice given by the physiotherapist, all in large print.

Falls reduction was a key intervention for Mira and was multifactorial and multidisciplinary in its approach. Strength and balance training with the physiotherapist, alongside advice about footwear and preventing falls during daily activities from the OT, with medication advice by the doctor, all helped to reduce her risk of further falls.

Mira was discharged home after 2 weeks on a rehabilitation ward, to continue her rehabilitation in her own home, with support from the community reablement service.

SUMMARY POINTS

- Occupational therapy uses meaningful activities to help people gain or regain skills, strength and confidence to carry out the occupations they wish to do
- Goals set within rehabilitation should be practical and important to the person; this enables them to engage in the rehabilitation process
- Different approaches are used by OTs during rehabilitation, including cognitive assessment, functional assessment, equipment provision and education
- Rehabilitation interventions include practising transferable skills and modifying activities using different techniques or equipment, to increase independence

MCQs

Q1. What does an occupational therapist do?
   a. Provide equipment
   b. Use meaningful activities to help people overcome effects of disability
   c. Educate about falls prevention
   d. Carry out cognitive assessments
   e. All of the above
Q2. How can an occupational therapist aid rehabilitation for an older person?
   a. Increase a person's confidence in carrying out daily activities
   b. Teach alternative techniques for getting washed and dressed
   c. Advise on the impact of cognitive difficulties on functional activities
   d. Ensure rehabilitation goals are those which are most important to the person
   e. All of the above

REFERENCES

AOTA (American Occupational Therapy Association). (2002). Occupational therapy practice framework: domain and process. *American Journal of Occupational Therapy*, *26*, 609–639.

RCOT (Royal College of Occupational Therapists). (2019). What occupational therapy? *Royal College of Occupational Therapists*. [viewed 26 April 2019]. Retrieved from https://www.rcot.co.uk/about-occupational-therapy/what-is-occupational-therapy (Accessed 26 April 2019).

14

Nursing Patients Through Rehabilitation

Cliff Kilgore

LEARNING OBJECTIVES

- Explain why nursing is important within rehabilitation
- Describe the role of the registered nurse within rehabilitation settings
- Describe the interventions provided by nurses

CASE

Ruby is an 89-year-old lady referred for rehabilitation after she fractured her pubic ramus (part of the pelvis) in a fall at home. She was treated with pain relief and advised to mobilise.

Ruby was accepted for initial rehabilitation in an in-patient rehabilitation unit for part of her rehab before being transferred to the rehabilitation team based in the community for home rehab.

The initial assessment by the rehabilitation nurse identified the following:

Ruby lives on her own in a two-storey house in a centrally located part of town. Her husband died 2 years ago and she had started to struggle with her activities of daily living (ADLs) in recent months before her fall.

She has a past medical history of heart failure, chronic kidney disease stage 3 and falls but has remained independent at home and did not require any regular care provision before her fracture. Ruby's family visits regularly but she has not asked for their help. She is determined to remain independent although she does acknowledge that she needs rehabilitation.

The assessing nurse screened Ruby for frailty based on her level two weeks prior to her fall, to help with monitoring her recovery and assessing her need for support. They checked blood pressure, temperature, pulse, respiration rate and oxygen saturation levels in their initial assessment. This provided a baseline for future monitoring in case Ruby became unwell during her rehabilitation. The nurse also identified worsening of Ruby's heart failure symptoms which include shortness of breath during activity. Ruby said this had started since her fracture and hospital stay.

The nurse discussed her falls history with her and this was not the first fall although she had not broken any bones before. The nurse also discussed the risks of being in hospital and the reduced mobility she would have experienced after her injury.

By this point, Ruby was walking with a frame but had not used any walking aids prior to the fall. Her pain was controlled but the nurse identified that Ruby had not walked very much since her fall and therefore explained possible pain that may occur during rehabilitation as she would be more active.

Plan:

The nurse used their analysis of the assessment information based on experience and knowledge to determine a plan of care and rehabilitation for Ruby.

This included:

- A review of Ruby's heart failure by a doctor or advanced practitioner
- A falls assessment which would include an assessment at home by the home rehabilitation team
- Suggested rehabilitation goals were discussed by the nurse and Ruby, focusing on what she felt she needed to achieve to live independently at home. This was done with guidance from the nurse on expected recovery timescale from a pubic ramus fracture and took into account Ruby's long-term conditions.
- Education was required for Ruby in regard to recovery from a fracture and maintaining bone health in future.
- Pain monitoring and management throughout rehabilitation
- Regular reviews of Ruby's progress were included in the rehabilitation programme with agreement that when it was felt safe to do so, she would continue her rehabilitation at home with the home team.

SUMMARY

A comprehensive assessment was completed on Ruby's transfer to the rehabilitation service and this used pre- and post-admission information and also Ruby's own aims to help decide on her rehab goals. The nurse used information from Ruby's past medical history and also her own knowledge of frailty, heart failure and pain management to determine what course of action to take in regard to monitoring. The rehabilitation programme provided a seamless progression from inpatient rehab to home rehab with clear progression steps for Ruby, and she made a good recovery.

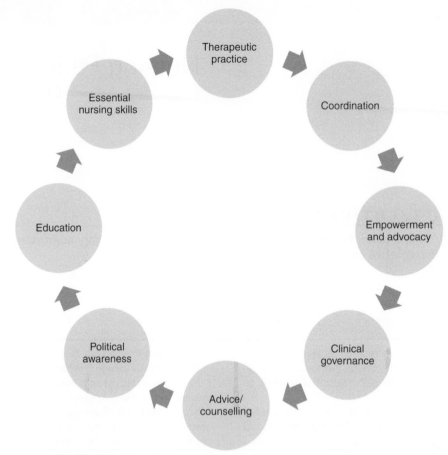

FIG. 14.1   Categories where rehabilitation nurses can influence care.

WHY ARE NURSES IMPORTANT FOR PATIENTS HAVING REHABILITATION?

Nurses are the largest professional group within the rehabilitation team and are vital to the recovery of patients after a healthcare crisis. Nurses act both as advocate and educator for patients ensuring that they maximise their rehabilitation as they try to recover after an illness or injury. Achieving optimisation and improving quality of life are key factors and because of this rehabilitation nursing has to be a dynamic, continuous process that focuses on improving what an older person can do to achieve optimal independence. A framework identifies eight categories where rehabilitation nurses can influence care (see Fig. 14.1) (RCN, 2007).

Nurses are key to delivering patient-centred care, as they build professional relationships with patients within the rehabilitation setting. Patients recognise the role that nurses have, particularly when it comes to ensuring that their daily needs are met. However, the nurse also has an important role in coaching, encouraging and promoting independence for the patient. It is the frequent nursing contact that enables this, referred to as the therapeutic relationship (Tyrrell et al., 2012). In a hospital rehabilitation setting, nurses provide a 24-hour-a-day, 7-day-a-week presence.

Although rehabilitation nursing focuses on recovery and improvement for patients, it is also crucial that they understand the potential of deterioration in older people's health. Nurses will often use information gathered from other health professionals and family or carers to help identify early deterioration, which may lead to longer hospital stay and also inhibits rehabilitation. This will mean working together with the therapy team to jointly recognise signs of deterioration in function and cognition and listening to family concerns regarding any difference that they see in the patient's well-being. Ensuring that concerns are escalated at the right time will mean that they have to weigh information critically and make a decision that is safe and right for the patient (Wolf, 2012). Protocols are often applied with clear pathways of escalation to doctors or advanced clinical practitioners.

LOOKING AFTER OLDER PEOPLE DURING REHABILITATION

Nurses working with older people need a wide range of skills and knowledge to be able to make sound clinical judgements and ensure that appropriate care is delivered (Burke & Doody, 2012). Older people often require rehabilitation after many different types of healthcare crisis, and nurses require expert knowledge in a wide range of clinical conditions, some of which will be complex. Dealing with uncertainty is a core competence for the nurse supporting an older person's rehabilitation as this patient group is likely to present with a multitude of healthcare variables. Using 'critical thinking' is crucial to how knowledge is applied.

It is important to understand the additional risks that older people have after a health crisis and particularly those living with frailty. For example, early identification of age-related changes and risk factors for falls during rehabilitation is essential to prevent older people from further deterioration (Gouveia et al., 2016). The nurse will understand the intrinsic factors that may result in someone falling and examine ways of minimising these without detracting from the aims of functional rehabilitation. Extended periods of inactivity, with the inevitable loss of muscle bulk, strength and fitness, can lead to an increased risk of falls; the nurse will work with other members of the multidisciplinary team to reduce this risk (Kneafsey, Clifford, & Greenfield, 2013).

The simple but effective 'Get up, get dressed and get moving' campaign in the UK (see Chapter 21 Avoiding Deconditioning) has led to dramatic changes (NHS Improvement, 2017). Fear of falling has been identified as an obstacle for rehabilitation, and any condition that has led to prolonged immobility is likely to affect strength and balance in an older person.

GATHERING INFORMATION ABOUT PATIENTS

Gathering information is fundamental to the start of the nursing process but when considering rehabilitation, it is crucial to understand the individual's pre-admission levels. Clarity on what a person could do before their illness or injury enables the rehabilitation process to focus on a patient's aim or goal and helps the nurse to compare what is normal and abnormal (Kahneman, 2011). For example, an 80-year-old walking 50 m using a walking stick may appear to be mobile, but if the same patient informs the nurse that they were playing 18 holes of golf 2 weeks ago, then this may bring a different rehabilitation goal. However, there are times when gaining information about previous levels requires additional information from family or friends, known as 'collateral history'. This may be necessary due to a person's inability to recall accurate information such as in dementia or as a result of a delirium (a sudden confusional state). Either way the aim is to personalise the rehabilitation programme both in regard to achieving what is needed for the patient to make a reasonable recovery and to balance the risks of trying to achieve these goals (Coutts, 2014).

AGREEING GOALS

After the nurse gathers information on previous level of function, it is important to mutually agree which goals would be achievable based on professional judgement and the commitment of the older person to achieving these goals (Burke &

Doody, 2012). This is often done in conjunction with the entire multidisciplinary team. It is important for the nurse to be honest and realistic in regard to the disability that comes with certain health conditions. However, there are times when the nurse will need to provide encouragement to what can be achieved after an illness or injury based on their expertise. There are obvious key elements to a person's function that are important to any assessment. How someone is currently able to perform their ADLs provides a benchmark to what success looks like and this in turn informs the patient's individual goals. This in reality is where the nursing treatment actually starts and is often something that is an interactive and cyclical process (Burke & Doody, 2012). Key elements for the nurse in this role are providing psychological and emotional support, encouraging the patient to achieve maximum independence and functional ability through coaching, providing education on essentials such as what good fluid intake looks like and the importance of nutrition in recovery and rehabilitation as well as responding to issues such as pain (Burke & Doody, 2012; Perry et al., 2012).

INDIVIDUALISING CARE

Older people are not homogeneous as human beings or how they respond to similar illness, injury or subsequent rehabilitation. Anecdotally nurses will often recount examples of a patient that reduces their complex goals of rehabilitation to a simple task such as 'being able to walk the dog' or 'I want to be able to meet my friends'. It is therefore important for the nurse to consider what an older person believes, desires and needs in order to promote successful rehabilitation outcomes. In order to do this the relationship between the patient and the nurse is vital. Tyrrell et al. (2012) suggest that patients undergoing rehabilitation often work better with nurses that provide the 'correct fit' to what the patient is trying to achieve. This supports the notion that providing 'good' rehabilitation is about the nurse adapting their approach to patients and ensuring that everything in the therapeutic relationship is done with kindness and consideration for what the patient wants.

COMMUNICATION

Nursing is often seen as pivotal within the rehabilitation team when considering coordination between patient, family and other professional staff, and is vital to effective team working (Burke & Doody, 2012; Perry et al., 2012; RCN, 2007). This is not surprising, as it is often nurses who are ever-present in patients' rehabilitation experience. Nursing plays a significant part in ensuring that factors affecting patient care and rehabilitation are successfully communicated. Everything that is gained in the nursing process is based on excellent communication skills. Throughout the older person's rehabilitation experience, from the initial meeting and assessment and throughout the transitional process to planning the final discharge, the communication process is key (Burke & Doody, 2012).

SUMMARY POINTS

- Rehabilitation nursing is a dynamic, continuous process that focuses on improving what an older person can do to achieve optimal independence
- Personalising rehabilitation is key to success
- Nurses are fundamental in influencing the rehabilitation process
- Good communication by nurses is a vital component in the rehabilitation of older people

MCQs

Q.1 Why are nurses important in rehabilitation?
   a. They ensure the patient's needs are met
   b. They act as a coach for the patient
   c. They monitor for patient deterioration
   d. They individualise care
   e. All of the above

Q.2 To support rehabilitation nurses need:
   a. To tell patients to decide their goals by themselves
   b. A wide range of skills and knowledge
   c. To try their best and hope they get it right
   d. To minimise a patient's use of painkillers
   e. To avoid helping patients with their daily activities

Q.3 Which one of the following is part of the nursing role in rehabilitation?
   a. Understand that all older people are the same
   b. Recognise that older people don't know what is good for them
   c. Understand that older people have specific goals to achieve in rehab
   d. Remember that older people are usually not interested in recovering
   e. Caution all patients not to walk without assistance

REFERENCES

Burke, K., & Doody, O. (2012). Nurses' perceptions of their roles in rehabilitation of the older person. *Nursing Older People, 24*(2), 33–38.

Coutts, B. (2014). The complex decision making needed in significant event analysis. *Primary Healthcare, 24*(2), 26–30.

Gouveia, B. R., Jardim, H. G., Martins, M. M., Gouveia, É. R., de Freitas, D. L., Maia, J. A., & Rose, D. J. (2016). An evaluation of a nursing led rehabilitation programme to improve balance and reduce risk of community dwelling older people: a randomised controlled trial. *International Journal of Nursing Studies, 56*, 1–8.

Kahneman, D. (2011). *Thinking fast and slow*. London: Penguin Books.

Kneafsey, R., Clifford, C., & Greenfield, S. (2013). What is the nursing team involvement in maintaining the mobility of older adults in hospital? *International Journal of Nursing Studies, 50*, 1617–1629.

NHS Improvement. (2017). Helping patients to get up and get moving. Retrieved from https://improvement.nhs.uk/resources/helping-patients-get-up-and-get-moving/ (Accessed 30 August 2019).

Perry, L., Hamilton, S., Williams, J., & Jones, S. (2012). Nursing interventions for improving nutritional status and outcomes of stroke patients: descriptive reviews of processes and outcomes. *Worldviews on Evidence-Based Nursing, 10*(1), 17–40.

Royal College of Nursing. (2007). Maximising independence: the role of the nurse in supporting the rehabilitation of older people. Retrieved from https://numerons.files.wordpress.com/2012/04/4the-role-of-the-nurse.pdf (Accessed 27 March 2019).

Tyrrell, E., Levack, W., Ritchie, L., & Keeling, S. (2012). Nursing contribution to the rehabilitation of older patients; patient and family perspectives. *Journal of Advanced Nursing, 68*(11), 2466–2476.

Wolf, L. (2012). An integrated, ethically driven environment model of clinical decision making in emergency settings. *International Journal of Nursing, 24*(1), 49–53.

15

Speech Therapy: Communication and Swallowing

Sarah Duggan & Emma Finch

LEARNING OBJECTIVES

- Explain the role of the speech and language therapist (SLT) when working with an older person
- Describe normal swallowing and dysphagia
- Outline the process of communication

- Identify conditions that may lead to dysphagia and/or communication difficulties
- Describe elements of the assessments completed by an SLT

INTRODUCTION

Speech and language therapists (SLTs, also known as speech language pathologists in some areas) are experts in swallowing and communication. The ability to safely eat and drink and to communicate with ease is of utmost importance to a person's day to day life.

SWALLOWING

Swallowing involves the coordination of more than 40 muscles and six cranial nerves. There are motor and sensory components to swallowing (movement and sensation). It is a surprisingly complex process and is split into four main phases. Eating and drinking is an important aspect of daily life and socialisation. Fig. 15.1 demonstrates the structures involved in swallowing.

Pre-Oral

Includes all the steps involved in getting the food/drink/medication (referred to as a bolus) into the oral cavity. This utilises multiple senses, e.g. smelling and recognising the bolus, and physically transporting the bolus to the mouth.

Oral Phase

It starts with the bolus entering the oral cavity. It is chewed, manipulated and transported to the back of the mouth before the swallow is initiated.

Pharyngeal Phase

It begins when the bolus reaches the back of the tongue. The larynx elevates which starts a series of protective mechanisms to stop the bolus from entering the airway. The epiglottis (a flap of cartilage at the top of the airway) covers the airway, the vocal cords come together and breathing is momentarily paused to protect the lungs. The muscles in the pharynx (the throat) contract and push the bolus through the upper oesophageal sphincter (a band of muscle at the entrance to the oesophagus, a muscular tube leading to the stomach).

Oesophageal Phase

The muscles of the oesophagus contract and relax propelling the bolus into the stomach (known as peristalsis).

All these movements need to be well coordinated for a safe and efficient swallow. It is imperative that the muscles involved have adequate strength and that the person can sense if any material enters the airway or remains in the pharynx after swallowing. If any part of the above stages is impaired, the person will experience dysphagia (swallowing difficulty).

Aspiration is the medical term used when a bolus enters the airway instead of the oesophagus. If a person's sensation is intact, they will cough and attempt to clear the material from their airway. However, a high percentage of older people who have dysphagia aspirate silently, i.e. there will be no overt signs to indicate aspiration has occurred (Kikuchi et al., 1994). Silent aspiration is known to be an important mechanism for the development of pneumonia in older adults (Teramoto et al., 2008) but not all people who aspirate will develop pneumonia (O'Keeffe, 2018).

Potential Indicators of Dysphagia

There are many signs that may indicate that dysphagia is present. However, the presence of some of the symptoms below in isolation may not necessarily indicate dysphagia. The overall presentation should be considered when determining whether a person requires a swallowing evaluation. If dysphagia and/or aspiration are suspected, a referral to SLT is indicated.

- Food and/or drinks gathering in oral cavity during a meal.
- Difficulty chewing or manipulating food.
- Coughing or excessive throat clearing post swallow.
- Choking episodes.
- Complaints of food sticking.
- 'Wet' or 'gurgly' vocal quality after swallowing.
- Low oxygen level associated with eating and drinking.
- Recurrent or unresolving chest infections.
- A condition that predisposes you to dysphagia.

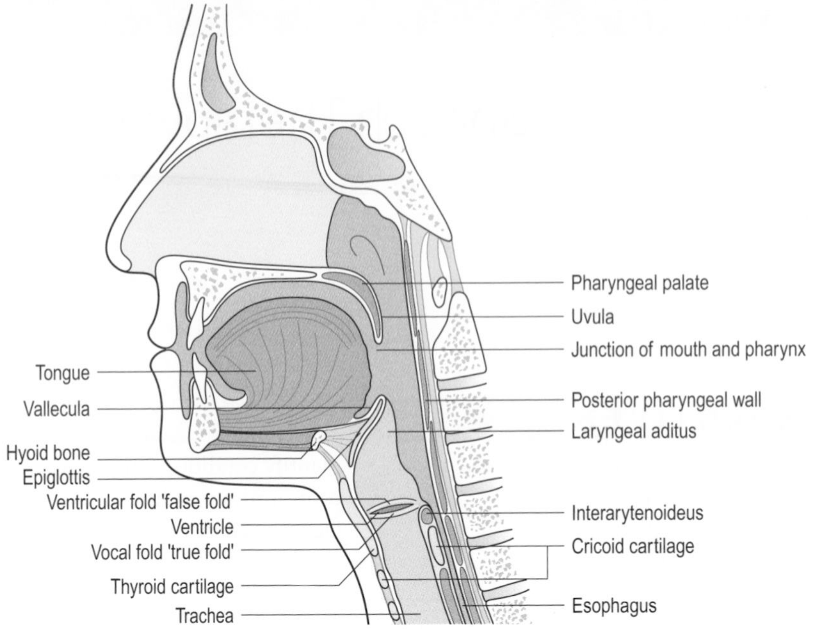
Pharyngeal palate
Uvula
Junction of mouth and pharynx
Posterior pharyngeal wall
Laryngeal aditus
Interarytenoideus
Cricoid cartilage
Esophagus
Tongue
Vallecula
Hyoid bone
Epiglottis
Ventricular fold 'false fold'
Ventricle
Vocal fold 'true fold'
Thyroid cartilage
Trachea

FIG. 15.1 Lateral view of the anatomy of the head and neck pertinent to swallowing. (From Bosma JF, Donner MW, Tanaka E, et al. Anatomy of the pharynx, pertinent to swallowing. *Dysphagia* 1986;1:24.)

Clinical Swallowing Examination

This is a comprehensive swallowing assessment undertaken by the SLT (see Table 15.1).

CASE 1

Gerry is a 90-year-old gentleman who was brought to hospital with shortness of breath and a productive cough. He has chronic obstructive pulmonary disease (COPD), osteoarthritis and hypertension. He was treated for pneumonia.

He was referred to SLT as nursing staff had noticed that he was coughing after mealtimes. He had never been seen by SLT before and denied any swallowing difficulties.

Instrumental Assessments of Swallowing

Following Clinical Swallowing Examination (CSE), the SLT may complete an instrumental assessment of swallowing. These include:

Videofluoroscopy

This is a dynamic x-ray examination of swallow function performed by the SLT with the radiologist and/or radiographer in the radiology department. It involves swallowing varying consistencies of food and drinks mixed with barium to assess the biomechanics of swallowing. Barium is a radio-opaque material that shows up on an x-ray, therefore the SLT can view the bolus in real time when swallowing (see Fig. 15.3). A videofluoroscopy may be carried out to further evaluate for suspected silent aspiration, trial various strategies, manoeuvres and postures to determine their effectiveness in improving swallow safety and efficiency or to guide a specific swallow rehabilitation programme.

Fibreoptic Endoscopic Evaluation of Swallowing

Fibreoptic Endoscopic Evaluation of Swallowing (FEES) (Langmore, Kenneth, & Olsen, 1988) involves placement of a small, flexible scope into the nose to provide a direct view of the larynx and pharynx (see Fig. 15.4).

The SLT will typically administer various drink consistencies and food textures to objectively assess the swallow. A FEES is carried out for the same reasons as a videofluoroscopy mentioned above. It has the advantage of being carried out at the person's bedside.

Following the assimilation of all collected information and assessment results, an individualised dysphagia management plan will be put in place. The SLT may commence a dysphagia rehabilitation programme as deemed appropriate. See Chapters 43 and 44 for more information on dysphagia rehabilitation.

CASE 1 Continued

SLT completed a CSE with Gerry. He was noted to occasionally cough during and after a meal. A videofluoroscopy was completed which showed silent aspiration of thin drinks (level 0) and reduced efficiency of pharyngeal musculature that led to a build-up of residue post swallow.

Dysphagia Management Plan

Drink/food modifications: Level 1 thickened drinks and regular food

Compensatory: Single sips of drinks. Take regular sips of drinks during meal

Rehabilitation: Exercises focusing on pharyngeal strengthening

Education: Family trained to thicken drinks. Educate re: nature and signs of dysphagia

Consequences of Dysphagia

There are many consequences of dysphagia which range from milder effects to serious, life-threatening consequences.

TABLE 15.1   Components of the clinical swallowing examination.

Case history	- Comprehensive medical history; in particular: Diseases/diagnoses associated with dysphagia Respiratory status (past and current) Nutritional status Medications Social history Patient and carer's accounts of dysphagia Eating and drinking preferences
Oromotor assessment	- Assessment of movement and sensation of the face, lips, tongue and jaw - Oral health - Dentition - Vocal quality - Cough integrity
Cognitive and communication screen	- Memory - Insight into difficulties - Communicative ability - Vision and hearing
Oral trials	If appropriate, the SLT will administer a variety of drink and food consistencies and assess for signs of difficulties in the oral and pharyngeal stages of swallowing. These consistencies will be in line with International Dysphagia Standardisation of Diet Initiative (IDDSI) (see Fig. 15.2). The SLT may trial some strategies to optimise swallow safety and efficiency, e.g. • Reducing distractions at mealtimes • Self-feeding strategies, e.g. the feeding assistant will physically help direct the person's hand to their mouth • Alternating solids and sips (fluid wash) • Increasing sensory input, e.g. strong flavours, temperatures • Altering bolus size
Dysphagia management plan	Based on the CSE, the SLT makes a recommendation regarding the suitability of continuing oral intake, specific mealtime guidelines including food and drink consistencies and any strategies as above. The SLT will refer for instrumental assessment of swallowing if indicated.

Longer Hospital Stays

Evidence indicates that people with aspiration pneumonia spend a longer time recovering in hospital (Lanspa et al., 2015).

Malnutrition and Dehydration

For many older people, it is known that there can be a reduction in their oral intake. Therefore, it is not surprising that many older people with dysphagia struggle to meet their daily nutrition and hydration requirements. Malnutrition may bring about further loss of muscle mass and function, which may itself contribute to worsening of the dysphagia (Wirth et al., 2016).

Quality of Life

Healthcare professionals often focus solely on the implications of dysphagia on a person's physical health, frequently overlooking the psychosocial consequences. Some evidence suggests that aspects such as fear, embarrassment and frustration caused by the symptoms of dysphagia are more important to the older person and their caregivers (Martino, Beaton, & Diamant, 2009).

Carer Burden/Stress

Dysphagia can contribute to increased caregiver burden and stress. A recent systematic review by Namasivayam-MacDonald and Shune (2018) concluded that the presence of dysphagia in community-dwelling older adults is a factor leading to an increased burden among caregivers. Clinicians should look at ways to develop interventions to support caregivers as part of routine dysphagia care.

Mortality

There are varying statistics regarding mortality associated with dysphagia. Falcone et al. (2012) found that frail older adults with aspiration pneumonia were more likely to die within 30 days of presentation to hospital than older adults who did not have aspiration pneumonia.

Choking is also a contributing factor to dysphagia-related mortality in older adults (Wu et al., 2015).

Difficulties with Medication Intake

A recent study investigated the ability to swallow pills in people with Parkinson's disease (PD). Significant problems with swallowing medications were found to be common (in 28% of participants) and that this may influence the clinical response to oral medication (Buhmann et al., 2019). It is important to assess an older person's ability to swallow their medication.

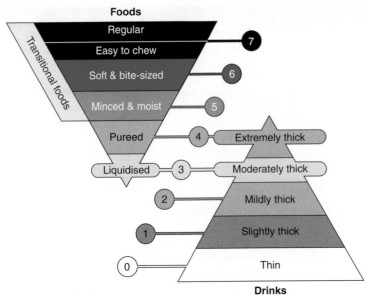

FIG. 15.2 The International Dysphagia Diet Standardisation Initiative Framework (IDDSI) © The International Dysphagia Diet Standardisation Initiative 2016 @https://iddsi.org/framework/. Attribution is NOT PERMITTED for derivative works incorporating any alterations to the IDDSI Framework that extend beyond language translation.

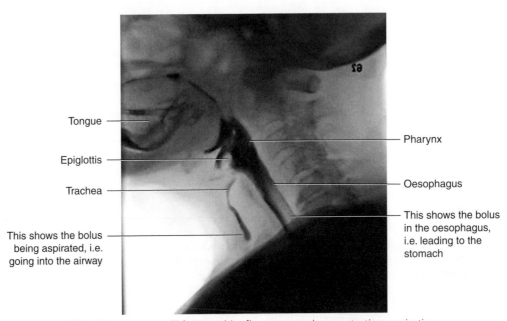

FIG. 15.3 Image still from a videofluoroscopy demonstrating aspiration.

COMMUNICATION

CASE 2

Helen is an 81-year-old lady with a diagnosis of PD. She was recently admitted to hospital due to a fall at home. She was referred to SLT for assistance in capacity assessment. The team was struggling to make decisions with Helen about discharge destination. The referral for SLT stated that she had 'reduced hearing and a quiet voice'.

Communication is a two-way process involving the understanding and portraying of a message between a listener and a speaker. Fig. 15.5, a communication chain, is a simplified representation of this complex process.

As all the areas and connections are interlinked, a person may have difficulty in one or many of the areas. Communication is broken down further into the domains listed below. It is important to understand these distinctions as these areas may be targeted when an older person is undergoing rehabilitation. These will be discussed in more detail in Chapter 43.

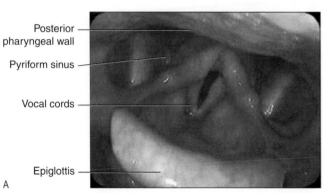

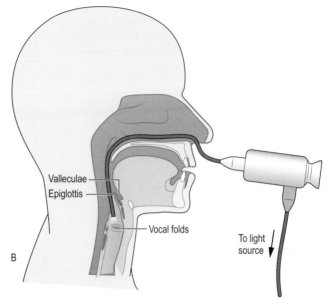

Posterior pharyngeal wall

Pyriform sinus

Vocal cords

Epiglottis

A

Valleculae
Epiglottis

Vocal folds

To light source

B

FIG. 15.4 (A) Superior view during FEES examination showing pharyngeal and laryngeal structures. (B) Illustration of FEES procedure (with kind permission from Dr Susan Langmore).

Specific Communication Difficulties

Voice

A sound that is produced when air from the lungs vibrates the vocal cords in the larynx. The voice can vary in pitch, volume or tone.

A voice disorder is known as *dysphonia*. Signs of dysphonia include a hoarse, breathy and/or rough quality to the voice, strain in the voice, weak or low volume voice and sudden breaks in or fading of voice.

Speech

Requires pressure from the lungs to generate sound in the larynx and subsequent coordination of the muscles in the vocal tract into the correct positions to articulate sounds and words.

Difficulty with any of the following speech subsystems due to neuromuscular weakness is known as *dysarthria*: articulation, resonance (airflow through nose and mouth), prosody (naturalness and intonation patterns) and respiration (breath support for speech).

Language

Refers to the actual words we use and how they relate to each other. This includes receptive language (understanding) and expressive language (language output), and encompasses verbal and written language.

Language difficulty caused by brain disease or damage is known as *aphasia* or *dysphasia*. See Chapter 43 for more information.

Non-Verbal Communication

These are the essential ways that we communicate. This includes facial expression, tone of voice, body language, proximity and gesture.

Pragmatics

Refers to the ability to understand the rules about appropriate communication, e.g. knowing when it is appropriate to speak, changing communication style depending on the situation or listener and turn-taking.

Cognition

A number of cognitive skills are essential for effective communication, i.e. attention, memory, sequencing, reasoning and planning skills.

A referral to SLT is indicated in the following situations:
- Communication difficulty is noted to be impacting on an older person's daily functioning.
- If there is a new onset of a communication difficulty.
- If there is change in a pre-existing communication difficulty.

Assessment

Communication assessment is complex and multifaceted and each assessment will be tailored to the individual. The International Classification of Functioning, Disability and Health Framework (ICF) shows the different aspects that will be considered for each individual (Fig. 15.6).

CASE 2 Continued

Helen was referred to audiology, who provided a hearing aid. A full SLT assessment showed that she had moderate to severe dysarthria associated with her PD. This was affecting her ability to communicate her wishes to her sister and the multidisciplinary team. As her voice was weak and her speech imprecise, it was difficult for people to hear and understand what she was saying. This affected her ability to show that she was capable of making a decision to return home. SLT provided a voice amplifier which allowed her to voice her wishes and led to a safe discharge home.

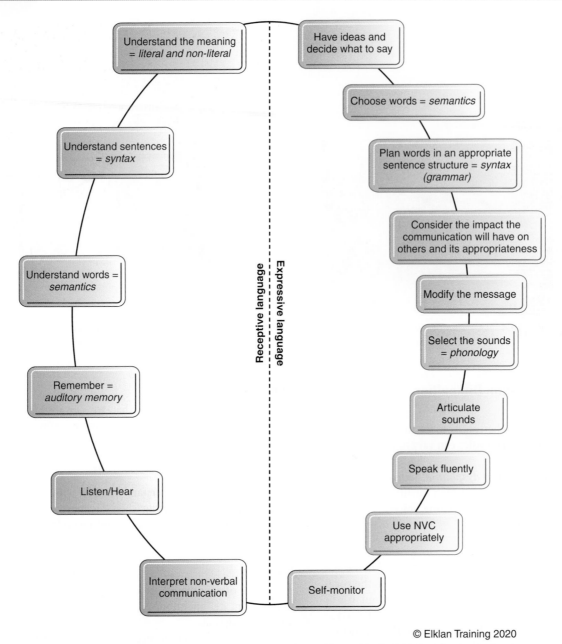

© Elklan Training 2020

FIG. 15.5   Communication chain. (Adapted from Afasic (2019) with permission.)

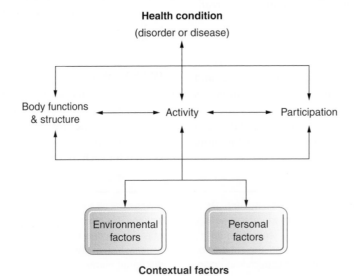

FIG. 15.6   The ICF from World Health Organisation (World Health Organisation, 2001).

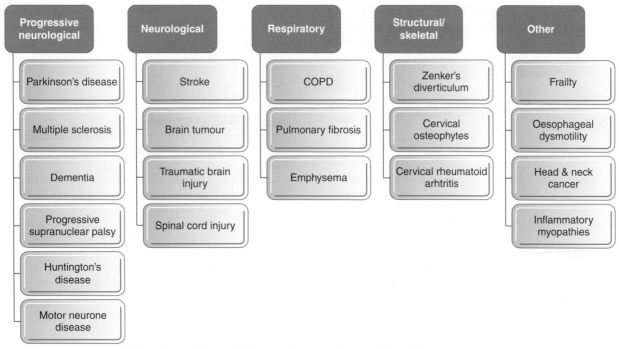

FIG. 15.7 List of conditions which may be associated with swallowing or communication difficulties.

An assessment will include informal or standardised assessments of communication to measure impairments. It must include consideration of how the impairment is affecting a person's ability to participate in their daily activities. Personal factors such as educational levels and cultural considerations, as well as environmental factors including communication partners and daily communication needs, have to be considered.

Consequences of a Communication Difficulty

There are a myriad of potential consequences for someone with a communication difficulty. It is clear that someone living with a communication difficulty may experience a reduction in their quality of life. Consequences may also include social isolation, increased dependency on others or difficulty making their wishes known including when considering future decisions about their own care. It may also lead to potential increased lengths of stay in hospital or poorer outcomes while in hospital. Research has shown that people with com-

munication difficulties associated with impairments of language, speech or voice are three times more likely to experience adverse events in hospital. Some evidence also suggests that difficulty communicating is a causal factor in falls for some people (Hemsley et al., 2019).

A study conducted in 2018 showed that adults with communication impairment experienced more difficulties with accessing healthcare, which sometimes led to a delay in receiving necessary care (Stransky, Jensen, & Morris, 2018).

Specific Conditions

There are number of different medical conditions that are common in older people and are associated with an increased risk of developing swallowing and/or communication difficulties (see Fig. 15.7).

It is worth noting that even in the absence of one of these conditions associated with dysphagia, there are multiple other factors that may predispose an older person to dysphagia. These will be discussed in Chapter 44.

SUMMARY POINTS

SLTs play an integral role in the management of both swallowing and communication difficulties. Early referral to a SLT service is essential to minimise any adverse outcomes associated with both. Dysphagia is a common and serious issue that may be experienced by the older person for a variety of rea-

sons. The consequences of dysphagia include malnutrition, dehydration, frequent hospital admissions, reduction in quality of life and higher mortality. Communication is a complex process, and difficulties with communication can lead to a significant reduction in quality of life.

MCQs

Q.1 Aspiration refers to:
  a. Food particles entering the lungs
  b. Saliva or secretions entering the lungs
  c. Fluids entering the lungs
  d. All of the above

Q.2 A referral to SLT is indicated for which of these cases:
  a. A man with PD who has dysphonia and can't be heard
  b. A lady with advanced dementia who is not following verbal directions for the MDT
  c. A man with COPD who is having recurrent chest infections despite multiple courses of antibiotics. There are no obvious signs of difficulty at mealtimes.
  d. All of the above

REFERENCES

Afasic. (2019). The communication chain. Retrieved from https://www.afasic.org.uk/about-talking/what-skills-are-involved/the-communication-chain/ [Accessed 30 April 2019].

Buhmann, C., Bihler, M., Emich, K., Hidding, U., Pötter-Nerger, M., Gerloff, C., Niessen, A., Flügel, T., Koseki, J., Nienstedt, J., & Pflug, C. (2019). Pill swallowing in Parkinson's disease: a prospective study based on flexible endoscopic evaluation of swallowing. *Parkinsonism and Related Disorders, 62*, 51–56.

Falcone, M., Blasi, F., Menichetti, F., Pea, F., & Violi, F. (2012). Pneumonia in frail older patients: an up to date. *Internal and Emergency Medicine, 7*(5), 415–424.

Hemsley, B., Steel, J., Worrall, L., Hill, S., Bryant, L., Johnston, L., Georgiou, A., & Balandin, S. (2019). A systematic review of falls in hospital for patients with communication disability: highlighting an invisible population. *Journal of Safety Research, 68*, 89–105.

International Dysphagia Diet Standardisation Initiative. (2016). What is the IDDSI Framework? Retrieved from http://iddsi.org/framework [Accessed 30 April 2019].

Kikuchi, R., Watabe, N., Konno, T., Mishina, N., Sekizawa, K., & Sasaki, H. (1994). High incidence of silent aspiration in elderly patients with community-acquired pneumonia. *American Journal of Respiratory and Critical Care Medicine, 150*(1), 251–253.

Langmore, S., Kenneth, S., & Olsen, N. (1988). Fiberoptic endoscopic examination of swallowing safety: a new procedure. *Dysphagia, 2*(4), 216–219.

Lanspa, M., Peyrani, P., Wiemken, T., Wilson, E., Ramirez, J., & Dean, N. (2015). Characteristics associated with clinician diagnosis of aspiration pneumonia: a descriptive study of afflicted patients and their outcomes. *Journal of Hospital Medicine, 10*(2), 90–96.

Martino, R., Beaton, D., & Diamant, N. E. (2009). Using different perspectives to generate items for a new scale measuring medical outcomes of dysphagia (MOD). *Journal of Clinical Epidemiology, 62*(5), 518–526.

Namasivayam-MacDonald, A., & Shune, S. (2018). The burden of dysphagia on family caregivers of the elderly: a systematic review. *Geriatrics, 3*(2), 30.

O'Keeffe, S. (2018). Use of modified diets to prevent aspiration in oropharyngeal dysphagia: is current practice justified? *BMC Geriatrics, 18*(1), 167.

Stransky, M., Jensen, K., & Morris, M. (2018). Adults with communication disabilities experience poorer health and healthcare outcomes compared to persons without communication disabilities. *Journal of General Internal Medicine, 33*(12), 2147–2155.

Teramoto, S., Fukuchi, Y., Sasaki, H., Sato, K., Sekizawa, K., & Matsuse, T. (2008). High incidence of aspiration pneumonia in community- and hospital-acquired pneumonia in hospitalized patients: a multicenter, prospective study in Japan. *Journal of the American Geriatrics Society, 56*(3), 577–579.

Wirth, R., Dziewas, R., Beck, A., Clave, P., Heppner, H., Langmore, S., Leischker, A., Martino, R., Pluschinski, P., Rösler, A., Shaker, R., Warnecke, T., Sieber, C., Volkert, D., & Hamdy, S. (2016). Oropharyngeal dysphagia in older persons; from pathophysiology to adequate intervention: a review and summary of an international expert meeting. *Clinical Interventions in Aging, 11*, 189–208.

World Health Organization. (2001). *International classification of functioning, disability and health*. ICF. Geneva: World Health Organization.

Wu, W. S., Sung, K., Cheng, T., & Lu, T. (2015). Associations between chronic diseases and choking deaths among older adults in the USA: a cross-sectional study using multiple cause mortality data from 2009 to 2013. *BMJ Open, 5*(11), e009464.

FURTHER READING

Balzer, K. (2000). Drug-induced dysphagia. *International Journal of MS Care, 2*(1), 40–50.

Liu, F., Ghaffur, A., Bains, J., & Hamdy, S. (2016). Acceptability of oral solid medicines in older adults with and without dysphagia: a nested pilot validation questionnaire based observational study. *International Journal of Pharmaceutics, 512*(2), 374–381.

Smithard, D. (2016). Dysphagia: a geriatric giant? *Medical and Clinical Reviews, 2*(1), 5.

Tilda.tcd.ie. (2019). Oral health and wellbeing in older adults in Ireland. Retrieved from https://tilda.tcd.ie/publications/reports/pdf/Report_OralHealth.pdf [Accessed 1 May 2019].

16

Psychological Input

Ciara Preston

LEARNING OBJECTIVES

- Explain the role of clinical psychology in rehabilitation of older people
- Describe how a clinical psychologist assesses problems and constructs treatment plans

- Explain how a clinical psychologist delivers evidence-based psychological therapy interventions to older people

CASE

Judith, a 74-year-old retired teacher, was admitted to an inpatient neurorehabilitation unit after sustaining a traumatic brain injury (TBI) in a car accident. She was disorientated, declined care and shouted at staff, which family described as out of character.

The unit's clinical psychologist interviewed Judith and her family, completed a detailed neuropsychological assessment of her cognitive function, assessed her mood, observed her behaviour in different settings and consulted with staff.

Assessment findings were consistent with a significant decline in Judith's verbal memory for new information and executive function compared to her prior abilities. She experienced significant anxiety, and her shouting was associated with confusion, fear and an inability to regulate her behaviour.

The clinical psychologist designed a rehabilitation programme that included memory-based compensatory strategies, anxiety management techniques, changes to Judith's daily routine and the way staff and family interacted with her and psychoeducation for her family about TBI. The psychologist also provided family therapy, invited the family to a support group and offered staff supervision. Programme evaluation revealed improvements in Judith's orientation, mood and behaviour, in her relatives' understanding of her presentation and reduced familial distress.

WHAT IS A CLINICAL PSYCHOLOGIST?

Clinical psychologists are professionals working in mental and physical healthcare who are trained in the scientific study of human behaviour, thought and emotion and have extensive practical experience in clinical settings. Psychologists help people understand why they think, feel and behave as they do and encourage them to draw on their strengths, to use psychological strategies and to make life changes in order to feel happier, more in control and less distressed.

Clinical psychologists use a variety of methods and instruments to assess people's difficulties and needs. They use this information (by reference to psychological theories, models and research) to help understand and formulate hypotheses about how they arise and are maintained. This is shared with the patient, relatives and others working in the rehabilitation process.

This information, along with assessments of the person's abilities, strengths and other characteristics, is used to develop and deliver evidence-based psychological therapy, treatment or interventions designed to help people resolve or manage psychological difficulties. When delivering therapies, the clinical psychologist may work with the patient individually, in groups and with families. As part of the multidisciplinary team (MDT), clinical psychologists share their assessment findings and treatment recommendations with team members and help develop psychologically informed MDT rehabilitation programmes. Clinical psychologists employ research methods to evaluate the effectiveness of psychological interventions, improve and innovate new interventions and contribute to the scientific understanding of human experience. They also train and supervise members of the MDT in psychological approaches that can inform their practice.

WHY MIGHT OLDER ADULTS NEED THE HELP OF A CLINICAL PSYCHOLOGIST?

As people live longer, increasing needs for care arise in relation to not only physical problems, but also age-related 'neurocognitive', psychological and behavioural problems. These include changes in intellectual and thinking skills (e.g. difficulties with learning and memory), the emergence of uncharacteristic, risky or socially inappropriate behaviour and emotional needs. Mental health conditions may also arise alongside age-related health issues and life stressors, including difficulties in adjusting to an unwelcome diagnosis, loss of function or enforced life changes.

All these issues affect not only the patient but also families, carers and the staff team and can delay achievement of rehabilitation goals and discharge into the community (Joint Commissioning Panel for Mental Health, 2013). It is important, therefore, to offer patients and families help with

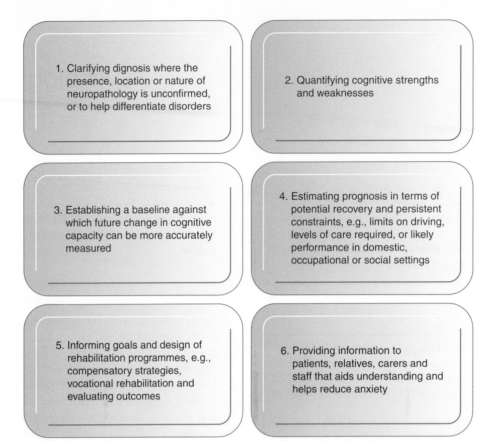

1. Clarifying dignosis where the presence, location or nature of neuropathology is unconfirmed, or to help differentiate disorders

2. Quantifying cognitive strengths and weaknesses

3. Establishing a baseline against which future change in cognitive capacity can be more accurately measured

4. Estimating prognosis in terms of potential recovery and persistent constraints, e.g., limits on driving, levels of care required, or likely performance in domestic, occupational or social settings

5. Informing goals and design of rehabilitation programmes, e.g., compensatory strategies, vocational rehabilitation and evaluating outcomes

6. Providing information to patients, relatives, carers and staff that aids understanding and helps reduce anxiety

FIG. 16.1 The uses of neuropsychological assessment in older adult rehabilitation.

their psychological and emotional needs as part of the holistic 'illness experience' (DoH, 2001; WHO, 2001) and clinical psychologists have an essential role to play in this.

WHAT DOES A CLINICAL PSYCHOLOGIST DO?

The nature and presentation of psychological problems and needs varies across the age range, and clinical psychologists consider work with older adults to be a speciality. When helping older adults understand and manage their difficulties, clinical psychologists therefore draw on specialist knowledge, training and experience to inform the way they assess and 'formulate' problems and needs, and design, plan and evaluate treatment and rehabilitation interventions.

Examples are considered below in relation to cognitive function, behaviour and emotional experience.

ASSESSMENT OF COGNITIVE FUNCTION

As people age, their functional capabilities change. Some reduction in the efficiency of cognitive function and thinking skills (e.g. problem solving, mental flexibility, memory) is common and normal. However, this can happen earlier than expected or to a more severe degree than that associated with typical ageing, e.g. in progressive conditions such as dementia, or sudden damage through acquired brain injury.

Clinical psychologists seek to accurately measure these changes and to understand the relationship between brain function and behaviour, using a wide range of specialised neuropsychological tests and observational and measurement techniques that require specific training and qualifications for their selection, administration and interpretation (Hebben & Milberg, 2009; Lezak et al., 2012) (see Fig. 16.1). The functions assessed using standardised tests include attention, intelligence, memory, executive function, social cognition, aphasia and language, motor skills and visuospatial function (Lezak et al., 2012). The psychologist ensures that the measures used are valid and reliable and that their findings are carefully interpreted taking account of information obtained by interview and observation, including that concerning pre-illness/injury function and mood.

Clinical psychologists may also undertake 'mental capacity assessments' to help establish whether, in the light of changed cognitive function, an older adult has the 'mental capacity' to make important decisions about, for example, where to live on discharge, or whether to consent to intervention (see Chapter 20 Brain Health and Mental Capacity).

COGNITIVE INTERVENTIONS

On the basis of their assessment findings, clinical psychologists then agree goals and targets for change with the patient, their families and other professionals, and design interventions to help achieve them. Attempts may, for example, be made to minimise the impact of cognitive change and promote optimum function through 'cognitive rehabilitation' programmes that commonly include compensatory strategies and environmental modifications. When working with memory difficulties, for example, these may include mnemonic, spaced retrieval and errorless learning techniques; the provision of written information normalising everyday forgetfulness; environmental adaptations (e.g. electrical timers, information boards) to prompt, remind and direct; and external memory aids such as diaries, computers, online assistants, digital recorders and mobile phones. In progressive conditions, particularly where cognitive decline constrains the use of internal memory strategies, clinical psychologists may also support interventions aiming to preserve cognitive function and reduce decline, including cognitive stimulation therapy (CST; Spector et al., 2001).

ASSESSMENT OF BEHAVIOUR

Changes in cognitive function can make it difficult for older adults to adapt to changing circumstances and may occasion behaviour that is inappropriate to the setting. Clinical psychologists are often contacted by staff or family members concerned about behaviour that is uncharacteristic and difficult to understand and manage, particularly when it poses risks to themselves or others. The psychologist will commonly complete behavioural assessments (for example, observing the precursors of the behaviour, the behaviour itself and its consequences), to help understand why it occurs and to inform the design of interventions to promote self-control and socially adaptive appropriate behaviour.

BEHAVIOURAL INTERVENTIONS

Understanding the cognitive, emotional and environmental factors that cause and maintain 'inappropriate' and 'uncharacteristic' behaviour can reduce distress, enhance empathy and tolerance of others when it occurs and promote a more constructive approach to its management. The clinical psychologist shares their hypotheses and understanding with staff and relatives, and recommends behavioural interventions and strategies. These can be used to reduce behaviour that is challenging to manage, and encourage socially appropriate alternatives (drawing on theories of learning, the way the environment and patterns of interaction can influence behaviour and other psychological models). The psychologist may also work individually with the patient, for example, using cognitive behavioural therapy techniques, to promote the self-control of unhelpful behaviour.

ASSESSMENT OF EMOTION, DISTRESS AND/OR MENTAL HEALTH DIFFICULTY

Adjusting to health changes can be challenging. For some, it is a temporary struggle, but for others it may trigger persistent psychological reactions that are distressing and disrupt

participation in meaningful activity. Mental health difficulties in older adult settings may include anxiety, depression, post-traumatic stress disorder (PTSD), obsessive compulsive disorder (OCD), psychosis and adjustment disorder, as well as internalised stigma associated with ageing and disability. Adjustment difficulties can also arise in relation to loss of occupation, reduced engagement in recreational activity, inability to drive and associated loss of independence, as well as personal mortality and challenges to religious beliefs. Pre-existing mental health difficulties can also be exacerbated by health decline and changes in cognitive function.

Psychological assessment of these experiences typically includes a detailed interview with the individual, self-completed rating questionnaires, direct observation and where appropriate, ratings completed by others who know the older adult well. In rehabilitation settings, assessment often involves observations of multidisciplinary sessions, for example, when anxiety associated with falling constrains progress in physiotherapy.

PSYCHOLOGICAL THERAPY INTERVENTIONS

Psychological therapy can take varied forms, dependent on the expertise of the clinical psychologist, type of presenting issues and the individual's characteristics. Typical models of therapy used include Cognitive Behavioural Therapy, Acceptance and Commitment Therapy, Compassion Focused Therapy, Mindfulness, Psychoanalysis, Behaviour Therapy and Systemic Therapy, with models such as Emotionally Focused Therapy being increasingly adapted to older adult rehabilitation.

Therapy is often individual, but can take the form of couples work and family therapy (including adult and child relatives). Clinical psychologists also provide group therapy and psychoeducational groups, where typically 5–10 people with a shared experience learn from the clinical psychologist and each other. They may also provide carer/relative support on an individual or group basis to promote understanding and adjustment to cognitive and behavioural changes in their loved one.

Hypotheses as to how and why a patient may be experiencing emotional difficulties can be helpfully shared with staff teams. Increasing empathy, understanding, compassion and communicating ways of supporting older adults in the emotional aspects of their rehabilitation are important in attaining rehabilitation goals.

EVALUATION, RESEARCH AND SERVICE DEVELOPMENT

The evaluation and governance of their activities, innovative research and service development are core elements of a clinical psychologist's role. Patients, relatives, carers or staff team members may be approached to take part in psychological research studies or evaluations of interventions, treatments or services they have used or worked for.

HOW DOES A CLINICAL PSYCHOLOGIST SUPPORT THE HEALTHCARE TEAM?

Clinical psychologists spend much of their time working 'indirectly' within older adult rehabilitation settings via the provision of consultation, teaching, training and supervision to staff from other disciplines. They have a significant role in consultation when highly complex ethical issues arise. It is common for patients to be referred for risk assessments when they have expressed suicidal ideation, are declining life-sustaining treatment or nutrition, or when staff have concerns about the safety of vulnerable individuals. Clinical psychologists work closely with colleagues in safeguarding, social, legal and housing services, the police, and third sector agencies such as charities in aiding teams to support patients.

SUMMARY POINTS

- Clinical psychology helps to reduce psychological distress and support achievement of rehabilitation goals, while continually learning about the human experience
- The role of the clinical psychologist in the rehabilitation of older adults is broad
- Clinical psychologists work with individuals, families and MDTs

MCQs

Q.1 Which of the following describes the role of a clinical psychologist?
  a. A physician working in geriatric medicine
  b. A healthcare professional providing psychological assessment and interventions
  c. A doctor who prescribes medication for mental health difficulties
  d. A specialist in physiotherapy

Q.2 Which of the following is a psychological model of therapy used by clinical psychologists?
  a. Cognitive Behavioural Therapy
  b. Acceptance and Commitment Therapy
  c. Compassion Focused Therapy
  d. All of the above

REFERENCES

Department of Health, HM Government. (2001). National service framework for older people. Retrieved from: www.dh.gov.uk.

Hebben, N., & Milberg, W. (2009). *Essentials of neuropsychological assessment.* New Jersey: John Wiley & Sons.

Joint Commissioning Panel for Mental Health. (2013). Guidance for commissioners of older people's mental health services. Retrieved from: www.jcpmh.info.

Lezak, M. D., Howieson, D. B., Bigler, E. D., & Tranel, D. (2012). *Neuropsychological assessment* (5th ed.). New York: Oxford University Press.

Spector, A., Orrell, M., Davies, S., & Woods, B. (2001). Can reality orientation be rehabilitated? Development and piloting of an evidence-based programme of cognition-based therapies for people with dementia. *Neuropsychological Rehabilitation, 11,* 377–397.

World Health Organisation. (2001). *International classification of functioning, disability and health.* Geneva: World Health Organisation.

FURTHER READING

Department of Constitutional Affairs. (2007). Mental Capacity Act, 2005. Code of Practice. London, TSO. Retrieved from: https://www.bps.org.uk/; http://www.psige.org/.

Laidlaw, K. (2014). *CBT for older people: an introduction* (1st ed.). London: SAGE Publications Ltd.

Llewelyn, S., & Murphy, D. J. (2014). *What is clinical psychology?* (5th ed.). New York: Oxford University Press.

McGrath, J. C. (2007). *Ethical practice in brain injury rehabilitation.* Oxford: Oxford University Press.

Newby, G., Coetzer, R., Daisley, A., & Weatherhead, S. (2013). *Practical neuropsychological rehabilitation in acquired brain injury: a guide for working clinicians (the brain injuries series)* (1st ed.). London: Karnac Books.

Wilson, B., & Betteridge, S. (2019). *Essentials of neuropsychological rehabilitation* (1st ed.). New York: The Guilford Press.

Wilson, B., Winegardner, J., van Heugten, C., & Ownsworth, T. (2017). *Neuropsychological rehabilitation: the international handbook* (1st ed.). London: Routledge.

Woods, R. T., & Clare, L. (2015). *Handbook of the clinical psychology of ageing* (2nd ed.). Chichester: Wiley-Blackwell.

Supporting Rehabilitation

17

Nutrition and Hydration

Naomi Bates & Laura Masterson

LEARNING OBJECTIVES

- Describe the role of nutrition and hydration in rehabilitation of the older person
- Explain how the dietitian can help the rehabilitation process
- Explain how to identify malnutrition and sarcopenia and the impact they can have on rehabilitation
- List potential causes of malnutrition and possible interventions

CASE

John is an 80-year-old man, who is widowed but lives independently at home on his own with good family support and home help daily. He is admitted to intensive care following a fall at home and diagnosed with a subdural haematoma (bleeding in the lining of the brain). He started nasogastric (NG) tube feeding because he was unconscious and couldn't eat. John's weight was approximately 72 kg on his admission to hospital.

During week 1 to 8, John was confused and agitated because of his head injury (a condition called delirium), and often pulled out the feeding tube during these episodes. A nasal bridle was placed on the feeding tube to secure it in order to try and prevent this, and he also needed close supervision on the ward. His swallow was impaired (dysphagia) meaning that food and fluids (any texture/grade) went into his lungs instead of his food pipe (oesophagus) causing recurrent aspiration pneumonia.

Weeks 8–16 of admission: John had surgery to reduce the pressure on his brain but he remained confused and continued to pull out his feeding tube regularly, and so lost weight (approximately 9 kg or 12% weight loss). Despite regular assessment of his swallow function by the speech and language therapist, John still needed tube feeding. No physiotherapy or occupational therapy gains were achieved during this period as he wasn't strong enough to participate in these sessions.

Week 16: as John continued to pull out his NG feeding tube, a more permanent feeding tube was inserted into his abdomen to meet his nutritional needs and to prevent repeated NG tube placements. By receiving adequate nutrition and hydration via this new feeding tube (RIG, radiologically inserted gastrostomy), John's weight gradually increased to 66 kg (3 kg/5% weight gain) over 8 weeks, and his strength and mobility improved. His delirium also gradually resolved.

Eight weeks after the RIG was placed (week 23 of admission), John was making good progress with his rehabilitation with occupational therapy, physiotherapy, and speech and language therapy. His strength, weight, swallow and cognitive function continued to improve. He started a soft diet (level 6) and thickened fluids (level 2). As his oral intake improved, his nutrition provision via the RIG gradually decreased.

Thirty-two weeks after admission, John was transferred to a rehabilitation facility with the aim of discharge home. At this time John was meeting his full requirements for nutrition and hydration orally and no longer needed additional nutrition through his feeding tube.

This case study highlights the importance of adequate nutrition and hydration and multidisciplinary team working in rehabilitation of the older person.

MALNUTRITION

Malnutrition is often a consequence of acute and/or chronic disease. Anorexia (poor appetite) of ageing when combined with catabolic disease (loss of muscle and fat tissue due to disease) rapidly leads to malnutrition. Malnutrition has clinical consequences such as muscle wasting, increased risk of infection, predisposition to falls and pressure ulcers, delayed recovery and reduced quality of life. It triples mortality in older patients in hospital and after discharge and costs more than £7.3 billion annually in the UK.

An older person could be considered at risk of malnutrition if their dietary intake is 50% less than their requirements for more than 3 days or if the patient has increased requirements (e.g. acute disease identified by raised inflammatory markers/C reactive protein) or reduced intake due to neuropsychology problems, chewing or swallowing problems (Volkert et al., 2018).

Sarcopenia, the loss of skeletal muscle mass and strength in combination with a decline in physical activity functionality and performance, affects up to 17.5% of older persons (Murphy et al., 2019). This excess loss of muscle and strength

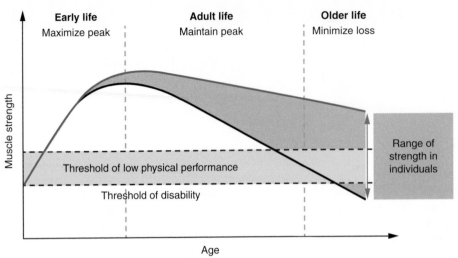

FIG. 17.1   Changes in muscle strength with age (From Cruz-Jentoft et al., 2019, with permission).

results in physical impairment, frailty, disability and dependence on others (Volkert et al., 2018). Fig. 17.1 illustrates the decline in muscle strength as the body ages. While lifestyle factors and genetics can increase the loss of muscle mass, nutrition and exercise can slow or potentially reverse this process (Cruz-Jentoft et al., 2019).

Obesity affects 18%–30% of the world population aged 65 years and older (Volkert et al., 2018). It often masks weight loss and sarcopenia. Regular nutrition screening therefore in all patients, not just those who visibly look depleted, should be part of routine care for the older person, in all settings. For more information on how sarcopenia or obesity can affect rehabilitation, see Chapter 34 Weight Loss and Overweight.

Routine nutrition screening is recommended for all older persons by trained health professionals using a validated screening tool (e.g. the Nutrition Screening Tool, the Mini Nutritional Assessment and the Malnutrition Universal Screening Tool). This will then identify if the person needs referral to a dietitian for nutritional advice and support.

DEHYDRATION

As well as malnutrition, dehydration is common in the older person. Approximately 30% of older adults with frailty and those in care are dehydrated (Volkert et al., 2018). The consequences of dehydration are reduced mental function, low blood pressure, dizziness, impaired kidney function and increased risk of falling. For adequate hydration the older person should aim to have 30 ml/kg daily with extra if they have increased losses of fluid e.g. temperature (pyrexia) or diarrhoea.

ROLE OF THE DIETITIAN

Dietitians are responsible for the nutritional management of individuals who are referred to them. Nutrition impacts on many aspects of patient health and well-being. Dietitians work in consultation with other healthcare professionals to ensure that the patient receives appropriate advice in line with their holistic treatment. A patient's dietary needs should be managed as part of their rehabilitation with the promotion of healthy eating habits.

ARTIFICIAL FEEDING ('TUBE FEEDING')

Diet is an important part of our daily lives, and having a meal is important socially and psychologically. However, there are times where feeding by mouth is not possible. Artificial feeding (via a feeding tube) may then be considered, but only if it is likely to improve the patient's outcome and quality of life. This is where links with the multidisciplinary team and goal setting are essential.

Artificial feeding is either enteral or parenteral. Enteral tube feeding includes:

1. NG tube: inserted through the nose, down the back of the throat into the oesophagus and into the stomach. It is primarily used for short-term tube feeding. It can be uncomfortable, and patients with delirium may not tolerate it well. They can fall out relatively easily and are sometimes secured to help with this; however, this can cause injury if the tube is pulled on.

2. Gastrostomy: either a percutaneous endoscopic gastrostomy (PEG tube) or a RIG tube. PEG insertion needs a procedure, usually under sedation, to insert a tube through the oesophagus into the stomach that exits directly through the abdominal wall. This carries more risk than an NG tube insertion, but they can be kept in long term. They are generally better tolerated in patients who have delirium, but again can fall out or be pulled out. Reinsertion is relatively easy. Because there is a hole in the skin where a PEG tube is inserted, there can be a risk of infection.

A RIG is similar to a PEG but inserted using x-ray guidance, and sedation is not needed.

Parenteral tube feeding bypasses the gut and provides nutrients directly to the blood via a large vein. It should only be used when other feeding routes are not possible, for example when the gut is not working. Each patient needs to be individually assessed by a dietitian to ensure the benefit outweighs the risks.

The patient's wishes are always a priority, and decisions regarding artificial feeding should be made with them and if appropriate their family or carer.

HOW DIETITIANS CAN SUPPORT PATIENTS IN REHABILITATION

Dietitians undertake a nutritional assessment using an accredited Nutrition Care Process (Field & Hand, 2015) which includes Nutrition Focused Physical Findings (White et al., 2012). This enables the dietitian to categorise the level of malnutrition and set a nutrition care plan in line with its cause. Table 17.1 lists some potential causes of malnutrition and interventions that may be used.

It is useful if carers and family are involved in the patient's care. Linking with them helps to empower their involvement in the patient's rehabilitation. Food is part of daily life and should be a social experience. Family eating with the patient and giving assistance at mealtimes has been shown to increase patient dietary intake. It also allows the carer to help with meal choices and identify meal preferences with the patient where needed.

FOOD FORTIFICATION

If you have lost weight and are experiencing malnutrition adding extra energy and protein to your diet may help. Table 17.2 shows some ways to do this.

The importance of healthy nutrition cannot be understated, especially in the rehabilitation setting. The Resources section at the end of this book provides healthy eating advice, and guidance on important nutrients. These can help to support the rehabilitation process.

TABLE 17.1 Potential causes of malnutrition and reasonable interventions (amended from Volkert et al., 2018).

CAUSES OF MALNUTRITION	INTERVENTIONS
Chewing Problems	Oral care, dental treatment, texture modification
Swallowing Problems (dysphagia)	Speech and language therapist assessment for texture modification
Impaired Upper Body Function/Restricted Mobility/Immobility	Physiotherapy (resistance training group exercises), occupational therapy, assistance with meals, shopping and providing cooking aids and finger foods
Cognitive Impairment	Supervision and assistance with meals (includes prompting or contrasting coloured crockery). Shopping and cooking aids. Eating in a dining room instead of at the bedside in an institution
Depressive Mood, Depression	Adequate medical treatment, eating with others/shared meals. Pleasant environment, group therapy, occupational therapy
Loneliness, Social Isolation	Eating with others
Poverty	Social programmes
Acute Disease, Chronic Pain	Medical treatment
Restricted Diets	Education

TABLE 17.2 Fortification of food.

FOOD	HOW TO FORTIFY
Potatoes and Vegetables	Add melted cheese, cream cheese, butter or cream
Soup and Sauces	Make up with full fat milk, add cheese or cream
Milk	Use in sauces and drinks. See recipe for high protein milk
Bread	Add plenty of full fat butter, margarine, mayonnaise, honey, cream cheese, jam, peanut butter
Dessert	Add cream, evaporated milk, condensed milk, sugar, jam or honey
Breakfast Cereals	Add yoghurt, cream, high protein milk, honey, dried fruit, sugar
Fruit	Chop fruit and eat with full fat yoghurt, cream, custard, ice cream Add to milkshake

SUMMARY POINTS

- Nutritional assessment and regular screening are important parts of the rehabilitation process for older people
- If nutritional advice or input is needed, referral should be made to a registered dietitian
- A healthy balanced diet with regular exercise is important to maintain muscle strength

MCQs

Q.1 The role of the dietitian in rehabilitation of older people is to:
- **a.** Be responsible for the nutritional management of patients referred to them
- **b.** Ensure that all patients are considered for tube feeding
- **c.** Provide calcium supplements for everyone over 65 years of age
- **d.** Discourage patients from fortifying their food

Q.2 Malnutrition is relevant to individuals who
- **a.** Are underweight, have a poor or reduced dietary intake due to appetite or other causes e.g. impaired swallow
- **b.** Have increased dietary requirements due to acute illness
- **c.** Are overweight with significant unintentional weight loss
- **d.** All of the above

Q.3 Artificial feeding is not appropriate in
- **a.** Patients who are unable to meet their nutritional requirements orally
- **b.** Patients who are undergoing active rehabilitation
- **c.** Malnourished patients for whom artificial feeding would not improve their medical outcome or quality of life, e.g. palliative or in end stage of their disease
- **d.** Malnourished patients who have delirium

REFERENCES

Bennett, A. (2016). *Good nutrition for the older Person.* MINDI. Retrieved from: https://www.indi.ie/healthy-ageing/509-good-nutrition-for-the-older-person.html (Accessed 28 May 2020).

Cruz-Jentoft, A. J., Bahat, G., Bauer, J., Boirie, Y., Bruyère, O., Cederholm, T., Cooper, C., Landi, F., Rolland, Y., Sayer, A. A., Schneider, S. M., Sieber, C. C., Topinkova, E., Vandewoude, M., Visser, M., & Zamboni, M. Writing Group for the European Working Group on Sarcopenia in Older People 2 (EWGSOP2), and the Extended Group for EWGSOP2. (2019). Sarcopenia: revised European consensus on definition and diagnosis. *Age Ageing, 48*(1), 16–31.

Field, L. B., & Hand, R. K. (2015). Differentiating malnutrition screening and assessment: a nutrition care process perspective. *Journal of the Academy of Nutrition and Dietetics, 115*(5), 824–828.

Murphy, C. H., McMorrow, A. M., Flanagan, E. M., Cummins, H., McCarthy, S. N., McGowan, M. J., Rafferty, S., Egan, B., De Vito, G., Corish, C. A., Roche, H. M., et al. (2019). SUN-LB651: prevalence of sarcopenia in community-dwelling older adults in Ireland: comparison of EWGSOP1 and EWGSOP2 definitions. *Clinical Nutrition, 38*, S301.

Volkert, D., Beck, A. M., Cederholm, T., Cruz-Jentoft, A., Goisser, S., Hooper, L., Kiesswetter, E., Maggio, M., Raynaud-Simon, A., Sieber, C. C., Sobotka, L., van Asselt, D., Wirth, R., & Bischoff, S. C. (2018). ESPEN guideline on clinical nutrition and hydration in geriatrics. *Clinical Nutrition, 38*, 10–47.

White, J.V., Guenter, P., Jensen, G., Malone, A., & Schofield, M. Academy Malnutrition Work Group; A.S.P.E.N. Malnutrition Task Force; A.S.P.E.N. Board of Directors (2012). Consensus statement of the Academy of Nutrition and Dietetics/American Society for Parenteral and Enteral Nutrition: Characteristics recommended for the identification and documentation of adult malnutrition (undernutrition). *Journal of the Academy of Nutrition and Dietetics, 112*(5), 730-738.

FURTHER READING

Litchford. M. D. (2012). *Nutrition focused physical assessment: making clinical connections* (pp. 21-57, 138-141,173-200). Greensboro, NC: CASE Software & Books.

18

Social Work

Carol de Wilde

LEARNING OBJECTIVES

- Explain what social work is
- Describe the role of the social worker in rehabilitation of the older person
- Explain the social work assessment process
- Outline some possible social work interventions

CASE

Paul is a 69-year-old man who has had a stroke. He has been left with limited mobility on his left side and some cognitive impairment. Paul lives in a two-storey house with his wife Carmel. They have three adult children: two live locally but have their own young families and one lives abroad. In the house, the bedroom and bathroom are upstairs.

Paul was previously independent with all activities of daily living, liked to keep active and enjoyed socialising with Carmel and with friends. Carmel is in good health. Rehabilitation potential is unclear.

WHAT IS SOCIAL WORK?

Social work is a profession that aims to enhance social functioning and overall well-being. It also promotes social justice by challenging discrimination and respecting diversity, cultures and values of others. The British Association of Social Workers (2017) states 'Social workers work with individuals and families to help improve outcomes in their lives. This may be helping protect vulnerable people from harm or abuse or supporting people to live independently … act as advocates … often work in multidisciplinary teams'. Social workers take a holistic view of people and this influences the range of interventions available to the profession.

Social workers can work in a variety of settings, including hospitals, community care, rehabilitation centres, child and adolescent services, adult safeguarding and mental health. The types of interventions that can be provided include counselling and family work, planning discharge from hospital, group work, crisis intervention, problem solving, advocacy and community work.

SOCIAL WORK IN REHABILITATION

Social workers can work with clients in rehabilitation in hospital, rehab centre or community settings. This work is hugely integrated with the full multidisciplinary team (MDT). The social worker often takes up a coordination role within the team to facilitate communication and plan for discharge.

There are many interventions that can be provided by the social worker in a rehabilitation setting. A comprehensive psychosocial assessment will be able to highlight which interventions are needed and appropriate. For this type of assessment, information can be gathered from the patient, their medical chart, the family and any other relevant people. The information should indicate the patient's age, why they were admitted to the hospital, their systemic supports in the nuclear family, extended family and the wider community, current abilities, environmental structures at home, strengths, goals and hopes for the future. The assessment should conclude with an agreed plan of action. This could be to contact family for a collateral history (their perspective on all relevant issues), to provide emotional support, to refer to community services or to organise a care planning meeting or to commence discharge planning amongst other things. In rehabilitation settings the social work role should include provision of emotional support to the patient and the family regarding what has changed for them and how this has impacted on them, their relationships and their wishes. The social worker should also encourage advance care planning and support around this. The social work role involves working collaboratively with the patient and family to maximise quality of life while maintaining the integrity of the individual and advocating for their wishes.

SAFEGUARDING

A social worker's role always includes the safeguarding of vulnerable adults and children. There are a number of types of abuse that one must be aware of and look out for (see example in Fig. 18.1). They are physical abuse (slapping, hitting, pushing, restraint), sexual abuse (sexual acts to which the person has not consented or could not consent), psychological abuse (threats of harm, humiliation, blaming, isolation, no access to services), financial abuse (theft, fraud, exploitation, pressure around wills), institutional abuse (poor care standards, rigid routines, inadequate responses to complex needs), neglect (ignoring

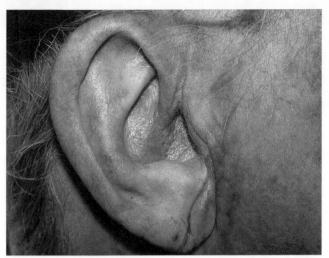

FIG. 18.1 Bruising on the ear, as seen in this abused older woman, is unusual location for accidental bruising. (From Palmer M, Brodell RT, Mostow EN. Elder abuse: dermatologic clues and critical solutions. *J Am Acad Dermatol.* 2013; 68(2):e37–42, with permission.)

needs, failure to provide access to services, withholding necessities of life like warmth or medication) and discriminatory abuse (ageism, racism, sexism). The abuse can sometimes be very nuanced and hard to pinpoint so it is important to have a local process for identifying, reporting and preventing elder abuse (see Fig. 18.2). If in doubt it is best to discuss with the social worker on the team, who will help to put in place a plan. Safeguarding can be an issue within rehabilitation particularly when there is a cognitive impairment or the person was previously vulnerable. Safeguarding also crosses settings, e.g. in an older adults' rehabilitation unit it may be possible to identify a safeguarding issue for children who are being looked after by an older person with cognitive impairment.

CARE PLANNING MEETINGS

Care Planning Meetings are covered in depth in Chapter 67. If used correctly and appropriately, they can provide a voice for the patient within a system that can be overwhelming and distressing. They can prevent the patient being an 'afterthought' as happens at times when families take the lead in decision making and the patient is left behind. The social worker must find the voice of the patient and try to encourage the patient to use this voice. This can be written down or communicated in an appropriate manner if the patient's actual voice is not able to verbalise their wishes. If necessary the social worker may ask the speech and language therapist to assist with communication techniques to facilitate effective communication. At times the social worker must really advocate for the patient in these meetings. Families most often want what they think is best for their loved one but if the patient has mental capacity to make a decision, it is important that this is facilitated as far as practicable. It can also happen that the MDT can get caught in collusion with the family regarding 'what is best for the patient'. The social worker must also advocate for the patient with their colleagues.

SUPPORT FOR ADJUSTMENT

Social workers can take a lead role in working with a patient and their family to readjust to the new norm. In rehabilitation work, roles often need to be redefined as the old roles are no longer relevant or possible due to disability. The social worker can explore the impact of physical changes, emotional changes and relationship changes. Depression and anxiety are not uncommon in the rehabilitation setting. The social worker can work with the patient around their feelings and emotions and look at what can be done to help. In individual work with the patient, the social worker should discuss the impact of physical limitations on physical intimacy in the relationship – what was the norm and what will be the likely impact in the future. Being open and able to initiate this conversation is very important as it is something that often gets forgotten. A disability, e.g. stroke, can profoundly impact how sexuality is experienced by the patient and their partner, physically and emotionally. Each part of the couple can have concerns or questions so initiating this discussion can help them both. The person may find that for example they now have little interest in sex, or their sex drive has increased or they are concerned about their new physical appearance. The partner could be concerned that they will hurt the person or that their needs may not be met.

Cognitive changes must also be explored by the social worker. What is the impact on the person, their family, their lives? What can be done to assist and plan for the future? If rehabilitation is likely to only cause limited improvements to the person's functioning, the social worker can help to look at what resources in the community will be necessary to enable the individual to maintain their dignity and remain as independent as possible.

PLANNING FOR THE FUTURE

Social workers should always discuss future care planning with their clients. Anyone over the age of 50 years should have a look at planning for their future, deciding what their wishes would be in different circumstances, discussing with loved ones and documenting your wishes. Unfortunately, this is often not the case and it is a stroke or other illness that forces people to eventually look at these issues. The social worker can provide information on future care planning and may be able to recommend some documentation that can assist people in having these conversations and writing down what their wishes are. There are helpful documents available in most countries that cover a number of items, including emergency contact information, care preferences, spiritual/religious beliefs, advance healthcare directives, legal and financial information, and wishes around death and dying. See Chapter 74 Advance Care Planning for more information.

More immediately the patient may need assistance with referral to community services for help at home while in the process of rehabilitation, or indefinitely. The social worker can also provide information and facilitate discussion regarding care homes and how the process works with the patient and their families. The social worker must always keep in mind that the patient is their client and they should advocate

Subjective
The following statements may be a red flag indicating further investigation:

Abandonment:	I am all alone. I have no one who cares for me.
Physical abuse:	They hurt me. Please don't tell anyone about the injury. Stories that do not correlate to the type of injury and/or physical signs and symptoms.
Exploitation:	I don't know what happened to my money. I can no longer afford ...I have misplaced my jewelry or my money. I don't understand what happened.
Neglect:	My caregiver is so busy, it is not their fault that they don't have time to feed me, get my medications, or change my diaper.
Psychological Abuse:	I don't want to complain, my son/daughter yell if I complain. Please don't make fun of me.
Self-Neglect:	I'm fine, I don't feel like taking my medications or taking care of myself. I'd don't need to bathe much, I'm clean enough as I am.

Objective

Physical manifestation	Psychological manifestation	Sociological/environment manifestation
• Bruising in various stages of healing • Contractures • Falls • Dehydration • Fractures in various stages of healing • Lacerations • Diarrhoea • Faecal impaction • Malnutrition • Inappropriate use of medications • Poor hygiene • Sexual abuse signs • Pressure ulcers • Urine burns • Delirium	Assess for caregiver and patient • Anxiety • Anxiety toward CG* • Anger by patient toward CG* • Depression • Fearfulness • Impatience toward CG • Irritability toward CG • Nervousness • Nervousness toward CG • CG impatience toward patient • CG irritability toward patient	• Recent inability to pay bills • Left alone in emergency room • Nonadherence to medication • Repeated ER admissions • Repeated hospital admissions

*CG=Caregiver

Assessment	Plan
Patient in immediate danger from abuse or neglect	• Refer to emergency services and adult protective services (APS)
Unexplained or inconsistent explanations for physical findings, suspicious for mistreatment	• Refer to APS and emergency services if recent sexual abuse to gather forensic evidence
Diminished decision-making ability (risk of self-neglect)	• Utilize health care proxy, durable power of attorney if available • Refer to APS if no family or friend available • Contact primary care provider or referral to evaluate cognitive impairment
Not suspicious of elder abuse or neglect	• Complete routine medical exam • Refer to other health care providers if needed

FIG. 18.2 Subjective, objective, assessment, and plan (SOAP) process for identifying, reporting and preventing elder abuse. (From Burnett J, Achenbaum WA, Murphy KP. Prevention and early identification of elder abuse. *Clin Geriatr Med.* 2014; 30(4):743–59, with permission.)

for their wishes. The social worker often takes a central role in discharge planning and this process is discussed further in Chapter 66 Discharge Planning: When, How and Who?

Case: Assessment

The social worker met with Paul for a psychosocial assessment after stroke. Prior to the meeting, the social worker gathered information from the MDT and the medical chart. While Paul has some cognitive impairment, he still has capacity to make decisions regarding his care and discharge decisions. Therefore the initial conversation centred on clearly explaining the role of the social worker and asking Paul for consent to complete the assessment. The social worker used clear and explicit language and conducted the assessment in a quiet room without visual or auditory distractions.

Paul was asked about his previous level of functioning, confirmed his environment at home (as documented by the occupational therapist), and gave details on his wife Carmel and their adult children. As it was still unclear what the lasting impact of the stroke would be on Paul physically and cognitively, the social worker allowed space and time and asked open-ended questions to enable Paul to talk about the emotional impact of the stroke on him and any concerns that he had. Due to his previous independent level of function, he was really invested in the rehabilitation programme. He was concerned as he felt Carmel had been distant since the stroke and it was troubling him. He had tried to talk to her about it but she had stated she was ok. He consented for the social worker to contact Carmel. During the assessment Paul became tearful but was unable to name why. The social worker actively listened and remained with Paul during his tears. She did not try to make him feel better or soothe him; she let him think and speak as much as he was able and willing. This was important to establish a relationship of trust and open communication that would influence their future interactions.

When the social worker spoke to Carmel she stated that she was distressed. She described how hard it was to see Paul incapacitated when she was used to him being active and caring and 'in charge'. When the social worker asked her to describe more about this, Carmel stated she felt lonely. The social worker then asked tactfully about Paul and Carmel's previous intimacy, both physical and emotional. It became clear that Paul and Carmel were very tactile and liked to hold hands and embrace a lot while in their home but this had not been 'the done thing' outside of the home. This connection was now missing. The social worker asked Carmel to reflect on this and they would discuss it at their next meeting.

Case: Intervention

The social worker worked with Paul around the loss of independence that was impacting on him emotionally and psychologically. They looked at Paul's previous coping mechanisms and how they could be applied to this situation. They discussed discharge options; Paul's wish was to return home as soon as possible and he would accept home support services if they were necessary. On the social worker's next meeting with Carmel they reflected on the previous discussion on loneliness and how it was impacting on Carmel and her relationship with Paul. They discussed how she and Paul could connect on their previous level of holding hands and embracing in the new environment of the hospital. Carmel felt uncomfortable as she hadn't discussed this with Paul and didn't want to put any pressure on him. The social worker offered to facilitate this conversation. The social worker then worked with Paul and Carmel around the impact the stroke had on their lives in general and some more specifics. They were both able to say they missed feeling close and connected, and that the only reason they weren't more affectionate outside the home was because they were not used to it. They made a task-centred plan to look at incorporating holding hands, being close to each other and being able to sit together to watch television in the evenings while in hospital. The outcome of this was that their relationship resumed fully and communication between them improved.

Regarding discharge planning, Carmel was initially reluctant regarding the referral to community services. She did not like the idea of strangers coming into the house to assist Paul with getting up in the morning and showering. During an intervention with the social worker this was explored and Paul was encouraged to voice his wishes that he could have help to remain as independent as possible. Carmel reluctantly agreed for the referral to be made and to trial community services coming into the home. The social worker made the referral to community services with information gathered from the full MDT regarding Paul's current care needs.

SUMMARY POINTS

- Social work is a wide-ranging profession that works in many locations, including rehabilitation
- Social workers often work as part of a multidisciplinary team and coordinate Care Planning Meetings or discharge planning
- Social workers work with people on an emotional level and often use strengths- and systems-based social work theories
- Social workers link with community services to ensure the patient has what is necessary for discharge
- Social workers are trained to facilitate communication between people and to support these interventions

MCQs

Q.1 Which one of the following is true about social work?
- a. It aims to enhance social functioning and overall well-being
- b. It promotes social justice by challenging discrimination
- c. It helps protect vulnerable people from harm
- d. It works in a variety of different settings
- e. All of the above

Q.2 Which one of the following is true about the social work assessment process?
- a. Interaction with the family is not necessary
- b. Assessments are generally open ended without a particular plan
- c. Emotional needs are not part of the assessment
- d. A comprehensive psychosocial assessment is performed
- e. Older people only need brief assessments

REFERENCES

British Association of Social Workers. (2017). Social work careers. Retrieved from https://www.basw.co.uk/social-work-careers/ (Accessed 23 September 2019).

FURTHER READING

AgeUK. 2019. Factsheet 78 Safeguarding older people from abuse and neglect. Retrieved from https://www.ageuk.org.uk/ globalassets/age-uk/documents/factsheets/fs78_safeguarding_older_people_from_abuse_fcs.pdf (Accessed 23 September 2019).

19

The Patient Story

Kit Byatt

LEARNING OBJECTIVES

- Explain why knowing the patient as an individual is important
- Explain what can inhibit or thwart the therapeutic relationship supporting this
- Identify a tool you can use to get to know the patient better in depth ('This is me')

- Identify a tool to check cognitive function (IQCODE)
- Identify a tool to encourage the patient to participate actively in decision-making (BRAN)

This chapter takes a different approach from others. It considers the idea that knowing our patients as individuals is really important. Rather than looking at scientific evidence, the chapter is written based on many years of personal experience of caring for older people. It is primarily written for health professionals, but anyone who has contact with patients should find the approach provided to be beneficial. I plan to focus on two key aspects central to your relationship with your patient. The first is helping you to know your patient better. The second is what you can do to help the continuity of care in their rehabilitation. Finally, I give some practical tips.

THE INDIVIDUAL

I want you to consider these thumbnail sketches of two interestingly contrasting personae. Both are widows in their early eighties, living in the same quiet cul-de-sac in a leafy suburb.

Mrs A

A retired teacher, then councillor of 15 years, whose view was that if something needed to be done, just get on and do it. She organised family holidays abroad, and latterly trips with her husband all over the UK.

Membership of several local voluntary groups and governorship of a local school bore testimony to her social commitment. Her mother was a musician; she herself always enjoyed playing the piano. She attended the Three Choirs Festival annually with her husband until he died.

She had always loved words and kept a 'word search' puzzle book in her handbag to fill spare minutes. She also had a great sense of humour, revelling in making the most outrageous puns. She organised herself meticulously with her Filofax, always being punctual.

Invariably immaculately smartly turned out, she drove herself to the cathedral each Sunday and was warmly welcomed by the clergy and her many friends in the congregation. Afterwards, she went to the same restaurant for Sunday lunch, being looked after as if a family member. She also took her professional children out for lunch there when they visited. She died peacefully at home, her children by her side.

Mrs B

The widow of a teacher, her parents divorced during the war; she was subsequently sent off to boarding school, having to spend exactly half of each holiday with each parent, in order to be 'fair'. This left a life-long legacy of pain saying goodbyes to people.

She met her husband at university. His father was not wealthy so they had to make their own way. Mrs B left before her degree to go with her husband to his first teaching post in the city where they lived for the rest of their lives.

Having been brought up in post-war austerity, she learned to 'scrimp and save' and 'make do and mend'. A dutiful and practical housewife, she enjoyed maintaining the fabric of the home, keeping it attractive and orderly. She worked hard to bring the children up to achieve the best they could.

The family enjoyed the thrills and spills of family camping during summer holidays. After university, her children left to develop their careers, ending up several hours away.

Mrs B latterly had difficulty speaking from a rare dementia (primary progressive aphasia), only diagnosed after her husband's death. Luckily she had supportive neighbours who helped her and looked out for her in between her children's visits.

What mental images do you have of these two survivors?

What rehabilitation approach would you have envisaged using if they fractured their wrist?

What might be the reasons to vary your approach?

How might this affect your attitude, your communication with her and her family, and your management strategies and tactics?

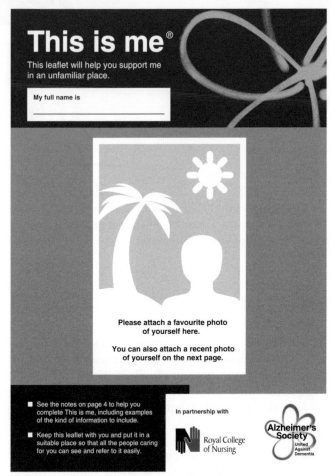

FIG. 19.1 'This is me', a simple leaflet for anyone receiving professional care who is living with dementia or experiencing delirium or other communication difficulties (Reproduced with permission from Alzheimer's Society).

It may come as a surprise that these personae both inhabited the same individual. All aspects mentioned informed the person she was, and how she behaved. Some of her skills were well preserved – she still drove safely and ran her house well – but her language skills were badly affected. All of us have many facets: some public, some private and some unknown until we reach a crisis.

We easily form a view based on partial data. Sadly, management decisions are not only often based on these, but are also informed by prejudice and projected presumptions. We are all complex beings with varying reactions and behaviours. These depend on which aspects of our personality are in the ascendancy at the time. We are not always logical, rational or internally consistent. For example, a widow in her nineties had lived a full life. She spent her final two years in a residential home because of physical frailty, although mentally intact. She confirmed with her GP she did not want any life-sustaining measures if she became unwell. Each night she prayed not to wake up next morning; she simply wanted to re-join her husband. One night she developed a chest infection and was prescribed antibiotics. She took them, thereby probably saving her life. When I asked her why, she said 'The staff here are lovely; I didn't want to let them down.'

I remember the change on the faces of some medical students when I pointed out that the frail old man in the end bed had been a Battle of Britain Spitfire pilot. When teaching doctors, I reminded them of two epigrams of Sir William Osler (possibly the pre-eminent 20th century physician):

'It is much more important to know what sort of a patient has a disease than what sort of a disease a patient has.'

'The good physician treats the disease; the great physician treats the patient who has the disease.'

(John, 2013)

We know that two people with exactly the same illness can be affected quite differently by it. If you gain insight into the motivations of your patient, you are in a much stronger position to help them achieve their objectives. Working towards what they *really* want is much more likely to succeed than trying to encourage them towards a different goal, not of their choosing.

CONTINUITY OF CARE

One thing most patients and healthcare colleagues value is relationship. When present, this is where human, *transformational*, things happen. The patient feels inspired and engaged; the healthcare professional derives fulfilment from seeing the best outcome in the circumstances. The corollary is that trust, inseparable from vulnerability and critical for good shared decision making (Hall et al., 2001), depends on a good relationship. This takes time. Unfortunately, continuity of care is at a premium in healthcare today. There are two big obstacles.

The first is staff numbers. Even in OECD (Organization for Economic Cooperation and Development) countries, this is a problem. For example, in the British NHS approximately 1 post in 11 is unfilled currently (The King's Fund, 2019). However, other countries have far fewer healthcare professionals per head of population than the UK (Gapminder.org, 2019). At best, this results in delays or disruption; at worst, patients just don't receive treatment.

The second obstacle is shift work for doctors and nurses. This causes unpredictable appearances of individuals within a team during the working week, even when there is a full complement of staff.

What Can You Do To Mitigate These Problems?

Some well-organised patients with long-term conditions maintain a printed summary of their medical details. This is invaluable for the healthcare team. A list of diagnoses, problems, allergies, medications (with doses) and specialists involved is a great start. Knowing their preferences and priorities is also invaluable for anything more than brief stays to allow person-centred care. For example: 'I like tea with milk and one sugar; I never drink coffee.' This can be systematised with a form, ideally kept near the patient. Several forms have been devised and used. The simplest sort is just one side of A4, for example 'Nine Important Things About Me' (see Resources section). A number of organisations have developed hospital (or healthcare) 'passports' along these lines (Easy Health, 2010). A much more comprehensive form has been developed by the UK Alzheimer's Society, called 'This is me' (Fig. 19.1). It was originally designed for people with dementia, but is a great *aide mémoire* for all (Alzheimer's Society, 2019). Family members, or others knowing the patient well, can help if the patient cannot (for example, with language, memory or learning difficulties). If they have any pets, record their names. These are often the most important focus of a patient's life.

If there is concern about a patient's cognitive abilities, the IQCODE is a simple, reliable and cross-culturally applicable tool in secondary care – even if delirium is present (Harrison et al., 2013). It asks someone who knows the patient well whether there has been any change in several of the patient's simple activities of daily living, compared to 10 years earlier. In effect, it's a systematic way of building up a picture of any change in a patient's cognitive function over time, across several domains – a structured way of taking a 'collateral history'.

HELPING YOU TO HELP YOUR PATIENTS

'Choosing Wisely' is a collaboration between patients and healthcare professionals to improve communications and aid decision making. They suggest four key questions for patients to ask (see Resources section, Box 1) (Choosing Wisely, 2016). It's worth considering the answers and pre-emptively sharing them with your patient if they don't ask. If you can't answer any, you've just identified an educational need for your continuing professional development.

Atul Gawande is an American surgeon who has written about improving healthcare. He observed 'I was confusing care with treatment' (Gawande, 2015). He suggests for patient-centred care, healthcare workers should ask five questions (see Resources section, Box 2).

Finally, an excellent article outlined the five questions that every patient has, but never asks (Whyte, 2018). Why not pre-emptively answer these, too (see Resources section, Box 3)?

SUMMARY POINTS

- Knowing your patient's real hopes, fears and priorities will enable you to help them better
- Tools are available to aid you with this
- Patients are human – we can all be preoccupied, illogical or inconsistent at times
- Inhabiting your patient's world, or at least seeing it from the inside, can help you to help them

MCQs

Q.1 Which one of the following statements is true?
   a. It is possible to get an evaluation of a patient's cognitive function even if they have delirium
   b. It is possible to help a patient express their preferences and priorities
   c. It is impossible to know a patient's goals of therapy without asking
   d. In general, patients with the same conditions can have very different outcomes
   e. All of the above

Q.2 For which of the following are published structured tools available?
   a. Screening for dementia
   b. Helping a patient engage with their treatment
   c. Expressing a patient's underlying concerns about the clinician and treatment
   d. Helping the staff to know a patient's preferences and priorities
   e. All of the above

REFERENCES

Alzheimer's Society. (2019). This is me ® [online] Retrieved from: https://www.alzheimers.org.uk/sites/default/files/2019-03/Alzheimers-Society_NEW_This-is-me-booklet_190318.pdf (Accessed 15 June 2020).

Choosing Wisely UK. (2016). Questions to ask your doctor. [online] Retrieved from: http://www.choosingwisely.co.uk/i-am-a-patient-carer/questions-ask-doctor/ (Accessed 15 June 2020).

Easy Health. (2010). Hospital passports (leaflets). [online] Retrieved from: https://www.easyhealth.org.uk/index.php/health-leaflets-and-videos/hospital-passports/ (Accessed 15 June 2020).

Hall, M. A., Dugan, E., Zheng, B., & Mishra, A. K. (2001). Trust in physicians and medical institutions: what is it, can it be measured, and does it matter? *The Milbank Quarterly, 79*(4), 613–639.

John, M. (2013). From Osler to the cone technique. *HSR Proceedings in Intensive Care & Cardiovascular Anesthesia, 5*(1), 57–58.

Gapminder.org. (2019). Gapminder Tools. [online] Retrieved from: https://www.gapminder.org/tools/#$state$marker$axis_x$which=medical_doctors_per_1000_people&spaceRef:null;;;&chart-type=barrank (Accessed 15 June 2020).

Gawande, A. (2015). *Being mortal: medicine and what matters in the end.* New York, NY: Picador.

Harrison, J.K., Fearon, P., Noel-Storr, A.H., McShane, R., Stott, D.J., & Quinn, T.J. (2015). IQCODE for the diagnosis of dementia within a secondary care setting. *Cochrane Database of Systematic Reviews.* www.cochranelibrary.com/cdsr/doi/10.1002/14651858.CD010772.pub2/full.

The King's Fund. (2019). The NHS crisis of caring for staff. [online] Retrieved from: https://www.kingsfund.org.uk/blog/2019/03/nhs-crisis-caring (Accessed 15 June 2020).

Whyte, J. (2018). Five questions that every patient has but never asks. *JAMA Neurology, 75*(8), 911.

20

Brain Health and Mental Capacity

Paul McElwaine & Shane O'Hanlon

LEARNING OBJECTIVES

- Explain the concept of brain health and its importance in ageing well and building resilience
- Describe current evidence for interventions to promote brain health

- Explain how mental capacity is assessed

INTRODUCTION

In this chapter, the concept of maintaining good overall brain health will be explored. The human brain has over 100 billion nerves cells and is not well understood. The different elements considered important in brain health will change depending on age and circumstance, but the building blocks remain the same. Brain health should be treated as a rainy-day fund, one which is grown throughout life. It is never too early to look at ways of improving brain health and equally it is never too late. It is important that people actively think about ways they can improve and protect their brain health. This will establish a cognitive reserve which can be drawn down when needed in times of ill health (Stern, 2012). Brain health should be supported through robust health promotion and education, giving people the best opportunity to make good decisions with regards to their overall health. The evidence base is still evolving, as shown in Fig. 20.1.

Also explored in this chapter is the topic of mental capacity. This concept is central to patient autonomy and although the legal situation changes from country to country, the basics of assessment are similar. Rehabilitation teams need to be aware of how brain health can affect mental capacity and should be alert to fluctuations. Optimisation is sometimes possible, and it is important to recognise that patients should be supported as much as possible to express their wishes and preferences and that these should be central to the rehabilitation process.

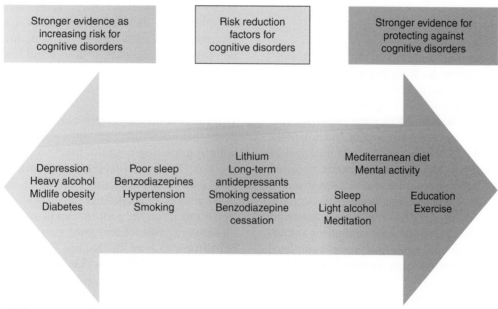

FIG. 20.1 Health-promoting strategies for the ageing brain. (From Chen ST, Volle D, Jalil J, Wu P, Small GW. Health-promoting strategies for the aging brain. *Am J Geriatr Psychiatry.* 2019;27(3):213–36, with permission).

BRAIN HEALTH

Brain health depends on a complex interplay of factors, with likely a sum of individual components optimising benefit, rather than any single intervention (Ngandu et al., 2015). The pragmatic approach would view treating the brain like a muscle. In order to maintain optimum function, the muscle needs to be exercised and challenged, whether that be thought processing, speech or working memory. The optimum type and dose of an intervention may be unknown but adopting an 'any is better than none' approach is reasonable, coupled with a 'use it or lose' philosophy.

The brain is adaptable; the term 'neuroplasticity' refers to the ability of the brain to adapt to environmental change, respond to injury and to acquire novel information by modifying neural connectivity and function. The more input the brain receives the better, the more functions it can perform. The following are suggested areas that may help to maintain or challenge the brain's neuroplasticity (Vance et al., 2010).

COGNITIVE RESERVE

Cognitive reserve has been described as 'the ability to withstand acquired changes in the brain due to neurodegenerative and vascular diseases and head trauma without developing symptoms or signs of disease' (Fratiglioni & Wang, 2007). It is sensible to look for ways to enhance and encourage cognitive reserve in earlier life. The structure and function of the brain are inseparable, so reserve aims to help the brain be efficient, flexible, and have increased capacity and compensation when needed. Building cognitive reserve helps maintain function in the face of accumulating brain pathology and may lower the risk of dementia (Tow et al., 2016). Indicators of cognitive reserve include educational attainment and socioeconomic background, and modifiable factors as outlined below including physical activity and cognitively stimulating activities.

Physical Activity

The benefit of regular physical activity on general health and specifically brain health is clear. Recent guidelines recommend that all older adults should perform moderate intensity physical activity for at least 30 minutes a day, at least five times per week, above usual routine levels of activity (Piercy et al., 2018). Legitimate concern exists that modern living leads to a sedentary lifestyle and reduces people's daily levels of exercise in whatever form that takes. A combination of aerobic, flexibility, balance and strengthening activities should provide the platform to age well.

Rapidly developing wearable technologies such as fitness trackers have huge potential. These devices have the capabilities to provide information which can potentially identify people at risk of falls, stroke and possibly highlight frailty in older people. The limitations are in the acceptance of the technology, and it is unclear if these devices lead to consistent increases in activity in older people.

Group exercise interventions have clear benefit covering several key areas of brain health. Being active with a group provides not only strength and conditioning, improving cardiovascular status, but also improves mental well-being and provides social interaction.

Nutrition and Supplements

A huge amount of research has explored the benefits of different diets or supplements on both existing disease and prevention of disease. Generally, no single agent exists which has shown benefit in isolation. Specific supplements such as antioxidants and omega-3 polyunsaturated fatty acids have shown no clear benefit by themselves particularly on cognition (Andrieu et al., 2017). The emphasis is better directed on eating an overall balanced diet that is rich in fruit, vegetables and fish, and has a reduced reliance on meat and dairy. The benefit of a Mediterranean diet (see Resources section for details) in cardiovascular disease risk reduction is well established; Fig. 20.2 shows potential mechanisms by which it could protect against cardiovascular disease. There is considerable overlap between cardiovascular disease and brain health, so the Mediterranean diet is a positive choice (Scarmeas et al., 2009; Valls-Pedret et al., 2015). The interaction between cardiovascular disease and brain health is discussed later in the chapter.

Sleep

Why humans need to sleep is not fully understood. It is believed that maintaining a healthy sleep pattern is important both in protecting cognitive function and restoring loss of function (Xie et al., 2013). It is hypothesised that sleep is a period where the body can promote brain plasticity. Even in the absence of a definitive understanding, poor sleep can clearly impact on the performance of an individual. There is inconsistent evidence that poor sleep can predict cognitive impairment in later life. Studies have shown that duration of sleep, both too little (less than 6 hours) or too much sleep (greater than 8 hours), may have a negative impact on memory function (Ramos et al., 2013; Xu et al., 2014). Promoting a good pattern of sleep hygiene is an overlooked element of daily living especially in rehabilitation. A common-sense approach which is practical and takes consideration of the

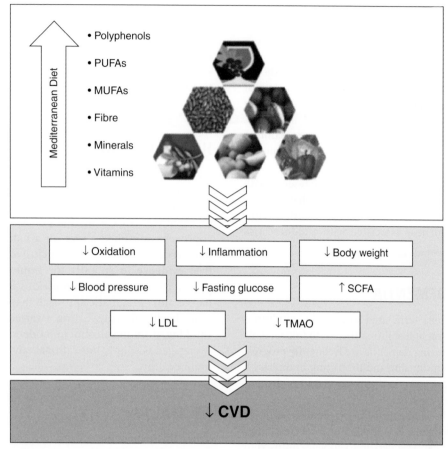

FIG. 20.2 Potential mechanisms by which a Mediterranean diet could protect against cardiovascular disease. (From Salas-Salvadó J, Becerra-Tomás N, García-Gavilán JF, Bulló M, Barrubés L. Mediterranean diet and cardiovascular disease prevention: what do we know? *Prog Cardiovasc Dis.* 2018;61(1):62–7, with permission).

sleeping environment should be adopted. Chapter 32 Sleep and Fatigue describes how sleep impacts on rehabilitation in more detail.

Social Engagement

Social engagement refers to maintenance of social connections and participation in social activities. It can be viewed in terms of quantity, the size and frequency of contact, and the quality of contact, such as emotional support provided. More frequent participation in social activities and a higher level of perceived social support have been shown to be associated with higher level of cognitive functioning (Holtzman et al., 2004). Social engagement is often linked to other areas of brain health such as physical activity, but its benefit should not be undervalued as it can support areas of positive lifestyle choices such as diet, exercise and smoking cessation. The evidence supports the neuroprotective effect social engagement can have into later life (Fratiglioni, Paillard-Borg, & Winblad, 2004).

Cognitively Stimulating Activity

Cognitively stimulating activities are those that challenge elements of mental processing such as concentration or memory in an engaging and often enjoyable way. Cognitively stimulating activities may benefit cognition and reduce dementia risk and promote recovery from brain injury. Cognitive training can improve older adults' performance on cognitive tasks, but whether it translates to daily function is less clear (Kelly et al., 2014). The activity could be related to work experiences, learning a new skill, participating in a mentally challenging leisure activity, and exploring music and the arts. The activity can help to maintain essential functions such as memory, language, reasoning, thinking and attention.

Research evidence suggests that training in a cognitive task will improve ability in that task, but unless it is a skill that is useful in daily living then the benefit is minimal (Ball et al., 2002). Commercial cognitive training programmes or 'Brain Games' do not have a strong evidence base, and in most cases just improve skills at the game and do not translate as improved cognitive ability. Variety in activities may have the greatest benefit.

Mental Well-Being

Mental well-being, as defined by the World Health Organization, 'is a state where a person realises their own potential, can cope with the normal stresses of life, can work productively and fruitfully, and is able to contribute to their community' (World Health Organization, 2004). Mental health is maintained through investing in the mental capital that both cognitive and emotional intelligence brings through the ability to learn and be resilient in the face of challenges. This should be coupled with an understanding of the dynamic state of mental well-being that a person requires to perform within relationships and communities (Beddington et al., 2008). Greater appreciation of wellness is being seen in programmes for children in schools. This may translate to better resilience into later life.

Mental illness can have an effect on cognitive reserve, with an association between depression and dementia having been long described (Chen et al., 2019). In bipolar disorder, maintenance lithium treatment is associated with a reduced risk of dementia.

DELIRIUM AND DEMENTIA

Dementia is an umbrella term used to describe conditions that cause a decline in mental ability sufficient to impact daily life. The conditions causing dementia are frequently progressive at varying rates. Optimising and protecting brain health is of fundamental importance in the management of dementia.

Brain health can be challenged during illness, more often as people age. Delirium is a sudden and severe change in brain function that causes a person to appear confused or disoriented, or to have difficulties maintaining focus, thinking clearly, and remembering recent events, typically with a fluctuating course. It is a sign of an underlying problem, has multiple potential causes and is associated with poor outcomes. It can be a sign of cognitive problems in future, with a greater than fivefold increased rate of incident dementia if a person has an episode of delirium (Witlox et al., 2010). It can limit recovery and is distressing to both the individual and family, friends and carers. Recognition is the key to reduce the risk.

People with dementia are more prone to developing delirium than those with normal baseline cognition. When delirium occurs in people who are fit, the outcomes are worse (Dani et al., 2018). This suggests that a more severe precipitant is present, such as a very serious illness. Both dementia and delirium are explored in more detail in Chapter 30 Cognitive Problems.

SMOKING, ALCOHOL AND VASCULAR RISK

Smoking should be avoided, and alcohol taken in moderation. Both smoking and alcohol dependence are risk factors for late-life cognitive impairment. Prevention and management of vascular risk factors is essential to maintaining brain health and promoting recovery. Identification of hypertension (high blood pressure) and its control has been shown to reduce not only conditions such as heart disease and stroke but also types of cognitive decline including dementia (Peters et al., 2008). Obesity, diabetes and cigarette smoking should all be targeted in preventative health strategies. The interplay between vascular health and cognition should be apparent, and the evidence supports modification of these risk factors as early as possible but in particular middle age.

HEALTH PROMOTION

As well as the personal choices people must make around their brain health, the onus is also on policy makers to provide the environment and opportunity for people to make the right choices. Changes in policies to adopt some of the approaches outlined above on a national level have been hampered by waiting for conclusive randomised control trial evidence to support the implementation. However, this inertia may have repercussions in the future and perhaps a more pragmatic approach may help improve overall brain health globally. Eating a varied diet, exercising, not smoking, drinking alcohol in moderation and being socially engaged is simple but rational advice to age well and be brain healthy.

MENTAL CAPACITY

'Does this patient have capacity?' is a question commonly heard in the rehabilitation setting. Mental capacity is the ability to understand the nature and consequences of a decision in the context of available choices at the time the decision is to be made. It should be noted that it is specific to a decision; for example, someone could have capacity to decide about whether they want to have bloods taken but not have capacity to decide about their discharge plan.

There is a presumption that people have mental capacity to make decisions, unless demonstrated otherwise. Some conditions such as dementia may mean that people can be shown to lack capacity. If there are reasonable grounds to suggest that the person lacks capacity to make the decision, then a formal assessment should be undertaken.

The process for assessing capacity has been set out in law in several countries, and approaches to it can vary. The legislation used in the UK is a sensible approach and is as follows (Department of Health, 2005):

1. Can the person understand the information necessary to make the decision?
2. Can they retain the information for long enough to make the decision?
3. Can they weigh up the information in order to make the decision?
4. Can they communicate the decision by any means?

Because capacity can fluctuate, it should ideally be assessed only when the patient is at their best. For example, if they are unwell, then they should be given time to recover – the assessment should be delayed until the person regains capacity. Similarly, if there are barriers to demonstrating capacity (e.g. no hearing aid, or difficulty with speech), these should be optimised where possible. Communication does not have to be spoken, and could also be with gesture or yes/no answers indicated using a tool. The input of speech and language therapists can be extremely valuable in some cases.

It is extremely important that patients are provided with information in a manner that they can understand. They should also be given time to absorb the information, and support offered from an advocate if needed.

Once a patient has demonstrated that they have capacity to make a decision, then they are entitled to do so (assuming it is legal) even if to the healthcare professional it seems an unwise decision.

If a patient lacks capacity to make a decision, the approach to decision making differs in different countries. Some such as the UK use a 'best interests' decision, whereas in the United States a 'substituted judgement' system can be found. Ireland has adopted a 'will and preference' approach.

CASE CONCLUSION

When Femi was initially assessed by the doctor, there was no time to gain more information about why he had delirium. However, given that Femi was fit, he is likely to have good cognitive reserve. His delirium has a worse outcome as it probably indicates a very significant illness. This point can be missed by some health professionals who assume that all older people are prone to confusion. When Femi's mental capacity to decide about self-discharge was assessed, it was felt that he did not understand the risks nor could he weigh them up. He was therefore declared not to have capacity to leave the hospital.

Femi was given sedation as it was felt he was a risk to himself and others when he became agitated. This is a last resort as other approaches such as distraction and reassurance often work initially in delirium. An emergency CT of his head demonstrated a large subdural haemorrhage (bleed in the lining of the brain), and this was the reason why he became delirious. He had surgery that evening to evacuate the bleeding and made an excellent recovery. Two weeks later he was discharged home and had regained his cognitive baseline when reviewed in clinic a month later.

SUMMARY POINTS

- Brain health is developed throughout life, and the more investment in cognitive reserve the better
- A multimodal approach to maintaining brain health is suggested including regular physical activity, social engagement, healthy nutrition, adequate quality sleep, cognitive stimulating activities and targeting of vascular risk factors
- Mental capacity is the ability to understand the nature and consequences of a decision in the context of available choices at the time the decision is to be made
- There is a presumption that everyone has capacity to make decisions, unless there is a reason to displace this or a capacity assessment for a specific decision has been made
- Mental capacity should be assessed when patients have been optimised where possible, using local laws or guidance

MCQs

Q.1 Which of the following is true about brain health?
  a. Social engagement does not have a neuroprotective effect into later life
  b. Too much sleep may have a negative impact on memory function
  c. Cognitive training has clear benefits on daily memory function
  d. Having an episode of delirium carries no increased risk of later dementia
  e. The American diet has been shown to reduce cardiovascular risk

Q.2 Which one of the following is true about mental capacity?
  a. Formal assessment should be undertaken for all medical decisions
  b. Capacity does not change from one day to the next
  c. Someone who cannot speak cannot have mental capacity to make a decision
  d. There is a presumption that everyone has mental capacity
  e. Patients are not allowed to make decisions that seem unwise

REFERENCES

Andrieu, S., Guyonnet, S., Coley, N., Cantet, C., Bonnefoy, M., Bordes, S., Bories, L., Cufi, M. N., Dantoine, T., Dartigues, J. F., Desclaux, F., Gabelle, A., Gasnier, Y., Pesce, A., Sudres, K., Touchon, J., Robert, P., Rouaud, O., Legrand, P., Payoux, P., Caubere, J. P., Weiner, M., Carrié, I., Ousset, P. J., & Vellas, B. MAPT Study Group. (2017). Effect of long-term omega 3 polyunsaturated fatty acid supplementation with or without multidomain intervention on cognitive function in elderly adults with memory complaints (MAPT): a randomised, placebo-controlled trial. *The Lancet Neurology, 16*(5), 377–389.

Ball, K., Berch, D. B., Helmers, K. F., Jobe, J. B., Leveck, M. D., Marsiske, M., Morris, J. N., Rebok, G. W., Smith, D. M., Tennstedt, S. L., Unverzagt, F. W., & Willis, S. L. (2002). Effects of cognitive training interventions with older adults: a randomized controlled trial. *JAMA, 288*(18), 2271–2281.

Beddington, J., Cooper, C. L., Field, J., Goswami, U., Huppert, F. A., Jenkins, R., Jones, H. S., Kirkwood, T. B. L., Sahakian, B. J., & Thomas, S. M. (2008). The mental wealth of nations. *Nature, 455*, 1057–1060.

Chen, S. T., Volle, D., Jalil, J., Wu, P., & Small, G. W. (2019). Health-promoting strategies for the aging brain. *American Journal of Geriatric Psychiatry, 27*(3), 213–236.

Dani, M., Owen, L. H., Jackson, T. A., Rockwood, K., Sampson, E. L., & Davis, D. (2018). Delirium, frailty, and mortality: interactions in a prospective study of hospitalized older people. *The Journals of Gerontology Series A, Biological Sciences and Medical Sciences, 73*(3), 415–418.

Department of Health. (2005). *Mental capacity act.* London: HMSO.

Fratiglioni, L., Paillard-Borg, S., & Winblad, B. (2004). An active and socially integrated lifestyle in late life might protect against dementia. *The Lancet Neurology, 3*(6), 343–353.

Fratiglioni, L., & Wang, H. X. (2007). Brain reserve hypothesis in dementia. *Journal of Alzheimer's Disease, 12*, 11–22.

Holtzman, R. E., Rebok, G. W., Saczynski, J. S., Kouzis, A. C., Wilcox Doyle, K., & Eaton, W. W. (2004). Social network characteristics and cognition in middle-aged and older adults. *The Journals of Gerontology: Series B, 59*(6), P278–P284.

Kelly, M. E., Loughrey, D., Lawlor, B. A., Robertson, I. H., Walsh, C., & Brennan, S. (2014). The impact of cognitive training and mental stimulation on cognitive and everyday functioning of healthy older adults: a systematic review and meta-analysis. *Ageing Research Reviews, 15*, 28–43.

Ngandu, T., Lehtisalo, J., Solomon, A., Levälahti, E., Ahtiluoto, S., Antikainen, R., Bäckman, L., Hänninen, T., Jula, A., Laatikainen, T., Lindström, J., Mangialasche, F., Paajanen, T., Pajala, S., Peltonen, M., Rauramaa, R., Stigsdotter-Neely, A., Strandberg, T., Tuomilehto, J., Soininen, H., & Kivipelto, M. (2015). A 2 year multidomain intervention of diet, exercise, cognitive training, and vascular risk monitoring versus control to prevent cognitive decline in at-risk elderly people (FINGER): a randomised controlled trial. *The Lancet, 385*(9984), 2255–2263.

Peters, R., Beckett, N., Forette, F., Tuomilehto, J., Clarke, R., Ritchie, C., Ritchie, C., Waldman, A., Walton, I., Poulter, R., Ma, S., Comsa, M., Burch, L., Fletcher, A., & Bulpitt, C. HYVET investigators. (2008). Incident dementia and blood pressure lowering in the Hypertension in the Very Elderly Trial cognitive function assessment (HYVET-COG): a double-blind, placebo controlled trial. *The Lancet Neurology, 7*(8), 683–689.

Piercy, K. L., Troiano, R. P., Ballard, R. M., Carlson, S. A., Fulton, J. E., Galuska, D. A., George, S. M., & Olson, R. D. (2018). The physical activity guidelines for Americans. *JAMA, 320*(19), 2020–2028.

Ramos, A. R., Dong, C., Elkind, M. S., Boden-Albala, B., Sacco, R. L., Rundek, T., & Wright, C. B. (2013). Association between sleep duration and the mini-mental score: the Northern Manhattan study. *Journal of Clinical Sleep Medicine, 9*(7), 669–673.

Scarmeas, N., Stern, Y., Mayeux, R., Manly, J. J., Schupf, N., & Luchsinger, J. A. (2009). Mediterranean diet and mild cognitive impairment. *Archives of Neurology, 66*(2), 216–225.

Stern, Y. (2012). Cognitive reserve in ageing and Alzheimer's disease. *The Lancet Neurology., 11*(11), 1006–1012.

Tow, A., Holtzer, R., Wang, C., Sharan, A., Kim, S. J., Gladstein, A., Blum, Y., & Verghese, J. (2016). Cognitive reserve and postoperative delirium in older adults. *Journal of the American Geriatrics Society, 64*(6), 1341–1346.

Vance, D. E., Roberson, A. J., McGuinness, T. M., & Fazeli, P. L. (2010). How neuroplasticity and cognitive reserve protect cognitive functioning. *Journal of Psychosocial Nursing and Mental Health Services, 48*(4), 23–30.

Valls-Pedret, C., Sala-Vila, A., Serra-Mir, M., Corella, D., De la Torre, R., Martínez-González, M. Á., Martínez-Lapiscina, E. H., Fitó, M., Pérez-Heras, A., Salas-Salvadó, J., Estruch, R., & Ros, E. (2015). Mediterranean diet and age-related cognitive decline: a randomized clinical trial. *JAMA Internal Medicine, 175*(7), 1094–1103.

World Health Organization. (2004). Promoting mental health: concepts, emerging evidence, practice: Summary report.

Xie, L., Kang, H., Xu, Q., Chen, M. J., Liao, Y., Thiyagarajan, M., O'Donnell, J., Christensen, D. J., Nicholson, C., Iliff, J. J., Takano, T., Deane, R., & Nedergaard, M. (2013). Sleep drives metabolite clearance from the adult brain. *Science, 342*(6156), 373–377.

Xu, L., Jiang, C. Q., Lam, T. H., Zhang, W. S., Cherny, S. S., Thomas, G. N., & Cheng, K. K. (2014). Sleep duration and memory in the elderly Chinese: longitudinal analysis of the Guangzhou Biobank Cohort Study. *Sleep, 37*(11), 1737–1744.

Witlox, J., Eurelings, L. S. M., de Jonghe, J. F. M., Kalisvaart, K. J., Eikelenboom, P., & van Gool, W. A. (2010). Delirium in elderly patients and the risk of postdischarge mortality, institutionalization, and dementia: a meta-analysis. *JAMA, 304*(4), 443–451.

21

Avoiding Deconditioning

Amit Arora & Brian Dolan OBE

LEARNING OBJECTIVES

- Describe the clinical syndrome of deconditioning and explain why it is harmful

- Identify opportunities to help patients to get up, get dressed and get moving

CASE

Arthur is a 78-year-old man who was admitted to hospital with a lower respiratory tract infection. At home, he had been independently mobile with a Zimmer frame. However, he was felt to be a 'high falls risk' as he fell in the emergency department, and as a result was told not to walk without having supervision. Due to staff shortages he found it very difficult to go anywhere, feeling like he was 'constantly told to sit back down'. He was not referred to the physiotherapist during his stay. After a week in hospital his infection had resolved and he was told he could go home, but he was unable to stand up from a chair without assistance.

INTRODUCTION

While known about for many decades, particularly among geriatricians and physiotherapists, in recent years there has been a resurgence of awareness among health professionals and even the public about deconditioning and its consequences. In part, this is because of a coalescence of the work of organisations like the British Geriatrics Society, individual clinicians, campaigns led by the authors, and the public becoming more conscious of the impact of lack of mobility and protracted hospital stays, especially among older people.

WHAT IS DECONDITIONING?

Hanson et al. (2019) define deconditioning as 'a complex process of physiological change that can affect multiple body systems and often results in functional decline'. In a clinical context, deconditioning (which is also called hospital-acquired functional decline) is much more than muscle tone and fitness. As our understanding of human physiology in times of imposed bed rest has developed, it highlights that this is more a syndrome rather than a condition and a different definition can therefore be considered. Deconditioning syndrome comprises physical, psychological and functional decline that occurs as a result of prolonged bed rest and associated loss of muscle strength, commonly experienced through hospitalisation (see Fig. 21.1 for an information leaflet from the hospital where the deconditioning campaign was introduced). Though it can affect people of any age, the effect on older people can be more rapid, severe, and can often be irreversible (Arora, 2017a).

THE HARMS OF BED REST

As relatively recently as the 1970s, bed rest was commonly prescribed as a medical therapy for a variety of conditions such as tuberculosis and strokes (Allen, Glasziou, & Del Mar, 1999). Bed rest was thought to not only aid the healing process but also expedite the recovery time (Fortney, Schneider, & Greenleaf, 2011). However, there is now robust evidence that inactivity, bed rest and even a sedentary lifestyle can have detrimental effects on body physiology and function (Gordon, Grimmer, & Barras 2019; Hanson et al., 2019; Kortebein, 2009). Prevalence estimates report older hospitalised patients can spend anything up to 95% of their time in bed or chair, during their hospitalisation. Deconditioning can often start within the first day of hospitalisation (see Box 21.1) and possibly whilst patients are still on a trolley in the emergency department and interventions such as intravenous infusion, catheterisation, bedrails, nasogastric tube, etc, may precipitate deconditioning even sooner.

Deconditioning syndrome, a consequence of immobility, is therefore a complex physiological process that results in a multisystem deterioration in function. This phenomenon can result in a significant reduction in bone mass, muscle mass and durability as well as demotivation, swallowing difficulties, confusion and an increased reliance on others.

The physiological effects of bed rest are summarised in Box 21.1.

The effects of inappropriately prolonged hospitalisation are summarised in Box 21.2.

Deconditioning syndrome is not limited to hospitalised patients; it can also occur in care homes and even in an individual's own home.

Although deconditioning as a concept is not novel, the term has become more used and understood since the 2016 launch in the UK of the 'National Deconditioning Prevention and Awareness Campaign: Get Up, Get Dressed, Get Moving' (Arora, 2017a, b) and the International #endpjparalysis campaign (Dolan, 2017).

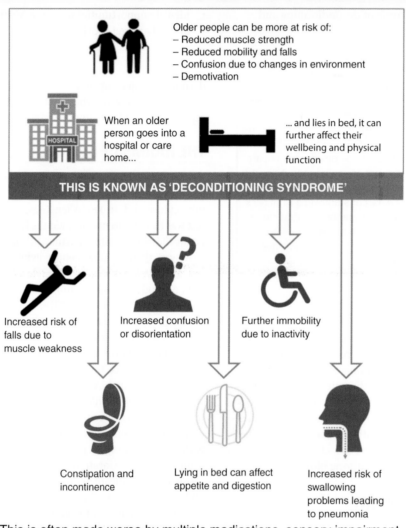

A Campaign For Deconditioning Awareness – "Sit up... Get dressed... Keep on moving..."

PREVENTING DECONDITIONING AND ENABLING INDEPENDENCE FOR OLDER PEOPLE

Older people can be more at risk of:
– Reduced muscle strength
– Reduced mobility and falls
– Confusion due to changes in environment
– Demotivation

When an older person goes into a hospital or care home...

... and lies in bed, it can further affect their wellbeing and physical function

THIS IS KNOWN AS 'DECONDITIONING SYNDROME'

Increased risk of falls due to muscle weakness

Increased confusion or disorientation

Further immobility due to inactivity

Constipation and incontinence

Lying in bed can affect appetite and digestion

Increased risk of swallowing problems leading to pneumonia

This is often made worse by multiple medications, sensory impairment, dementia and current illness

YOUR MUSCLES / YOUR STRENGTH / YOUR ABILITIES - USE THEM OR LOSE THEM

British Geriatrics Society
Improving healthcare for older people

University Hospitals of North Midlands
Department for Older Adults   NHS Trust

FIG. 21.1 Information leaflet on deconditioning (© University Hospitals of North Midlands NHS Trust 2016).

BOX 21.1 Physiological Effects of Bed Rest

Impact of bed rest in first 24 hours:
Reduced muscle power by 2%–5%
Reduced circulatory volume by up to 5%

Impact in the first 7 days:
Reduced circulatory volume by up to 25%
Reduced VO2 max by up to 8%–15%
Reduced muscle strength by up to 5%–10%
Reduced functional residual capacity (FRC) by up to 15%–30%
Reduced skin integrity
Reduced dignity, self-confidence, independence, choice and quality

BOX 21.2 Harms Associated with Inappropriately Prolonged Hospitalisation

Conventional safety incidents – iatrogenic infections including diarrhea, methicillin-resistant *Staphylococcal aureus* (MRSA) and pneumonias, thromboembolism, etc.
Deconditioning syndrome
Delirium
Immobility
Incontinence
Loss of self-esteem
Poorly planned discharge
Delayed care transitions/coordination/communication
Premature institutionalisation
Premature decisions about future care needs in wrong setting

IMPACT OF DECONDITIONING

Deconditioning can have a dramatic impact on the hospitalised older population, especially those with frailty. The combination of an acute medical or surgical condition with pre-existing poor functional reserves can result in prolonged immobility. The addition of sleep disturbance, nutritional deficiencies and relative inactivity will intensify the detrimental effects of deconditioning (Falvey, Mangione, & Stevens-Lapsley, 2015; Walthall, Jackson, & Dolan, 2019).

There is evidence that activity and exercise help in recovery, and therefore can contribute to reduced length of stay in hospitals and improve fitness potentially impacting on self-care, independence and care needs (Cortes, Delgado, & Esparza, 2019). The evidence around strategies for mass implementation has been relatively more sparse.

DECONDITIONING: AN OLD CHESTNUT OR A NEW MEDICAL DIAGNOSIS?

Hippocrates (430–370 BCE) originally proposed that 'in every movement of the body, whenever one begins to endure pain, it will be relieved by rest' (Hippocrates, 1849). However, shortly after suggesting rest as a medical therapy, he noticed that prolonged inactivity led to a significant decline in both strength and exercise performance (Chadwick & Mann, 1950). Thus, even as early as Hippocrates the potential detrimental effects of bed rest were partially understood. Long after Hippocrates, there is reference to harms of bed rest. In the 1867 edition of 'Hymns Ancient and Modern' (No. 23, Verse 3), it states:

'Teach me to live that I may dread, The grave as little as my bed'

(Cottage, 2016).

In 1947, Dr Richard Asher drew parallels between graves and beds as a means to increase awareness of 'The Dangers of Going to Bed' (Asher, 1947). He famously extolled:

'Teach us to live that we may dread, Unnecessary time in bed.
  Get people up and we may save, Our patients from an early grave'.

Since then, our scientific understanding and appreciation of deconditioning has substantially improved and it is now recognised that this complex process has the potential to disrupt almost every organ system (Box 21.1). Despite this long-standing appreciation of multisystem effects, the importance of addressing deconditioning has somehow not received the due recognition or priority in recent times. Box 21.3 demonstrates how staff can help patients prevent some of the harmful effects of hospitalisation and prevent deconditioning. Fig. 21.2 shows how to support and encourage movement.

BOX 21.3 What Can Staff Do to Prevent Deconditioning

Encourage/assist patients:
- To sit out in a chair
- To dress in their own clothes
- To walk to the toilet
- Cut patient's toenails where appropriate
- Encourage and support patients to perform activities of daily living (ADLs) which they will be performing at their home like shaving, dressing, etc. when feasible.
- Walk as much as possible – with or without support
- Transfer from bed to chair and chair to stand and walk
- Transfer from toilet seat
- Walk/wheel patients to toilet rather than bedside commode, etc.
- Cut food and eat independently where possible
- Avoid delirium, constipation
- Appropriate pain relief, mobilisation, promote ADLs, medication review (START/STOPP criteria)
- Avoid unnecessary catheters, cannula, tubes to aid independence and self-reliance/confidence to return home
- Measure hospital associated harms

Provide patients:
- Their reading glasses
- Their hearing aids
- Dentures if they use them
- Large print leaflets
- Clock and calendar in each bay and room
- Chairs and beds of appropriate height
- Appropriate walking equipment
- Signpost toilets
- Encourage families to bring patient's own clothes, shoes, etc.

A Campaign For Deconditioning Awareness – "Sit up... Get dressed... Keep on moving..."
Prolonged bed rest in older people can lead to substantial loss of muscle strength and physical activity
Assess
Comprehensive Geriatric Assessment
A comprehensive assessment should be completed to determine normal capabilities
A risk assessment should be completed
Glasses, hearing aids, clock and calendar should be accessible
Support
Are there appropriate mobility aids available? Is it the right size and reachable?
Walking to the toilet helps to prepare for going home. Is the catheter really needed?
Sitting out of bed helps (when possible). Can you get out of your chair?
Encourage
Feed or take fluids independently
Wash and dress independently in own clothes
Keep moving arms and legs even in a bed or chair
Thinking about how to support and encourage movement helps to:
– Reduce the risk of harm from falls, infection, thrombosis and delirium
– Reduce length of stay in hospital
– Reduce the likelihood of having an increase in their future care needs
Sit up... Get dressed... Keep on moving...
YOUR MUSCLES / YOUR STRENGTH / YOUR ABILITIES - USE THEM OR LOSE THEM
BGS
British Geriatrics Society
Improving healthcare for older people
University Hospitals of North Midlands NHS
Department for Older Adults
NHS Trust
© 2016 University Hospitals of North Midlands NHS Trust. All rights reserved.

FIG. 21.2 Ways to support and encourage movement (© University Hospitals of North Midlands NHS Trust 2016).

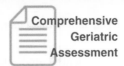

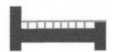

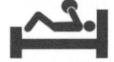

BOX 21.4   Barriers to Preventing Deconditioning in Hospitals

- Focus is generally on resolving the acute problem
- Less attention to underlying risk of functional decline
- Environment is not designed for enhancing function in older people
- Staff may encourage sedentary behaviour to prevent falls
- Patient and relatives expectations and beliefs
- Staff shortages and time pressures
- Some staff may feel it is 'someone else's job'
- Staff may feel this reduces time to complete essential paperwork
- Lack of awareness particularly within medical schools
- Inadequate staffing levels to promote activity in hospitals
- Lack of appropriate infrastructure – day rooms, laundry machines
- Relatives often unable to assist and bring clothes, shoes, etc. to hospitals
- Acute issues take priority
- Lack of awareness amongst staff and patients/families of harms associated with inappropriately prolonged hospitalization and bed rest in hospitals
- Fear of falls
- Lack of reporting mechanisms re: deconditioning

Regular physical exercise is known to reduce the risk associated with developing a wide variety of conditions ranging from cardiovascular disease, colorectal cancer, joint diseases to depression. In addition, various studies have demonstrated that sarcopenia, muscular atrophy and weakness, typical musculoskeletal features of ageing and deconditioning have the potential for partial reversibility through regular aerobic and resistance exercise. Thus, regular exercise has the ability to not only improve quality of life but could also prevent premature deaths from conditions such as cardiovascular disease (de Labra et al., 2015; Hanson et al., 2019; Migeotte et al., 2017).

This can partly be applied to patients in hospital that may remain immobile in hospitals. The reasons why patients sometimes can lie in bed with inappropriate bed rest are mentioned in Box 21.4.

There is also increasing evidence from telomere studies and mitochondrial studies in ageing that exercise in all ages helps. Similar evidence has emerged from space flight studies of human physiology, though these were performed in younger and healthier people, which have substantially aided our understanding of deconditioning. It highlights that regular activity and exercise could reverse the biological

and clinical characteristics of ageing and deconditioning (Maggioni et al., 2018).

PREVENTING DECONDITIONING

Driving Changes

The 'National Deconditioning Awareness and Prevention Campaign (UK) - Get Up, Get Dressed, Get Moving' and #EndPJParalysis have generated widespread support nationally and internationally as an approach to prevent the detrimental effects caused by deconditioning in hospitals, care homes and those living alone (Arora, 2017c; Chankova, 2018).

Next Steps

Methods to prevent deconditioning could involve multiple approaches. These could include creating individualised care plans for activity and exercise, deconditioning care bundles, measuring deconditioning and reporting harm, incorporating deconditioning in all root cause analysis, prescribing personalised exercises depending upon individuals' abilities, educating staff and the public, busting myths and highlighting facts; and some of these have been tried with varying successes.

To further raise awareness, it is essential that education on deconditioning syndrome is incorporated into all healthcare professionals' curricula and supported by charities and patient groups. A move to include importance of physical activity is currently underway with all UK medical, nursing and pharmacy schools. It remains to be seen how the prevention of deconditioning work may be better integrated nationally and despite staffing shortages, whether adequate training and deconditioning awareness will be enough to tackle this important challenge.

CONCLUSION

With a rapidly shifting population demographic, deconditioning syndrome must be addressed more robustly across the board. It has significant implications not least on quality of life, dignity and mortality but also in the number of occupied hospital beds and in reducing healthcare-associated unintended harms. All groups of staff including receptionists, therapists, porters, healthcare assistants, nurses, doctors and others have an important role in patient care and therefore in preventing deconditioning. The current challenge lies in implementing and creating new and effective strategies to prevent deconditioning in hospitals and care homes.

Older people deserve no less.

SUMMARY POINTS

- Deconditioning is a potentially very harmful syndrome that results from physical inactivity
- It can be precipitated even after a brief period of immobility, particularly in hospital, and in older people with frailty
- Wider awareness of deconditioning among health professionals and the public can help to reduce its occurrence

- Campaigns such as the 'National Deconditioning Awareness and Prevention Campaign - Get Up, Get Dressed, Get Moving' and #EndPJParalysis are effective tools to reduce deconditioning

MCQs

Q.1 Which of the following is true about mobility?

    a. Bed rest is an effective treatment for older people recovering from illness

    b. Deconditioning is a normal part of ageing and cannot be avoided

    c. Sleep disturbances, nutritional deficiencies and relative inactivity will intensify the detrimental effects of deconditioning

    d. Deconditioning is a syndrome of physical, psychological and functional decline

    e. Deconditioning does not affect other organ systems outside of the musculoskeletal system

Q.2 Which of these options is an appropriate intervention to help reduce deconditioning?

    a. National campaigns to promote awareness of deconditioning

    b. Empowering non-clinical staff such as receptionists and porters to motivate patients to mobilise

    c. Including deconditioning in the undergraduate curriculum for health staff

    d. Introducing care bundles for prevention of deconditioning

    e. All of the above

REFERENCES

Allen, C., Glasziou, P., & Del Mar, C. (1999). Bed rest: a potentially harmful treatment needing more careful evaluation. *The Lancet*, *354*(9186), 1229–1233.

Arora, A. (2017a). Deconditioning syndrome awareness and prevention campaign: why is everyone talking about it? Retrieved from: https://www.bgs.org.uk/blog/sit-up-get-dressed-keep-moving-the-campaign-everyone-is-talking-about (Accessed 8 September 2019).

Arora, A. (2017b). Deconditioning awareness. Retrieved from: https://www.bgs.org.uk/resources/deconditioning-awareness (Accessed 8 September 2019).

Arora, A. (2017c). Time to move: get up, get dressed and keep moving. Retrieved from: https://www.england.nhs.uk/blog/amit-arora/ (Accessed 8 September 2019).

Asher, R. A. J. (1947). The dangers of going to bed. *British Medical Journal*, *2*(4536), 967–968.

Chadwick, J., & Mann, W. N. (1950). *The medical works of Hippocrates*. Oxford: Blackwell.

Chankova, S. (2018). Why Britain's hospitals are waging war on pyjamas. *The Economist*. June 14. Retrieved from: https://www.economist.com/britain/2018/06/14/why-britains-hospitals-are-waging-a-war-on-pyjamas (Accessed 8 September 2019).

Cortes, O. L., Delgado, S., & Esparza, M. (2019). Systematic review and meta-analysis of experimental studies: in-hospital mobilization for patients admitted for medical treatment. *Journal of Advanced Nursing*, *75*(6), 1823–1837.

Cottage, R. M. (2016). *The writers of Hymns Ancient and Modern*. Norderstedt, Germany: Hansebooks.

de Labra, C., Guimaraes-Pinheiro, C., Maseda, A., Lorenzo, T., & Millán-Calenti, J. C. (2015). Effects of physical exercise interventions in frail older adults: a systematic review of randomized controlled trials. *BMC Geriatrics*, *15*, 154.

Dolan, B. (2017). Mindset shift on PJ paralysis. *Nursing Standard*, *31*(47), 32.

Falvey, J. R., Mangione, K. K., & Stevens-Lapsley, J. E. (2015). Rethinking hospital-associated deconditioning: proposed paradigm shift. *Physical Therapy*, *95*, 1307–1315.

Fortney, S. M., Schneider, V. S., & Greenleaf, J. E. (2011). *The physiology of bed rest*. London: John Wiley & Sons Inc.

Gordon, S., Grimmer, K. A., & Barras, S. (2019). Assessment for incipient hospital-acquired deconditioning in acute hospital settings: a systematic literature review. *Journal of Rehabilitation Medicine*, *51*, 397–404.

Hanson, S., Jones, A., Lane, K., & Penhale, B. (2019). Evidence briefing: hospital-associated deconditioning (HAD). Norwich: University of East Anglia. Retrieved from: https://ueaeprints.uea.ac.uk/id/eprint/71832/1/Evidence_Briefing_HADS_Approved_FINAL_version.pdf.

Hippocrates (1849). *The genuine works of Hippocrates*. London: The Sydenham Society.

Kortebein, P. (2009). Rehabilitation for hospital-associated deconditioning. *American Journal of Physical Medicine & Rehabilitation*, *88*(1), 66–77.

Maggioni, M. A., Castiglioni, P., Merati, G., Brauns, K., Gunga, H. C., Mendt, S., ..., & Stahn, A. C. (2018). High-intensity exercise mitigates cardiovascular deconditioning during long-duration bed rest. *Frontiers in Physiology*, *9*, 1553.

Migeotte, P. F., Monfils, J., Landreani, F., Funtova, I. I., Tank, J., Van De Borne, P., & Caiani, E. G. (2017). Cardiac strength deconditioning after the 60-days head-down bed-rest assessed by heart kinetic energy wearable monitoring. *European Heart Journal*, *38*(suppl 1), 60.

Walthall, H., Jackson, D., & Dolan, B. (2019). Trapped in care: recognising and responding to frailty as a cause of delayed transfers of care. *Journal of Clinical Nursing*, *28*, 5–6.

22

Measuring Progress with Rehabilitation

Yi-Yen Karen Kee

LEARNING OBJECTIVES

- Identify ways of measuring a patient's progress with rehabilitation
- List some of the outcome measures used in clinical practice
- Explain the importance of communicating progress with patients and families

CASE

Gertrude is an 80-year-old woman who is admitted for rehabilitation after a stroke. She has mild left-sided weakness and needs the assistance of one person for most of her activities of daily living (ADLs). Her modified Barthel Index was 20/20 at baseline, but she now scores 11/20. Her modified Rankin score at baseline was 0, but is now 4. Her goal is to get back to normal, and to be able to look after her cat Roger.

WHY DO WE MEASURE PROGRESS?

Measuring a patient's progress is one of the most important tenets of rehabilitation medicine. On an individual patient level, charting progress provides feedback to a patient on how he or she is performing. It allows clinicians to monitor the effects of rehabilitation and help clinicians gauge the speed of a patient's recovery as well as help predict the overall prognosis of a patient.

The ability to measure progress with rehabilitation is also crucial when it comes to clinical research. The use of standardised measures enables clinicians to compare new and different rehabilitation techniques.

There are times when the tools we use to measure progress with rehabilitation may not be sensitive enough to measure the small changes that patients and families see. The outcome measures that are used in clinical practice measure precise functional outcomes which can be different to what families focus on. Families may notice subtle changes which our tools cannot measure. For example, families will notice a patient's ability to smile and react after a large stroke but this may not be consistent enough for a speech therapist to further a patient's communicative ability.

Most multidisciplinary teams (MDT) meet on a weekly basis and will use a variety of measures to monitor a patient's progress. Teams may also have a separate goal setting meeting where new goals are set with patients (see Chapter 10 Setting Rehabilitation Goals). Clinicians use these two processes to see if patients are progressing in the right trajectory.

It can be difficult when patients do not show the progress that they want to make. There are times when patients do not achieve the goals that are set. Measurements of various outcomes may show that patients have plateaued in the rehabilitation process. Patients and their families need to be reassured that these are not necessarily negative outcomes but rather that the process of rehabilitation may no longer be appropriate or beneficial. These are often difficult conversations to have but vital in order to ensure that patients are being cared for in the most appropriate settings. During these discussions, therapists often suggest that they equip families and carers with a range of exercises that can be done outside the hospital setting. Relatives and patients should also be made aware of the importance of having a reassessment of rehabilitation potential if the patient does show a change in their circumstances.

HOW PROGRESS IS MEASURED

Progress with rehabilitation can be measured in various ways. Traditionally, most teams would use well-established and validated tools known as outcome measures. There is a range of outcome measures available to clinicians to use. They can be divided into generic outcome measures or disease-specific outcome measures. There are also outcome measures which are based on patient-centred goals. Goal-orientated outcome measures such as Goal-Attainment Scaling (GAS) look at what patients hope to achieve during rehabilitation and seek to use the goals to measure rehabilitation progress. Lastly, patient-reported outcome measures (PROMs) are outcome measures based on questionnaires completed by patients rather than measures obtained by clinicians. This chapter does not comprehensively detail all the outcome measures that are used in clinical practice but rather gives some examples of the various measures in routine use.

Generic Outcome Measures

These outcome measures tend to measure a patient's general performance in functional tasks. They tend to evaluate a person's functional ability to perform various activities that they may carry out in day to day life. There are a large number of these outcome measures that are used. Listed below are some of the more common scales that therapists use.

The Barthel Index (Barthel & Mahoney, 1965)

This measures performance in various ADLs: feeding, transferring from bed to chair, ability to wash oneself, getting on and off the toilet, ability to carry out grooming tasks, dressing, mobility, climbing stairs, bladder and bowel continence. It is one of the most widely used outcome measures in clinical practice.

Scores can be interpreted as follows:
- 80–100 = Independent
- 60–79 = Needs minimal help with ADLs
- 40–59 = Partially dependent
- 20–39 = Very dependent
- <20 = Totally dependent

The Barthel Index measures what patients are actually doing rather than what they can do.

The Modified Barthel Index

Collin et al. (1988) simplified the scoring and created the more widely used modified Barthel Index which has a total score of 20. Scores range from 0 to 2 or 3 for each activity, and it is easier and quicker to administer than the 100-point Barthel Index. Similar to the Barthel Index, patients can be categorised into various levels of disabilities dependent on the score. A score of <4 indicates total dependence, while a score of <12 indicates some element of dependence.

Functional Independence Measure/Functional Assessment Measure

The Functional Independence Measure (FIM) (Linacre et al., 1994) is another outcome measure that looks at a patient's level of disability. The FIM is more detailed than the Barthel score as it includes not only motor function but looks at cognitive function as well.

The motor subscale includes eating, grooming, bathing, dressing (upper body), dressing (lower body), toileting, bladder management, bowel management, transfers (bed/chair), transfers (toilet), transfers (bath/shower), walk/wheelchair and stairs. The cognition subscale includes comprehension, expression, social interaction, problem solving and memory.

Each item has a score between 1 and 7. The higher the score, the more independent the patient is.
1 Total assistance with helper
2 Maximal assistance with helper
3 Moderate assistance with helper
4 Minimal assistance with helper
5 Supervision or setup with helper
6 Modified independence with no helper
7 Complete independence with no helper

The Functional Assessment Measure (FAM) is another outcome measure that was initially developed by Hall et al. (1993) and modified by Turner-Stokes et al. (1999) to take into account other areas that the FIM did not measure, such as community functioning measures. The FAM does not stand alone but adds another 12 measures. Some of these measures do overlap and it is essential that that FAM is done in conjunction with the FIM.

Therapy Outcome Measures (Enderby, John, & Petheram, 2006)

This outcome measure is based on the International Classification of Function (Üstün et al., 2003) (ICF) which gives us a better framework of understanding how impairments affect patients.

The Therapy Outcome Measures (TOMs) has four separate domains:
1. Impairment
2. Activity/ Disability
3. Participation/ Handicap
4. Well-being/ Distress

Each of the dimensions is rated on a six-point ordinal rating scale: 0 being the severe end and 5 being what is normal for a given person's age, sex and culture. Fig. 22.1 shows the rating in more detail.

The TOMs has been used in across a variety of settings, from acute hospital across into the community. It can be used by various professional groups and takes a more holistic approach at looking at how a patient is progressing with rehabilitation. One benefit of using the TOMs is that even if patients do not show any improvements in their impairment, e.g. their weakness may not have improved, they can improve on other domains such as participation through the use of compensatory techniques or equipment. It is also useful to highlight issues such as a patient's mood as this can impact on how the patient progresses with rehabilitation.

Disease-Specific Outcome Measures

Some outcome measures assess issues relevant to a particular patient group and monitor the impact of a specific disease; for example, the Arthritis Impact Measurement Scale (Meenan, Gertman, & Mason, 1980) and the Ashworth Spasticity Scale (Bohannon & Smith, 1987). These scales tend to be unidisciplined and measure one specific aspect of a person's illness. There are also some disease-specific scales that take into account more general function in a patient.

The modified Rankin Scale and the Timed Up and Go test are two of the examples of more commonly used disease-specific scales used in geriatric rehabilitation.

Modified Rankin Scale

This scale is frequently used for measuring ADLs in people who have suffered a stroke or other cause of neurological disability

Profound		Severe		Severe/ Moderate		Moderate		Mild		Normal
0	0.5	1	1.5	2	2.5	3	3.5	4	4.5	5

FIG. 22.1 TOMs Ordinal Scale (Enderby, 2006).

(Rankin, 1957). It was modified to its current form by Warlow (Van Swieten et al., 1988).

The scale runs from 0 to 6:

0 = No symptoms.

1 = No significant disability, able to carry out all usual activities, despite some symptoms.

2 = Slight disability. Able to look after own affairs without assistance but unable to carry out all previous activities.

3 = Moderate disability. Requires some help, but able to walk unassisted.

4 = Moderately severe disability. Unable to attend to own bodily needs without assistance, and unable to walk unassisted.

5 = Severe disability. Requires constant nursing care and attention, bedridden, incontinent.

6 = Dead.

Timed Up and Go Test

The Timed Up and Go test is a simple outcome measure used to test a patient's mobility – it uses the time taken for a patient to rise from a chair, walk 3 m, turn around and walk back to the chair and sit down (Podsiadlo & Richardson, 1991). This test was initially used to assess the risk of falls in an older population (Mathias, Nayak, & Isaacs, 1986). It is especially useful in patients with Parkinson's disease. A normal score has been suggested to be between 11 and 20 seconds, but different cut-offs have been used in different groups and for different purposes (Podsiadlo & Richardson, 1991).

Goal-Orientated Outcome Measures

These are another set of outcome measures that are used in rehabilitation centres. Here, the therapists set goals for the patients. Achievement of the goals determine the scores that patients receive.

Goal Attainment Scale

GAS is a method of scoring the extent to which a patient has achieved a particular goal during rehabilitation. Here, each patient is their own outcome measure, but the scoring is done in a way to allow statistical analysis.

GAS combines the process of goal setting and evaluation. It encourages patients to be more involved in the setting of goals. There is some evidence that the use of GAS in itself can have a positive therapeutic value (Williams & Stieg, 1986). GAS is a useful tool to demonstrate how patients are or are not achieving their goals.

Each patient goal is rated on a five-point scale: 0 is the score for the patient achieving the expected level. If they achieve more than the expected outcome, they score +1 (somewhat more) or +2 (much more). If they achieve less than the expected outcome, they score –1 (somewhat less) or –2 (much less). The goal outcome score is then combined into a single aggregated T-score (Turner-Stokes, 2009).

GAS consists of a five-point procedure:

1. Identify the goals – these should be set using the SMART principle (see Chapter 10 Setting Rehabilitation Goals).
2. Weigh the goals (optional) – ask patients to rank the goals in order of importance.
3. Define expected outcome – scoring it as previously stated.
4. Scoring baseline.
5. Goal attainment scoring – calculating the score at an appointed review date.

Fig. 22.2 summarises the process of GAS.

Patient-Reported Outcome Measures

PROMs are increasingly used in clinical practice. They are validated patient questionnaires that seek to measure how patients feel about the effects of their treatment. The outcomes that are measured are perspectives from patients rather

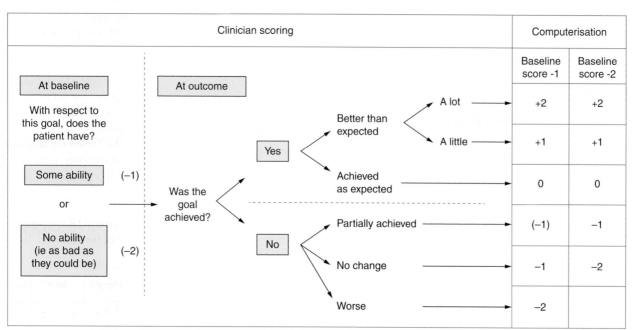

FIG. 22.2 Process of GAS (Turner-Stokes, 2009).

than observations from clinicians. Although they are known as an outcome measure, they measure a patient's health – by comparing a patient's perception of their illness/health at different times (Black, 2013).

There is also a range of PROMs that can be used – disease-specific PROMs created to look at a particular condition, for example the Oxford Hip Score (Dawson et al., 1996), or more generic PROMs looking at quality-of-life measures such as the EuroQol EQ-5D (Haigh et al., 2001).

Cognitive impairment may limit patients' ability to complete the PROMs, and there are various proxy tools that can be used. Various caregiver PROMs have been developed such as the CarerQol-7D (Brouwer et al., 2006) which is useful to measure the impact of illness on caregivers. Researchers have combined various PROMs to create a more specific PROM looking at issues in geriatric care (Lutomski et al., 2013). This particular PROM has been further developed into a shorter version which is easier to administer (Hofman et al., 2014).

COMMUNICATING PROGRESS WITH REHABILITATION

The rehabilitation journey can be a very stressful time for patients and their families. Frequently, patients and their families fear that the rehabilitation process is a pass or fail process. Effective communication is vital in order to help them navigate through the rehabilitation process. Often, the MDT can be made up of a large number of therapists and it may be difficult for people to know who to approach for information.

Most rehabilitation teams use a key-working system to help with effective communication. A keyworker is a person who, with the patient's consent and agreement, takes a key role in coordinating the patient's care and promotes continuity, ensuring the patient knows who to access for information and advice. The keyworker should be a member of the MDT who is involved in the patient's care. The British Society of Rehabilitation Medicine Guidelines highlight the importance of having a keyworker in rehabilitation teams (Turner-Stokes & Ward, 2009). Most teams mandate that the keyworker provides regular updates to families, normally on a weekly basis. This provides the patient and their families with a timely opportunity to ask any questions regarding a patient's rehabilitation progress.

It is also good practice to have wider family meetings with various members of the rehabilitation team, as there are instances when the keyworker may not be able to provide all the relevant information requested by patients and families. These meetings frequently occur later in a patient's journey with the team, but it may be useful to have early family meetings where expectations of a patient's initial rehabilitation goals can be explored. These meetings are helpful when planning a patient's discharge from a rehabilitation team.

Having the outcome measures to hand at these family meetings provides a good discussion platform for planning the next steps in a patient's journey. It is much easier to celebrate the achievements of patients when they have attained their rehabilitation goals and shown improvements in their outcome measures. Teams find it much more challenging for patients and their families when goals are not achieved, and patients are not improving. However, sensitive and thoughtful communications throughout the patient's journey will help.

SUMMARY POINTS

- The use of outcome measures is a way of charting a patient's progress with rehabilitation
- The choice of outcome measure used is dependent on the type of patient being rehabilitated, and their goals
- Weekly MDT meetings are often the best way of discussing patient progress
- Key working can help improve communications with patients and their families
- Good communication will help patients and families to understand the rehabilitation process

MCQs

Q.1 Which statement is correct about outcome measures?
  a. The Barthel Index measures what the patient can do
  b. The FIM/FAM do not need to be used together
  c. PROMs are a measure by clinicians
  d. Goal Attainment Scaling can be done without setting any goals
  e. The Timed Up and Go measures ability to stand from a chair

Q.2 Which statement is correct about rehabilitation?
  a. Rehabilitation is a pass/fail process
  b. Communication within the team is the most important part of rehabilitation
  c. The use of outcome measures can aid family discussions
  d. Rehabilitation goals and outcome measures are not related
  e. Families don't need any updates if rehabilitation is going well

REFERENCES

Barthel, D., & Mahoney, F. (1965). Functional evaluation: the Barthel Index. *Maryland State Medical Journal, 14,* 61–65.

Black, N. (2013). Patient reported outcome measures may transform healthcare. *British Medical Journal, 346,* f167.

Bohannon, R. W., & Smith, M. B. (1987). Interrater reliability of a modified Ashworth scale of muscle spasticity. *Physical Therapy, 67,* 206–207.

Brouwer, W. B. F., van Exel, N. J. A., van Gorp, B., & Redekop, W. K. (2006). The CarerQol instrument: a new instrument to measure care-related quality of life of informal caregivers for use in economic evaluations. *Quality of Life Research, 15*, 1005–1021.

Collin, C., Wade, D. T., Davies, S., & Horne, V. (1988). The Barthel ADL Index: a reliability study. *International Disability Studies, 10*, 61–63.

Dawson, J., Fitzpatrick, R., Carr, A., & Murray, D. (1996). Questionnaire on the perceptions of patients about total hip replacement. *The Journal of Bone and Joint Surgery British Volume, 78*, 185–190.

Enderby, P., John, A., & Petheram, B. (2006). *Therapy outcome measures for rehabilitation professionals* (2nd edn.). John Wiley & Sons.

Haigh, R., Tennant, A., Biering-Sørensen, F., Grimby, G., Marincek, C., Phillips, S., …, & Thonnard, J. L. (2001). The use of outcome measures in physical medicine and rehabilitation within Europe. *Journal of Rehabilitation Medicine, 33*(6), 273–278.

Hall KM, Gordon WA, Zasler ND. (1993). Characteristics and comparisons of functional assessment indices: Disability Rating Scale, Functional Independence Measure, and Functional Assessment Measure. *J Head Trauma Rehabil,* 8(2): 60–74.

Hofman, C. S., Makai, P., Boter, H., Buurman, B. M., de Craen, A. J., Olde Rikkert, M. G., Donders, R. A., & Melis, R. J. (2014). Establishing a composite endpoint for measuring the effectiveness of geriatric interventions based on older persons' and informal caregivers' preference weights: a vignette study. *BMC Geriatrics, 14*(1), 51.

Linacre, J. M., Heinemann, A. W., Wright, B. D., Granger, C. V., & Hamilton, B. B. (1994). The structure and stability of the Functional Independence Measure. *Archives of Physical Medicine and Rehabilitation, 75*, 127–132.

Lutomski, J. E., Baars, M. A., Schalk, B. W., Boter, H., Buurman, B. M., den Elzen, W. P., …, & Melis, R. J. F. (2013). The development of the Older Persons and Informal Caregivers

Survey Minimum DataSet (TOPICS-MDS): a large-scale data sharing initiative. *PLoS One, 8*, e81673.

Mathias, S., Nayak, U. S., & Isaacs, B. (1986). Balance in elderly patients: the "get-up and go" test. *Archives of Physical Medicine and Rehabilitation, 67*, 387–389.

Meenan, R., Gertman, P., & Mason, J. (1980). Measuring health status in arthritis. The arthritis impact measurement scales. *Arthritis and Rheumatism, 23*, 146–152.

Podsiadlo, J. D., & Richardson, S. (1991). The timed Up & Go: A test of basic functional mobility for frail elderly persons. *Journal of the American Geriatrics Society, 39*, 142–148.

Rankin, J. (1957). Cerebral vascular accidents in patients over the age of 60: II. Prognosis. *Scottish Medical Journal, 2*, 200–215.

Turner-Stokes L, Nyein K, Turner-Stokes T, Gatehouse C. (1999). The UK FIM+ FAM: development and evaluation. *Clinical Rehabilitation,* 13(4): 277–87.

Turner-Stokes, L. (2009). Goal attainment scaling (GAS) in rehabilitation: a practical guide. *Clinical Rehabilitation, 23*, 362–370.

Turner-Stokes, L., & Ward, C. (2009). *BSRM standards for rehabilitation services mapped on to the national service framework for long-term conditions.* London: BSRM.

Üstün, T. B., Chatterji, S., Bickenbach, J., Kostanjsek, N., & Schneider, M. (2003). The International Classification of Functioning, Disability and Health: a new tool for understanding disability and health. *Disability and Rehabilitation, 25*, 565–571.

Van Swieten, J. C., Koudstaal, P. J., Visser, M. C., Schouten, H. J., & van Gijn, J. (1988). Interobserver agreement for the assessment of handicap in stroke patients. *Stroke, 19*, 604–607.

Williams, R. C., & Stieg, R. L. (1986). Validity and therapeutic efficacy of individual patient goal attainment procedures in a chronic pain treatment center. *Clinical Journal of Pain, 49*, 219–228.

FURTHER READING

Gupta, A. (2008). *Measurement scales used in elderly care.* Oxford: Radcliffe Publishing Ltd.

COPM. The Canadian Occupational Performance Measure (no date). Retrieved from www.thecopm.ca.

Goal Attainment Scoring Resources. Retrieved from https://www.kcl.ac.uk/cicelysaunders/resources/tools/gas.

23

Keeping People Engaged in Rehabilitation

Shane O'Hanlon & Jenny Basran

LEARNING OBJECTIVES

- Explain the concepts of adherence, motivation and engagement
- Describe ways to maintain and improve motivation in older people during rehabilitation

INTRODUCTION

When rehabilitation goes well, it is a fantastic, effective and transformative process. However, sometimes things are not straightforward; goals can seem far away or unachievable, and it can be common for people to struggle. This can lead to a period of difficulty where patients are not able to gain the most out of rehabilitation. If patient motivation is low, there is a danger that it may be viewed by staff as a 'patient problem'. Staff need to be careful not to label patients as 'not engaging' as this may affect the behaviour of all professionals and in turn, the patient. Healthcare providers should understand how engagement occurs, and that they have a vital role to play in helping to keep people motivated and engaged in their rehabilitation.

ADHERENCE

Many health professionals will be familiar with the term compliance, defined as 'the extent to which the patient's behaviour matches the prescriber's recommendations' (Chakrabarti, 2014). The problem with this concept is that it is entirely one sided – the healthcare professional decides what is best for the patient and tells them to do it. In an era of shared decision making, it is important that such paternalism is left behind. Adherence refers to a process, in which the appropriate treatment is decided after a proper discussion with the patient. It also implies that the patient is under no compulsion to accept a particular treatment, and is not to be held solely responsible for the occurrence of non-adherence (Chakrabarti, 2014). As described in Chapter 10, goalsetting in rehabilitation should be a shared process between patient and provider.

There are many factors that influence adherence in rehabilitation, depending on the setting, the intervention and the population. Sjösten et al. (2007) found that among older people in the community attending group exercises, the strongest predictors of adherence were lower age, low self-perceived risk of falling at home and better functional ability. Stineman (2011) found that on-site exercise for older people had better adherence than home exercise, and that depression negatively affected adherence. There is no doubt that mood can impact rehabilitation, but there are several other reasons – for example medical illness, unsuitable goals, difficulty with the process/environment, amongst many other factors. Keeping people engaged in rehabilitation is a challenge, and when difficulties arise it is important to understand why.

MOTIVATION

Motivation has been identified as an important factor in older adults' recovery from disability (Geelen & Soons, 1996; Resnick, 1998). It consists of two components: an inner urge (or desire) and an action resulting from it (Resnick, 1999). Resnick (1999) interviewed 77 older adults undergoing rehabilitation to understand the factors that influence the efficacy beliefs that motivate them. Eleven major themes were identified – see Table 23.1 for a summary. Some practical suggestions leading from this are as follows: keep pain under control, provide encouragement, practise person-centred care, link with positive role models, provide goals and progress reports, and facilitate expression of spirituality. Motivating factors will vary from person to person, and it is important to get to know what drives someone on an individual level.

ENGAGEMENT

In a review of the literature by Bright et al. (2015), it was found that the process of engagement centred on the development of a connection between the patient and clinician or patient and service, while the state of engagement was an internal state experienced by the patient expressed via a number of observable behaviours. The development of 'a mutually trusting relationship or "connection" between the two parties in the therapeutic encounter' was crucial. This idea of creating a 'true partnership' has been acknowledged to be a challenge, but one that is important to achieve (Chen et al., 2016; Chen, Xiao, & De Bellis, 2016). Another critical concept is responsiveness to the patient, seeing them as a person rather than a diagnosis. This reflects the importance of person-centred care,

117

TABLE 23.1   Factors influencing motivation of older people in rehabilitation (Adapted from Resnick, 2002).

FACTOR	DETAILS
Personal expectations	Beliefs about ability and outcomes
Personality	Basic personality (e.g. being 'determined') helped with motivation
Role models	Seeing others in rehabilitation
Verbal encouragement	From staff, family and friends promotes optimism
Progress	Seeing progress strengthened beliefs about ability
Past experiences	Previous exposure to rehabilitation helped
Spirituality	Faith was reported to influence belief in ability
Physical sensations	Pain and other symptoms impacted negatively
Social supports	A connection with the outside world helped
Individualised care	Recognition of patient as unique person
Goals	Having goals helped motivate

discussed in detail in Chapter 1 Person-Centred Care. The related concept of each patient having their own story is explored in Chapter 19 The Patient Story. A summary of factors that health professionals need to consider to achieve successful engagement is shown in Box 23.1.

Engagement is not a binary process; there is a continuum along which patients may travel as engagement improves (see Fig. 23.1). This travel can happen in both directions, so it is important to be aware of how patients are feeling as well as performing in rehabilitation. For example, adjustment to a new disability may come at a later stage than expected, triggered by difficulty doing something that a patient expected would be easily achieved. These 'bumps in the road' are common in rehabilitation, and need to be faced as a team.

INTERVENTIONS

The first intervention should be to sit down and have a conversation. Patients may not be aware that they are perceived to be having difficulty with engagement. The use of regular meetings or updates to communicate progress with goals can help, and for this to happen there must be a clear rehabilitation plan. When people experience that they develop a mutually shared rehabilitation process, based on a rehabilitation plan, they became more engaged in their rehabilitation and

BOX 23.1   Important Actions for Health Professionals to Help Achieve Successful Patient Engagement

Showing interest in the patient
Being attentive
Being respectful
Doing more than just the basics
Showing empathy
Being knowledgeable
Being credible
Being engaged themselves
Being passionate about their job

gain a better understanding of their participation during the process (Lexell, Lexell, & Larsson-Lund, 2016).

It is also important to remember that people with cognitive impairment or conditions that can affect insight such as Parkinson's disease, may not understand that there

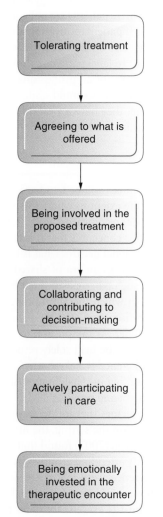

FIG. 23.1   Continuum of engagement.

is a mismatch between therapists' expectations or hopes and their own impression. Clear two-way communication needs to occur to clarify the situation. Advice should also be sought from a speech and language therapist if there are any difficulties with communication.

Once it has been discussed and acknowledged, possible solutions can be explored if there is agreement. As with other elements of rehabilitation, this should be a shared decision-making process. It may be helpful to look at some of the following options, depending on the patient's needs:

- Simple interventions such as ensuring comfortable clothes and shoes, presence of hearing aids and glasses if needed.
- Ensuring the timing of rehabilitation sessions suits the patient's needs and does not clash with mealtimes, personal care or time with loved ones (these are opportunities for rehabilitation interventions in themselves). Agreeing a weekly timetable and providing a copy to the patient is often very useful.
- Check that pain relief has been provided if necessary, and that it is effective.
- Ensure that the person feels they have been listened to, and that any concerns have been addressed.
- Ask families to bring in items related to hobbies or interests, to help patients to have a diversion to look forward to.
- Explore the concept of 'possible selves' – the way in which individuals think about themselves and their future, which may be motivational.
- Cognitive behaviour therapy has been recommended as a motivational tool that improves self-efficacy and has been associated with a lower level of dropout from exercise classes.
- Motivational interviewing has been shown to be associated with an increase in physical activity in older people with heart failure (Brodie & Inoue, 2005).

While strong research evidence is lacking for many interventions, ultimately an individualised patient-centred approach seems likely to be the best method. The importance of hope should not be underestimated; part of the human condition is to dream that things will get better and this can help to keep people engaged. One way to help patients

BOX 23.2 A Sporting Metaphor That Can Help People to Differentiate Goals and Hopes

In this "game" we can see our goal at the other end of the pitch; it's within reach. However our hope is that we win the league – something we cannot see, but thinking about it gives us encouragement, even though it may not happen in the end.

visualise the difference between goals and hopes is using a metaphor, such as that in Box 23.2.

Family

As mentioned in Chapter 7 What Can Patients and Families Do to Help with Rehabilitation?, family members have an important role to play in keeping people motivated. Bogardus et al. (2004) found that caregiver agreement with recommendations predicted adherence to recommendations, suggesting that the rehab team should spend time ensuring carers understand and 'buy in' to the rehabilitation plan. The concept of shared decision making is also important here, and it highlights the need for goalsetting to take on board not just the professional's recommendations but also the aims of the patient and their family. Family members also have a useful role in helping their relative to understand what they are working on in rehab, and why.

Gamification

Gamification and virtual reality are being explored as ways to help people stay active and motivated during or after rehabilitation. Exergames are active video games which combine game play with physical exercise and may also incorporate types of virtual reality simulations. These have the potential to help with motivation and engagement. They have been shown to improve balance, pain and fear of falling in people aged 55 years or older (Stanmore et al., 2019). Fig. 23.2 shows an example of a virtual reality-based exercise programme.

SUMMARY POINTS

- Difficulties with engagement during rehabilitation can come about for many reasons
- Patients should not be expected to resolve issues with engagement or motivation by themselves
- Health professionals have a duty to work with patients to construct a solution together
- Possible interventions include simple patient-centred measures, cognitive behaviour therapy and motivational interviewing

MCQs

Q.1 Regarding adherence, motivation and engagement, which of the following is true?
   a. Adherence is the ability of a patient to do what they are told
   b. Motivation consists of an inner urge and a stimulus to create this
   c. Engagement exists on a continuum rather than a binary level
   d. Engagement consists of a connection between a patient and their family
   e. Motivating factors are consistent from one person to another

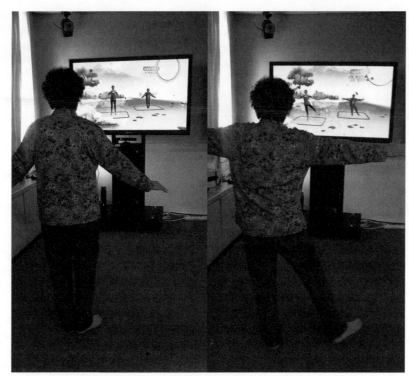

FIG. 23.2 An unsupervised virtual reality-based exercise programme that has been shown to improve hip muscle strength and balance in older adults. (From Kim J, Son J, Ko N, Yoon B. Unsupervised virtual reality-based exercise program improves hip muscle strength and balance control in older adults: a pilot study. *Arch Phys Med Rehabil*. 2013;94(5):937–43, with permission).

Q.2 Which of the following factors influence motivation?

a. Having goals

b. Previous exposure to rehabilitation

c. Seeing others rehabilitate

d. Belief about ability

e. All of the above

REFERENCES

Bogardus, S. T., Jr., Bradley, E. H., Williams, C. S., Maciejewski, P. K., Gallo, W. T., & Inouye, S. K. (2004). Achieving goals in geriatric assessment: role of caregiver agreement and adherence to recommendations. *Journal of the American Geriatrics Society*, *52*(1), 99–105.

Bright, F. A., Kayes, N. M., Worrall, L., & McPherson, K. M. (2015). A conceptual review of engagement in health-care and rehabilitation. *Disability and Rehabilitation*, *37*(8), 643–654.

Brodie, D. A., & Inoue, A. (2005). Motivational interviewing to promote physical activity for people with chronic heart failure. *Journal of Advanced Nursing*, *50*(5), 518–527.

Chakrabarti, S. (2014). What's in a name? Compliance, adherence and concordance in chronic psychiatric disorders. *World Journal of Psychiatry*, *22*(2), 30–36 4.

Chen, L., Xiao, L. D., & De Bellis, A. (2016). First-time stroke survivors and caregivers' perceptions of being engaged in rehabilitation. *Journal of Advanced Nursing*, *72*(1), 73–84.

Geelen, R., & Soons, P. (1996). Rehabilitation: an 'everyday' motivation model. *Patient Education and Counseling*, *28*, 69–77.

Lexell, E. M., Lexell, J., & Larsson-Lund, M. (2016). The rehabilitation plan can support clients' active engagement and facilitate the process of change – experiences from people with late effects of polio participating in a rehabilitation programme. *Disability and Rehabilitation*, *38*(4), 329–336.

Resnick, B. (1998). Self-efficacy in geriatric rehabilitation. *Journal of Gerontological Nursing*, *7*, 1–11.

Resnick, B. (1999). Motivation to perform activities of daily living in the institutionalized older adult: can a leopard change its spots? *Journal of Advanced Nursing*, *1*(4), 792–799.

Sjösten, N. M., Salonoja, M., Piirtola, M., et al. (2007). A multifactorial fall prevention programme in the community-dwelling aged: predictors of adherence. *European Journal of Public Health*, *17*(5), 464–470.

Stanmore, E. K., Mavroeidi, A., de Jong, L. D., Skelton, D. A., Sutton, C. J., Benedetto, V., ..., & Todd, C. (2019). The effectiveness and cost-effectiveness of strength and balance Exergames to reduce falls risk for people aged 55 years and older in UK assisted living facilities: a multi-centre, cluster randomised controlled trial. *BMC Medicine*, *17*(1), 49.

Stineman, M. G., Strumpf, N., Kurichi, J. E., Charles, J., Grisso, J. A., & Jayadevappa, R. (2011). Attempts to reach the oldest and frailest: recruitment, adherence, and retention of urban elderly persons to a falls reduction exercise program. *Gerontologist*, *51*(Suppl 1), S59–S72.

24

The Rehabilitation Environment & Culture

Marie Smith & Lisa Cogan

LEARNING OBJECTIVES

- Describe the rehabilitation environment
- Explain the importance of an outdoor and indoor environment

- Illustrate the impact of enrichment and socialisation on the rehabilitation environment

CASE

Anna is an 82-year-old lady who tripped at home and fractured her right humerus. She was brought to the emergency department for the investigation. She was admitted by the medical team and was transferred to a ward. Anna was in a lot of pain and she wanted to sleep. However, the busyness on the ward contributed to the noise and did not help Anna to rest. Anna required assistance with transferring from a bed to a chair and she found this challenging as she had to wait for the staff to help her out of bed. To add to her frustration, she couldn't enjoy the view through the hospital window because the only thing that she could see was grey buildings.

INTRODUCTION

The environment in a rehabilitation healthcare setting plays an important role in the delivery of patient care; it can have negative or positive impact on patients, the family and treatment outcomes (Rosbergen et al., 2019). Pryor (2000) highlights that creation of a rehabilitation environment should consider external and internal design. The external design should include the adequate location of the building, usage and availability of space, and location of facilities within the building.

There have been a number of frameworks that try to describe and characterise the important parts of healthcare design. For example, Gesler (cited in Lindenmayer et al., 2007), the health geographer, speaks about the concept of 'Therapeutic landscape' that could be included in the healthcare design. The concept includes the physical environment, the social environment and the symbolic environment. Ulrich (1991) points out that the rehabilitation environment should not focus only on functionality and cost, but also on creating a stress-free environment. The concept of a stress-free or a healing environment indicates that the physical environment in a healthcare setting can help patients to either recover quicker or help them to adapt better to their current medical condition. On the other hand, an environment that is not psychologically supportive can have negative consequences on patient health, presenting as increased anxiety, delirium, elevated blood pressure and the increased intake of pain medications.

INDOOR ENVIRONMENT

The healthcare environment in an inpatient setting should be friendly, safe and should respect autonomy, privacy, sense of control and the independence of the patient.

Personalised space is important for patients because it promotes social and spiritual connection between the staff and patients. However, to create a personal space on a Nightingale ward can be challenging. Patients who are staying on a Nightingale ward are using curtains to create a sense of personal space but very often these patients report a low sense of privacy. Ideally, a single room is the choice of most patients; however, some patients are in favour of shared accommodation as they like to have the opportunity to socialise with other patients.

Often rehabilitation settings are not purpose built. Many are located in community hospitals which traditionally provided long term nursing care on Nightingale style units. However, it is still possible to enhance the environment of these units to enable rehabilitation. The availability of a ward dining room where patients can share their meals and socialise with each other is important. Other initiatives include the introduction of a 'Rainbow Route' which is a visual display of colours for participants to walk to. These use the long corridors within older style hospital settings.

Opportunities for socialisation could be created by providing an open plan, central and visible area that encourages engagement and leisure activities and can address a both the patient's and their family's needs (Fig. 24.1). The activity area should be central to the ward and easily accessible by all patients. However, 'one size does not fit all' therefore

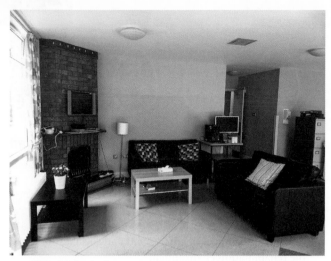

FIG. 24.1   Indoor space to encourage engagement.

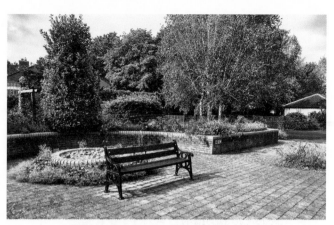

FIG. 24.2   Outdoor hospital garden.

a discreet private area for quiet time may be preferred by some patients and families (Killington et al., 2019). The availability of a coffee shop where patients can go with their family or friends can offer some respite and sense of normality.

In the study presented by Killington et al (2019), patients expressed that access to the facilities is important for them and that it fosters independence. In particular, access to the kitchen and gym facilities at the weekend or outside working hours was an important feature. This can be a challenge to facilitate due to the safety risks of using the equipment unsupervised. Some patients voiced their opinion regarding the insufficient number of basic facilities such as bathroom and toilets and that this could affect their physiological well-being (Ulrich, 1991). The study also highlights the importance of a pleasant décor and clear signage to give directions to facilities. What's more, the lack of clear signage and a noisy environment can often reduce the patient's sense of control and increase stress. Further examples that can help increase a patient's sense of control are televisions in patient and visitor areas, plus a sense of control over lighting and heating and access to gardens and grounds. Encouraging patients to use headphones when watching television reduces the noise on the ward.

Equipment is a key enabler to rehabilitation. Many patients are at risk of pressure ulcers and need specialised seating and cushions to mitigate against this. The availability of supported seating allows patients to sit out during the day. If the patient is non-weight bearing or cannot support their weight, often a wheelchair is necessary. This helps promote their independence and freedom to leave the ward. The availability of powered mobility (powerchair) in patients who are cognitively capable can further foster independence. Patients need to be encouraged and facilitated to dress in their own clothes or clothes that they can easily move around in. Proper footwear is also important. If a patient is dressed in their own clothes, they are more likely to walk around and feel more confident and restore their sense of self.

OUTDOOR/NATURE ENVIRONMENT

Easy access to an outdoor environment is one of the priorities for patients and it positively affects their well-being. Generally patients value a facility that has easy access to beautiful gardens and courtyards (visible from the ward and near the ward) (Fig. 24.2). It gives them the opportunity to meet the family outside a clinical environment. An undercover space to shade in summer and shelter in winter is also appreciated by patients. Frequently nature plays an important role for patients in an inpatient setting. It can help patients recover from attention fatigue that occurs after attending an intense rehabilitation therapy session.

Nature is considered to be multisensory as it includes responses to sounds, smells and visual content. The visual exposure to trees, water and nature can help a patient recover more quickly from stress. Views of everyday nature scenes in comparison to urban scenes are more effective in promoting patient recovery. Nature can facilitate positive feelings and reduce the presence of negative feelings such as anger, fear or sadness. Exposure to nature for a short time, even 10 minutes, can have positive effect on well-being.

Prolonged nature views from the window or a view of an aquarium can have a beneficial healthcare impact on patients and can reduce anxiety and discomfort (Fig. 24.3). In addition, patients who are exposed to pictures of water, flowers or rural landscapes often experience less anxiety in comparison to the exposure of abstract pictures, which are sometimes associated with high anxiety, especially in patients with cognitive impairment.

ENRICHED ENVIRONMENT

An environment that is enriching can increase social, physical and cognitive activities in a rehabilitation setting and can also impact positively on a patient's mood. Patients are also less likely to spend time inactive, alone and are less likely to sleep during the day.

An enriched environment not only facilitates patient activity but also encourages families to drive the activity for the patient, while at the same time supporting the staff in creating a stimulating environment. For example, the use

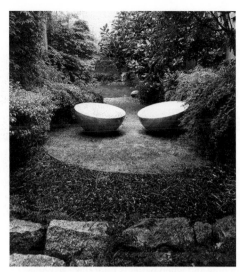

FIG. 24.3   A view from the window.

of equipment such as a computer tablet loaded with therapy apps, music, books, newspapers, games and puzzles according to patients' needs and wishes can be distributed in communal areas. Communal enrichment also involves the provision of an area with easy access to a computer or Wi-Fi that enables patients to have contact with family or with their community such as banks or businesses. Enrichment activities can also be stored at the patient's bedside to allow a patient to move them and use them in other areas. Scheduled group therapies, such as activities or education provided by a therapist, or self-directed activities that encourage the patient to use outside therapy sessions can contribute to enriching the environment.

Information brochures for families on how to support the patient are also an essential part of creating an enriching environment (Janssen et al., 2014; Rosbergen et al., 2019).

SOCIALISATION FACILITATED BY THE ENVIRONMENT

The previous section highlighted the fact that some patients prefer shared accommodation as it reduces their sense of isolation and loneliness. However, if a facility only has single rooms, then it is important to provide a space where patients can meet to relax in a social environment.

In providing such a space patients can meet and discuss their individual journeys, while at the same time facilitating a culture of motivational peer support.

Moreover, peer support helps a patient stay focused, while at the same time empowering them to engage with the rehabilitation process. It is not only patients but also families

who can receive support and understanding from other patients and families that 'I am not alone in this situation' (Ulrich, 1991).

Patients with strong social support experience less stress and feel better in themselves. Studies have also shown that there is an association with lower rates of illness and quicker recovery time. Helping patients to see their pets while they are in the hospital can reduce anxiety and increase mood (Rosbergen et al., 2019). Accessible hospital parking for friends and family as well as flexible visiting times can promote social engagement with the patient.

There are some strategies that can facilitate such social interaction, e.g. providing overnight accommodation for families who are traveling long distances. Another example is the layout of a sitting room that can either foster or hinder social interaction; for instance, in a day room, social interaction can be reduced if chairs are arranged side by side, especially along the walls of the room. Additionally, heavy and unmovable furniture can lessen social interaction in comparison to easily movable furniture that can be arranged in small groupings.

OTHER POSITIVE DISTRACTIONS

A patient's well-being is increased if the environment includes positive stimulation at a moderate level. High-level stimulation such as loud sounds, bright colours or intense lighting can make patients more stressed. On the other hand, low stimulation can produce boredom where patients may focus more on stressful thoughts. For instance, if there are few windows in a facility patients often feel anxious and depressed. On the other hand, the effect of sunlight coming through the window can have a positive effect on length of stay of the patient in the hospital while at the same time reducing their stress and pain levels.

In addition, certain types of sound, music and the use of essential oils can be beneficial for a patient's well-being.

CASE

After some time at the hospital, the medical team recommended that Anna should participate in a rehabilitation programme. She was transferred to the rehabilitation hospital where she stayed for 4 weeks. The hospital was much quieter and had a number of different spaces where she could spend time in private with her family. Moreover, there was a beautiful view of the garden from the dining room. But most of all she appreciated the easy access to the green area that she could enjoy with her family.

SUMMARY POINTS

- The physical environment in a healthcare setting can have a significant effect on the well-being and recovery of a patient
- The healthcare environment should not only focus on functional design but also on creating a psychologically supportive environment

- Nature and an enriching indoor environment can facilitate social interaction and a supportive culture

MCQs

Q.1 A healthcare environment that is psychologically supportive can be described as:
   a. A healing environment
   b. A functional environment
   c. A special environment
   d. Environmental design

Q.2 Socialisation enriched by environment supports a
culture of:
   a. Inclusion
   b. Peer support
   c. Individualism
   d. The organisation

REFERENCES

Janssen, H., Ada, L., Bernhardt, J., McElduff, P., Pollack, M., Nilsson, M., & Spratt, N. (2014). An enriched environment increases activity in stroke patients undergoing rehabilitation in a mixed rehabilitation unit: a pilot non-randomized controlled trial. *Disability and Rehabilitation, 36*, 255–262.

Killington, M., Fyfe, D., Patching, A., Habib, P., McNamara, A., Kay, R., Kochiyil, V., & Crotty, M. (2019). Rehabilitation environments: service users' perspective. *Health Expectations, 22*, 396–404.

Lindenmeyer, A., Hearnshaw, H., Sturt, J., Ormerod, R., & Aitchison, G. (2007). Assessment of the benefits of user involvement in health research from the Warwick Diabetes Care Research User Group: a qualitative case study. *Health Expectations, 10*(3), 268–277.

Pryor, J. (2000). Creating a rehabilitative milieu. *Rehabilitation Nursing Journal, 25*(4), 141–144.

Rosbergen, I., Grimley, R., Hayward, K., & Bauer, S. (2019). The impact of environmental enrichment in an acute stroke unit on how and when patients undertake activities. *Clinical Rehabilitation, 33*, 784–795.

Ulrich, R. (1991). Effects of interior design on wellness: theory and recent scientific research. *Journal of Healthcare Interior Design, 3*, 97–109.

FURTHER READING

Dijkstra, K., Pieterse, M., & Pruyn, A. (2006). Physical environmental stimuli that turn healthcare facilities into healing environments through psychologically mediated effects: systematic review. *Journal of Advanced Nursing, 56*(2), 166–181.

O'Connor, M., O'Brien, A., Bloomer, M., et al. (2012). The environment of inpatient healthcare delivery and its influence on the outcome of care. *Health Environments Research and Design Journal, 6*(1), 104–115.

Common Issues During Rehabilitation

25

Pain

Marissa C Galicia-Castillo

LEARNING OBJECTIVES

- Describe the basic physiology of pain sensation and explain how ageing can affect this
- Provide a framework for assessment of pain in older people

- Explain the principles of non-pharmacological and pharmacological management of pain in older people, both acute and chronic

CASE

Jayden is a 76-year-old male with a past medical history of hypertension and degenerative joint disease of his left hip who presents to the hospital for a left total hip arthroplasty (hip replacement). Surgery went well without any immediate complications. However, on postop day 3, he developed delirium and all of his pain medications were discontinued with the thought that the medications were the cause of his delirium. He was prescribed paracetamol 650 mg Q6 PRN (as required) for pain. He was transferred to a skilled nursing facility for rehabilitation as he lived alone with limited support. On the first day of rehabilitation, he refused to participate, noting his pain was 10/10. He was then prescribed oxycodone 2.5 mg every 4 hours as needed due to the concern about the development of delirium as he had in the hospital. He noted some improvement, but was still limiting participation in therapy. By the third day of his rehabilitative stay, he started participating, but still had significant pain. Nursing staff brought their concern to the physician and the pain regimen was changed to scheduled paracetamol every 8 hours with an additional oxycodone 5 mg one to two tablets every 4 hours as needed and prior to therapy. He was also prescribed a bowel regimen of Senna two tablets at bedtime. This pain regimen allowed him to participate fully in therapy, and pain was better controlled. Because of his pain, he lost 3 days of valuable in-facility rehabilitation before he was discharged home alone. He ultimately returned home with outpatient therapy.

Jayden's case highlights the importance of an effective pain management regimen for a successful rehabilitative stay. There is a fine balance between good pain control and the adverse effects of pain medications.

PHYSIOLOGY OF PAIN

Initially, an injury (stimuli) is experienced by nociceptors in the peripheral nervous system. The stimulus is transmitted to the dorsal root ganglion in the spinal cord. The signal is then sent up to the thalamus in the brain by the spinothalamic tract (ascending pathway) and then to the somatosensory cortex where pain is then perceived. The descending pathway is important in the modulation of pain as well. Neurotransmitters are activated during this process that can affect the pain pathways. Fig. 25.1 illustrates the pathways.

Pain should never be considered a natural part of the ageing process. However, pain perception appears to change with age. These changes may be related to changes in the pain pathway or neurotransmitters that affect their perception of pain. One possible mechanism is a decrease in pain receptors at the skin, but there is no consensus in studies. There may be a decrease in the function of pain receptors. Impairment of the conduction velocities in the fibres of the central nervous system as well as the loss of neurons at the dorsal horns may also be involved. Further research is needed to better understand the changes that occur with pain as we age.

In the rehabilitative environment, the older adult may experience both chronic and acute pain depending on the older adult's pre-existing comorbidities as well as any new injury necessitating the rehabilitative stay. The experience of pain has numerous components including physical, psychological, social and spiritual. Acute pain is a physiological response that alerts us to potential danger. There are two major types of pain: nociceptive and neuropathic. Nociceptive pain is caused by an injury to the body and generally improves with the healing of the injury. Neuropathic pain is caused by abnormalities in the system that carries and interprets pain and is typically felt as a burning, tingling, shooting or electric sensation. Chronic or persistent pain is defined as pain that continues beyond the expected time for healing. This pain lasts for at least 3 to 6 months. For some patients in rehabilitation, there will be a need to consider both acute and persistent pain.

ASSESSMENT

Pain assessment is integral to providing effective pain management. Ideally, pain assessment should focus on an interdisciplinary manner. There is no objective measure for pain. The pain experience is also multidimensional – sensory, emotions, psychological and cultural. Because there is no objective measure for pain, it is difficult to measure the effectiveness of analgesic interventions. A comprehensive pain

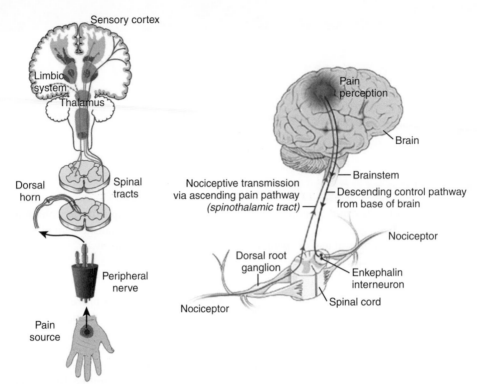

FIG. 25.1 Nerve pathways involved in transmission of pain (left side) and modulation of pain (right side). (From Davis P, Cladis F. *Smith's anesthesia for infants and children*, 9th edn. Elsevier; 2017, with permission).

assessment includes a robust description of the pain: location and quality, radiation, aggravating and alleviating factors, timing, duration, functional goals and intensity. It may be helpful to offer descriptors for your patients to choose if they are having difficulty describing their pain, such as sharp, dull, squeezing, throbbing, sore or colicky. It is difficult to capture all of these aspects in a unidimensional tool. However, these tools are quick, easy to use and provide rapid feedback about effectiveness of treatment.

The Verbal Descriptor Scale (simple descriptive pain intensity scale) uses spoken descriptions: 'no pain', 'mild pain', 'moderate pain', 'severe pain', 'very severe pain' and 'worst pain possible'. The most common is the Numeric Rating Scale which can be used graphically or verbally. Patients are asked to rate the intensity of their pain with '0' indicating and '10' indicating the worst pain imaginable (see Fig. 25.2).

A visual analogue scale such as the Wong Baker Faces Pain Scale is helpful as it is very patient-friendly (Fig. 25.3). While commonly used in the paediatric setting, it has also been tested in older people (Agit et al., 2018).

NON-PHARMACOLOGICAL TREATMENTS

Non-pharmacological treatments may be used in place of or in addition to pharmacological therapies. These treatments can be divided into physical interventions and psychoeducational interventions. Physical interventions include physical therapy, massage, ice, heat, chiropractic manipulation and acupuncture. Psychoeducational interventions include cognitive behavioural therapy (CBT), patient education and meditation.

PHARMACOLOGICAL TREATMENTS

For older patients who have rehabilitative needs, non-pharmacological treatments may not be adequate to control pain and it becomes necessary to utilise pharmacological strategies. In most cases, non-opioid formulations are preferred to opioids. However, it is important to recognise that non-opioid medications are limited and opioids need to be utilised. The strategy best used to maximise pain control and minimise adverse effects is to use the lowest effective dose and slowly increase to achieve pain management with the least amount of adverse effects.

Non-Opioids
Paracetamol (Also Known As Acetaminophen)
Paracetamol is the first-line treatment in the management of pain in the older adult due to its greater safety profile when compared to other medications. The exact mechanism of action is not known. Paracetamol may involve messengers of inflammation and pain, or there may be some effect on neurotransmission. There is not enough supporting evidence to explain paracetamol's actions. Paracetamol does not have any anti-inflammatory effects. When used, the maximum amount of paracetamol should be less than 4 g in a 24-hour period (3 g in some countries, or certain patient populations). It should be noted that paracetamol is a component of many over-the-counter combination

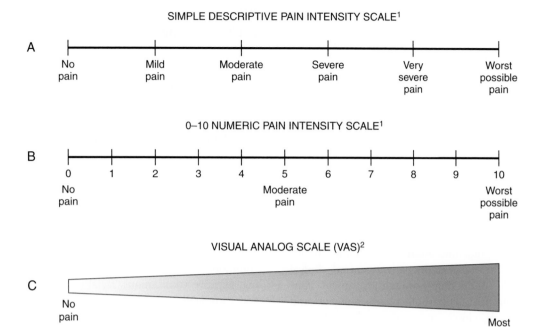

SIMPLE DESCRIPTIVE PAIN INTENSITY SCALE[1]

A

| No pain | Mild pain | Moderate pain | Severe pain | Very severe pain | Worst possible pain |

0–10 NUMERIC PAIN INTENSITY SCALE[1]

B

0   1   2   3   4   5   6   7   8   9   10

No pain   Moderate pain   Worst possible pain

VISUAL ANALOG SCALE (VAS)[2]

C

No pain   Most pain

[1]If used as a graphic rating scale, a 10-cm baseline is recommended.
[2]A 10-cm baseline is recommended for VAS scales.

FIG. 25.2 Examples of pain scales. (From Swartz M. *Textbook of physical diagnosis*, 7th edn. Elsevier; 2014, with permission).

medications and is important to look at all sources of paracetamol have to be specifically reviewed. Typical regimens with paracetamol are 500 mg every 6 hours or 650 to 1000 mg every 8 hours.

Non-Steroidal Anti-Inflammatory Analgesics

In the older adult, non-steroidal anti-inflammatory drugs (NSAIDs) should not be used for long-term pain control. Some common NSAIDs are ibuprofen and diclofenac. NSAIDs should only be used for up to 1 to 2 weeks due to the potential side effects, such as stomach ulcers, hypertension

and kidney impairment, especially in those who have chronic kidney disease, gastropathy and cardiovascular disease.

Adjuvants

Adjuvant (meaning 'add-on') medications include antidepressants and anticonvulsants. Muscle relaxants are also considered adjuvant medications; however, in the older adult they should be avoided due to side effects that include sedation, dizziness, anticholinergic effects and weakness.

Antidepressants are helpful in the setting of persistent pain. This drug class includes selective serotonin reuptake

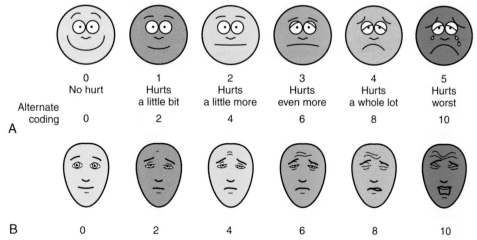

| | 0 No hurt | 1 Hurts a little bit | 2 Hurts a little more | 3 Hurts even more | 4 Hurts a whole lot | 5 Hurts worst |
| Alternate coding | 0 | 2 | 4 | 6 | 8 | 10 |

A

B   0   2   4   6   8   10

FIG. 25.3 Wong Baker Faces Pain Scale. (From Cote C, Lerman J, Anderson B A. *Practice of anesthesia for infants and children*, 6th edn, Elsevier; 2019, with permission.)

inhibitors (SSRIs), selective noradrenalin reuptake inhibitors (SNRIs) and tricyclic antidepressants (TCAs). Due to the high side effect profile and potential for drug interactions, TCAs should be avoided. SSRIs and SNRIs are preferred; however, it should be noted that SSRIs may be associated with a higher fall risk than TCAs.

Anticonvulsants, such as pregabalin and gabapentin, may be helpful in the treatment of neuropathic pain. The common adverse effects for this class of medications include dizziness, drowsiness and fatigue.

Opioids

Due to the concerns of increased opioid use disorder, overdose and death, the US Centers for Disease Control and Prevention has published guidelines for prescribing of opioids (CDC, 2016). These guidelines address prescribing opioids for chronic pain. The focus is on patient-centred clinical practices to include conducting thorough assessment, considering all possible treatments (both pharmacological and non-pharmacological), closely monitoring risks and safely discontinuing opioids.

To avoid adverse effects, it is important to follow the Geriatrics mantra – Start low, Go slow, but use enough.

When choosing an opioid, it is important to consider route of administration, time of onset, duration of action, interactions with other medications, coexisting medical conditions and sensitivity to side effects. Some common side effects from opioids include sedation, dizziness, nausea, vomiting, constipation, physical dependence, tolerance and respiratory depression (which is dose dependent). The ideal route in the rehabilitative setting is oral. Reasonable choices for opioids are oxycodone, morphine and hydromorphone. Oxycodone is sometimes the opioid of choice for older adults due to its short half-life, and it produces no toxic metabolites.

For patients who have renal dysfunction (glomerular filtration rate, <30 ml/min), opioids that are renally cleared should be used with caution. Morphine which produces active metabolites that are renally cleared should be avoided. When dosing opioids, the usual dose should be reduced in the older adult. One strategy is to decrease the initial dose one would give a 40-year-old patient by 25% for a 60-year-old patient and by 50% for an 80-year-old patient. However, the dosing interval should remain the same – Q 4 hours PRN.

SPECIAL POPULATIONS: PATIENTS WITH COGNITIVE IMPAIRMENT

Pain management in older adults with dementia is challenging with little scientific data. Patients with mild to moderate dementia who communicate verbally may provide a reliable report on their perception of pain. The challenge is for those patients who are non-verbal. Similarly in patients with delirium, they may not ask for pain relief due to disorientation or poor attention, so it can be difficult to ensure adequate pain relief.

With ageing, there may be coexistence of sensory and/or cognitive impairment that present a challenge in the older adult. It should be noted that many unidimensional pain tools, including the Numeric Rating Scale, have been validated in older adults. For those patients with cognitive impairment, the tool Pain Assessment in Advanced Dementia (PAINAD) is the most commonly used. The patient is evaluated to monitor breathing, negative vocalizations, facial expressions, body language and consolability. These are all domains that the American Geriatrics Society encourages. The Abbey Pain Scale, which also looks at similar characteristics, is commonly used; however, there is a lack of evidence for its reliability and validity.

PRACTICAL ADVICE

When managing pain, no matter the setting, it is important to manage patient and family expectations. Complete pain relief is uncommon. The treatment goals for pain should focus on improvement of function and quality of life. Pain can be a major obstacle in promoting rehabilitation in an older adult. When pain is a major factor, start with a scheduled paracetamol and provide some opioids for breakthrough pain and incidental pain. Oxycodone 5 mg one to two tablets every 4 hours as needed and prior to therapy can be effective. When prescribing opioids, it is imperative a bowel regimen is also prescribed.

Remember the following:
- Start with non-opioid medications
- Use of scheduled medication
- Close monitoring of adverse effects vs pain relief
- If it is unclear whether an older adult with cognitive impairment is in pain, a trial of pain medication is reasonable.

During this process constant re-evaluation in a multidisciplinary approach is necessary to make adjustments as needed to assure a successful rehabilitative stay.

SUMMARY POINTS

- Pain has to be managed well to promote and support participation in rehabilitation
- When considering pain management start low, go slow, but use enough

- Start with paracetamol – don't be afraid to schedule
- When using an opioid, bowel regimen should be co-prescribed

MCQs

Q.1 Which of the following is the ideal route for administration of pain medications?
  a. Intravenous
  b. Oral
  c. Transdermal
  d. Intramuscular

Q.2 Which medication should be avoided in patients who have kidney impairment?
   a. Oxycodone
   b. Morphine
   c. Paracetamol
   d. Sertraline

Q.3 Which one of the following is NOT an adjuvant medication?
   a. Serotonin reuptake inhibitors
   b. Tricyclic antidepressants
   c. Anticonvulsants
   d. Non-steroidal anti-inflammatory analgesics

REFERENCES

Agit, A., Balci, C., Yavuz, B. B., Cankurtaran, E., Kuyumcu, M. E., Halil, M., Arıogul, S., & Cankurtaran, M. (2018). An iceberg phenomenon in dementia: pain. *Journal of Geriatric Psychiatry and Neurology, 31*(4), 186–193.

Centers for Disease Control and Prevention Public Health Service U S Department Of Health and Human Services. (2016). Guideline for prescribing opioids for chronic pain. *Journal of Pain & Palliative Care Pharmacotherapy, 30*(2), 138–140.

26

Muscle and Joint Problems

Sheila Ryan & Roisin Purcell

LEARNING OBJECTIVES

- Describe how a healthy joint works
- Describe how to recognise common joint and muscle conditions in older people
- Identify best management of these conditions, particularly non-pharmacological management

---

CASE

Rod has rheumatoid arthritis (RA) and osteoarthritis (OA). He is admitted for rehabilitation following a non-injurious fall at home.

He complains of worsening pain in both hands and left knee over the preceding 9 months. He reports having difficulty with walking and has had several falls due to his 'knee giving way'.

He has had increasing difficulty with activities of daily living. One year ago he enjoyed walking 30 minutes daily. He has gained 3 kg in weight. His RA is reasonably well controlled but he gets a flare every few months.

Examination reveals that he is walking with a marked limp. He has a swollen left knee, swollen and tender areas over the small joints of both hands with mild deformities, widespread muscle loss and decreased painful range of movement in his left shoulder.

HEALTHY JOINT STRUCTURE

In order for a joint to work properly there are three things to consider:

1. the physical **anatomy** of the joint,
2. the degree of **support** from the tendons and ligaments, and
3. the **strength** of the muscles surrounding the joint.

Problems in **any** of these areas can lead to issues with how the joint functions, potentially causing discomfort and difficulty. Problems in all three areas carry a much higher risk of pain and dysfunction and present challenges during the rehabilitation process.

Anatomy of a Joint

In a normal healthy joint such as that of the knee in Fig. 26.1, the two surfaces of the bones that form the joint are smooth and covered in cartilage. The joint itself is surrounded by a synovial membrane. The thick layer of cartilage reduces the friction between the two surfaces, allowing the bones to glide on each other easily. This creates smooth and comfortable movement. The membrane around the joint protects the joint surfaces and produces synovial fluid that lubricates the joint and keeps it healthy. Both OA and RA cause changes to the anatomy of the joint, creating issues with the function of that joint.

Support of a Joint

In addition to the physical architecture of the bones, joints also receive secondary support from the ligaments and tendons surrounding the joint, evident in Fig. 26.1.

Ligaments are flat fibrous bands that connect one bone to another and act as reinforced 'scaffolding' for the joint, helping it to 'track' properly during movement.

Tendons are tough bands of collagen tissue, connecting muscle to bone. They serve to transmit the forces from a muscle through to the bone in order to move it.

Both ligaments and tendons can be affected by degenerative (normal age-related changes) and inflammatory conditions, posing risks to the joint's stability and function. As the joint surface changes in response to a degenerative process, more pressure is placed on the ligaments to reinforce the joint and 'hold' it in place. If the ligament system has no previous injury and remains intact, this is usually sufficient to maintain joint stability.

However, in advanced degeneration e.g. OA, the surface can deform to the point where the mechanical stress on the ligaments exceeds their limit and tears of the fibres can occur. This can not only cause pain (depending on the degree of the tear) but creates further uncontrolled movement at the joint, leading to instability and difficulty with function. A similar process occurs in RA where the abnormal swelling in the joint stretches the joint capsule and the ligaments beyond their tensile capacity. Once stretched to this point, ligaments are not able to recover their former shape and strength and thus can develop varying degrees of laxity.

As well as this, the ligament and tendon tissue itself can be affected in inflammatory conditions such as RA and if left untreated can cause tissue breakdown leading to complete rupture and instability of the joint.

Clinically this situation is most evident in the hands (causing significant deformity and dysfunction with manual

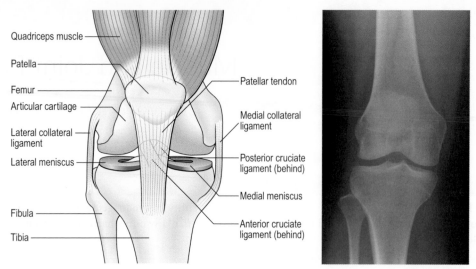

FIG. 26.1   Knee anatomy. (From White TO, Mackenzie S, Gray A. *McRae's Orthopaedic Trauma and Emergency Fracture Management*, 3rd edn. Elsevier; 2015, with permission.)

tasks), feet (causing deformity and difficulty walking) and knees (creating instability when weight bearing and increased risk of falling).

Strength of Muscles Around a Joint

Impairments such as muscle weakness, slowing of movement and early muscle fatigue are common features in the older person. Natural strength decline typically starts during the third decade of life and accelerates during the sixth and seventh decades (Marcell, 2003). As a result, many older people expose their joints to excessive strains simply as a result of impaired muscle function. These abnormal forces can accelerate the degenerative process outlined earlier and contribute to joint pain and functional difficulty. This contributes to a 'vicious cycle' of inactivity, where the person avoids any manual tasks, and becomes gradually weaker and less able as a result, which further increases pain, avoidance, etc. This creates a spiral of rapid deconditioning which can often result in injury, most commonly by way of a fall. Subsequent prolonged inactivity during and after hospitalisation can lead to the rapid decline of the muscular system, making recovery difficult and the outcomes of rehabilitation poorer (Kortebein et al., 2008).

COMMON JOINT AND MUSCLE CONDITIONS IN OLDER PEOPLE

There are over 200 rheumatological conditions (common diseases affecting tendons, ligaments, bones and muscles), including:

Osteoarthritis (OA) is the most common joint disorder and accounts for more disability in older people than any other disease. It is a slow, non-inflammatory disorder that typically affects the joints of the hands, spine, and weight-bearing joints (hips, knees, first metatarsophalangeal [MTP] joint) of the lower limb. In OA, the cartilage layer breaks down

and causes the bones to rub up against each other, creating friction. Other features include osteophyte (spur) formation and subchondral remodelling and hypertrophy (sclerosis). OA can affect how the joint moves, making it stiff and rigid. It can be associated with joint pain, particularly after activity, stiffness after immobility, crepitus (crackling) and reduced range of movement.

Rheumatoid arthritis (RA) is the most common chronic inflammatory arthritis. The cause is unknown but it is related to an abnormal function of a person's immune system. In RA, the synovial membrane (inner lining of joints) becomes inflamed (synovitis), causing swelling, pain and stiffness. Over time, ongoing inflammation in the joint can cause erosions of the joint surface, creating a deformity. Symmetrical synovitis of the small joints of the hands and the wrists is common. Specialist medications called disease-modifying antirheumatic drugs (DMARDs) are used to control this abnormal inflammatory immune response and help to slow the progression of the disease. Early and aggressive therapy with DMARDs should target low disease activity for optimal outcomes (Anderson et al., 2000). Patients have accelerated atherosclerosis (build-up of plaque that narrows arteries) making management of vascular risk factors (e.g. smoking, high blood pressure) an important feature (Aviña-Zubieta et al., 2008). Extra-articular (outside the joint) manifestations also require careful management. Some areas that can be affected include the eyes (scleritis, episcleritis), the lungs (pleuritis, interstitial lung disease), the skin (vasculitis, subcutaneous nodules), the heart (pericarditis, myocarditis) and the nerves (peripheral neuropathy).

Gout is a disease where the deposition of urate crystals occurs as a result of excessive urate in the blood (hyperuricemia). Recurrent flares of inflammatory arthritis are common, along with chronic joint pain (arthropathy), deposits of urate crystals (tophi), kidney stones and kidney impairment. The diagnosis of gout is best achieved by examining synovial fluid under a microscope and confirming the presence of the crystals. As gout is associated with diet, obesity and the metabolic syndrome, dietary and lifestyle modifications are important. Management also includes a review of prescribed medications to determine if they are contributing (e.g. diuretics such as frusemide or bendroflumethiazide; low-dose aspirin, levodopa).

First-line treatment of an acute flare of gout is often non-steroidal anti-inflammatory drugs (NSAIDs). However, many older people cannot tolerate these drugs due to their side effect profile, and alternatives such as colchicine or steroids are preferentially used. Urate-lowering therapy (allopurinol) should not be started until after complete resolution of the acute gouty attack, nor should it be stopped if an acute gouty attack occurs while the patient is on allopurinol (Khanna et al., 2012; Qaseem, Harris, & Forciea, 2017).

Polymyalgia rheumatica (PMR) is a common inflammatory disorder in older people. Patients present with subacute onset of severe pain and stiffness, often in the shoulders or thighs, and a high ESR (erythrocyte sedimentation rate) on blood testing. Treatment with steroids at a dose of 15–20 mg/day usually results in a rapid and dramatic improvement.

Sarcopenia is a progressive and generalised skeletal muscle disorder involving the accelerated loss of muscle mass and function that can be associated with poor outcomes, including falls, functional decline, frailty and mortality. It is often associated with rheumatological conditions. It can occur at any age but is most frequently seen in older people. Research is ongoing to explore how best to understand, treat and prevent sarcopenia, mainly with nutrition and resistance training (Marcell, 2003).

NON-PHARMACOLOGICAL MANAGEMENT OF RHEUMATOLOGICAL CONDITIONS IN OLDER PEOPLE

It is important to be aware of the disease process at work as it will have implications on the management plan. For example, an exercise programme for an older person with OA or RA might need to include stretching and movement exercises in a sitting or lying position initially, in order to get the joint moving comfortably before progressing to weight-bearing positions. Table 26.1 outlines management in specific conditions.

TABLE 26.1 Common joint and muscle problems.

CONDITION	PRESENTATION	MANAGEMENT
Rheumatoid arthritis flare	Associated with flare of disease activity. Visible swelling and increased temperature at joint, associated with pain and stiffness especially following prolonged inactivity	Cold therapy, anti-inflammatory medication, gentle movement through available range and avoidance of prolonged positions. May require medication review
Degenerative meniscus tear	Develops over years. Presents in older people without history of injury. Knee may catch or lock. Pain on turning or pivoting	Short-term over-the-counter pain medication. Strengthening exercises to develop muscle strength and control around knee joint
Popliteal cyst (Baker's cyst)	Swelling behind knee, knee pain, inability to fully bend the joint	Rest, ice, compress and elevate. Range of movement and strengthening exercises
Rotator cuff tear	Can be acute following injury but usually associated with a degenerative process in the older person. Pain, weakness and difficulty with movement	Progressive exercise-based rehabilitation programme guided by a physiotherapist (Ainsworth, Lewis, & Conboy, 2009)
Adhesive capsulitis (e.g. frozen shoulder)	Develops over time, associated initially with pain, progressively worsening stiffness and marked loss of movement	Often self-limiting and will resolve with time. Range of movement exercises to maintain range as best as possible and over-the-counter pain medication to manage symptoms. May benefit from ultrasound-guided intra-articular (into the joint) injection (Neviaser & Hannafin, 2010)
Bursitis	Often can occur after prolonged pressure on superficial joints, e.g. on elbow or kneeling. Pain and localised swelling	Joint protection strategies. Cold therapy. Exercises to maintain range
Tendinopathy	Localised pain often related to overloading. Frequently stiff at night and early in morning, symptoms can initially ease with movement but worsen with further activity. Exists on a continuum from mild to severe symptoms (Rees, Maffulli, & Cook, 2009)	Progressive exercise-based rehabilitation programme guided by a physiotherapist

Physical Exercise is an Essential Component in the Management of Rheumatological Conditions

- **Aerobic activity** is important to improve cardiovascular fitness. Swimming, walking, stationary bicycling, elliptical training and treadmill walking are all recommended activities for people with rheumatological conditions. As with any new physical activity programme, activity levels should be suited to the person's existing fitness level and physical capacity and increased gradually. For example, this might mean starting initially with a walk twice a day for 15 minutes at a time and gradually increasing this to a brisk walk for 30 minutes over time. The aim is to reach an intensity which is sufficient to elevate the heart rate to 75% of maximum (220 minus age) for 20–40 minutes (Garber et al., 2011; Riebe et al., 2018; Roddy et al., 2005).
- **Strength or resistance training** is highly recommended, particularly in people with knee OA and those with sarcopenia. Studies examining the effects of resistance training on OA show improvements in pain and function (Garber et al., 2011; Riebe et al., 2018; Roddy et al., 2005). Exercise in partial- or low load-bearing positions initially, e.g. in a water environment or on a stationary bike, can be especially beneficial for a patient to engage in strengthening exercise without putting their ligaments or tendons under excessive load. Once able to take further weight through the joint, people should be progressed to a controlled weight-bearing programme.
- **Balance retraining** is an essential component in rehabilitation of older people with muscle and joint problems (for more information, see Chapter 12 Physiotherapy: How It Works).

Symptom management is important to facilitate exercise and physical activity. Whilst ice and heat can be safely used interchangeably for an osteoarthritic joint, the use of heat in an actively swollen RA joint is advised against as it will bring further blood flow to the area, increasing the swelling, adding to the symptoms. Cryotherapy (cold application) is the recommended management for a joint experiencing an acute flare of disease activity. This can be easily applied by placing a cold pack over the joint for periods of no more than 15 minutes and never directly on the skin itself.

Used appropriately, heat can have several beneficial effects. It can increase tendon and joint capsule extensibility, reduce muscle spasm, provide analgesic affect, increase tissue blood flow and increase tissue metabolism. Superficial joints are easy to heat with hot packs, paraffin wax, radiant heat and certain topical creams. Heat can be applied both before and after physical activity to help manage any mild discomfort that is normal to occur during exercise.

Relative rest for appropriate periods of time is an essential part of the rehabilitation process. Although rest periods can be beneficial for recovery and symptom management, prolonged rest for RA is not recommended as extended periods of inactivity will increase the inflammatory response, creating further symptoms for the patient. Prolonged periods of inactivity, particularly bed rest, can have significant negative effects on a patient's overall muscle strength and endurance and should be avoided (Kortebein et al., 2008).

Education around techniques to optimise function and reduce harm is important. For example, explaining to a patient with symptomatic knee OA that the best way to go up the stairs is to lead with the good leg and lead with the bad leg coming down (up to heaven, down to hell).

Education around avoiding extremes of movement and assistive devices (splints, walking aids) to reduce abnormal stresses on ligaments are very useful to protect and maintain ligamentous integrity.

Explaining and demonstrating how to effectively use a mobility aid is important. If using a single crutch or walking stick, the handle of the aid should be at the same height as the patient's wrist and should be used in the opposite side to the leg that is symptomatic (e.g. swollen and inflamed right knee causing poor balance and a limp, use stick in left hand).

A rehabilitation programme should consider:

1. The extent of pain, inflammation, weakness and deformity
2. General medical condition and stage of disease
3. The activities that the patient enjoys
4. Cognition

Goals of a rehabilitation programme:

1. Maintain or improve range of movement
2. Prevent contractures
3. Increase strength and enhance endurance
4. Maintain or improve function in personal, professional and community life
5. Improve overall sense of well-being
6. Self-management
7. Understand the need and value of regular exercise (an exercise prescription)

PHARMACOLOGICAL MANAGEMENT

Pain management is essential to optimise outcomes for people with joint and muscle conditions, particularly arthritis. Non-pharmacological management is hugely important but often needs to occur in combination with medications.

The approach to pharmacological management is 'Start low (lowest dose possible), go slow (small increments if needed to optimise response) and review regularly (ideally daily)'. As mentioned, oral NSAIDs are best avoided in older people; however, topical (e.g. cream or gel) non-steroidal preparations are often used with good effect.

Although there is debate about the evidence for its use in arthritis, regular paracetamol is recommended first line as its side effect profile is good. Sometimes low-dose opiates (e.g. codeine) may need to be used (Zhang et al., 2007, 2008).

Intra-articular injections of steroids are sometimes considered for those with significant pain, an effusion and minimal structural damage (Zhang et al., 2007, 2008).

MANAGEMENT PLAN FOR ROD

- Bloods tests to evaluate the activity of RA.
- Medication review and optimisation. Consider adjustments to the disease-modifying agents given activity suggesting synovitis in the hands.
- Symptomatic treatment could include a trial of ice to left knee OA.
- Provision of walking stick in right hand to support left knee, thereby reducing painful loading temporarily and reducing the risk of falling.
- Hand exercise programme to target impairments. Advice on rest and functional positions for hands. Assess for the use of splints.

- Hand exercise programme to target impairments. Advice on rest and functional positions for hands. Assess for the use of splints.
- Graduated return to walking programme.
- As symptoms resolve and function improves, focus should move to higher level muscle strengthening and dynamic balance work.
- Education and advice about weight management, flares, role of medication and appropriate regular physical activity levels.

SUMMARY POINTS

- Muscle and joint problems are common in the older person
- A multidisciplinary approach to management is recommended
- Consider non-pharmacological approaches
- Exercise in chronic rheumatological conditions should be seen as a prescribed essential treatment

MCQs

Q.1 Which one of the following is the usual treatment for gout?
  a. Review of medication
  b. Colchicine
  c. Steroids
  d. Exercise
  e. All of the above

Q.2 Heat treatment should not be used to:
  a. Manage pain in chronic OA of the knee
  b. Relieve spasm and muscular pain in the back
  c. Reduce acute rheumatoid inflammation
  d. All of the above

Q.3 The best approach to manage pain of osteoarthritis in older people is:
  a. Bed rest
  b. Non-steroidal anti-inflammatory medications
  c. High-dose opiate medication
  d. None of the above

REFERENCES

Ainsworth, R., Lewis, J., & Conboy, V. (2009). A prospective randomized placebo controlled clinical trial of a rehabilitation programme for patients with a diagnosis of massive rotator cuff tears of the shoulder. *Shoulder & Elbow*, *1*(1), 55–60.

Anderson, J. J., Wells, G., Verhoeven, A. C., & Felson, D. T. (2000). Factors predicting response to treatment in rheumatoid arthritis: the importance of disease duration. *Arthritis and Rheumatism*, *43*(1), 22–29.

Aviña-Zubieta, J. A., Choi, H. K., Sadatsafavi, M., Etminan, M., Esdaile, J. M., & Lacaille, D. (2008). Risk of cardiovascular mortality in patients with rheumatoid arthritis: a meta-analysis of observational studies. *Arthritis and Rheumatism*, *59*(12), 1690–1697.

Garber, C. E., Blissmer, B., Deschenes, M. R., Franklin, B. A., Lamonte, M. J., Lee, I. M., Nieman, D. C., & Swain, D. P. (2011). American College of Sports Medicine position stand. Quantity and quality of exercise for developing and maintaining cardiorespiratory, musculoskeletal, and neuromotor fitness in apparently healthy adults: guidance for prescribing exercise. *Medicine and Science in Sports and Exercise*, *43*(7), 1334–1359.

Khanna, D., Khanna, P. P., Fitzgerald, J. D., Singh, M. K., Bae, S., Neogi, T., …, & Terkeltaub, R. (2012). American College of Rheumatology guidelines for the management of gout. Part 2. Therapy and anti-inflammatory prophylaxis of acute gouty arthritis. *Arthritis Care and Research*, *64*(10), 1447–1461.

Kortebein, P., Symons, T. B., Ferrando, A., Paddon-Jones, D., Ronsen, O., Protas, E., …, & Evans, W. J. (2008). Functional impact of 10 days bed rest in healthy older adults. *The Journals of Gerontology A: Biological Sciences and Medical Sciences*, *63*(10), 1076–1081.

Marcell, T. (2003). Sarcopenia: causes, consequences and preventions. *The Journals of Gerontology A: Biological Sciences and Medical Sciences*, *58*(10), 911–916.

Neviaser, A. S., & Hannafin, J. A. (2010). Adhesive capsulitis: a review of current treatment. *American Journal of Sports Medicine*, *38*(11), 2346–2356.

Qaseem, A., Harris, R. P., & Forciea, M. A. (2017). Management of acute and recurrent gout: a clinical practice guideline from the American College of Physicians. *Annals of Internal Medicine*, *166*(1), 58–68.

Rees, J. D., Maffulli, N., & Cook, J. (2009). Management of tendinopathy. *American Journal of Sports Medicine*, *37*(9), 1855–1867.

Riebe, D., Ehrman, J., Liguori, G., & Magal, M. (2018). *ACSM's guidelines for exercise testing and prescription* (10th edn.). Philadelphia: Wolters Kluwer.

Roddy, E., Zhang, W., Doherty, M., Arden, N. K., Barlow, J., Birrell, F., …, & Richards, S. (2005). Evidence-based recommendations for the role of exercise in the management of osteoarthritis of the hip and knee – the MOVE consensus. *Rheumatology*, *44*(1), 67–73.

Zhang, W., Doherty, M., Leeb, B. F., Alekseeva, L., Arden, N. K., Bijlsma, J. W., …, & Zimmermann-Górska, I. (2007). EULAR evidence based recommendations for the management of hand osteoarthritis: report of a Task Force of the EULAR Standing Committee for International Clinical Studies Including Therapeutics (ESCISIT). *Annals of the Rheumatic Diseases, 66*(3), 377–388.

Zhang, W., Moskowitz, R. W., Nuki, G., Abramson, S., Altman, R. D., Arden, N., …, & Tugwell, P. (2008). OARSI recommendations for the management of hip and knee osteoarthritis, part II: OARSI evidence-based, expert consensus guidelines. *Osteoarthritis and Cartilage, 16*(2), 137–162.

27

Posture

Timothy L. Kauffman

LEARNING OBJECTIVES

- Explain deleterious age-related postural changes and how they impact functional mobility
- Describe the complex interactions of connective tissues and the neuromusculoskeletal systems that contribute to postural control
- Outline how to recognise the potential for improvement in posture

CASE

Emily, a 79-year-old female, complains of moderate to severe back pain, worse in the thoracolumbosacral areas but she also commonly gets upper back, neck and bilateral shoulder pain. She has not experienced any recent trauma. Her symptoms impair her walking and sleep and have diminished her quality of life. She presents with a significant medical history of osteoporosis with fractures of several ribs and multiple thoracic and lumbar vertebral compressions. She also has a moderate spinal kyphoscoliosis with her lower ribs painfully resting on her iliac crests. She is alert, oriented, lives alone and drives. Her goals are to decrease pain, improve her mobility, stop further postural degradations and avoid further fractures.

INTRODUCTION

Age-related postural changes are ubiquitous and almost never addressed by healthcare providers yet are critical to mobility and quality of life. Posture is the alignment of body parts in relationship to one another at any given moment. Posture involves complex interactions between bones, joints, connective tissue, skeletal muscles and the nervous system, both central and peripheral (Pauelsen et al., 2018b). The complexity of these interactions is compounded when one considers the variety of human balance, motor control and movement in relation to gravity and may be a factor in falls. Furthermore, with the passage of time, each person undergoes change resulting from microtrauma, frank injuries and the effects of disease on the neuromusculoskeletal system which result in the common and unique variations of ageing posture.

Posture is appropriately assessed using a grid or plumb line, with the patient in a static standing position; however, within the ageing population, this becomes more difficult because of the age-associated increase in postural sway. This can be seen in the two photos in Fig. 27.1 of a 98-year-old man taken only moments apart. The postural control mechanisms produce minor shifts in weight in order to avoid fatigue, excessive tissue compression and venous stasis. Hence, a photographic assessment of posture represents a fixed instant of a postural set. Thus, posture is actually a relative condition requiring full body integration and both static and dynamic balance control, as shown in Fig. 27.2.

Multiple factors are involved in common age-related postural changes. These factors may be pathological, degenerative or traumatic, or may result from primary musculoskeletal changes, primary neurological changes or a combination of diminutions in the neuromusculoskeletal system.

Degenerative joint disease is a common age-related pathology involving bony and joint surface changes (see Chapter 26 Muscle and joint problems). The osteophytes that result from arthritis may prevent normal joint motion, cause pain and possibly encroach on nerves with a subsequent radiculopathy ('pinched nerve') that includes muscle weakness and imbalance. Postural adjustments may be the result of attempts to unload weight from an osteophyte in order to reduce pain or to accommodate a radiculopathy/neuropathy (Muchna et al., 2018).

AXIAL AND APPENDICULAR SKELETAL CHANGES

The common age-associated postural changes in the axial skeleton and their clinical implications are enumerated in Table 27.1 and may be seen in Figs 27.3 and 27.4. The idiosyncratic effects of 20 years of ageing can be seen by comparing the images of the 78-year-old man in Figs 27.3B and 27.4B with the photographs in Figs 27.1 and 27.5, which were taken when the man was 98 years old. In the lateral view, note the large increases in trunk kyphosis (outward curvature of the spine) and hip flexion. By comparing images of the posterior view at different ages (Figs 27.4B and 27.5), the kyphoscoliosis

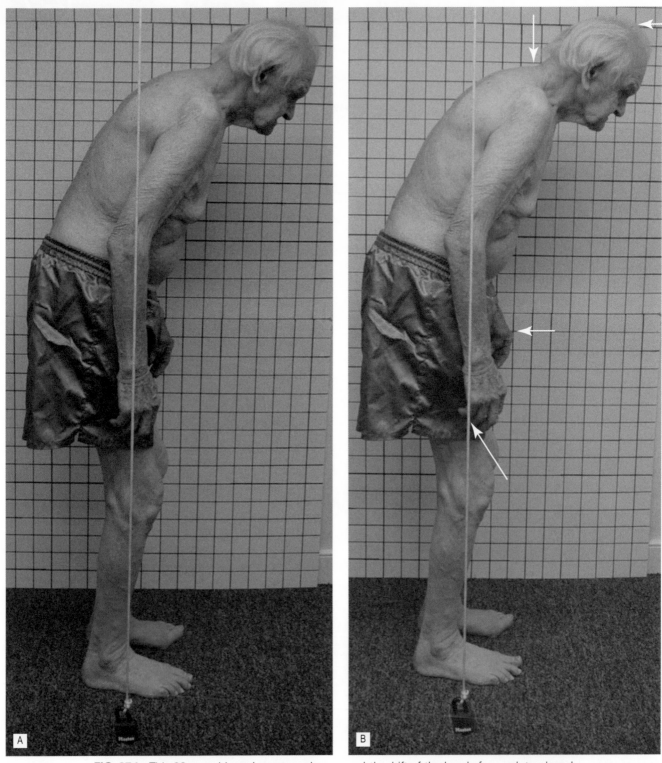

FIG. 27.1 This 98-year-old man's posture shows a subtle shift of the hands forward, trunk and head more erect and right great toe extension. The photos were taken less than 1 second apart.

(a combination of kyphosis and lateral curvature (scoliosis) of the spine) with upper extremity extension, increased hip and knee flexion and loss of muscle mass in all four extremities and trunk are evident. A different individual, aged 93 years and shown in Fig. 27.3C, also demonstrates extension of the upper extremities. The 98-year-old man's postural set (Figs 27.1

and 27.5) may be affected by his complaints of right hip pain, and decreased sensation and strength in the lower extremities. He lives in assisted living and uses a wheeled walker for most ambulation.

It is important to note that not all of these changes should be classified as being faulty or abnormal. Some of the

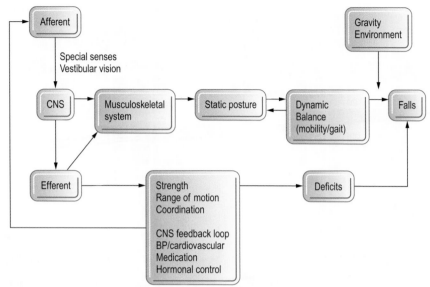

FIG. 27.2 Factors affecting posture and falls. Multiple interactive forces govern static posture and dynamic balance. *BP*, Blood pressure; *CNS*, central nervous system. (From Kauffman T. Impact of ageing-related musculoskeletal and postural changes on falls. *Top Geriatr Rehabil.* 1990;5:34–43.)

adjustments may be normal compensatory changes resulting from other neuromusculoskeletal alterations in the spine, extremities or central control mechanisms (Barreyet al., 2011). For example, the head-forward position, especially when there is an increased extension of the upper cervical spine, may be the result of the body's attempts to counter a dorsal kyphosis caused by wedged thoracic vertebrae.

The effect of osteoporosis in the vertebrae on posture and vice versa is profound, with an abundance of recognised and silent fractures and probable microfractures (see Chapter 38 Bone Health and Chapter 46 Vertebral and Lower Limb Fractures and Surgery). Katzman et al. (2012) found hyperkyphosis, an exaggerated anterior concavity or 'dowager's hump' to be associated with older age, less

body weight, lower spine bone mineral density and spine muscle density.

Spinal spondylosis is found in the vast majority of people by the age of 55 years. This may include deterioration of the spinal facet joints, loss of vertebral height, narrowing of the spinal canal or neural foramina, loss of intervertebral disc space, anterior lipping, formation of bony bridges and calcification of the periarticular connective tissue. Clinically, these changes may cause pain and reduction in spinal motions, especially the subtle rotation motions involved in segmental rolling and the normal reciprocal pattern of the extremities in normal gait. The sit-to-stand motion may be more difficult because of the loss of coordinated spine flexion and extension.

TABLE 27.1	Age-associated postural axial skeletal changes and their clinical implications.
AXIAL SKELETAL CHANGES	**CLINICAL IMPLICATIONS**
Head forward	Shifts centre of mass forward; may increase dizziness because of a compromised basilar artery
Dorsal kyphosis	Reduces trunk motions for breathing and motor responses; encourages scapular protraction; may provoke shoulder pathologies
Flat lumbar spine	Reduces trunk/hip extension for gait strides
Occasional kyphosis of lumbar spine	Results from compression of vertebral bodies; not reversible
Increased lordosis (least common)	Results in tightness of trunk/hip extensors; weakened abdominals
Posterior pelvic tilt	Results from prolonged sitting; reduces trunk/hip extension for gait strides
Scoliosis	May alter balance, breathing and extremity motions

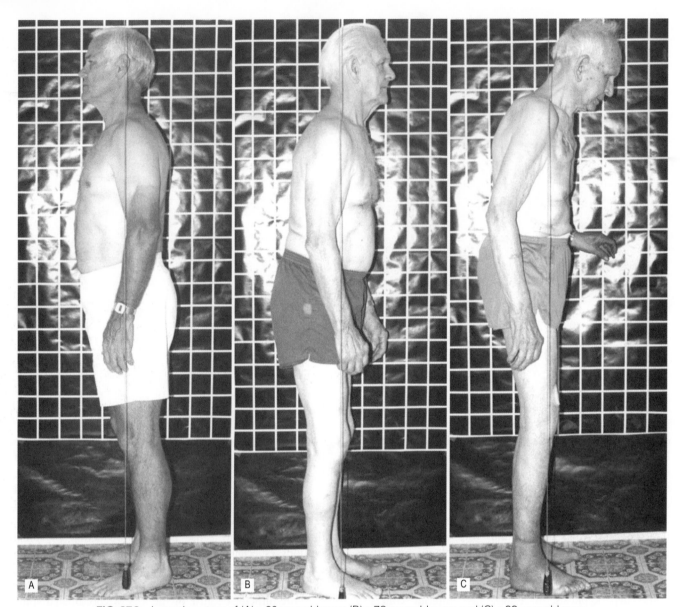

FIG. 27.3   Lateral posture of (A) a 60-year-old man; (B) a 78-year-old man; and (C) a 93-year-old man.

In the appendicular skeleton, numerous combinations of changes occur as a result of a lifetime of wear and tear, habit, trauma and pathology in the neuromusculoskeletal system. These changes result in the unique postural features of ageing individuals. The common age-associated extremity changes and clinical implications are enumerated in Table 27.2 and may be seen in Figs 27.3 and 27.4.

SOFT TISSUE

Postural changes caused by soft-tissue alterations may be a result of previous injuries that have lengthened or tightened tendons, ligaments and joint capsules. Collagen, a major component of skin, tendons, cartilage and connective tissue, may become increasingly stiff because of cross-linkage between fibres. Elastin is another major fibrous component of connective tissue found in skin, ligaments, blood vessels and lungs. With increasing age, elastin is supplanted by pseudoelastin, which is a partially degraded collagen or faulty elastin protein.

Additional soft-tissue changes that may lead to postural alterations can be found in the muscle. The muscle length may be increased or decreased. There is a loss of muscle fibres, which is likely to result in reduced strength. Type II muscle fibres are denervated and reinnervated as type I as ageing progresses (Ditroilo et al., 2012), thus altering the fibre relationship, possibly influencing postural control responses and mechanisms. In addition, there is an increase in non-contractile tissue because of deposition of fat and collagen, causing the muscle to become increasingly stiff. Muscle tone may increase, decrease or vary because of changes in nervous system control.

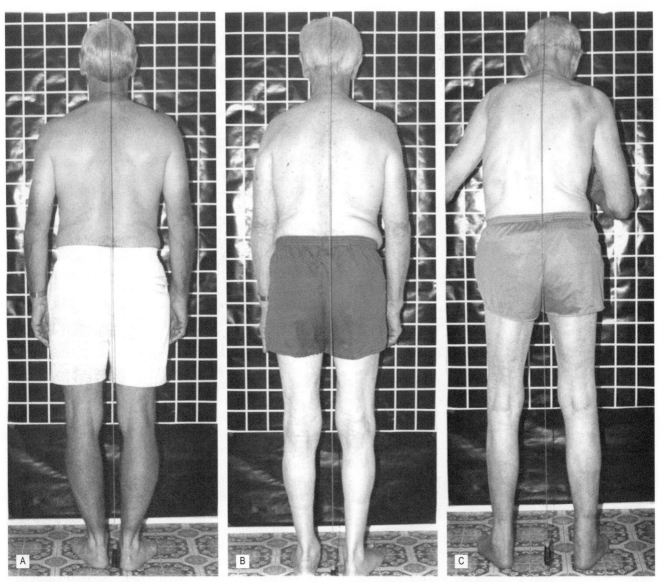

FIG. 27.4   Posterior posture of (A) a 60-year-old man; (B) a 78-year-old man; and (C) a 93-year-old man.

CLINICAL CONSIDERATIONS

Falls are significant problems for older people and may represent a failure of the neuromusculoskeletal posture control system as well as falls-related concerns like fear of falling (Pauelsen et al., 2018a). Centrally, the basal ganglia and cerebellum have important roles in modulating posture. Backward disequilibrium is associated with vascular lesions in the brain, normal pressure hydrocephalus and hypertonia of extensor muscles (Manckoundia et al., 2008). In response to postural perturbations, older persons used an increased active stiffness and damping (reduces oscillations) to control sway when compared to younger subjects, and this may represent degradation in sensory and motor function (Cenciarini et al., 2010).

The occiput to the wall is a simple and easy clinical assessment of upright posture. It is done by having a person standing with back to a wall or doorframe and measuring the distance of the occiput to the wall. It has been associated with vertebral fractures (Ziebart et al., 2019). Another, albeit a poorly researched clinical assessment of posture is the rib to iliac crest measurement. More than two fingers of the examiner from the patient's iliac crest to the lower ribs may be normal. In this writer's experience, when the ribs rest on the iliac crest, the patient has minimal to severe pain and may have encroachment on the abdominal cavity making food intake difficult.

In the older population, posture should be assessed not only in standing and sitting positions but also in bed, especially in a patient confined to bed because of injury or illness. It is particularly important to prevent pressure areas, and special care should be taken to avoid muscle imbalances resulting from prolonged positioning. Areas of concern are the triceps surae, hip and knee flexors, and hip abductors and adductors, especially after hip surgery. It is common for the patient to assume a supine but side-bent posture that may lead to muscle

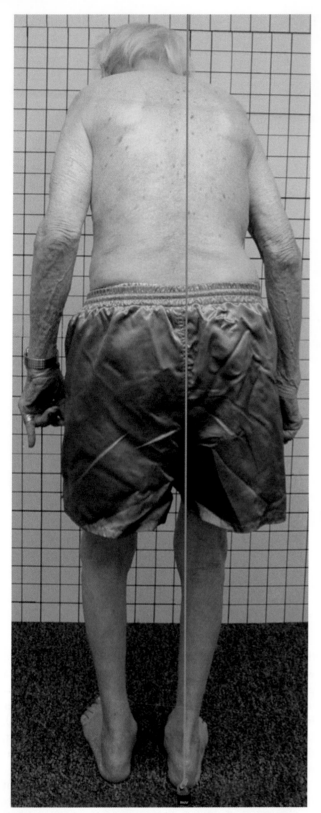

FIG. 27.5   Postural changes are quite evident in this 98-year-old man when compared with his posture 20 years earlier (Fig. 27.4B). This degree of change is unique to this individual but is common in ageing individuals. Note the kyphoscoliosis with extension of the upper extremities, increased hip and knee flexion and loss of muscle mass in all four extremities and trunk.

imbalance. The patient who side bends toward the operative side will suffer a contralateral hip abductor lengthening and an ipsilateral hip abductor shortening. The converse is true for the patient who side bends away from the operative side. These muscle imbalances will become significant during rehabilitation when the patient attempts to regain independent ambulation and may contribute to a Trendelenburg gait.

Ryan and Fried (1997) found that kyphosis was associated with slower speeds of gait and stair climbing and difficulties with reaching or heavy lifting in community dwellers between the ages of 59 and 89 years.

Hyperkyphosis measured in the supine position in 1578 older community dwelling males and females was significantly associated in a stepwise manner with declining self-reported function for bending, walking, climbing and rising from a chair. Grip strength was also significantly associated with this postural change; the greater the kyphosis, the less strength (Kado et al., 2005). Slower speeds were reported by Katzman, Vittinghoff, and Kado (2011) on the Timed Up and Go Test for persons with greater kyphotic angles. But, it is essential to know that Katzman et al. (2017) reported that spine strengthening exercise and postural training reduced radiographic and clinical measures of spinal kyphosis.

Most important are reports of diminished pulmonary function and increased risk of death related to osteoporosis and the forward bent posture resulting from vertebral compression fractures (Leech et al., 1990). Surgical vertebral augmentation has been shown to decrease mortality rate after vertebral compression fracture (Kurra et al., 2018).

Brown, Sinacore, and Host (1995) demonstrated the important relationship between the strength of postural muscles in the lower extremities and functional tasks, including walking, stair climbing and getting up from a chair. Weakness of calf muscles coupled with insufficient strength of the scapulothoracic stabilisers can contribute to increased kyphotic posture and loss of balance, especially when reaching forward with the upper extremities.

Clinical intervention should be undertaken in the case of postural changes if they cause pain, impair function or are likely to lead to future impairment. The typical interventions listed in Box 27.1 are not listed in order of importance. One or all of the interventions may be appropriate, depending upon the clinical assessment and the individual patient's condition and prognosis.

BOX 27.1   Clinical Interventions for Postural Changes Related to Pain or Dysfunction

1. Brace, support, immobilise, protect
2. Heat, cold, electrical stimulation
3. Therapeutic exercise to enhance respiratory capacity, functional muscle strength, tone, length, coordination, balance, appropriate interface between agonist and antagonist and postural retraining
4. Balance retraining and falls reduction
5. Medications
6. Surgery

TABLE 27.2 Age-associated postural extremity changes and their clinical implications.

EXTREMITY SKELETAL CHANGES	CLINICAL IMPLICATIONS
Scapular protraction or abduction	Alters normal scapulohumeral rhythm, leading to painful shoulder conditions
Tightness/contractures in elbow flexion, wrist ulnar deviation, finger flexion	Reduces reach and hand function
Hip flexion contractures (loss of hip extension to neutral or 0°)	Reduces stride length; may increase energy cost of mobility and may increase postural control requirements, especially if change is unilateral
Knee flexion contractures (loss of knee extension to neutral or 0°)	Reduces stride length and gait push-off; may increase energy cost of mobility and may increase postural control requirements, especially if change is unilateral
Varus/valgus changes at hip, knee, ankle	Reduces stride length and gait push-off; may increase energy cost of mobility and may increase postural control requirements especially if change is unilateral. Usually is a cause of pain because of mechanical deformation and strain on musculoskeletal tissues

SUMMARY POINTS

- Common postural changes occur with increasing age, but their characteristics are unique to each individual
- Although not present in a young healthy adult, the new postural alignments are not necessarily faulty but may increase falls risk and pulmonary dysfunction
- Posture may indicate normal compensation for degradation in the neuromusculoskeletal alignment or a loss of control of any of its component parts
- Many of these changes have taken place slowly over decades and may not be ameliorated easily, if at all

MCQs

Q.1 What are the most common age-related postural changes in the axial skeleton?
   a. Flat spine
   b. Head forward, dorsal kyphosis and loss of lumbar lordosis
   c. Increased lumbar lordosis
   d. Anterior wedging of the cervicothoracic vertebral bodies
Q.2 What controls age-related posture?
   a. The central nervous system
   b. Joint anatomy
   c. Peripheral nervous system
   d. Complex interactions of connective tissues and the neuromusculoskeletal systems

   e. a and b
   f. Dissolution of collagen fibrils
Q.3 Why is postural assessment an important component of care in the ageing patient?
   a. Postural sway may be a factor in falls risk
   b. Abnormal postural changes may be associated with pain
   c. Kyphotic changes in the spine are associated with declining functional mobility and reduced pulmonary function
   d. Posture improvements can be gained with proper intervention
   e. All of the above

REFERENCES

Barrey, C., Roussouly, P., Perrin, G., & Le Huec, J. C. (2011). Sagittal balance disorders in severe degenerative spine. Can we identify the compensatory mechanisms? *European Spine Journal, 20*(suppl 5), 626–633.

Brown, M., Sinacore, D., & Host, H. (1995). The relationship of strength to function in the older adult. *The Journals of Gerontology Series A Biological Sciences and Medical Sciences, 50,* 55–59.

Cenciarini, M., Loughlin, P., Sparto, P., & Redfern, M. S. (2010). Stiffness and damping in posture control increase with age. *IEEE Transactions on Biomedical Engineering, 57,* 267–275.

Ditroilo, M., Cully, L., Boreham, C., & De Vito, G. (2012). Assessment of musculo-articular and muscle stiffness in young and older men. *Muscle Nerve, 46,* 559–565.

Kado, D., Huang, M., Barrett-Connor, E., & Greendale, G. A. (2005). Hyperkyphotic posture and poor physical functional ability in older community-dwelling men and women: the Rancho Bernardo Study. *The Journals of Gerontology Series A Biological Sciences and Medical Sciences, 60*(5), 633–637.

Katzman, W., Cawthon, P., Hicks, G., et al. (2012). Association of spinal muscle composition and prevalence of hyperkyphosis in healthy community-dwelling older men and women. *The Journals of Gerontology Series A Biological Sciences and Medical Sciences, 67,* 191–195.

Katzman, W., Vittinghoff, E., & Kado, D. M. (2011). Age-related hyperkyphosis, independent of spinal osteoporosis, is associated with impaired mobility in older community-dwelling women. *Osteoporosis International, 22*, 85–90.

Katzman, W., Vittinghoff, E., Lin, F., et al. (2017). Targeted spine strengthening exercise and posture training program to reduce hyperkyphosis in older adults: results from the study of hyper-kyphosis, exercise, and function (SHEAF) randomized controlled trial. *Osteoporosis International, 28*, 2831–2841.

Leech, J., Dulberg, C., Kellie, S., Pattee, L., & Gay, J. (1990). Relationship of lung function to severity of osteoporosis in women. *American Review of Respiratory Disease, 141*, 68–71.

Manckoundia, P., Mourey, F., Perennou, D., & Pfitzenmeyer, P. (2008). Backward disequilibrium in elderly subjects. *Clinical Interventions in Aging, 3*, 667–672.

Muchna, A., Najafi, B., Wendel, C., Schwenk, M., Armstrong, D., & Mohler, J. (2018). Foot problems in older adults: associations with incident falls, fraility syndrome, and sensor-derived gait, balance, and physical activity measures. *Journal of the American Podiatric Medical Association, 108*, 126–139.

Pauelsen, M., Nyberg, L., Roijezon, U., & Vikman, I. (2018a). Both psychological factors and physical performance are associated with fall-related concerns. *Aging Clinical and Experimental Research, 30*, 1079–1085.

Pauelsen, M., Vikman, I., Strandkvist, V. J., Larsson, A., & Roijezon, U. (2018b). Decline in sensorimotor systems explains reduced falls self-efficacy. *Journal of Electromyography and Kinesiology, 42*, 104–110.

Ryan, S., & Fried, L. (1997). The impact of kyphosis on daily functioning. *Journal of the American Geriatrics Society, 45*, 1479–1486.

Ziebart, C., Adachi, J., Ashe, M., et al. (2019). Exploring the association between number, severity, location of fracture, and occiput to wall distance. *Archives of Osteoporosis, 14*, 27.

28

Falls, Dizziness and Funny Turns

Robbie Bourke, Giulia Rivasi & Rose Anne Kenny

LEARNING OBJECTIVES

- List the common causes of falls, dizziness and 'funny turns' in the rehabilitation setting
- Explain the initial evaluation for falls and dizziness occurring during rehabilitation
- Identify which patients may need specialist referral
- Describe strategies for falls prevention
- Explain the benefits of rehabilitation for falls and dizziness prevention and treatment

CASE

James is an 81-year-old gentleman who was recently an inpatient in the acute hospital following a fall that resulted in a pubic ramus fracture. His background history is significant for hypertension, left total hip replacement following fracture, recurrent falls, mild cognitive impairment, benign prostatic hyperplasia and possible transient ischaemic attack (TIA). His current medications include atorvastatin, atenolol, bendroflumethiazide, perindopril, zopiclone and tamsulosin. The circumstances surrounding his fall are unclear. It was unwitnessed and he can't recall the event. He has been falling frequently and reports a 'terrible dizziness' that can come over him when standing. He refers to the events as 'my TIAs'. During the first day in rehab, he has several 'near misses' characterised by unsteadiness on standing up or after prolonged standing.

INTRODUCTION

A 'funny turn' is a term frequently used by patients to describe anything from unsteady episodes, presyncope or syncope to TIAs. In this chapter, we will focus on falls, dizziness and syncope. These are three distinct yet often interrelated issues facing older people.

Falls

A fall is an unexpected event in which the participant comes to rest on the ground, floor or lower level without known loss of consciousness (Panel on Prevention of Falls in Older Persons; AGS/BGS, 2011). Falls are very common with 32%–42% of over 75s falling at least once a year. The annual incidence rate in long-term care settings is 30%–50%, with 40% of those falling recurrently. Patients with dementia fall 10 times more frequently. A total of 40%–60% of falls lead to some injury and up to 1% of falls in older people result in hip fracture (Kenny, Romero-Ortuno, & Cogan, 2013).

Dizziness

Dizziness is one of the most common complaints in older adults and can result in serious functional deficits and a negative impact on quality of life. Patients frequently report dizziness as a symptom associated with both syncope and falls. Dizziness can be categorised as vertiginous or non-vertiginous (Fig. 28.1).

Vertigo is an illusion of movement that usually (but not always) has a rotatory component. People who experience vertigo often have a sensation of turning or being tilted. Patients report that the spinning occurs inside the head or that the external environment is spinning. The different causes of dizziness are shown in Table 28.1.

Syncope

Syncope is a transient loss of consciousness due to a reduced blood supply to the brain. It is characterised by a rapid onset, short duration and spontaneous complete recovery. It can often manifest as what could be called a 'faint'. This definition excludes epileptic seizures, concussion and psychogenic pseudo-syncope (Brignole et al., 2018). Syncope is a common symptom, experienced by up to 30% of healthy adults at least once in their lifetime. The main causes of syncope are listed in Table 28.2.

Orthostatic Intolerance

Orthostatic intolerance (OI) syndromes refer to symptoms which occur moving from sitting or lying to standing. It is generally assumed to be caused by a reduced blood supply to the brain due to a blood pressure (BP) drop on standing (Brignole, 2007).

Symptoms associated with OI include the following:
- Dizziness and lightheadedness (presyncope)
- Visual disturbances (blurring, colour changes, enhanced brightness, darkening or blackening and tunnel vision)
- Hearing disturbances (impaired hearing, crackles and tinnitus)
- Neck pain (occipital/paracervical and shoulder region)
- Weakness

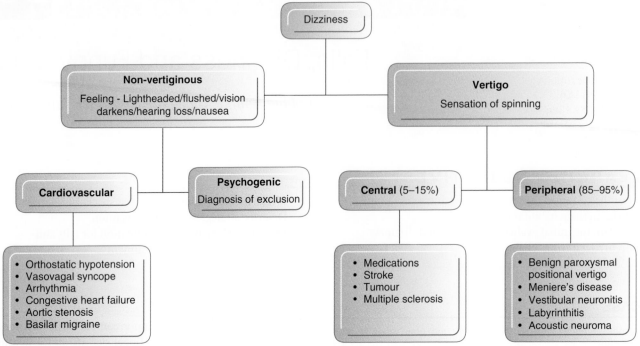

FIG. 28.1 Classification and main causes of dizziness.

FALLS, SYNCOPE AND DIZZINESS OCCURRING DURING REHABILITATION IN OLDER PATIENTS

'Bed rest' can lead to loss of muscle function, strength and volume (sarcopenia). However, there is also deconditioning in the cardiovascular system leading to higher rates of falls and OI (Goswami et al., 2017). Consequently, falls are common in the rehabilitation setting (Sherrington et al., 2010), where older patients tend to have problems with both mobility and transfers.

Whether a patient has had a fall or a syncopal event, it is essential to assess them for any 'red flag' features that may require urgent review from a cardiologist/geriatrician or syncope expert.

Initial Evaluation Following a Fall or Syncopal Event

If a patient has had a fall or a syncopal event, the initial emergency response should follow the principles of basic trauma life support. A *primary survey* should be conducted assessing **A**irway, **B**reathing and **C**irculation, followed by assessment of **D**isability (i.e. level of consciousness and targeted neurological examination) and **E**xposure (e.g. signs indicative of injury such as externally rotated and shortened leg typical of a hip fracture). The *secondary survey* consists of an AMPLE history including **A**llergies, **M**edications (with special attention to culprit medications), **P**ast medical history, **L**ast meal and **E**vents prior to injury.

A full report of the circumstances and symptoms surrounding the fall is important. This is best broken down into events before, during and after the fall. This approach can provide vital clues to point to a specific aetiology or narrow down the differential diagnosis. Witness reports are essential since 25%–30% of older patients with syncope have amnesia for loss of consciousness and present as unexplained falls (Kenny et al., 2012).

Falls may also be due to transient loss of consciousness. Therefore, in patients with unexplained falls the diagnostic management should be the same as that for unexplained syncope (Fig. 28.2).

An ECG (electrocardiograph – 'heart tracing') should be performed in all cases.

Risk Stratification for Syncope

The clinical history is essential to ascertain the presence of low- or high-risk features, the latter also known as 'red flags' (Table 28.3). Three key questions should be addressed during the initial evaluation:

1. Is loss of consciousness attributable to syncope?
2. Is heart disease present?
3. Are there important clinical features in the history and physical examination, which suggest the aetiology?

An important issue in patients with unexplained syncope is whether structural heart disease or an abnormal ECG are present; both are associated with a higher risk of arrhythmias and a higher mortality at 1 year (Brignole et al., 2018). In these patients, additional cardiac evaluation is recommended (Kenny & Bhangu, 2016). These patients would be candidates for rehabilitation but would be considered higher risk and would benefit from identification and treatment of any potential underlying cause. In patients without heart disease, evaluation for OI and neurally mediated causes should be considered.

TABLE 28.1 Different causes of dizziness.

CAUSES OF DIZZINESS	SUBTYPES	DIAGNOSIS
Peripheral vestibular disorder (PVD) **Vestibular dysfunction involving vestibular end organs and/or the vestibular nerve**	**Benign paroxysmal positional vertigo (BPPV)** – brief episodes of vertigo precipitated by rapid change of head position **Vestibular neuronitis** – prolonged severe vertigo (acute onset), head movement may exacerbate, may be associated with nausea, nystagmus and postural imbalance. Usually no effect on hearing **Meniere's disease** – initial sensation of ear fullness and reduction in hearing. Tinnitus may be present, followed by rotational vertigo, postural imbalance, nystagmus, nausea and vomiting. Symptoms can persist for 30 minutes to 24 hours	Clinical and Hallpike test Clinical and HINTS exam (exam to differentiate central to peripheral cause) Clinical exam
Orthostatic intolerance syndromes	**Initial OH** – a 20 mmHg fall in systolic BP during the first 2 minutes of standing, with reproduction of symptoms (often seen in primary autonomic failure) **Progressive orthostatic hypotension (OH)** – slow progressive decrease in systolic BP (together with compensatory heart rate increase) upon the assumption of a standing position (most common – seen in older people)	Lying and standing BP/active stand Tilt table testing
Arrhythmia	**Bradyarrhythmias** – sinus pauses of greater than 2 seconds, prolonged sinus bradycardia, slow atrial fibrillation **Tachyarrhythmia** – supraventricular tachycardia, ventricular tachycardia associated with symptoms	Cardiac rhythm monitoring - ECG - Cardiac event recorder or Holter - Implantable loop recorder
Carotid sinus hypersensitivity	**Vasodepressor** – 50 mmHg fall in systolic BP following unilateral carotid sinus massage for 5 seconds, with symptom reproduction in either supine or upright positions. Combined cardioinhibitory and vasodepressor responses are 'mixed' responses **Cardioinhibitory** – ventricular pause >3 seconds or asystole	Carotid sinus massage
Vasovagal (reflex) syncope	See Table 28.2 - hypotension (**vasodepressor**) - and/or bradycardia (**cardioinhibitory**)	Tilt table testing
Central neurological disorders	Stroke Cervical spondylosis Basilar artery migraine	MRI brain imaging

TABLE 28.2 Main causes of syncope.

Classification of syncope			
Reflex syncope (neutrally mediated)	Vasovagal - Orthostatic - Emotional	Situational - Specific situations - Swallow - Cough	Carotid sinus syndrome
Orthostatic intolerance	Drug induced - Diuretics - Vasodilators	Volume depletion - Bleeding - Vomiting - Diarrhoea	Autonomic - Primary (PD/MSA/LBD) - Secondary (DM/amyloid)
Cardiac syncope	Bradyarrythmia - Sinus node dysfunction - AV conduction	Tachyarrhythmia - SVT - Ventricular	Structural cardiac - Valvular - MI

AV, Atrioventricular; *LBD*, Lewy body dementia; *MI*, myocardial infarction; *MSA*, multiple systems atrophy; *PD*, Parkinson's disease; *SVT*, supraventricular tachycardia.

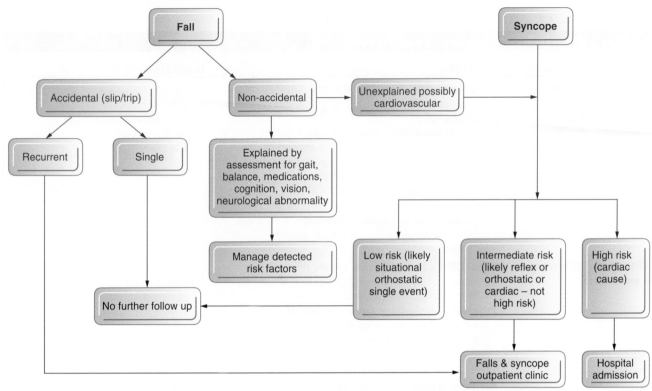

FIG. 28.2 Care pathway for risk stratification of falls and syncope. As unexplained falls may be due to transient loss of consciousness, the diagnostic management should be the same as that for unexplained syncope.

TABLE 28.3 Main syncope features for risk stratification, including 'red flags'.

High-Risk Features (Red Flags)	Low-Risk Features
Syncopal event	
Seated or supine event	Prodrome typical of orthostatic intolerance/VVS (lightheaded, warmth, sweaty, nausea)
New onset chest discomfort, breathlessness	
Palpitation before/during/after event	Prolonged standing
Family history of sudden cardiac death	Standing from supine/sitting position
Short prodrome (<10 seconds)	Unpleasant stimulus (sight/smell/pain)
	Triggered by cough/micturition/defecation
ECG Findings	
Abnormal ECG	Normal ECG
Acute ischaemic event	
Bradyarrythmias <40 ± AF	
VT	
Heart block patterns	
Abnormal QTC (long or short)	
Brugada patterns	
Clinical Exam	
Unexplained hypotension <90 mmHg systolic	Normal exam
Undiagnosed murmur	
Persistent daytime bradycardia <40	
Suggestion of GI bleed	

VT, ventricular tachycardia; *VVS,* vasovagal syncope.

Main Causes of Falls, Syncope and Dizziness During Rehabilitation

Accidental Falls Favoured by Comorbidities, Gait and Balance Disorders. The causes of a fall can be classified according to risk factors (Kenny et al., 2012).

- *Intrinsic* (to do with the patient) causes include muscle weakness, balance and/or gait disorders, cognitive impairment, low BP, visual deficits and infection.
- *Extrinsic* (related to other factors) causes include medications, environmental factors such as poor lighting and loose carpets.

We must appreciate the interactive and synergistic effects between risk factors. There is almost always more than one possible attributable cause for a fall (Brignole et al., 2018); therefore a comprehensive risk factor assessment and modification of all known risk factors is recommended for falls prevention (AGS/BGS guidelines, 2009).

Always consider osteoporosis/bone protection following a fall.

Orthostatic Intolerance

OI frequently results from deconditioning that relates to both loss of muscle bulk (the mechanical pump in the legs to help increase venous return) and cardiovascular deconditioning. The most effective intervention is rehabilitation and reconditioning exercises.

Vestibular Causes

The vestibular causes of falls are outlined in Table 28.1.

In a patient presenting with acute vertigo, it is important to consider an acute stroke as a possible diagnosis.

Useful Tests in the Rehabilitation Setting

Lying and standing blood pressure and heart rate measurement. To assess any postural drop in BP and appropriateness of heart rate response. The patient should be supine for at least 5 minutes prior. The longer they remain supine, the greater the BP drop. BP is then checked while lying and then standing at 1 and 3 minutes. It is best to perform the test in the morning or after the main meal because it is more likely to detect transient changes at these times. If there is no BP drop but the history is still suspicious for OI, repeat the measures.

24-hour ambulatory blood pressure monitoring (ABPM). To diagnose and monitor high and low BP behaviour over a longer recording period. In these patients, ABPM allows the assessment of overall hyper/hypotension, nocturnal hypertension, postprandial hypotension, and exercise- and drug-induced hypotension.

Dix-Hallpike manoeuvre. In suspected cases of benign paroxysmal positional vertigo (BPPV), this can be a useful diagnostic test. See Chapter 52 Vestibular Rehabilitation for more details.

TREATMENT STRATEGIES

Prevention is the mainstay of treatment for falls and syncope; however, in patients with suspected cardiogenic syncope an urgent referral for specialist input is advisable.

In patients with BPPV, repositioning manoeuvres represent the first-line treatment. The Epley manoeuvre (Epley, 1992) is the most widely used and can be performed by trained therapists if there is a positive Dix-Hallpike.

In patients suffering from dizziness due to chronic vestibular disorders, vestibular rehabilitation may be considered.

PREVENTION

Orthostatic Intolerance

Older adults undergoing rehabilitation frequently present with low BP and/or OI, which are related to deconditioning, reduced muscle mass and medical conditions. In this context, non-pharmacological interventions are helpful to treat or prevent OI.

The first step consists of reducing/stopping medications that can lower BP. Particular attention should be paid to drugs that increase fluid output (e.g. diuretics), cause vasodilatation (widening of blood vessels) or slow the heart rate (e.g. beta blockers). The non-pharmacological approach also includes lifestyle measures to counteract conditions enhancing OI such as increasing fluid and salt intake.

Medication to increase BP can be considered in severe forms of orthostatic hypotension, in addition to lifestyle measures. In these patients, referral to a Falls and Syncope Service should be considered, to assess the underlying causes of hypotension.

Falls Prevention

The first step in falls prevention is a risk assessment aimed at identifying those at risk of falling and most likely to benefit from fall-prevention interventions. Individual risk factors should be investigated, defining each patient's risk profile. An individualised multifactorial intervention strategy can be implemented (AID approach, Fig. 28.3).

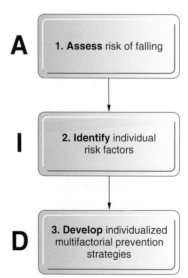

FIG. 28.3   Falls prevention flow-chart – AID approach. Falls prevention begins with risk Assessment (A). Subsequently, individuals' risk factors should be Identified (I), to Develop tailored multifactorial intervention strategies addressing those issues in which individuals need to be supported (D).

The two main approaches to identify older people at risk of falling are single physical performance tests and risk scores. Physical performance tests mainly evaluate gait (walking pattern) and balance and may also be useful to direct exercise interventions. Falls risk scores usually assess the presence of the most relevant risk factors for falls, e.g. mobility, a history of falls and/or stroke, recent hospitalisation and fear of falling. A simple risk score for rehabilitation – the *Predict FIRST* (Prediction of Falls in Rehabilitation Settings Tool) – has been proposed by Sherrington et al. (2010), including some of the main risk factors such as medications, history of falling and balance impairment. Fallers have an average of four possible risk factors, and a multifactorial approach, treating all modifiable risk factors, is recommended.

Evidence concerning the value of scores and physical performance tests is conflicting, and there is no agreement on which tool is most appropriate. The American Geriatrics Society/British Geriatrics Society guidelines suggest a simple falls risk assessment algorithm, comprising both screening questions and a physical performance test (Fig. 28.4).

This approach could be applied in rehabilitation given it is practical and easy to use. As it combines two different tools, it increases the overall predictive accuracy.

Falls risk factors and their specific intervention strategies are summarised in the **Resources section 'Falls risk factors and interventions'**. Multifactorial interventions represent the most effective strategy to reduce falling in all the healthcare settings, including rehabilitation. Education and behavioural counselling for both patients and their families are also important and represent an essential component of any multifactorial intervention. Education should raise awareness about falls risk factors and interventions that reduce the risk, including exercise, to encourage patients and families to play an active role in prevention.

Medications Review and Deprescribing

It is essential to remember that syncope, falls and dizziness are frequently caused by or exacerbated by medications (see Resources section: 'Medications associated with an increased risk of falls').

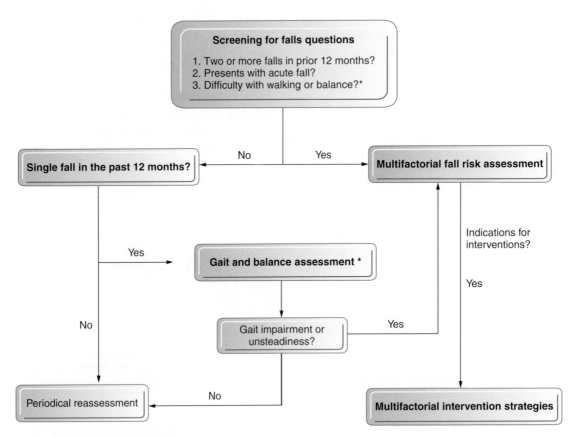

* to be assessed using simple screening test, such as the TUG test or the BERG balance scale

FIG. 28.4 Screening algorithm for fall risk assessment, modified from the American Geriatrics Society/British Geriatrics Society guidelines. If the answer to any of the screening questions is positive, a multifactorial falls risk assessment should be provided to identify individual risk factors and target appropriate interventions. In addition, older patients reporting a single fall in the past year should undergo gait and balance assessment, since the fall may be the sign of difficulties or unsteadiness in walking or standing. If the gait and balance tests reveal a poor performance, then a multifactorial fall risk assessment should be given. For details on multifactorial falls risk assessment and intervention strategies, see Table 28.3.

A systematic medication review should be routinely conducted in older adults. The risk of both falls and syncope increases with polypharmacy (i.e. ≥4 regular medications), due to a higher probability of drug interactions and toxicity. Older people are sensitive to antihypertensives and are more prone to syncope and hypotensive episodes. Newer recommendations for aggressive treatment of hypertension do not apply universally. Systolic values <130 mmHg should be avoided in this population and a systolic target of 140–150 mmHg should be considered in individuals with OI and/or falls risk factors, to minimise the risk of hypotension-related adverse events (Sexton et al., 2017).

REHABILITATION AS A TREATMENT STRATEGY IN SYNCOPE, FALLS AND DIZZINESS

Rehabilitation has a well-established role in treating and preventing falls, syncope and dizziness. Exercise is crucial to counteract deconditioning and sarcopenia, and helps improve muscle function, gait and balance performance. Exercise may increase confidence and reduce the fear of falling that frequently leads to activity restriction and physical decline. Rehabilitation is helpful for functional ability and physical performance and may improve bone density, reducing the risk of fall-related fractures.

Exercise Programmes

Exercise programmes should be goal directed and incorporate both single modality exercise and multicomponent activity, which combines two or more types of exercise involving muscle strengthening, balance training and aerobic physical activity. Multicomponent activity provides a more comprehensive approach to increase physical capacity and promote greater improvement in physical function and reduces sarcopenia.

Both community group and home-based exercise programmes may be beneficial. Home-based programmes may be suitable for patients who have limited capacity to travel to outpatient services. When feasible, group exercise should be preferred, given the recognised benefits of social participation on patients' well-being.

Falls

Strong evidence supports exercise interventions to reduce falls and their injurious consequences and exercise programmes are recommended as part of falls prevention strategies. A successful falls prevention exercise programme must include a combination of strength, coordination, gait and balance training. Pilates and Tai Chi are also useful.

- Balance and strength training (Sherrington et al., 2017)
  Programmes involving a challenge to balance are among the most effective interventions for falls prevention. Activities should include progressively difficult postures that gradually reduce the base of support (e.g. semi-tandem, tandem or one-legged stand); dynamic movements that move the centre of gravity (e.g. tandem walk, circle turns); exercise stressing postural muscle groups (e.g. toe stands) and modulating sensory input (e.g. standing with eyes closed). Muscle strengthening counteracts sarcopenia and improves standing balance (lower extremities muscle strengthening).
- Tai Chi (Blake & Hawley, 2012)
  Tai Chi is a multicomponent activity consisting of slow, rhythmic movements that emphasise balance, flexibility, coordination and posture control. Psychological benefits include improvement in balance confidence and fear of falling. Finally, as a group exercise it promotes social engagement. Tai Chi reduces falls risk.
- Pilates (Bullo et al., 2015)
  Pilates incorporates movement patterns from gymnastics, martial arts, yoga and dance. It enhances muscle endurance, flexibility and strength, particularly in the lower limbs, thus improving both static and dynamic balance, even after a short intervention. Pilates may be useful in reducing falls risk and improving functional capacity, and a positive impact on mood and quality of life has been reported.

Dizziness and Vestibular Disorders

For a detailed discussion, see Chapter 52 Vestibular Rehabilitation.

Dizziness and Orthostatic Intolerance

In the context of OI, rehabilitation is aimed at improving the effectiveness of the 'muscle pump', which usually helps blood that has pooled in the leg veins to return to the heart. Activation and strengthening of lower limb muscles improves dizziness caused by low BP (Dent et al., 2018). Initially, reclining exercises that are not gravitationally challenging are preferable to the upright ones, e.g. recumbent cycling or rowing. Patients could also be advised to perform water exercise, since the pressure of the water may help to improve venous return. Additionally, protein supplementation or a protein-rich diet should be considered in older adults with sarcopenia; this should be combined with physical activity (Dent et al., 2018).

CANDIDATES FOR REHABILITATION

An overview of the indications for rehabilitation in OI, dizziness and falls is illustrated in Table 28.4.

TIMING AND WARNINGS OF REHABILITATION

Rehabilitation should be started as soon as possible, particularly during or after hospitalisation. Deconditioning rapidly develops even after a short duration of bed rest and exercise to promote reconditioning should be provided promptly to inpatients.

TABLE 28.4 Clinical features of candidates to rehabilitation and specific exercise strategies.

Patients' Clinical Profile	Exercise Programme
Subjects with *orthostatic intolerance*, particularly if frail and deconditioned or with poor muscle mass	Lower body muscle strengthening
Subjects with a *history of falls*	Multicomponent activity programme Tai Chi
Subjects with at *high risk for falls* due to gait impairment or poor physical performance*	Multicomponent activity programme Tai Chi
Subjects with *fear of falling* and poor balance confidence	Tai Chi
Balance impairment	Balance training Tai Chi, Pilates
Non-orthostatic dizziness and balance disorders	Vestibular rehabilitation Tai Chi
Unilateral and bilateral peripheral *vestibular dysfunction*	Vestibular rehabilitation
Non-orthostatic dizziness of uncertain aetiology (no documented vestibular deficits)	Empirical trial with vestibular rehabilitation
*Residual dizziness after treatment of benign paroxysmal vertigo***	Vestibular rehabilitation

*With a view to *preventing falls*, physical performance tests, e.g. the Short Physical Performance Battery or Timed Up and Go test, may be used to identify people who are more likely to benefit from moderate intensity exercise programmes.
**In patients with *benign paroxysmal vertigo*, repositioning manoeuvres represent the first line treatment. Vestibular rehabilitation can be considered in patients with residual symptoms, in order to prompt functional recovery.

There are no contraindications to rehab, only some warnings. Exercise is feasible and beneficial in all older adults, provided that it is appropriate to their health profile, physical capabilities and needs. Intensity and duration should be low at the beginning and activity should be increased gradually over time, according to the individual's tolerance.

CASE CONCLUSION

James has **OI**, a common presentation in older adults. The case illustrates the difficulties in diagnosis due to uncertain history and the many ways that polypharmacy can worsen the problem (dehydration, BP lowering).

The rehabilitation team stopped all antihypertensive medications, instituted a reconditioning exercise programme and increased his fluid intake, to improve balance and standing BP and to reduce the risk of dizziness and falls.

SUMMARY POINTS

- A careful history will usually determine the cause of a person's dizziness or syncopal event
- Falls prevention is one of the most important elements of rehabilitation and presents health professionals with numerous opportunities to help minimise the risk of falling
- Syncope is common and we must recognise 'red flags'
- 1/3 of syncope presents as a fall particularly in older patients; therefore beware 'unexplained' falls
- Multifactorial causes are the rule rather than exception

MCQs

Q.1 Which of the following is considered to be a 'red flag' in a syncopal event?
  a. Event occurred after prolonged standing
  b. Event triggered by passing urine
  c. Event occurred while seated
  d. Patient suffered a broken bone
Q.2 Which of the following statements is true?
  a. Falls in older adults have a single identifiable cause

  b. 30% of healthy adults will experience a syncopal event in their life
  c. A person who suffers a fracture as a result of a fall is not suitable for rehabilitation
  d. Intensive blood pressure control (<130/80 mmHg) should be targeted in all adults in the rehabilitation setting

REFERENCES

American Geriatrics Society 2015 Beers Criteria Update Expert Panel. (2015). American Geriatrics Society 2015 Updated Beers Criteria for potentially inappropriate medication use in older adults. *Journal of the American Geriatrics Society, 63*(11), 2227–2246.

Blake, H., & Hawley, H. (2012). Effects of Tai Chi exercise on physical and psychological health of older people. *Current Aging Science, 5*(1), 19–27.

Brignole, M. (2007). The syndromes of orthostatic intolerance. *E-Journal of the ESC Council for Cardiology Practice, 6*, 5.

Brignole, M., Moya, A., de Lange, F. J., et al. (2018). 2018 ESC Guidelines for the diagnosis and management of syncope. *European Heart Journal, 39*(21), 1883–1948.

Bullo, V., Bergamin, M., Gobbo, S., Sieverdes, J. C., Zaccaria, M., Neunhaeuserer, D., & Ermolao, A. (2015). The effects of Pilates exercise training on physical fitness and wellbeing in the elderly: a systematic review for future exercise prescription. *Preventive Medicine, 75*, 1–11.

Dent, E., Morley, J. E., Cruz-Jentoft, A. J., et al. (2018). International clinical practice guidelines for sarcopenia (ICFSR): screening, diagnosis and management. *The Journal of Nutrition, Health & Aging, 22*(10), 1148–1161.

Epley, J. M. (1992). The canalith repositioning procedure– for treatment of benign paroxysmal positional vertigo. *Otolaryngology–Head and Neck Surgery, 107*(3), 399–404.

Goswami, N., Blaber, A. P., Hinghofer-Szalkay, H., & Montani, J. P. (2017). Orthostatic intolerance in older persons: etiology and countermeasures. *Frontiers of Physiology, 8*, 803.

Kenny, R. A., & Bhangu, J. (2016). Syncope. In H. Fillet, K. Rockwood, & J. B. Young (Eds.), *Brocklehurst textbook of geriatric medicine & gerontology* (8th edn, pp. 335–347). Philadelphia: Elsevier.

Kenny, R. A., Romero-Ortuno, R., & Cogan, L. (2013). *Falls. Medicine, 41*(1), 24–28.

Panel on Prevention of Falls in Older Persons, American Geriatrics Society and British Geriatrics Society. (2011). Summary of the Updated American Geriatrics Society/British Geriatrics Society clinical practice guideline for prevention of falls in older persons. *Journal of the American Geriatrics Society, 59*(1), 148–157.

Sexton, D. J., Canney, M., O'Connell, M. D. L., Moore, P., Little, M. A., O'Seaghdha, C. M., & Kenny, R. A. (2017). Injurious falls and syncope in older community-dwelling adults meeting inclusion criteria for SPRINT. *JAMA Internal Medicine, 177*(9), 1385–1387.

Sherrington, C., Michaleff, Z. A., Fairhall, N., Paul, S. S., et al. (2017). Exercise to prevent falls in older adults: an updated systematic review and meta-analysis. *British Journal of Sports Medicine, 51*(24), 1750–1758.

Sherrington, C., Lord, S. R., Close, J. C., et al. (2010). Development of a tool for prediction of falls in rehabilitation settings (Predict_FIRST): a prospective cohort study. *Journal of Rehabilitation Medicine, 42*(5), 482–488.

FURTHER READING

Ambrose, A. F., Paul, G., & Hausdorff, J. M. (2013). Risk factors for falls among older adults: a review of the literature. *Maturitas, 75*(1), 51–61.

Berg, K. O., Wood-Dauphinee, S. L., Williams, J. I., & Maki, B. (1992). Measuring balance in the elderly: validation of an instrument. *Canadian Journal of Public Health, 83*(Suppl 2), S7–S11.

Bolding, D. J., & Corman, E. (2019). Falls in the geriatric patient. *Clinics in Geriatric Medicine, 35*(1), 115–126.

Gates, S., Smith, L. A., Fisher, J. D., & Lamb, S. E. (2008). Systematic review of accuracy of screening instruments for predicting fall risk among independently living older adults. *The Journal of Rehabilitation Research and Development, 45*(8), 1105–1116.

Goldberg, A., Chavis, M., Watkins, J., & Wilson, T. (2012). The five-times-sit-to-stand test: validity, reliability and detectable change in older females. *Aging Clinical and Experimental Research, 24*(4), 339–344.

Guirguis-Blake, J. M., Michael, Y. L., Perdue, L. A., Coppola, E. L., & Beil, T. L. (2018). Interventions to prevent falls in older adults: updated evidence report and systematic review for the US Preventive Services Task Force. *JAMA, 319*(16), 1705–1716.

Guralnik, J. M., Simonsick, E. M., Ferrucci, L., Glynn, R. J., Berkman, L. F., Blazer, D. G., Scherr, P. A., & Wallace, R. B. (1994). A short physical performance battery assessing lower extremity function: association with self-reported disability and prediction of mortality and nursing home admission. *Journal of Gerontology, 49*, M85–94.

Hill, K. D., & Wee, R. (2012). Psychotropic drug-induced falls in older people: a review of interventions aimed at reducing the problem. *Drugs Aging, 29*(1), 15–30.

Hirase, T., Inokuchi, S., Matsusaka, N., Nakahara, K., & Okita, M. (2014). A modified fall risk assessment tool that is specific to physical function predicts falls in community-dwelling elderly people. *Journal of Geriatric Physical Therapy, 37*(4), 159–165.

Mathias, S., Nayak, U., & Isaacs, B. (1986). Balance in elderly patients: the "getup and go" test. *Archives of Physical Medicine and Rehabilitation, 67*, 387–389.

Park, S. H. (2018). Tools for assessing fall risk in the elderly: a systematic review and meta-analysis. *Aging Clinical and Experimental Research, 30*(1), 1–16.

Seppala, L. J., van der Velde, N., Masud, T., et al. (2019). EuGMS Task and Finish group on Fall-Risk-Increasing Drugs (FRIDs): position on knowledge dissemination, management, and future research. *Drugs Aging, 36*, 299–307.

Tinetti, M. E. (1986). Performance-oriented assessment of mobility problems in elderly patients. *Journal of the American Geriatrics Society, 34*(2), 119–126.

Tricco, A. C., Thomas, S. M., Veroniki, A. A., et al. (2017). Comparisons of interventions for preventing falls in older adults: a systematic review and meta-analysis. *JAMA, 318*(17), 1687–1699.

Whitney, S. L. (2014). Dizziness. In L. T. Kauffman, R. Scott, J. O. Barr, & M. L. Moran (Eds.), *A comprehensive guide to geriatric rehabilitation* (3rd edn, pp. 426–433). Edinburgh: Churchill Livingstone/Elsevier.

Whitney, S. L., Alghwiri, A. A., & Alghadir, A. (2016). An overview of vestibular rehabilitation. *Handbook of Clinical Neurology, 137*, 187–205.

29

Anxiety and Depression

Rosalind Kings & Adrian Vyse

LEARNING OBJECTIVES

- Describe how anxiety and depression present in older people
- Explain how to employ practical methods and strategies to engage patients with anxiety and depression in the rehabilitation setting

- Identify medical treatment options for anxiety and depression

Questions to Think About

What do you understand by the words anxiety and depression? Why might patients undergoing rehabilitation become anxious or depressed?

BACKGROUND

Depression is a common and serious mood disorder. Older adults have a 12% lifetime risk of a major depressive episode (Andreas et al., 2017). People who suffer from depression experience persistent and pervasive feelings of sadness and hopelessness, and lose interest in activities they once enjoyed. Depression can be common in the rehabilitation situation, particularly as there may be a very pertinent feeling of loss.

Anxiety is also very common in the general population, affecting 26% of older adults (Andreas et al., 2017), and in patients undergoing rehabilitation. It can present in multiple ways, being related to one specific circumstance, event or object (a phobia), or more generalised and affect the whole of life (generalised anxiety disorder, GAD).

Both anxiety and depression can present with physical or biological symptoms. Typically for depression these include lack of appetite, weight loss, lethargy and insomnia. In anxiety, heightened awareness, palpitations and insomnia are common. However, any physical symptom including pain can be caused by anxiety or depression, and healthcare workers need to be aware of this when investigating and treating people.

HOW DEPRESSION AND ANXIETY CAN AFFECT REHABILITATION

Depression and anxiety (especially fear of falling) during rehabilitation are associated with poorer recovery of independence in mobility and activities of daily living (washing, dressing, meal preparation, etc.) (Denkinger et al., 2010; Shahab et al., 2017). The difficulties that are encountered in engaging people with depression and anxiety can lead to negative statements from staff such as 'unable to comply with therapy', 'not engaging in therapy sessions' and 'no rehab potential' (Bamford et al., 2018). This effect may well be amplified when the patient has underlying cognitive impairment. However, there is a growing body of evidence that physical activity and engagement in meaningful occupation can be beneficial in aiding recovery from depression and anxiety (Mulholland & Jackson, 2018; Rosenbaum et al., 2015), and therefore a more holistic approach to rehabilitation that encompasses mind and body should be adopted (Mulholland & Jackson, 2018; Rosenbaum et al., 2015).

Engaging people in physical activity who may have a combination of cognitive impairment, depression and anxiety can be challenging for the multidisciplinary team (MDT). Thorough Comprehensive Geriatric Assessment (CGA) should underpin management (Stott & Quinn, 2017) and should be combined with a person-centred approach to engagement (Etkind et al., 2019; NHS, 2014). The MDT should then aim to tailor a treatment and rehabilitation plan to the individual's cognitive, mental health and physical needs (Bamford et al., 2018; Mitchell & Angnelli, 2015; Kitwood, 1997).

HOW TO IDENTIFY ANXIETY OR DEPRESSION IN A REHABILITATION SETTING

Screening tools for anxiety and depression in a rehabilitation setting can be useful, although the most reliable way to recognise them is to have a 'high index of suspicion', that is, for healthcare professionals to have them in the back of their mind as a possibility in each patient, particularly those who are struggling to progress with rehabilitation.

There are several screening tools available for both anxiety and depression. Examples include HADS (Hospital Anxiety and Depression Scale), a 14-item questionnaire (seven relating to anxiety and seven to depression), which gives a score for both anxiety and depression (Zigmond & Snaith, 1983), and the GDS (Geriatric Depression Scale) which gives a score out of 30 for depression (Yesavage et al., 1982). However, often a simple question such as 'do you feel depressed?' can be the easiest way of finding out or getting some idea of whether there is a problem.

Any screening tool used may give an indication of anxiety and/or depression but will not give a diagnosis. For this the patient will need a full assessment involving a discussion around how they are feeling and what is troubling them, and a physical examination to rule out other causes of these feelings. It may also involve investigations such as blood tests. A psychiatrist or another member of the mental health team may also be asked to review the patient.

TREATMENT OPTIONS FOR ANXIETY AND DEPRESSION

Treatment of anxiety and depression should involve the entire MDT, including psychologists if possible. Patients require a coordinated, multidisciplinary and patient-centred treatment plan, looking holistically at the patient and involving them and their family. Psychological therapies can be useful either on their own or in addition to pharmacological treatment but unfortunately, access to these talking therapies in acute hospitals and in intermediate care centres remains extremely limited in many health services. Patients who are cognitively impaired can sometimes struggle with the level of complexity required to engage in psychological therapies; however, it should not be ruled out as some patients with cognitive impairment will benefit significantly.

If it is felt that pharmacological therapy would be beneficial, this may be commenced in tandem with psychological therapies and ongoing rehabilitation. Antidepressant drugs can be effective in treating moderate to severe depression, particularly that associated with psychomotor and physiological changes (such as loss of appetite and sleep disturbance). Improvement in sleep is usually the first benefit of therapy, which can also help to improve anxiety. The antidepressant effect of these drugs often takes 4–6 weeks to gain full effect.

There are several groups of antidepressants, the most common of which are the selective serotonin reuptake inhibitors (SSRIs) which include citalopram, sertraline and paroxetine; tricyclic and related antidepressants such as amitriptyline, clomipramine, dosulepin and trazodone; and the monoamine oxidase inhibitors (MAOIs) which are used less often now due to multiple side effects and interactions with food and with other drugs (Royal Pharmaceutical Society, 2019). A number of additional antidepressant drugs, such as mirtazapine, cannot be accommodated easily into this classification, but may be seen in practice. SSRIs are better tolerated than other classes of antidepressants and are safer in overdose so are usually used as first-line therapy when antidepressants are recommended. Many antidepressants also have anxiolytic (anxiety relieving) properties and so they can be useful in treating both depression and anxiety.

Anxiolytics or sedatives should be used with caution (particularly in older people) and only short term, as dependence and tolerance can occur and there is significant evidence that they increase the risk of falls (Seppala et al., 2018).

Antipsychotics and ECT (electroconvulsive therapy) are also sometimes used in severe depression with psychotic features, with good effect.

Enabling people with major depression or severe anxiety to engage in physical activity takes patience and persistence. Goals should initially be short term and as functionally based as possible. A clear history of the patient's likes and dislikes and normal motivators helps to tailor the goal setting process (Etkind et al., 2019), and using aids such as 'This is me' (Alzheimer's Society, 2017) can be helpful in understanding what is important to the person. Small meaningful goals that are achieved can aid the overall motivation to continue and can help to improve depression and anxiety.

Case 1

Michael was admitted to a psychiatry unit for major depressive illness. Due to minimal oral intake he was transferred to the acute hospital for nasogastric (NG) feeding and commenced a course of ECT for his depression. He had not walked for six weeks. During his stay, the rehabilitation therapists worked on building a relationship with him setting small goals initially around lifting his legs off the bed to relieve his heels and washing his face. His progress was initially slow with only intermittent engagement. As treatment continued, he started to see small improvements in muscle activity and movements and he regained some independence in washing. Slowly his mood, activity and engagement in meaningful activities improved. He started reading the paper and listening to music. He began eating meals and engaging with others. His NG tube was removed, physical improvements continued and he progressed from supervised exercises requiring lots of encouragement to completing an independent exercise programme. He developed the ability to stand and walk short distances. When his course of ECT was completed, he was moved to an intermediate care facility where he continued to improve and was successfully discharged to his flat with minimal support.

Question to Think About

What strategies can you think of to engage people who may be anxious or depressed?

FEAR OF FALLING

Fear of falling is associated with both anxiety disorders and depression, and can considerably impair quality of life. It is one of the most common manifestations of anxiety in older adults. In one study of 635 patients with a mean age of 80.6 years, 78% expressed a fear of falling (Gaxatte et al., 2011). Patients with fear of falling were not going out alone as much as the fearless group (see Fig. 29.1). Even low levels of anxiety around falling can limit activity, which further lowers confidence in walking ability. Consequently, the symptoms can worsen over time. It is important to provide

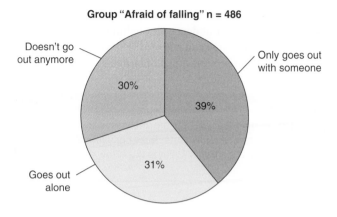

Group "Afraid of falling" n = 486

Doesn't go out anymore — 30%

Only goes out with someone — 39%

Goes out alone — 31%

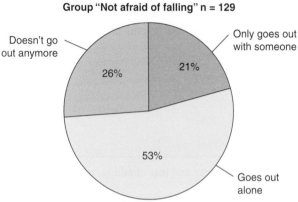

Group "Not afraid of falling" n = 129

Doesn't go out anymore — 26%

Only goes out with someone — 21%

Goes out alone — 53%

FIG. 29.1 Difference in going out habits between those with fear of falling and those who were not afraid of falling. (From Gaxatte, C, Nguyen T, Chourabi F, et al. Fear of falling as seen in the multidisciplinary falls consultation. *Ann Phys Rehabil Med.* 2011;54(4):248–58, with permission).

timely practical physiotherapy and occupational therapy to help change behaviours alongside any psychological and pharmacological treatment of their depression and anxiety (Bamford et al., 2018; Jahn, Zwergal, & Schniepp, 2010).

Anxiety can have a significant influence on human movements. There is a specific gait (walking pattern) associated with anxiety, with slower velocity, shorter step length, a broad base, longer time spent with both feet touching the ground simultaneously and a significantly smaller range of motion in the ankle, knee, and hip (Brown et al., 2002; Jahn et al., 2010; Scheets et al., 2015). In some threatening circumstances, a physical reaction can occur which causes exaggeration of postural sway, increased lower limb balance-correcting muscle activity and early onset of arm responses such as gripping or reaching for support (Cleworth et al., 2016; Scheets et al., 2015). In research situations these same reactions have been demonstrated by inducing a perception of a sheer drop in front of the subject and in older people these reactions can be seen when sitting on the edge of a bed or when attempting to move forward to stand, resulting in backwards leaning or fixing/pushing with the arms (Scheets et al., 2015).

These exaggerated responses can be observed after falls, or periods of immobility. In extreme cases, tonic immobility can occur, with patients fixing and extending arms, lower limbs and

trunk (Leite-Panissi, 2016; Kozlowska et al., 2015). Methods focusing on decreasing arousal and allowing normalisation of response can be helpful. This may include breathing exercises to slow respiration rate and regular exercise. Rehabilitation may need to be started in bed, the least threatening environment. Mindfulness and reassurance, emphasising compassion, hope and expectations for improvement may also help to decrease anxiety (Kozlowska et al., 2015). Cognitive behavioural therapy (CBT) can also be useful.

OTHER MANAGEMENT OPTIONS AND APPROACHES

Unfortunately, patients with severe anxiety often do not respond well to breathing exercises or mindfulness and reassurance, particularly if cognitive impairment is also present. They may also have little response to CBT (Kozlowska et al., 2015). In these situations, practical attempts can be made to alter the environment to decrease the perceived threat and allow activity to occur. Strategies can include space filling in front of the patient when attempting to sit or stand to decrease the perceived drop, for example, placing a high-backed chair in front of the patient, or using the bed perpendicular to the chair and then standing to lean on the bed. Other strategies can include stabilisation of joints to give positive proprioceptive feedback using supports such as abdominal binders or ankle foot orthoses (Scheets et al., 2015).

Minimising the number of staff interacting with the person and ensuring all handling is smooth, unhurried and kept to a minimum can also help. As far as possible, distractions from the task at hand should be minimised although this can be hard on a busy hospital ward. Relatives or carers can be helpful in providing positive support and encouragement in some cases; however, there are cases when their presence increases anxiety. It is also important to consider the least threatening environment in which rehabilitation can take place, preferably the patient's own home but if this is not possible, an intermediate care facility is often preferable to an acute ward.

Case 2

Christine was found by her carer on the floor following a fall. She was brought to the emergency department (ED) where a fracture was excluded and she was assessed by the therapy team aiming to discharge home. However, Christine was still in significant pain and was extremely anxious about the possibility of falling again, so required admission for pain control and ongoing therapy. Despite good muscle strength and coordination on testing, and constant reassurance from the therapist, on her first assessment Christine struggled to move into a stable sitting position and was unable to attempt standing, due to pushing backwards and 'fixing' with her arms.

During the following therapy session, the back of a high chair was positioned so as Christine moved to the edge of the bed the space in front of her was filled. A therapist was positioned either side providing encouragement and positive feedback but minimal physical assistance. Christine was able to sit independently on the edge of the bed and move into a position ready to stand. With verbal prompting, reassurance and some gentle physical facilitation, she was able to stand holding the back of the chair despite some initial backwards leaning.

Over a period of time, marching on the spot was added, a pulpit frame was introduced to replace the chair, and she managed to move from sitting to standing with verbal reassurances and minimal assistance. She was then able to access activities and meals at the communal table, motivating her further. Further progression used a walking frame with a towel over the front to fill the perceived space and the degree of assistance could be reduced. Christine continued to regain mobility and confidence throughout her hospital and rehabilitation unit stay and engaged well with a strength and balance programme, continuing at home.

Questions to Think About

What different responses in the multidisciplinary team do staff hear if they say a patients 'lacks confidence' compared to saying they 'are anxious'? Why is this? How can we change this bias?

SUMMARY POINTS

- Both anxiety and depression can have profound effects on rehabilitation and how people make progress
- A holistic approach augmented by good multidisciplinary work and patience gives an opportunity for improved rehabilitation outcomes
- Medication can also be helpful in treating anxiety and depression

MCQs

Q.1 Which one of the following is true about depression in older people?
  a. The initial approach should be telling people to 'cheer up'
  b. Medications are inevitably needed to help treat it
  c. Physical activity can be beneficial in aiding recovery
  d. Psychologist input should only be considered in severe cases
  e. A screening tool such as the GDS provides a definitive diagnosis

Q.2 Regarding anxiety and fear of falling, which one of these is true?
  a. Increased balance-correcting muscle activity is seen
  b. Cognitive behavioural therapy (CBT) has no role
  c. Patients should be encouraged to close their eyes and walk
  d. Anxiolytics (anxiety-relieving medications) should be used in the long-term
  e. Physiotherapy should focus on muscle strengthening exercises

REFERENCES

Alzheimer's Society. (2017). *This is me.* London: Alzheimer's Society.

Andreas, S., Schulz, H., Volkert, J., Dehoust, M., Sehner, S., Suling, A., …, & Härter, M. (2017). Prevalence of mental disorders in elderly people: the European MentDis_ICF65+ study. *The British Journal of Psychiatry, 210*(2), 125–131.

Bamford, C., Wheatley, A., Shaw, C., & Allan, L. M. (2018). Equipping staff with the skills to maximise recovery of people with dementia after an injurious fall. *Aging & Mental Health, 23,* 1524–1532.

Brown, L. A., Gage, W. H., Polych, M. A., Sleik, R. J., & Winder, T. R. (2002). Central set influences on gait. *Experimental Brain Research, 145*(3), 286–296.

Cleworth, T. W., Chua, R., Inglis, J. T., & Carpenter, M. G. (2016). Influence of virtual height exposure on postural reactions to support surface translations. *Gait & Posture, 47,* 96–102.

Denkinger, M. D., Igl, W., Lukas, A., Bader, A., Bailer, S., Franke, S., Denkinger, C. M., Nikolaus, T., & Jamour, M. (2010). Relationship between fear of falling and outcomes of an inpatient geriatric rehabilitation population—fear of the fear of falling. *Journal of the American Geriatrics Society, 58*(4), 664–673.

Etkind, S. N., Lovell, N., Nicholson, C. J., Higginson, I. J., & Murtagh, F. E. (2019). Finding a 'new normal' following acute illness: a qualitative study of influences on frail older people's care preferences. *Palliative Medicine, 33*(3), 301–311.

Gaxatte, C., Nguyen, T., Chourabi, F., Salleron, J., Pardessus, V., Delabrière, I., Thévenon, A., & Puisieux, F. (2011). Fear of falling as seen in the multidisciplinary falls consultation. *Annals of Physical and Rehabilitation Medicine, 54*(4), 248–258.

Jahn, K., Zwergal, A., & Schniepp, R. (2010). Gait disturbances in old age: classification, diagnosis, and treatment from a neurological perspective. *Deutsches Ärzteblatt International, 107*(17), 306.

Kitwood, T. (1997). *Dementia reconsidered: the person comes first.* Buckingham: Open University Press.

Kozlowska, K., Walker, P., McLean, L., & Carrive, P. (2015). Fear and the defense cascade: clinical implications and management. *Harvard Review of Psychiatry, 23*(4), 263.

Leite-Panissi, C. R. A. (2016). Tonic immobility behavior: a model to fear, anxiety or depression? *Progress in Neurobiology, 65,* 453–471.

Mitchell, G., & Agnelli, J. (2015). Person-centred care for people with dementia: Kitwood reconsidered. *Nursing Standard, 30*(7), 46.

Mulholland, F., & Jackson, J. (2018). The experience of older adults with anxiety and depression living in the community: aging, occupation and mental wellbeing. *British Journal of Occupational Therapy, 81*(11), 657–666.

NHS. (2014). Rehabilitation, reablement and recovery. Rehabilitation is everyone's business: principles and expectations for good adult rehabilitation. Wessex Strategic Clinical Networks. Retrieved from: https://www.networks.nhs.uk/nhs-networks/clinical-commissioning-community/documents/principles-and-expectations.

Rosenbaum, S., Tiedemann, A., Ward, P. B., Curtis, J., & Sherrington, C. (2015). Physical activity interventions: an essential component in recovery from mental illness. *British Journal of Sports Medicine, 49*, 1544–1545.

Royal Pharmaceutical Society of Great Britain. (2019). In *British national formulary* (Vol. 77). London, UK: Pharmaceutical Press.

Scheets, P. L., Sahrmann, S. A., Norton, B. J., Stith, J. S., & Crowner, B. E. (2015). What is backward disequilibrium and how do I treat it?: a complex patient case study. *Journal of Neurologic Physical Therapy, 39*(2), 119–126.

Seppala, L. J., Wermelink, A. M., de Vries, M., Ploegmakers, K. J., van de Glind, E. M., Daams, J. G., van der Velde, N., & ... EUGMS Task and Finish group on fall-risk-increasing drugs. (2018). Fall-risk-increasing drugs: a systematic review and meta-analysis: II. Psychotropics. *Journal of the American Medical Directors Association, 19*(4), 371.e11.

Shahab, S., Nicolici, D. F., Tang, A., Katz, P., & Mah, L. (2017). Depression predicts functional outcome in geriatric inpatient rehabilitation. *Archives of Physical Medicine and Rehabilitation, 98*(3), 500–507.

Stott, D. J., & Quinn, T. J. (2017). Principles of rehabilitation of older people. *Medicine, 45*(1), 1–5.

Yesavage, J. A., Brink, T. L., Rose, T. L., Lum, O., Huang, V., Adey, M., & Leirer, V. O. (1982). Development and validation of a geriatric depression screening scale: a preliminary report. *Journal of Psychiatric Research, 17*(1), 37–49.

Zigmond, A. S., & Snaith, R. P. (1983). The hospital anxiety and depression scale. *Acta Psychiatrica Scandinavica, 67*(6), 361–370.

30

Cognitive Problems

Thomas Jackson & Hannah Moorey

LEARNING OBJECTIVES

- Describe the assessment of cognitive problems in older people
- Explain how to diagnose dementia, mild cognitive impairment and delirium
- Describe how cognitive problems can impact on rehabilitation

---

CASE

Hetty is an 82-year-old lady admitted to hospital following a fall and hip fracture 1 week ago. She had a hemiarthroplasty on day 1 and has been transferred to the rehabilitation ward. On initial assessment she is withdrawn, not paying attention to instructions, and appears disorientated and 'confused'.

Her notes state she has 'dementia' and has been confused since admission, needing assistance with most tasks. She has mobilised a short distance using a frame with the assistance of one person. Previously she lived alone and mobilised with a stick around her single level flat, using a wheeled frame to go outside. She has a daughter who helps with instrumental activities of daily living (IADLs), but no formal care. Her daughter has been away, but is returning tomorrow.

She has a past medical history of hypertension and diabetes, but no previous diagnosis of dementia. She is currently taking painkillers (codeine) and her regular medications (metformin, bendroflumethiazide).

This case represents a common scenario when looking after older people in hospitals. Hetty has inadequately assessed cognitive problems – 'confusion'. There is often pressure in rehabilitation settings to state if people have 'rehab potential' so discharge planning can take place.

Confusion is a symptom, not a diagnosis.

The key is to get the diagnosis right. Confusion is a symptom, not a diagnosis. This may be acute delirium, or it may be a more long-term cognitive impairment such as dementia. It is impossible to offer best care without the right diagnosis.

Delirium is important to recognise as it is associated with a higher chance of dying, or being discharged to a nursing home. Crucially it is treatable in most cases, by addressing the underlying causes and allowing time for the condition to improve.

This chapter reviews the common causes of cognitive impairment (changes in thinking, memory, and brain function; see Box 30.1) seen in older people, and touches on some of the other rarer causes. We will aim to give a structure of assessment and management.

DEMENTIA AND MILD COGNITIVE IMPAIRMENT

Dementia is an umbrella term for chronic neurodegenerative diseases (diseases which cause irreparable degeneration or death of nerve cells), characterised by a progressive decline in cognition with an effect on everyday function. In contrast, mild cognitive impairment (MCI) is a condition where people have cognitive impairment, but not great enough to impact on their everyday function. Alzheimer's disease is the most common cause of dementia accounting for 60%–70% (World Health Organisation, 2017). Other causes include vascular dementia, mixed dementia, dementia with Lewy bodies (DLB), frontotemporal dementia and alcohol-related dementia.

It is important that practitioners are aware of the likelihood of encountering undiagnosed dementia during rehabilitation.

Dementia is common in people admitted to hospital, affecting up to 40% of acute hospital admissions (Sampson et al., 2009). Furthermore, patients with dementia are more likely to present with falls or hip fractures (Seitz et al., 2011), presentations where rehabilitation is often vital. In hospital, dementia is underrecognised, with up to half of those with dementia not having the diagnosis identified and noted by their clinical team (Sampson et al., 2009). It is important that all health staff are aware of the likelihood of encountering undiagnosed dementia during rehabilitation. There is debate over whether dementia should be diagnosed during a hospital admission and diagnosis in the UK is usually made by an old age psychiatrist in a memory clinic. However, it is important to recognise the possibility of a diagnosis to ensure the patient's needs are met during the admission and to

---

BOX 30.1 What Is Cognitive Impairment?

Cognitive impairment – a general term to describe impairment of brain function of varying severity and cause.

Dementia – a term for conditions that lead to a progressive decline in brain function that impacts on everyday function. Alzheimer's disease is the most common cause but there are others.

Mild cognitive impairment – impaired brain function that does not have an impact on everyday function.

Delirium – an acute condition where a person's thinking, memory and alertness are altered. It often occurs after an operation or with an infection.

---

consider initiating the diagnostic process. This may include (NICE, 2018):

- A thorough history from the patient and any friends or relatives.
- The Informant Questionnaire on Cognitive Decline in the Elderly (IQCODE) to aid taking a history from a relative (Jackson et al., 2016).
- A brief structured cognitive instrument such as the Mini-Cog (See Box 30.2) or 6 item cognitive impairment test (6CIT). If the patient is stable and time permits, a more thorough test such as the Addenbrookes Cognitive Examination (ACE).
- Relevant physical examination, blood tests and imaging.
- Referral to a memory clinic for full diagnosis and further management on discharge.

People with dementia can experience challenges when admitted to a hospital or a rehabilitation centre. The change in environment can be disorientating and distressing, and staff may find it difficult to recognise and address the person's needs (Michael, 2014). People with dementia are at higher risk of delirium, falls and of a deterioration in their cognitive and physical functioning during a hospital admission (Jackson et al., 2017). Some of the common challenges encountered include the following.

Pain Management

Pain is underrecognised in people with dementia as they may not be able to inform staff when they require pain medication (Lichtner et al., 2016). Pain in people with dementia may be identified by looking for a change in behaviour including aggressive or challenging behaviour, a change in appetite, body language, facial expression or vocalisation. A pain scale validated in dementia, such as the Abbey Pain Scale (Abbey et al., 2004), can be used to aid recognition (NICE, 2018). Good pain management is vital to ensure successful rehabilitation. People with dementia may benefit from regular, rather than as required, painkillers. More consistent pain relief may also be achieved with different forms or medications, such as patches.

Nutrition

Reasons for poor nutrition in people with dementia include reduced appetite, poor oral health, forgetting to eat, not recognising food or having difficulty cutting, chewing

---

BOX 30.2 The Mini-Cog.

The Mini-Cog Assessment Instrument for Dementia

The Mini-Cog assessment instrument combines an uncued three-item recall test with a clock-drawing test (CDT). The Mini-Cog can be administered in about 3 minutes, requires no special equipment and is relatively uninfluenced by level of education or language variations.

Administration

The test is administered as follows:

1. Instruct the patient to listen carefully to and remember three unrelated words and then to repeat the words.
2. Instruct the patient to draw the face of a clock, either on a blank sheet of paper or on a sheet with the clock circle already drawn on the page. After the patient puts the numbers on the clock face, ask him or her to draw the hands of the clock to read a specific time, such as 11:20. These instructions can be repeated, but no additional instructions should be given. Give the patient as much time as needed to complete the task. The CDT serves as the recall distractor.
3. Ask the patient to repeat the three previously presented words.

Scoring

Give 1 point for each recalled word after the CDT distractor. Score 1–3.

A score of 0 indicates positive screen for dementia.

A score of 1 or 2 with an abnormal CDT indicates positive screen for dementia.

A score of 1 or 2 with a normal CDT indicates negative screen for dementia.

A score of 3 indicates negative screen for dementia.

The CDT is considered normal if all numbers are present in the correct sequence and position, and the hands readably display the requested time.

From Ball J, Dains J, Flynn J, Solomon B, Stewart R Seidel's *Guide to Physical Examination*, 8th edn. Elsevier; 2019, with permission.

---

or swallowing food (Harwood, 2014). Psychiatric symptoms such as low mood, anxiety or delusions may also influence feeding. Avoiding malnutrition is important in a rehabilitation setting. A person-centred approach is key. Nutrition may be improved by ensuring staff have enough time to aid people with meals, encouraging involvement of family or carers, being flexible with mealtimes and food choices, and considering the dining environment including lighting and opportunity to interact with other people.

Behavioural and Psychological Symptoms in Dementia

Behavioural and psychological symptoms in dementia (BPSD) are symptoms common in people with dementia which are not directly related to memory (non-cognitive symptoms). They include depression, agitation, aggression, apathy and sleep disturbance, which may all impact on rehabilitation. A change in environment and unfamiliar staff may worsen symptoms. Prevalence of BPSD in patients with dementia undergoing rehabilitation post hip fracture is 31% (Shibasaki et al., 2018) and as high as 75% in people with dementia admitted to an acute hospital (Sampson et al., 2014). These symptoms are distressing for people with dementia and their carers. The cause is often multifactorial, and the first step in management is to consider possible causes: pain, lack of routine, understimulation (Tible et al., 2017). Antipsychotic medications may be used to manage symptoms, but only if patients are at risk of harm to themselves or others, or the symptoms are causing severe distress (NICE, 2018). It is important that a full discussion should be had with the patient and their family before starting a sedative such as an antipsychotic medication (e.g. risperidone), and they should be avoided in DLB disease as they may aggravate motor symptoms.

DELIRIUM

Delirium is a neuropsychiatric disorder characterised by acute changes in attention and cognition (Inouye, Westendorp, & Saczynski, 2014). It is a sudden change in a person's thinking, memory and alertness, usually seen after an operation, or when people have an infection. Delirium is common; 20% of older people who are admitted to hospital will have delirium at some point during their admission (Pendlebury et al., 2015) and it is a common postoperative complication in older people. Delirium can also affect people who are critically ill and admitted to intensive care units (Girard, Pandharipande, & Wesley Ely, 2008).

Delirium is associated with poor outcomes. People with delirium stay longer in hospital, are less likely to get back to their own home after being in hospital and are more likely to die (Witlox et al., 2010). Older people may have delirium when referred to a rehabilitation programme or develop it during rehabilitation. It is therefore important that everyone can recognise and diagnose delirium.

The key symptoms of delirium are (American Psychiatric Association, 2013):

- Disturbance of consciousness – people may have a reduced awareness of their environment and difficulty focusing their attention.
- Change in cognition – people may have problems with memory, be disorientated to time, place or person, have difficulty with language or perceptual disturbances such as hallucinations.

Symptoms develop over a short period and tend to fluctuate. Delirium may be directly caused by medical conditions or by medications, but the cause is often due to a combination of factors. A number of screening tools can be used, e.g., the 4AT test is quick, does not require any training and is validated in detecting delirium (Bellelli et al., 2014; SIGN, 2019) (see Box 30.3).

Symptoms of delirium usually improve with treatment of underlying causes. The TIME bundle is a practical framework for management (see Box 30.4). Delirium usually improves within 4 days, but in some people, delirium symptoms can persist for weeks, and even months (Cole et al., 2010). Sometimes people with delirium may not recover to the same level that they were functioning at before.

BOX 30.3   The 4AT

ALERTNESS

This includes patients who may be markedly drowsy (e.g. difficult to rouse and obviously sleepy during assessment) or agitated/hyperactive. Observe the patient. If asleep, attempt to wake with speech or gentle touch on the shoulder. Ask the patient to state their name and address to assist rating.

Normal (fully alert but not agitated) throughout assessment	0
Mild sleepiness for <10 seconds after waking, then normal	0
Clearly abnormal	4

AMT4

Age, date of birth, place (name of the hospital or building), current year

No mistakes	0
1 mistake	1
2 or more mistakes/untestable	2

ATTENTION

Ask the patient: 'Please tell me the months of the year in backwards order, starting at December.' To assist initial understanding one prompt of 'what is the month before December?' is permitted.

Months of the year backwards	Achieves 7 months or more correctly	0
	Starts but scores <7 months/ refuses to start	1
	Untestable (cannot start because unwell, drowsy, inattentive)	2

ACUTE CHANGE OR FLUCTUATING COURSE

Evidence of significant change or fluctuation in alertness, cognition, other mental function (eg paranoia, hallucinations) arising over the last 2 weeks and still evident in last 24 hours

No	0
Yes	4

4 or above: possible delirium ± cognitive impairment
1-3: possible cognitive impairment
0: delirium or cognitive impairment unlikely (but delirium still possible if [4] information incomplete)

From Bellelli G, Bruni A, Malerba M, et al. Geriatric multidimensional assessment for elderly patients with acute respiratory diseases. *Eur J Intern Med.* 2014, with permission.

People with dementia are at higher risk of getting delirium, but identifying delirium in these patients can be more difficult (Jackson et al., 2017). People with dementia are also at higher risk of worsened cognition following an episode of delirium.

OTHER CONDITIONS TO CONSIDER

Depression

Older people are at greater risk of depression, especially after an acute illness and hospital stay, where depression is associated with worse outcomes (Pederson et al., 2016; Rodda, Walker, & Carter, 2011). Depressive symptoms affect about

---

BOX 30.4   The TIME Bundle

Initiate TIME within 2 hours

T   Think exclude and treat possible triggers
Check observations/vital signs
Blood glucose
Medication history (identify new medications/change of dose/medication recently stopped)
Pain review (Abbey Pain Scale)
Assess for urinary retention
Assess for constipation

I   Investigate and intervene to correct underlying causes
Assess hydration and start fluid balance chart
Bloods (FBC, U&E, Ca, LFTs, CRP, Mg, glucose)
Look for symptoms/signs of infection (skin, chest, urine, CNS) and perform appropriate cultures/imaging depending on clinical assessment
ECG

M   Management plan
Initiate treatment of ALL underlying causes found above

E   Engage and explore (complete within 2 hours or if family/carer not present within 24 hours)
Engage with patient/family/carer – explore if this is usual behaviour. Ask: How would you like to be involved?
Explain diagnosis of delirium to patient and family/carers (use delirium leaflet)
Document diagnosis of delirium

Modified version from Healthcare Improvement Scotland - Improving the Care of Older People: Delirium Tool Kit, 2014, with permission

---

30% of older people in hospital. Importantly, older people are more likely to have cognitive impairment, or psychotic symptoms as part of their depression, than younger people, thus making depression an important diagnosis to consider (Schaakxs et al., 2018). The hypoactive subtype of delirium can appear similar to depression, as can dementia – indeed depression is often described as a 'pseudo-dementia' (something that mimics dementia) in older adults.

Brief screening tools are available, such as the Geriatric Depression Scale, but these are not as accurate in people with cognitive impairment (Dennis, Kadri, & Coffey, 2012). As always, the history and a careful examination are key to distinguishing depression from delirium and dementia. See Chapter 29 Anxiety and Depression for more details.

Dementia with Lewy Bodies

This is a rarer cause of dementia that has similar symptoms to delirium. It is characterised by fluctuating attentional deficits and visual hallucinations. It is progressive and patients with DLB develop motor symptoms similar to parkinsonism (increased muscle tone, reduced speed of movement and tremor) (McKeith et al., 2017). This is an important diagnosis to consider especially in people who appear very

slow to recover from delirium. It is important to recognise, but difficult to make a final diagnosis without more specialised brain scans. There is increasing evidence that some of the symptoms respond to treatment with cholinesterase inhibitors, which are memory enhancers usually used to help treat Alzheimer's dementia.

Charles Bonnet Syndrome

This is a condition of visual hallucinations, which is often the result of impaired vision (Schadlu, Schadlu, & Shepherd, 2009). It is a so-called visual release syndrome, where the visual cortex becomes overactive to compensate for the reduced stimuli from the diseased retina. The hallucinations are described as stereotypical – often involving small animal or human figures, and patients are rarely distressed by them. It is said to occur in the absence of cognitive impairment. Again, it is important to recognise as a diagnosis because reassurance to the patent can be very therapeutic.

SPECIFIC ISSUES AND INTERVENTIONS IN REHABILITATION

Delivering rehabilitation for people with cognitive impairment can be challenging. A qualitative study looking at perceptions of physiotherapists working with patients after hip fracture surgery reflects this (Hall et al., 2017). Some staff were not confident working with people with dementia and attitudes of staff could lead to patients being 'written off too early' and not appropriately referred. They felt frustrated that there was a lack of services for people with dementia and that they could be excluded from services. They also found the use of standardised outcomes and targets frustrating, as they felt they were not always appropriate for this patient group and restricted the use of patient-centred approaches.

DOES REHABILITATION FOR PATIENTS WITH DEMENTIA WORK?

Although challenging, the current limited evidence suggests that rehabilitation in this group may improve outcomes. Most studies have focused on rehabilitation following hip fracture. Overall, people with cognitive impairment achieve improved outcomes with rehabilitation following hip fracture and improvements may be comparable to patients without cognitive impairment (Allen et al., 2011). However, the results are difficult to interpret as the studies involve small samples, measure cognitive impairment in a variety of ways, do not always differentiate between dementia and delirium, use a variety of interventions in a number of settings and measure variable functional outcomes (Allen et al., 2011; Smith et al., 2015). Further high-quality research is needed to answer this question and evaluate which specific therapy interventions are most useful in patients with cognitive impairment. Although guidelines for specific rehabilitation interventions are lacking, it is clear that a flexible and innovative approach is needed when working with people with dementia. For example, if patients are unable to sustain attention during sessions, one longer session can be replaced by a number of shorter sessions distributed throughout the day. Rehabilitation can also be personalised by incorporating interests, e.g. by walking to see a football match with a patient who enjoys football (Hall et al., 2017).

DOES REHABILITATION FOR PATIENTS WITH DELIRIUM WORK?

Older people with delirium have worse outcomes, including a higher likelihood of being admitted to a nursing home on discharge from hospital. However, research into rehabilitation in delirium is limited. We do not know whether rehabilitation in patients with delirium can improve these outcomes, or even if exclusion from rehabilitation programmes may contribute to poor outcomes in these patients.

One study looked at rehabilitation following hip fracture in older patients with cognitive impairment and BPSD, where the definition of BPSD included delirium (Shibasaki et al., 2018). The group of patients where BPSD symptoms resolved during rehabilitation had good functional outcomes. This offers some support that patients with delirium may benefit from rehabilitation.

We do know that multicomponent interventions, which often involve physiotherapy and early mobilisation, can reduce the incidence of delirium in hospitalised non-ICU patients (Siddiqi et al., 2016). There is also evidence for the use of rehabilitation to prevent delirium in ICU patients. With the introduction of physiotherapists and occupational therapists to the ICU with a focus on early mobilisation a reduction in the number of days patients suffered with delirium was observed (Needham et al., 2010). A randomised controlled trial of early physiotherapy and occupational therapy input, combined with pausing drugs that cause sedation, in mechanically ventilated patients, led to shorter delirium duration and an increased likelihood of patients returning to independent functioning (Schweickert et al., 2009). In a study where older patients took part in early intensive occupational therapy, delirium incidence was only 3%, compared to 20% in the usual care group (Álvarez et al., 2017). The occupational therapy intervention included polysensory stimulation, positioning, cognitive stimulation, basic activities of daily living, stimulation of upper limb motor function and family participation.

Location of rehabilitation may also be important. In Australia, delirium incidence was lower in older patients who underwent a rehabilitation programme at home compared to those who stayed as inpatients on a geriatric rehabilitation ward (Caplan et al., 2006). There was no difference in function at the end of the programme between the two groups and patients were more satisfied with the home-based rehabilitation programme.

HOW CAN WE MANAGE RISK IN PATIENTS WITH COGNITIVE IMPAIRMENT IN REHABILITATION?

Rehabilitation can be considered an inherently risky activity, often involving encouraging people to function beyond their current ability. Managing risk in patients with cognitive impairment can be challenging as patients often lack capacity to make certain decisions (see Chapter 20 Brain Health and Mental Capacity), and practitioners may need to make decisions in their best interests. Healthcare staff may be overly cautious to minimise risk, which may ultimately disadvantage the patient. The UK Department of Health has advocated a risk enablement, or positive risk management, approach for people with dementia (Department of Health, 2010). The positive benefit of taking risks is balanced against the negative effects of attempting to avoid risk altogether. For example, in rehabilitation the risk of a patient with cognitive impairment falling when mobilising without a walking aid may be balanced against the frustration generated by preventing the patient from mobilising and the deconditioning. Risk enablement encourages a person-centred approach allowing people with cognitive impairment to maximise control. Involvement of the patient and carers is essential to understand the patient's biographical approach to risk and what is important to them. Risk enablement plans can be used in a rehabilitation setting to 'summarise the risks and benefits that have been identified, the likelihood that they will occur and their seriousness, or severity'(Department of Health, 2010). The 'actions to be taken by practitioners to promote risk enablement and to deal with adverse events should they occur' (Department of Health, 2010) should also be included.

CASE CONCLUSION

Referring back to our case, Hetty is presenting with 'confusion'. A delirium assessment using the 4AT identifies delirium, and this is supported by her daughter when she returns from holiday and describes her brain as usually 'working well, she's still got all her marbles'. An IQCODE-SF confirms this, so she is unlikely to have any unrecognised dementia or MCI.

Clinical examination and assessment shows she is constipated, with a low blood sodium level and these are treated. Her recent hip fracture and operation are also likely to be underlying causes of her delirium. The diagnosis is explained to Hetty (it's important for patients to know, too) and her daughter, and non-pharmacological strategies to improve delirium, such as mobility, are encouraged with the help of the whole multidisciplinary team. Within 4 days, her cognitive function has improved and she is progressing well with rehabilitation.

The risks in this case are that Hetty is given an incorrect diagnosis of dementia, with inappropriate lowering of rehabilitation expectations. This may lead to unnecessary institutionalisation.

Recommendations in this chapter aim to provide structure to the assessment and management of older people with cognitive problems during rehabilitation, thus avoiding the risks described above.

SUMMARY POINTS

- Cognitive impairment is common in older people, especially so in hospital settings. However, it is underdiagnosed, leading to poor care
- Delirium is a common, sudden change in cognition, often due to infection or surgery. It is poorly recognised by healthcare professionals, but causes worse outcomes
- Delirium is important to recognise because it is treatable and preventable
- Dementia is common in older people in hospital, but should not be seen as a barrier to rehabilitation

MCQs

Q.1 An 80-year-old woman is admitted from a residential home with pneumonia. Her pneumonia is treated, but she remains functionally impaired (she was independently mobile with a stick, but now requires the assistance of two people to transfer). The nurses report she is confused, and occasionally agitated. She calls out at night, and is not very good at following instructions. A 4AT is 8/12 (positive). Which of the following is the best working diagnosis?
  a. Probable dementia
  b. Behavioural and psychological symptoms of dementia (BPSD)
  c. Depression
  d. Delirium
  e. Alzheimer's disease

Q.2 A 74-year-old man presents to the emergency department following a fall at home. He has no bony injuries, but is unsteady on mobilising, disorientated and calling out to visual hallucinations. He is referred for rehabilitation.

His wife is present, and they are both worried as he has become progressively more forgetful over the last year. On further questioning he has then developed reduced mobility over the last 4 months, and has had a number of recent falls. Examination reveals mild increased tone in his right arm and a 'shuffling' gait. 4AT is 4/12 (positive), and you notice he has difficulty paying attention to your assessment.

Which is the most likely diagnosis:
  a. Alzheimer's disease
  b. Delirium
  c. Dementia with Lewy bodies
  d. Mild cognitive impairment
  e. Vascular dementia

REFERENCES

Abbey, J., Piller, N., De Bellis, A., Esterman, A., Parker, D., Giles, L., & Lowcay, B. (2004). The Abbey pain scale: a 1-minute numerical indicator for people with end-stage dementia. *International Journal of Palliative Nursing, 10*(1), 6–13.

Allen, J., Koziak, A., Buddingh, S., Liang, J., Buckingham, J., & Beaupre, L. A. (2011). Rehabilitation in patients with dementia following hip fracture: a systematic review. *Physiotherapy Canada, 64*(2), 190–201.

Álvarez, E. A., Garrido, M. A., Tobar, E. A., Prieto, S. A., Vergara, S. O., Briceño, C. D., & González, F. J. (2017). Occupational therapy for delirium management in elderly patients without mechanical ventilation in an intensive care unit: A pilot randomized clinical trial. *Journal of Critical Care, 37*, 85–90.

American Psychiatric Association. (2013). *Diagnostic and statistical manual of mental disorders: DSM-5.* American Psychiatric Publishing, Inc.

Bellelli, G., Morandi, A., Davis, D. H., Mazzola, P., Turco, R., Gentile, S., …, & MacLullich, A. M. (2014). Validation of the 4AT, a new instrument for rapid delirium screening: a study in 234 hospitalised older people. *Age and Ageing, 43*, 496–502.

Caplan, G. A., Coconis, J., Board, N., Sayers, A., & Woods, J. (2006). Does home treatment affect delirium? A randomised controlled trial of rehabilitation of elderly and care at home or usual treatment (The REACH-OUT trial). *Age and Ageing, 35*(1), 53–60.

Cole, M. G., Ciampi, A., Belzile, E., & Zhong, L. (2010). Persistent delirium in older hospital patients. *Current Opinion in Psychiatry, 23*(3), 250–254.

Dennis, M., Kadri, A., & Coffey, J. (2012). Depression in older people in the general hospital: a systematic review of screening instruments. *Age and Ageing, 41*(2), 148–154.

Department of Health. (2010). Nothing ventured, nothing gained: risk guidance for dementia. Retrieved from: https://www.gov.uk/government/publications/nothing-ventured-nothing-gained-risk-guidance-for-people-with-dementia.

Girard, T. D., Pandharipande, P. P., & Wesley Ely, E. (2008). Delirium in the intensive care unit. *Critical Care, 12*(suppl. 3), S3.

Hall, A., Watkins, R., Lang, I. A., Endacott, R., & Goodwin, V. A. (2017). The experiences of physiotherapists treating people with dementia who fracture their hip. *BMC Geriatrics, 17*(1), 91.

Harwood, R. (2014). Feeding decisions in advanced dementia. *The Journal of the Royal College of Physicians of Edinburgh, 44*(3), 232–237.

Inouye, S. K., Westendorp, R. G. J., & Saczynski, J. S. (2014). Delirium in elderly people. *The Lancet, 383*(9920), 911–922.

Jackson, T. A., MacLullich, A. M., Gladman, J. R. F., Lord, J. M., & Sheehan, B. (2016). Diagnostic test accuracy of informant-based tools to diagnose dementia in older hospital patients with delirium: a prospective cohort study. *Age and Ageing, 45*(4), 505–511.

Jackson, T. A., Gladman, J. R. F., Harwood, R. H., MacLullich, A. M. J., Sampson, E. L., Sheehan, B., & Davis, D. H. J. (2017).

Challenges and opportunities in understanding dementia and delirium in the acute hospital. *PLOS Medicine, 14*(3), e1002247.

Lichtner, V., Dowding, D., Allcock, N., Keady, J., Sampson, E. L., Briggs, M., …, & José Closs, S. (2016). The assessment and management of pain in patients with dementia in hospital settings: a multi-case exploratory study from a decision making perspective. *BMC Health Services Research, 16*(1), 427.

McKeith, I. G., Boeve, B. F., Dickson, D. W., Halliday, G., Taylor, J. P., Weintraub, D., …, & Kosaka, K. (2017). Diagnosis and management of dementia with Lewy bodies. *Neurology, 89*(1), 88–100.

Michael, M. (2014). Excellence in dementia care. In Murna, D., Barbara, B., (Eds). Maidenhead: McGraw Hill Education/Open University Press.

Needham, D. M., Korupolu, R., Zanni, J. M., Pradhan, P., Colantuoni, E., Palmer, J. B., Brower, R. G., & Fan, E. (2010). Early physical medicine and rehabilitation for patients with acute respiratory failure: a quality improvement project. *Archives of Physical Medicine and Rehabilitation, 91*(4), 536–542.

NICE. (2018). Dementia: assessment, management and support for people living with dementia support for people living with dementia and their carers and their carers NICE guideline. Retrieved from: https://www.nice.org.uk/guidance/ng97.

Pederson, J. L., Warkentin, L. M., Majumdar, S. R., & McAlister, F. A. (2016). Depressive symptoms are associated with higher rates of readmission or mortality after medical hospitalization: a systematic review and meta-analysis. *Journal of Hospital Medicine, 11*(5), 373–380.

Pendlebury, S. T., Lovett, N., Smith, S. C., Dutta, N., Bendon, C., Lloyd-Lavery, A., Mehta, Z., & Rothwell, P. M. (2015). Observational, longitudinal study of delirium in consecutive unselected acute medical admissions: age-specific rates and associated factors, mortality and re-admission. *BMJ Open, 5*(11), e007808.

Rodda, J., Walker, Z., & Carter, J. (2011). Depression in older adults. *BMJ, 343*, d5219.

Sampson, E. L., Blanchard, M. R., Jones, L., Tookman, A., & King, M. (2009). Dementia in the acute hospital: prospective cohort study of prevalence and mortality. *The British Journal of Psychiatry, 195*(1), 61–66.

Sampson, E. L., White, N., Leurent, B., Scott, S., Lord, K., Round, J., & Jones, L. (2014). Behavioural and psychiatric symptoms in people with dementia admitted to the acute hospital: prospective cohort study. *The British Journal of Psychiatry, 205*(3), 189–196.

Schaakxs, R., Comijs, H. C., Lamers, F., Kok, R. M., Beekman, A. T. F., & Penninx, B. W. J. H. (2018). Associations between age and the course of major depressive disorder: a 2-year longitudinal cohort study. *The Lancet Psychiatry, 5*(7), 581–590.

Schadlu, A. P., Schadlu, R., & Shepherd, J. B. (2009). Charles Bonnet syndrome: a review. *Current Opinion in Ophthalmology, 20*(3), 219–222.

Schweickert, W. D., Pohlman, M. C., Pohlman, A. S., Nigos, C., Pawlik, A. J., Esbrook, C. L., …, & Kress, J. P. (2009). Early physical and occupational therapy in mechanically ventilated, critically ill patients: a randomised controlled trial. *The Lancet, 373*(9678), 1874–1882.

Seitz, D. P., Adunuri, N., Gill, S. S., & Rochon, P. A. (2011). Prevalence of dementia and cognitive impairment among older adults with hip fractures. *Journal of the American Medical Directors Association, 12*(8), 556–564.

Shibasaki, K., Asahi, T., Mizobuchi, K., Akishita, M., & Ogawa, S. (2018). Rehabilitation strategy for hip fracture, focused on behavioral psychological symptoms of dementia for older people with cognitive impairment: a nationwide Japan rehabilitation database. *PLOS One, 13*(7), e0200143.

Siddiqi, N., Harrison, J. K., Clegg, A., Teale, E. A., Young, J., Taylor, J., & Simpkins, S. A. (2016). Interventions for preventing delirium in hospitalised non-ICU patients. *Cochrane Database of Systematic Reviews, 3*, CD005563.

SIGN. (2019). Risk reduction and management of delirium. A national clinical guideline. Retrieved from https://www.sign.ac.uk/assets/sign157.pdf.

Smith, T. O., Hameed, Y. A., Cross, J. L., Henderson, C., Sahota, O., & Fox, C. (2015). Enhanced rehabilitation and care models for adults with dementia following hip fracture surgery. *Cochrane Database of Systematic Reviews, 6*, CD010569.

Tible, O. P., Riese, F., Savaskan, E., & von Gunten, A. (2017). Best practice in the management of behavioural and psychological symptoms of dementia. *Therapeutic Advances in Neurological Disorders, 10*(8), 297–309.

Witlox, J., Eurelings, L. S. M., de Jonghe, J. F. M., Kalisvaart, K. J., Eikelenboom, P., & van Gool, W. A. (2010). Delirium in elderly patients and the risk of postdischarge mortality, institutionalization, and dementia: a meta-analysis. *JAMA, 304*(4), 443–451.

World Health Organisation. (2017). *Dementia*. Retrieved from: https://www.who.int/news-room/fact-sheets/detail/dementia (Accessed 3 May 2019).

31

Exercise Tolerance

Emily Ainger & Sean Ninan

LEARNING OBJECTIVES

- Describe how to determine a patient's normal exercise tolerance
- Identify factors that may affect exercise tolerance
- Identify physical and psychological factors that may affect exercise tolerance and outline strategies to optimise these factors
- Evaluate medications that may cause acute decline in exercise tolerance
- Explain how to evaluate a patient with acute decline in exercise tolerance

CASE

Jens is a 75-year-old man, who has recently had emergency surgery for a gallbladder infection (cholecystitis) having been unwell and off his legs for several days before admission. He initially made very good progress postoperatively, walking 20–30 m with a Zimmer frame and minimal supervision on the surgical ward. He has been transferred to a rehabilitation unit but seems to be becoming more fatigued and is now only able to walk 10 m with a Zimmer frame and close supervision due to unsteadiness. He wishes to return to his previous state of health and tells you that he 'used to walk for miles'.

Determining a patient's normal exercise tolerance involves a clinical judgement as to when they were last well so as to establish baseline performance. This can help in goal setting during rehabilitation. A not uncommon scenario when healthcare professionals ask the question 'How far can you normally walk?' is 'I used to walk for miles, doctor'. The task then is to figure out when the patient was last well and what true baseline performance is – we are interested in using the normal exercise tolerance to set appropriate rehabilitation goals. A useful rule of thumb for acute illness is to ask 'What were you like two weeks ago?', but in a subacute setting it may be that the patient has had a prolonged illness or a series of illnesses that have taken place over a longer period.

It is important, then, to consider the following:

1. How robust or frail is the patient when they are their normal self, taking 2 weeks ago as a guide for when this might have been, but considering that point of 'normal' may have been longer ago? Reduced exercise tolerance is one of the components for the phenotype of frailty. Patients with increasing severity of frailty may find it harder to recover from illnesses that have caused functional decline, as their physiological reserve is less (see Chapter 4 Frailty).

2. How severe and how 'reversible' was the illness? A large, disabling stroke may lead to incomplete recovery whereas immobility as a result of acute opioid (e.g. morphine) administration may be more easily reversible.

It is useful to compare 'normal' exercise tolerance and current exercise tolerance and consider what the patient's goals are with respect to future exercise tolerance.

In Jens's case, he was quite fit before his illness. Although it is true to say that he had previously walked for miles, in recent years he had started to slow down and actually had an exercise tolerance of 100 yards in the weeks and months prior to becoming unwell. He was independent with most activities of daily living within the house but his son used to help with cleaning and gardening and take him shopping every week. His other medical conditions are type 2 diabetes, hypertension and congestive cardiac failure. He would have been considered as 'mildly frail' prior to admission. His immediate postoperative course was complicated by a delirium precipitated by urinary retention and pain, but since then he had made steady progress, initially requiring the assistance of two staff to transfer but was walking 20–30 m with a Zimmer frame and minimal supervision. His goal is to progress to walking with a stick and to improve his exercise tolerance to as close to his previous baseline as possible.

While physiotherapy is key to improving exercise tolerance, other factors that need to be considered may include:

- Degree of frailty
- Comorbidities
- Deconditioning
- Obesity
- Depression
- Anxiety
- Motivation
- Fear of falling
- Acute illness
- Nutrition
- Pain
- Polypharmacy

A multifactorial approach will need to be taken to improve exercise tolerance, and a thorough search for contributory factors should be especially considered when patients are 'not progressing' as might be expected.

MEDICAL CONDITIONS THAT MAY AFFECT EXERCISE TOLERANCE

Conditions that may have a particular role to play in affecting exercise tolerance include osteoarthritis, chronic obstructive pulmonary disease (COPD), congestive cardiac failure, cognitive impairment and Parkinson's disease.

Osteoarthritis may be optimised by appropriate use of topical analgesia (painkillers), e.g. topical NSAIDs (non-steroidal anti-inflammatory drugs), or capsaicin and oral analgesia, e.g. NSAIDs or paracetamol. NSAIDs are generally best avoided in older people with frailty due to the risk of gastrointestinal side effects and acute kidney injury. Intra-articular steroids may provide short-term relief, e.g. 4–6 weeks, but benefits are not likely to be seen when repeated courses are given over a longer period.

Most patients with **COPD** need bronchodilator therapy and many patients will be on long-acting beta agonist (LABA), long-acting muscarinic antagonist (LAMA) or inhaled corticosteroid (ICS) inhalers. NICE guidance recommends the use of a LABA and a second inhaler if patients remain breathless or have exacerbations despite:

- having used or been offered treatment for tobacco dependence if they smoke,
- optimised non-pharmacological management and relevant vaccinations and
- using a short-acting bronchodilator (NICE, 2018).

Those patients with asthmatic features or features suggesting steroid responsiveness should be considered for dual therapy with LABA/ICS combination. Features to be considered include a diagnosis of asthma or of atopy, a higher blood eosinophil count, substantial variation in FEV1 (forced expiratory volume, the maximal amount of air you can exhale in one second) over time (at least 400 ml) or substantial diurnal variation in peak expiratory flow (at least 20%). Patients being considered for ICS therapy should be counselled for side effects, including an increased risk of pneumonia.

Patients without such features should be considered for dual LABA/LAMA therapy. All patients should have inhaler technique and adherence to therapy reviewed.

Congestive cardiac failure is another major condition that can affect exercise tolerance. Most patients will be on medications, including an ACE (angiotensin-converting enzyme) inhibitor/angiotensin receptor blocker and a beta-blocker. Patients with symptoms despite these treatments may be started on aldosterone antagonists, such as spironolactone. Heart failure specialists may use ivabradine for patients with persistent symptoms, or those intolerant to beta-blockers. Sacubitril-valsartan is a new drug which may be used in place of ACE inhibitors or angiotensin receptor blockers in patients on optimal therapy with reduced ejection fraction – this is a measure of how well the heart pumps blood to the rest of the body. It has been shown to reduce mortality and hospitalisation.

Symptom relief of fluid overload from congestive cardiac failure is achieved through diuretic ('water tablet') therapy. Monitoring weight is useful to judge response and knowledge of a patient's 'dry weight' can provide a useful target for therapy. Fluid restriction is not required for most patients with normal sodium levels.

Patients with cardiovascular disease may find that their exercise tolerance is limited by **angina** (chest pain due to reduced blood flow to the heart). It is important to establish how far they can walk before they develop symptoms of angina, and whether this has remained 'stable'. Patients may be on medications, such as beta-blockers, calcium-channel blockers or nitrates, to help prevent angina attacks. A short-acting nitrate spray may be taken when patients do develop symptoms of angina. Patients should be encouraged to maintain physical activity within the limits of their angina. If they are usually sedentary, then slowly building up activity over a long period of time is important. Patients who get anginal symptoms at rest or are experiencing worsening of symptoms should be reviewed by a physician to help optimise management and assess suitability for physical rehabilitation. Cardiac rehabilitation, a specialised programme of exercise and information sessions, including lifestyle advice (see Chapter 57 Cardiac Rehabilitation) is commonly offered to patients after myocardial infarction or percutaneous coronary intervention, but should also be considered for patients with stable angina where it may help with exercise capacity.

Patients with **Parkinson's disease** may have periods of reduced mobility. This may be due to acute illness as outlined below but consideration also needs to be given to their medication regimen. It is imperative that patients with Parkinson's disease get their medication on time. Diet should be examined – protein-rich meals may compete with absorption of medications. Those patients suffering motor fluctuations, 'off' periods or dyskinesias where there are involuntary movements should have a review of their medications.

A medical review is performed and it is discovered that Jens has clinical signs of congestive cardiac failure with a significant amount of fluid on his legs. This can affect mobility and exercise tolerance, and it is noted that his diuretics were stopped in hospital. Jens tells you that he has noticed his legs get more swollen over the past few weeks. He is started on diuretics with plans to monitor his progress with blood tests and regular measurement of his weight.

COGNITIVE AND PSYCHOLOGICAL FACTORS THAT MAY AFFECT EXERCISE TOLERANCE

When looking after patients with **cognitive impairment,** it is important to confirm normal exercise tolerance by taking a collateral history from an informant that knows them well. Be aware that patients with cognitive impairment may not express pain in the usual way or may forget they had it, and careful attention should be paid to facial expressions and pain observed during rehabilitation sessions. Pain should be assessed regularly using a tool such as the Abbey Pain Scale (Abbey et al., 2004). Analgesia may need to be prescribed

TABLE 31.1 Common medications that may cause cognitive problems.	
Tricyclic antidepressants e.g. amitriptyline Sedatives, e.g. diazepam Antipsychotics Hypnotics, e.g. zopiclone	Increase risk of falls. May contribute to delirium. Anticholinergic side effects
Opioid analgesia	May be required for pain but can also cause confusion and cognitive slowing. Use at lowest possible dose. Anticholinergic side effects
Medications for overactive bladder, e.g. oxybutynin	Anticholinergic side effects
Sedating antihistamines, e.g. hydroxyzine	Anticholinergic side effects. Increased risk of cognitive decline and slowing
Prochlorperazine	Anticholinergic side effects. Regular use can cause parkinsonian side effects
Metoclopramide	Potential parkinsonian side effects when used long term
Drugs for neuropathic pain, e.g. gabapentin or pregabalin	Anticholinergic side effects
H2 receptor antagonists, e.g. ranitidine	Increased risk of delirium

'prophylactically' either regularly or just before a therapy session. Involving caregivers in goal setting and during therapy sessions can be very useful.

Delirium may be a reason for an acute decline in functional ability. The condition is characterised by being more confused than normal, and inattention – difficulty in sustaining attention. Inattention can be observed when patients struggle to follow what you are saying, or drift off. It can also be more formally tested by asking patients to recite the months of the year backwards. Other signs of delirium can include disorganised thinking, rambling speech, being more tired and sleepy, eating less and walking less. Patients may also become hyperactive and distressed. They may experience hallucinations. Delirium characteristically fluctuates, with patients being more severely affected at certain times more than others. See Chapter 30 Cognitive Problems for more information on how delirium and cognitive impairment can affect rehabilitation.

Patients with undetected **low mood** may be labelled as 'not engaging' with therapy. Depression is associated with adverse outcomes in terms of functional recovery. While the older person with overt low mood may be easy to identify, older patients with low mood may present with fatigue, poor concentration, chronic pain, slowing of movements and feelings of guilt or worthlessness. It can be screened for using a tool such as the Geriatric Depression Scale (GDS) or two-question screen. Patients who 'screen positive' should have a further detailed assessment of their mood and be considered for treatments such as psychological interventions or antidepressant therapy. Chapter 29, Anxiety and Depression, provides more detail.

Jens does not have any evidence of delirium or cognitive impairment. He does admit to occasionally feeling fed up since the operation but overall his mood is good and he is well motivated to participate in rehabilitation.

POLYPHARMACY

Polypharmacy – being on multiple medications – may become problematic when medicines are prescribed inappropriately such that the intended benefit is unlikely to be realised, or the

combination of medications causes problems with unintended side effects, hazardous interactions or unacceptable pill burden. Frail older people are particularly at risk of side effects from medications. A transition to rehabilitation-based care is a good opportunity to review medications in detail. With respect to drugs that may affect exercise tolerance, medications such as sedatives, antipsychotics and hypnotics may cause generalised slowing, and increase the risk of falls. All such drugs should be reviewed, and discontinued if possible, to reduce the risk of falls.

A large number of drugs can precipitate or worsen delirium. Drugs with anticholinergic activity are associated with increased risk of cognitive decline and may cause delirium directly or contribute to it through causing constipation, urinary retention or blurred vision. Common culprits are listed in Table 31.1 above, although this list is not exhaustive.

Jens's medications were as follows: bisoprolol 2.5 mg once daily, indapamide 2.5 mg once daily, ramipril 5 mg once daily, metformin 500 mg twice daily, zopiclone 7.5 mg once daily, co-codamol (codeine + paracetamol) 30 mg/500mg two tablets twice daily. After discussion it was noted that Jens had started on zopiclone due to difficulty sleeping in a noisy ward environment and this was no longer an issue. His pain since his operation had also much improved. He agreed to stop the zopiclone and change his co-codamol to regular paracetamol with codeine available on an 'as required' basis.

ACUTE DECLINE IN EXERCISE TOLERANCE

Where exercise tolerance seems to decline quickly over a few days, a prompt full clinical evaluation is warranted to determine the reason why. This may include:
- Evaluation for acute illness through history and examination
- Basic investigations in selected cases commonly including
  - Blood tests – looking for e.g. anaemia, infection, or worsening kidney function
  - Chest X-ray – in selected cases where infection or fluid overload is suspected, although these may also be treated clinically

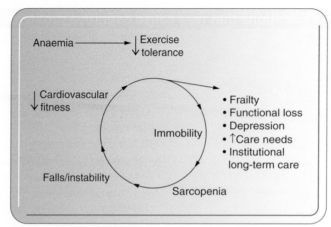

FIG. 31.1 Anaemia can cause a downward cycle, eventually leading to the conditions on the right. (From Robinson J. *Sleep Medicine Clinics*, vol. 8; 2013:241–53. *Am Geriatr Soc.* 2003;51(3 suppl):S14-7 with permission)

- Urine culture, bearing in mind that many older people will have 'positive' urine dipsticks and harmless bacteria in their urine so tests musts be interpreted alongside the presence of urinary symptoms or other evidence of infection
- Optimisation of major medical conditions as above
- Evaluation of psychological factors such as cognition and mood as above
- Evaluation of polypharmacy
- Evaluation of bowel function for constipation or faecal impaction
- Evaluation of urinary function for incontinence, urinary retention and inappropriate catheterisation
- Evaluation of pain
- Evaluation of hydration and nutrition.

Jens has a thorough assessment carried out and some routine blood tests performed. This detects a low haemoglobin level of 74 g/l. Subsequent haematinic tests (ferritin, vitamin b12 and folate) are normal, and it is noted that Jens had a normal haemoglobin before his surgery, had 2 units transfusion around the time of the operation but that his haemoglobin never returned to normal. A urine culture grows coliform bacteria but as he has no acute urinary symptoms, this is considered to be asymptomatic bacteriuria and not treated.

Significance and Management of Anaemia

Anaemia can have a profound effect on the functional abilities of older people. This commonly occurs over a long time, as the blood count drops slowly but progressively. Fig. 31.1 shows how this results in reduced exercise tolerance, leading in turn to relative immobility, muscle wasting (sarcopenia), falls and diminished cardiovascular fitness that further reduces exercise tolerance.

The threshold for transfusion is normally a haemoglobin of below 70 g/l with a target of 70–90 g/l. A degree of anaemia is common postoperatively or after an acute illness. Patients with anaemia should have this assessed, investigated appropriately and treated, depending on the cause.

However, patients with acute coronary syndrome or worsening heart failure may benefit from a more lenient threshold of 80 g/l with a target of 80–100 g/l. In situations where anaemia is present but not at the level requiring transfusions, and iron levels are low, intravenous iron can be given to help the body to produce more blood.

The pros and cons of blood transfusion are discussed with Jens, and he consents to having 2 units of blood transfused.

It can be seen that patients with reduced exercise tolerance may have a variety of contributing factors, including the underlying illness, comorbidities, acute illness, delirium and medication side effects. In Jens's case, he has had a significant illness that will take him time to recover from. However, his exercise tolerance has also been affected by decompensated heart failure, polypharmacy with sedative and opioid drugs, and anaemia. A thorough evaluation has been performed to identify and treat these issues.

Jens's exercise tolerance gradually improves, and he is eventually discharged to his own home environment with further therapy in place to further progress exercise tolerance.

SUMMARY POINTS

- A patient's normal exercise tolerance can be determined by asking when they were last well, taking 2 weeks ago as a guide for when this might have been, but considering that point of 'normal' may have been longer ago
- Normal exercise tolerance and the severity and 'reversibility' of the illness that has affected this should be considered when helping the patient to set goals
- Multiple factors may affect exercise tolerance, and management of contributory factors can help to optimise rehabilitation
- Many medications have the potential to affect exercise tolerance adversely, particularly those with anticholinergic activity
- An acute decline in exercise tolerance should prompt a systematic review of multiple potentially contributory factors to determine the causes

MCQs

Q.1 A patient's normal exercise tolerance can be determined by:
   a. Observing their mobility
   b. Asking them how far they could walk when last well
   c. Asking what is the furthest they have ever walked
   d. Asking them how far they could walk 6 months ago

Q.2 Which of the following is **not** a feature of delirium?
   a. Reduced mobility
   b. Tiredness and sleepiness
   c. Acute change in behaviour
   d. Progressive deterioration over months

Q.3 Which of the following investigations should **not be recommended** when working up acute decline in mobility?
   a. Full blood count
   b. Chest X-ray
   c. ECG
   d. Urine dipstick

REFERENCES

Abbey, J., Piller, N., De Bellis, A., Esterman, A., Parker, D., Giles, L., & Lowcay, B. (2004). The Abbey pain scale: a 1-minute numerical indicator for people with end-stage dementia. *International Journal of Palliative Nursing, 10*(1), 6–13.

NICE Guideline Updates Team (UK). (2018). *Chronic obstructive pulmonary disease in over 16s: diagnosis and management.* London: National Institute for Health and Care Excellence (UK).

32

Sleep and Fatigue

Andrew Scott, Marissa O'Callaghan & John Garvey

LEARNING OBJECTIVES

- Describe the role of sleep in the older person
- Outline sleep disorders that are common in the older person
- Identify features of insomnia, restless leg syndrome, obstructive sleep apnoea and parasomnias in the older person
- Create a plan for diagnosis and management of the common sleep disorders in the older person
- Explain how to recognise when fatigue might need a medical review

SLEEP IN THE OLDER PERSON

Humans spend one third of their life sleeping, yet it is not fully understood why we require sleep. Allowing the body to rest and heal is one theory, but this is offset by the fact that metabolic and neurological activity is in fact increased during sleep.

Older people will often report more difficulty in falling asleep and maintaining sleep compared to when they were younger. Numerous factors could account for this including normal physiological changes of sleep seen in older people, social factors such as stress, anxiety and mental health issues, comorbidities, medications and sleep disorders such as obstructive sleep apnoea (OSA), restless leg syndrome (RLS), insomnia and other sleep disorders.

In this chapter, we will outline how these common sleep disorders present, how they are diagnosed as well as how they are managed in the older person.

SLEEP HYGIENE

Rupert is a 78-year-old bachelor who is undergoing inpatient rehab in the seven-bedded long ward of the hospital. It is a busy place with frequent admissions and discharges. Rupert has always described himself as a night owl, often watching television late in the evening and he has found it even more difficult to fall asleep in the hospital environment. He has been in hospital for the last 4 weeks for rehabilitation after an infection complicated his planned hip replacement. He is becoming more and more concerned about how he will cope when he goes home as well as feeling anxious about his dog who is being cared for by a neighbour. Rupert frequently finds it difficult to wake up for breakfast in the mornings, and his tiredness is reducing his enthusiasm for participation in his rehab.

Hospitals and rehabilitation wards are far from the ideal place to get a good night's sleep. Frequent noises, artificial lighting, excessive heat or disturbances from other patients and even staff can all play a role in disrupting an individual's sleep pattern. This can reduce the ability of an older person to participate in rehabilitation. Compounded by these factors people could also have poor sleep hygiene to begin with and entering hospital only serves to exacerbate their already negative sleeping habits.

Most people require around 7 hours of sleep. Some will require less and some more to feel rested. It is important that people avoid things that disrupt sleep in the evenings such as excessive caffeine use, alcohol and nicotine. Bright lights and excess heat can make it difficult to initiate sleep and excess noise can make it challenging to initiate and maintain sleep. Partners of people with sleep problems will frequently complain of loss of sleep themselves. Nocturia (frequent night-time urination) may also cause considerable sleep disruption. This gets more common with age and there are many potential treatable causes. Nocturia can also be caused by OSA (Raheem et al., 2014). See Chapter 35 Bladder & bowel problems for more information on nocturia and other urinary disorders.

INSOMNIA

Insomnia is one of the most common sleep disorders in the general population. Women are more likely to report insomnia compared to men. Insomnia can be defined as a difficulty in falling asleep, staying asleep or waking up too early and not being able to go back to sleep, associated with excessive sleepiness during the day which impacts daily functions and this must occur despite having an adequate opportunity for sleep (American Academy of Sleep, 2014). To be described as chronic insomnia, these symptoms need to be ongoing for more than 3 months and occurring at least 3 times per week. Insomnia can lead to an increase in depression, cognitive impairment and impaired daytime performance.

A sleep diary and thorough history are used to make the diagnosis (Fig. 32.1). One should remember that OSA can sometimes mimic sleep disturbances being mistaken for insomnia and if any doubt a sleep study should be performed.

Sample		
Today's date	4/5/08	
1. What time did you get into bed?	10:15 p.m	
2. What time did you try to go to sleep?	11:30 p.m	
3. How long did it take you to fall asleep?	1 hour 15 min.	
4. How many times did you wake up, not counting your final awakening?	3 times	
5. In total, how long did these awakenings last?	1 hour 10 min.	
6. What time was your final awakening?	6:35 a.m	
7. What time did you get out of bed for the day?	7:20 a.m	
8. How would you rate the quality of your sleep?	☐ Very poor ☑ Poor ☐ Fair ☐ Good ☐ Very good	☐ Very poor ☐ Poor ☐ Fair ☐ Good ☐ Very good
9. Comments (if applicable)	I have a cold	

FIG. 32.1 Sleep diary template. (From Kryger M, Roth T, Dement W. *Principles and Practice of Sleep Medicine*, 6th edn, Elsevier; 2017, with permission).

Note that it is also not uncommon for people to have more than one sleep disorder! A useful screening tool used in primary care to diagnose insomnia and consider other sleep disorders is the Auckland Sleep Questionnaire (Arroll et al., 2011). This tool, although not validated for secondary care, could be useful for non-sleep specialists as an aide-memoire when considering a differential for sleep disorders in people with complaints of poor sleep and fatigue.

The main treatment for insomnia is cognitive behavioural therapy (CBT) and pharmacological interventions or a combination of the two (Morin et al., 2009). The two main CBT methods include stimulus control therapy and sleep restriction therapy. People need to associate the bed with sleep. If not sleepy, one should get up and perform a 'relaxing' task avoiding excessive artificial light until the desire to sleep returns. They should also keep to a routine of waking up at the same time despite lack of sleep and try to avoid naps during the day. A clinical psychologist with an interest in CBT for sleep would be an invaluable asset to any multidisciplinary team particularly in the rehab setting.

Traditionally short-term use of benzodiazepines (BZD) was used for initiating sleep, but their use is associated with dependence, excessive falls risk and drowsiness, especially in the older person. Their use is no longer routinely recommended. Z-drugs (zopiclone and zolpidem) can assist in sleep initiation and maintenance; while they also have reported risks (somnolence, dizziness, dry mouth, unpleasant taste), they are generally well tolerated. They are most successfully used as a short-term solution for insomnia (Sateia et al., 2017). Over-the-counter sedating antihistamines are not recommended in the long-term management of sleep disorders due to their anticholinergic side effects and possible association with dementia (Gray et al., 2015). Studies show that melatonin is a safe drug and while it has been shown to have some therapeutic benefits in patients with insomnia, it is not yet recommended in routine clinical practice (Sateia et al., 2017).

RESTLESS LEG SYNDROME

Nora is a 76-year-old lady who is undergoing rehab after recurrent falls at home. She has a background history of iron deficiency anaemia due to peptic ulcer disease and acid reflux. She has been complaining of an uncomfortable sensation in her legs when she is resting in the chair or in bed at night-time, which would only be relieved if she got up and moved about her room. It would frequently prevent her from going to sleep at night and she feels exhausted throughout the day and unable to participate in her physical rehabilitation programme.

RLS is a common condition which is manifested by an intensely uncomfortable urge to move the legs or less commonly the arms. This discomfort can prevent people from going to sleep and lead to significant sleep disturbances. RLS occurs more commonly in women compared with men. There is often a family history of restless legs (Allen et al., 2002). There is an increased incidence in people with iron deficiency anaemia (Allen et al., 2013), renal disease, pregnancy, peripheral neuropathy, neurodegenerative disorders and ageing.

RLS is a clinical diagnosis. Sleep studies/polysomnography are generally not required for the diagnosis but can be supportive when excessive periodic limb movements are detected in the right clinical context. Iron studies should be checked in all people with RLS as correcting low iron level can successfully treat the condition. The five diagnostic criteria that are necessary to make the diagnosis are shown in Table 32.1 (Allen et al., 2014).

Treatments include iron supplementation or intravenous replacement of iron when ferritin levels are less than 50 μg/L (Allen et al., 2011). Medications with a similar effect to dopamine, a chemical within the brain, can also be used to treat RLS. Patients should be aware of potential side effects of these

TABLE 32.1 Diagnostic criteria for RLS (adapted from Allen et al. with permission).
1. An urge to move the legs usually associated with an uncomfortable sensation in the legs
2. Begins or worsens during periods of rest, such as lying down or sitting
3. Partially or totally relieved by movement
4. Worse in the evenings or night-time compared to the day
5. The first four criteria are not fully accounted for by other medical or behavioural disorders (e.g. arthritis, positional discomfort, peripheral neuropathy, habitual foot tapping).

medications, most notably impulse disorders such as gambling, compulsive shopping or inappropriate sexual behaviours (Cornelius et al., 2010). It is also important to be vigilant for a state of so called 'augmentation', where the symptoms may start to occur earlier in the day or worsen after starting treatment, necessitating a change in dosage and timing of the dopaminergic medication. Often it will be necessary to change the class of medication used when augmentation occurs. Other treatments include pregabalin, gabapentin, BZD and long-acting opiates (Garcia-Borreguero et al., 2016).

OBSTRUCTIVE SLEEP APNOEA

Michael is a 76-year-old man with diabetes, hypertension and a body mass index (BMI) of 29 (overweight) who is undergoing inpatient rehab after a fall at home which resulted in an ankle fracture. Nursing staff have noted loud snoring and at times they became concerned because they thought that he had stopped breathing at night. He tells you that he has felt fatigued in the morning for years and frequently takes naps during the day. His excessive daytime tiredness has led him to stop driving due to a fear of falling asleep at the wheel due to a 'near miss' a number of years ago.

OSA is a potentially serious disorder which affects 3%–7% of adult men and 2%–5% of adult women (Garvey et al., 2015). OSA occurs when the throat muscles intermittently relax and completely or partially block the upper airway during sleep, with a consequent cessation/reduction of the airflow. These 'obstructive events' may lower the level of oxygen in the blood and cause a build-up of carbon dioxide. Your brain senses this impaired breathing and briefly rouses you from sleep so that you can reopen your airway. This awakening is usually so brief that you don't remember it. While there are several types of sleep apnoea, the most common is OSA.

The exact cause for OSA is not yet clear. It is generally believed to be multifactorial, consisting of a complex interplay between anatomic, neuromuscular factors and an underlying genetic predisposition toward the disease. Risk factors include snoring, male gender, middle age, menopause in women, obesity and craniofacial features such as a large neck circumference, retro- or micrognathia, nasal obstruction, enlarged tonsils/ adenoids, enlarged tongue (macroglossia) and low-lying soft palate (Spicuzza, Caruso, & Di Maria, 2015).

A noticeable sign of OSA is snoring or witnessed breath-holding while sleeping. Daytime sleepiness is reported in more than 80% of patients and occurs due to nocturnal sleep fragmentation. A questionnaire such as the Epworth Sleepiness Scale is helpful to assist with subjective assessment of daytime somnolence. As the disorder progresses, the sleepiness becomes increasingly dangerous, causing impaired performance at work and major work-related and road accidents. In addition, people experience behaviour changes, inability to concentrate, memory impairment and mood changes such as irritability and depression. This further impairs performance at work with a detrimental effect on quality of life. Furthermore, if OSA remains untreated, it can contribute towards heart disease and death (Bradley & Floras, 2009).

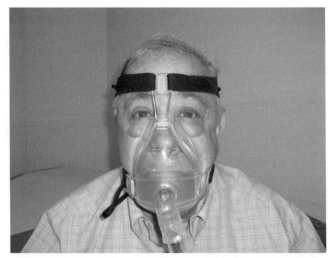

FIG. 32.2 Continuous positive airway pressure mask. (From Kryger M. *Atlas of Clinical Sleep Medicine*, 2nd edn. Elsevier; 2014, with permission).

The diagnosis of OSA is made through performance of a 'sleep study' or nocturnal polysomnography (PSG). During this test, the person is attached to equipment that monitors your heart, lung and brain activity, breathing patterns, arm and leg movements, and blood oxygen levels while asleep. This then detects the obstructive events and the associated changes in blood oxygen saturation (SaO_2) (American Academy of Sleep, 2014; Berry et al., 2012). The most commonly used index to define the severity of OSA is the Apnoea/Hypopnoea Index (AHI), calculated as the number of obstructive events per hour of sleep and obtained by nocturnal cardiorespiratory monitoring (Spicuzza et al., 2015).

The management of people with OSA requires a multi-disciplinary approach, and many treatment options are currently available. Continuous positive airway pressure (CPAP), available since the beginning of the 1980s, provides the most effective and commonly used treatment for mild, moderate and severe OSA (Fig. 32.2). This is a small machine that blows air under pressure into the mouth or nose. Alternative options include weight control, mandibular advancement devices and in some cases upper airway surgery (Spicuzza et al., 2015). During follow-up appointments, outcome indicators should be monitored. These include evaluation of resolution of sleepiness, patient and spousal satisfaction, adherence to therapy, avoidance of factors worsening disease, obtaining an adequate amount of sleep, practising proper sleep hygiene and weight loss for people who are overweight/ obese (Epstein et al., 2009).

PARASOMNIAS

Parasomnias are undesirable physical events or experiences that occur during sleep. Whilst there are numerous parasomnias, REM (rapid eye movement) sleep behaviour disorder (RBD) is the most relevant to the older person in the rehabilitation setting. This disorder most commonly occurs in males and is characterised by vigorous or violent movements during sleep which may result in injury to one-self or the bed partner. Typically, one will awaken easily and remember a dream associated with the behaviour. Shouting during sleep may also occur.

RBD can be idiopathic, but it can also be associated with the development of neurodegenerative disorders such as Parkinson's disease, multiple system atrophy and Lewy body dementia. RBD may manifest a decade prior to the onset of typical symptoms of these neurodegenerative disorders (Iranzo et al., 2006; Postuma et al., 2009).

RBD may be associated with other sleep disorders, such as narcolepsy, OSA and sleep deprivation. It can be caused or exacerbated by antidepressants (Postuma et al., 2013) and alcohol use (Yao et al., 2018). When one encounters a person with a history consistent with RBD, it should prompt a referral to a sleep physician and a neurologist to out rule nocturnal frontal lobe epilepsy which can mimic RBD or one of the above-mentioned neurodegenerative disorders.

Treatment involves preventing injury to the patient and bed partner by modifying the sleep environment as well as the use of medications such as clonazepam and melatonin.

OTHER MEDICAL CAUSES OF FATIGUE

Fatigue is a sensation of exhaustion during or after usual activities, or a feeling of inadequate energy to begin these activities. In national population surveys, 20%–30% of adults will report that they have significant fatigue at any given time (Cornuz, Guessous, & Favrat, 2006). The older person undergoing rehabilitation following a significant acute or chronic health issue is at high risk of fatigue.

Because the symptom of fatigue is often vague, clinical evaluation requires the consideration of distinct features such as associated symptoms, timing, precipitants, sleep quality, exercise capacity and sedation (Greenberg, 2002). Of course, symptoms predominantly related to sleep disruption should follow one of the investigative routes as outlined above. In the case of many others, a sleep disorder will not be the primary driver for the person's fatigue.

Common causes of fatigue in the older person can be broken into acute and chronic. Acute causes include infection, electrolyte imbalance, erratic blood glucose levels, anaemia and cardiac disease. Subacute or more chronic causes of fatigue include mental illness, thyroid problems, heart failure, malignancy, medications including neuropathic pain agents (gabapentin, pregabalin) and steroids, autoimmune diseases such as systemic lupus erythematosus and rheumatoid arthritis and many others.

If the person's fatigue is acute, a medical assessment is usually warranted to rule out and treat reversible causes. If the fatigue is of a more chronic nature, a medical assessment can still be beneficial if there is no clear cause for the person's fatigue. Chronic fatigue syndrome (CFS) is characterised by intense fatigue, with duration of over 6 months and associated with asthenia and easily induced tiredness that is not recovered after a night's sleep. The fatigue becomes so severe that it forces a 50% reduction in daily activities. It is a diagnosis of exclusion (Avellaneda Fernández et al., 2009).

SUMMARY POINTS

- There are normal physiological changes in sleeping patterns as we grow older, but in people who complain of poor-quality sleep and fatigue an underlying sleep disorder should be ruled out
- Insomnia is the most common sleep disorder and can have a significant impact on quality of life. The main treatment is cognitive behavioural therapy and adopting good sleep hygiene
- Restless leg syndrome is a common and bothersome condition. Iron levels should always be checked

- Obstructive sleep apnoea is underdiagnosed and has considerable health implications. It should be considered in people who are overweight, excessively sleepy and snore loudly
- Parasomnias and specifically REM behavioural disorders should prompt the consideration of an underlying neurodegenerative disorder that has yet to be diagnosed
- There are many other causes of fatigue including thyroid disease, diabetes, heart failure, diabetes, anaemia, depression and side effects from medications

MCQs

Q.1 Frank is an 82-year-old male with diabetes, coronary artery disease and osteoporosis who is undergoing inpatient rehabilitation following a fall which resulted in a left hip fracture. He is overweight with a BMI of 36. Every time he attends afternoon physiotherapy sessions, he is fast asleep and usually snoring loudly. Nursing staff report he is very restless at night. Frank tells you he cannot remember the last time he felt refreshed in the morning.

Which of the following is NOT an appropriate next step?
  a. Complete the Epworth Sleepiness scale with Frank
  b. Ask Frank if his legs are jumping at night

  c. Discuss sleep hygiene with Frank and ask him to keep a sleep diary
  d. Prescribe a benzodiazepine sleep medication

Q.2 Anne is a 67-year-old lady with rheumatoid arthritis, COPD and hypertension. She is undergoing inpatient rehabilitation following a prolonged admission (8 weeks) with an exacerbation of COPD requiring intubation and ventilation and an ICU stay. Since leaving the intensive care unit she has had 'terrible difficulty sleeping'. It is taking her hours to fall asleep and she wakes easily once asleep. She gets 2–3 hours of sleep on average a night. Anne has never been a great sleeper but usually watches a TV show from her bed until she falls asleep. She doesn't have this luxury while in hospital. She is a very outgoing lady and attended multiple social groups weekly with her husband prior to becoming unwell. She doesn't have the energy or interest in socialising over the last few weeks.

Which of the following is the most likely cause of Anne's insomnia?

a. Poor sleep hygiene
b. Polypharmacy
c. The hospital environment
d. All of the above

Q.3 Which of the following statements on the management of common sleep disorders is incorrect?

a. Intravenous iron replacement is recommended to treat persons with REM sleep behaviour disorder
b. CPAP is the gold standard treatment for polysomnography-confirmed obstructive sleep apnoea
c. Persons diagnosed with insomnia should be educated on good sleep hygiene and referred for cognitive behavioural therapy
d. Once ferritin levels are normal, persons with restless leg syndrome should be considered for dopamine-like medications

REFERENCES

Allen, R. P., Adler, C. H., Du, W., Butcher, A., Bregman, D. B., & Earley, C. J. (2011). Clinical efficacy and safety of IV ferric carboxymaltose (FCM) treatment of RLS: a multi-centred, placebo-controlled preliminary clinical trial. *Sleep Medicine, 12,* 906–913.

Allen, R. P., Auerbach, S., Bahrain, H., Auerbach, M., & Earley, C. J. (2013). The prevalence and impact of restless legs syndrome on patients with iron deficiency anemia. *Am J Hematol, 88,* 261–264.

Allen, R. P., La Buda, M. C., Becker, P., & Earley, C. J. (2002). Family history study of the restless legs syndrome. *Sleep Medicine, 3*(suppl), S3–S7.

Allen, R. P., Picchietti, D. L., Garcia-Borreguero, D., Ondo, W. G., Walters, A. S., Winkelman, J. W., ..., & Lee, H. B. (2014). Restless legs syndrome/Willis-Ekbom disease diagnostic criteria: updated International Restless Legs Syndrome Study Group (IRLSSG) consensus criteria--history, rationale, description, and significance. *Sleep Medicine, 15,* 860–873.

American Academy of Sleep Medicine. (2014). *International classification of sleep disorders.* Retrieved from: https://j2vjt3d-nbra3ps7ll1clb4q2-wpengine.netdna-ssl.com/wp-content/uploads/2019/05/ICSD3-TOC.pdf.

Arroll, B., Fernando, A., Falloon, K., Warman, G., & Goodyear-Smith, F. (2011). Development, validation (diagnostic accuracy) and audit of the Auckland Sleep Questionnaire: a new tool for diagnosing causes of sleep disorders in primary care. *Journal of Primary Health Care, 3,* 107–113.

Avellaneda Fernández, A., Pérez Martín, Á., Izquierdo Martínez, M., Arruti Bustillo, M., Barbado Hernández, F. J., de la Cruz Labrado, J., & Ramón Giménez, J. R. (2009). Chronic fatigue syndrome: aetiology, diagnosis and treatment. *BMC Psychiatry, 9,* S1.

Berry, R. B., Budhiraja, R., Gottlieb, D. J., Gozal, D., Iber, C., Kapur, V. K., & Tangredi, M. M. (2012). Rules for scoring respiratory events in sleep: update of the 2007 AASM Manual for the Scoring of Sleep and Associated Events. Deliberations of the Sleep Apnea Definitions Task Force of the American Academy of Sleep Medicine. *Journal of Clinical Sleep Medicine, 8,* 597–619.

Bradley, T. D., & Floras, J. S. (2009). Obstructive sleep apnoea and its cardiovascular consequences. *Lancet, 373,* 82–93.

Cornelius, J. R., Tippmann-Peikert, M., Slocumb, N. L., Frerichs, C. F., & Silber, M. H. (2010). Impulse control disorders with the use of dopaminergic agents in restless legs syndrome: a case-control study. *Sleep, 33,* 81–87.

Cornuz, J., Guessous, I., & Favrat, B. (2006). Fatigue: a practical approach to diagnosis in primary care. *CMAJ, 174,* 765–767.

Epstein, L. J., Kristo, D., Strollo, P. J., Jr., Friedman, N., Malhotra, A., Patil, S. P., ..., & Weinstein, M. D. (2009). Clinical guideline for the evaluation, management and long-term care of obstructive sleep apnea in adults. *Journal of Clinical Sleep Medicne, 5,* 263–276.

Garcia-Borreguero, D., Silber, M. H., Winkelman, J. W., Hogl, B., Bainbridge, J., Buchfuhrer, M., ..., & Allen, R. P. (2016). Guidelines for the first-line treatment of restless legs syndrome/Willis-Ekbom disease, prevention and treatment of dopaminergic augmentation: a combined task force of the IRLSSG, EURLSSG, and the RLS-foundation. *Sleep Medicine, 21,* 1–11.

Garvey, J. F., Pengo, M. F., Drakatos, P., & Kent, B. D. (2015). Epidemiological aspects of obstructive sleep apnea. *Journal of Thoracic Disease, 7,* 920–929.

Gray, S. L., Anderson, M. L., Dublin, S., Hanlon, J. T., Hubbard, R., Walker, R., Yu, O., Crane, P. K., & Larson, E. B. (2015). Cumulative use of strong anticholinergics and incident dementia: a prospective cohort study. *JAMA Internal Medicine, 175,* 401–407.

Greenberg, D. B. (2002). Clinical dimensions of fatigue. *Primary Care Companion to the Journal of Clinical Psychiatry, 4,* 90–93.

Iranzo, A., Molinuevo, J. L., Santamaria, J., Serradell, M., Marti, M. J., Valldeoriola, F., & Tolosa, E. (2006). Rapid-eye-movement sleep behaviour disorder as an early marker for a neurodegenerative disorder: a descriptive study. *Lancet Neurology, 5,* 572–577.

Morin, C. M., Vallieres, A., Guay, B., Ivers, H., Savard, J., Merette, C., Bastien, C., & Baillargeon, L. (2009). Cognitive behavioral therapy, singly and combined with medication, for persistent insomnia: a randomized controlled trial. *JAMA, 301,* 2005–2015.

Postuma, R. B., Gagnon, J. F., Tuineaig, M., Bertrand, J. A., Latreille, V., Desjardins, C., & Montplaisir, J. Y. (2013). Antidepressants and REM sleep behavior disorder: isolated side effect or neurodegenerative signal? *Sleep, 36,* 1579–1585.

Postuma, R. B., Gagnon, J. F., Vendette, M., Fantini, M. L., Massicotte-Marquez, J., & Montplaisir, J. (2009). Quantifying the risk of neurodegenerative disease in idiopathic REM sleep behavior disorder. *Neurology, 72,* 1296–1300.

Raheem, O. A., Orosco, R. K., Davidson, T. M., & Lakin, C. (2014). Clinical predictors of nocturia in the sleep apnea population. *Urology Annals, 6,* 31–35.

Sateia, M. J., Buysse, D. J., Krystal, A. D., Neubauer, D. N., & Heald, J. L. (2017). Clinical practice guideline for the pharmacologic treatment of chronic insomnia in adults: an American Academy of Sleep Medicine clinical practice guideline. *Journal of Clinical Sleep Medicine, 13,* 307–349.

Spicuzza, L., Caruso, D., & Di Maria, G. (2015). Obstructive sleep apnoea syndrome and its management. *Therapeutic Advances in Chronic Disease, 6,* 273–285.

Yao, C., Fereshtehnejad, S. M., Keezer, M. R., Wolfson, C., Pelletier, A., & Postuma, R. B. (2018). Risk factors for possible REM sleep behavior disorder: a CLSA population-based cohort study. *Neurology, 92,* e475–e485.

33

Oral Health

Taranjit Badh

LEARNING OBJECTIVES

- Explain the vital importance of maintaining optimal oral health for older people
- Describe the nature of oral health problems in older people
- Explain how to assist in supporting good oral health

CASE

Frank is a 75-year-old man with early dementia who was transferred to the rehab ward after a fall. He had recently been admitted to hospital as he had been refusing to eat on a regular basis. This had resulted in progressive weight loss and muscle weakness. Despite extensive investigation, no medical cause was found and he was referred for a trial of rehabilitation.

In the rehab ward, he is encouraged to regain his independence but still needs help with many activities due to weakness. He regularly points to his mouth and grimaces in pain when his teeth are attempted to be cleaned. Frank has no dental records and given that he has no surviving relatives and significant memory issues, his dental history could not be ascertained. After advice from his doctor and the local community dental service, Frank was seen as an emergency. He presented with severe dental problems: advanced gum disease and a number of broken teeth which were associated with dental abscesses. Although he was in the early stages of dementia he was able to consent for himself, and urgent treatment was carried out. Within a period of a few weeks, Frank was feeling a lot better, eating well and allowing his teeth to be cleaned.

INTRODUCTION

Despite increasing research into healthy ageing and improving independence in older age, there is relatively less emphasis on oral health problems, which have a significant impact on quality of life, nutritional intake and well-being in older age (Petersen & Yamamoto, 2005). The Global Burden of Disease 2010 Study showed that oral health problems accounted for 15 million disability-adjusted life years, implying an average health loss of 224 years per 100,000 population (Marcenes et al., 2013).

Due to population ageing, the burden of oral health problems increased from 1990 to 2010. This burden, particularly from periodontal (gum) disease and tooth loss, increases with age. A review of oral health conditions in older people highlighted the burden of conditions including tooth loss and dry mouth in older people (Murray Thomson, 2014). Although edentulism (complete loss of natural teeth) has declined in recent decades in several countries, a substantial number of older people are still edentulous (2.7 million in the UK, or one in five people over 65 years) (White et al., 2012) and partial tooth loss remains an important problem affecting eating and quality of life of older people.

Many older people live on their own, and for a number of reasons may suffer from mental as well as physical conditions. These problems are associated with loneliness, depression, poor diet and neglect of general personal hygiene, especially oral health. Diminishing manual dexterity plays a huge part in the deterioration of an older person's oral health. There are also specific issues for older people who are resident in nursing homes, with regards to variable standards of dental care provided (Curzon & Preston, 2004). Unfortunately, on presentation to a rehabilitation setting, the level of oral neglect can, on occasion, be irreversible.

THE IMPORTANCE OF ORAL HEALTH

Oral health is defined as 'the health of the mouth, teeth and associated structures and their functional viability' (Department of Health, 2005). Oral health affects general health, well-being and quality of life. Poor oral health can lead to pain, discomfort and an inability to chew food properly. Chronic oral health problems will inevitably lead to malnutrition, systemic illness and debilitating conditions that can be life-threatening. This is especially important for older people, who may be dependent on others for supportive care. Early detection where possible with instigation of oral hygiene, diet modification and treatment can limit these serious problems.

COMMON ORAL PROBLEMS IN OLDER PEOPLE

Dental Decay

This is the progressive destruction of teeth by acid, generated through bacterial plaque, which is present in every mouth. Three factors contribute to a susceptible tooth, bacteria, and dietary sugar. Bacteria in plaque metabolise dietary sugars to produce acid. Unless plaque is removed by regular brushing, the acid attacks and demineralises the tooth surface thus causing dental decay. Older people are more vulnerable to root surface decay because of gum recession.

Older people tend to have fewer natural teeth than younger people. Although the number of completely toothless (edentulous) people is projected to decrease (due to improving oral health) over the next 20–30 years, significant numbers who rely on dentures remain. People with some teeth, a high proportion of whom need to use dentures in combination with their natural teeth, can have a high susceptibility to dental decay. If dentures are not cleaned properly, food can trap around them, and settle on teeth, leading to dental decay.

Gum Disease

Increased retention of teeth into later life can increase the risk of gum disease.

Signs of gum disease include:
- Gums bleed on toothbrushing
- Red, swollen or tender gums
- Chronic bad breath or bad taste
- Loose teeth or teeth changing position when brushed.

Most adults experience gum disease at some point in time; it is still the major cause of tooth loss in adults. The main cause of gum inflammation and disease is inadequate removal of dental plaque, which accumulates at the margin between the tooth and gum. Bleeding gums are the first sign of gum disease and, if left untreated, will become more severe, lead to pain and eventual tooth loss.

Dry Mouth (Xerostomia)

Saliva has numerous important functions in maintaining oral health. It lubricates the mouth facilitating dietary intake, washing away food debris and neutralising acids. It also has important bacteriostatic and bactericidal properties. Salivary flow varies little with age in healthy people who are not taking medication. However, significant changes in saliva flow and composition are seen in the context of diseases associated with older age and the use of common drugs.

Having a dry mouth can be distressing; patients may complain of difficulty in eating, speaking and swallowing, reduced taste sensation and limited tolerance to dentures. There are also physical symptoms of bad breath, dryness, with cracking of the lips and corners of the mouth. This can lead to loss of appetite, and inadequate nutritional intake.

A dry mouth increases susceptibility to dental caries, gum disease and oral infections (Walls & Steele, 2004). The oral side effects of drugs are the most common cause of a dry mouth, with more than 500 medications implicated in

TABLE 33.1 Examples of drugs that can cause a side effect of dry mouth.

DRUG CLASSIFICATION	EXAMPLES
Anticholinergics	Scopolamine, solifenacin, tiotropium, tolterodine
Diuretics	Furosemide, spironolactone
Antihypertensives	Prazosin, clonidine, atenolol, propranolol
Antidepressants	Amitriptyline, doxepin, nortriptyline, escitalopram, fluoxetine, sertraline
Antihistamines	Fexofenadine, loratadine, cetirizine, levocetirizine, chlorpheniramine
Analgesics (pain medications) (particularly opiate based ones)	Codeine, fentanyl, morphine, hydrocodone, oxycodone
Sedatives	Alprazolam, diazepam, lorazepam
Cytotoxics	Azathioprine, cyclophosphamide, methotrexate

salivary gland dysfunction (see Table 33.1) (Porter, Scully, & Hegarty, 2004).

Denture Sore Mouth

This is a common disorder that affects denture wearers. It may be described as a chronic inflammation of the denture resting tissues. Denture sore mouth (DSM) is usually symptom-less, but can give rise to bleeding of the affected areas of mucosa, a burning sensation, halitosis, a bad taste and xerostomia.

Various studies have found that patients who are institutionalised are especially susceptible to DSM, possibly as a result of impaired immunity, overall general health, xerostomia, decreased motor function leading to an inability to carry out good oral hygiene and the reliance on others to carry out oral hygiene measures (Puryer, 2016).

EFFECTS OF LONG-TERM CONDITIONS

It is estimated that more than 100 systemic diseases have oral health manifestations (Haumschild & Haumschild, 2009). With increasing age it is more common for a person to experience the effects of a multiple chronic illnesses. Many of these may affect oral health and functioning or the ability of patients to maintain their oral hygiene. Links between severe gum disease, diabetes, ischaemic heart disease and chronic respiratory disease are relatively well known. The main conditions and their impact on oral health are listed in Table 33.2.

SUPPORTING ORAL HEALTH CARE

Every individual situation is unique; however, employment of a regular systematic and consistent approach to managing care should be utilised wherever possible.

TABLE 33.2 Commonest long-term conditions affecting oral health.

CONDITION	EFFECTS ON ORAL HEALTH
Diabetes	Increased susceptibility to DSM Altered taste Impaired healing after treatment Gum disease progresses more rapidly with poorer diabetic control
Parkinson's disease	Difficulty with self-care due to manual dexterity problems Increased risk of decay and gum disease Problems with retaining dentures/ looseness due to loss of neuromuscular control Drooling due to poor posture which can lead to dysphagia/swallowing problems
Stroke	Paralysis: leading to poor manual dexterity, impaired swallowing leading to dysphagia. Dysphagia can cause choking and aspiration pneumonia Communication problems: person may not understand what is being said and may have difficulty expressing needs and preferences (Singh & Hamdy, 2006)
Dementia	Memory loss: people may forget to clean teeth leading to increased decay and gum disease susceptibility. Dentures can be misplaced regularly Communication problems: may not be able to articulate sensation of pain. Behaviour changes: as dementia progresses, it may lead to aggression towards oral hygiene support
Osteoarthritis	May affect hands leading to limited manual dexterity
Respiratory disease	Leads to breathlessness, mouth breathing and dry mouth Increased risk of DSM.
Depression	Can lead to memory loss and general lack of motivation which can result in general personal hygiene neglect.
Thyroid disease	Can cause excessive tiredness and reduced motivation

Assessment and Recording Information

Healthcare teams will encounter unmet oral and dental health needs in patients in the rehabilitation setting. Members of the healthcare team should carry out an initial assessment within 24 hours of a person entering a rehabilitation facility. This will provide a baseline for the oral health of the patient. Oral assessments should be carried out at regular intervals to monitor the effectiveness of oral hygiene interventions and their impact on oral health during rehabilitation and recovery (Griffiths & Boyle, 2005).

A data recording sheet for oral assessment is being phased in by NHS England; see Further reading for details. Fig. 33.1 provides a visual guide to the appearance of the commonest oral health conditions that a patient may suffer from, along with a corresponding action plan. Fig. 33.2 shows what to look for when examining the mouth.

Routine Daily Procedures

The basic steps listed below are fundamental in managing oral health for older people.

CARE OF THE LIPS

Moisten a clean soft cloth or cotton wool with water and gently wipe the lips. Use a lubricant such as water-based lip balm to prevent any dryness and reduce the risk of sore painful lips.

Care of the Denture Wearing Patient

- Mark dentures with owner's name.
- Clean dentures with an individual toothbrush under cold water.
- Leave dentures in plain water overnight and then soak in dilute sodium hypochlorite for 20–30 minutes. Products such as denture cleaning tablets are available from pharmacies or dental practices. Metal component dentures can be soaked in chlorhexidine mouth wash.
- Rinse after every meal, as residual food debris under the denture can irritate the oral mucosa.
- Use a small amount of the person's preferred denture fixative and ensure this is brushed off at the end of the day, before dentures are placed into soak.

Care of Natural Teeth

- People who require assistance with oral care should have been identified through the initial assessment.
- Twice daily cleaning using a fluoride-based toothpaste should be employed. Use a manual or if the person can tolerate, an electric toothbrush which is more efficient at cleaning teeth. Alternately, a cloth wrapped around a finger can suffice if the person refuses a toothbrush.
- Additional oral hygiene products such as alcohol-free mouthwashes, sprays and gels can also be employed.
- Seat the person in a dining room type chair.
- From behind, the carer cradles the patients head against their body using an arm to provide neck support and reduce involuntary movements.
- Carefully and gently pull back the cheek with the non-brushing hand to aid access and vision.
- Brush the teeth using firm pressure but ensure the person is comfortable. Ensure all surfaces are cleaned.
- If a person can rinse, use a fluoride-based toothpaste; if they cannot, dampen the brush in fluoride mouthwash regularly instead as you brush.

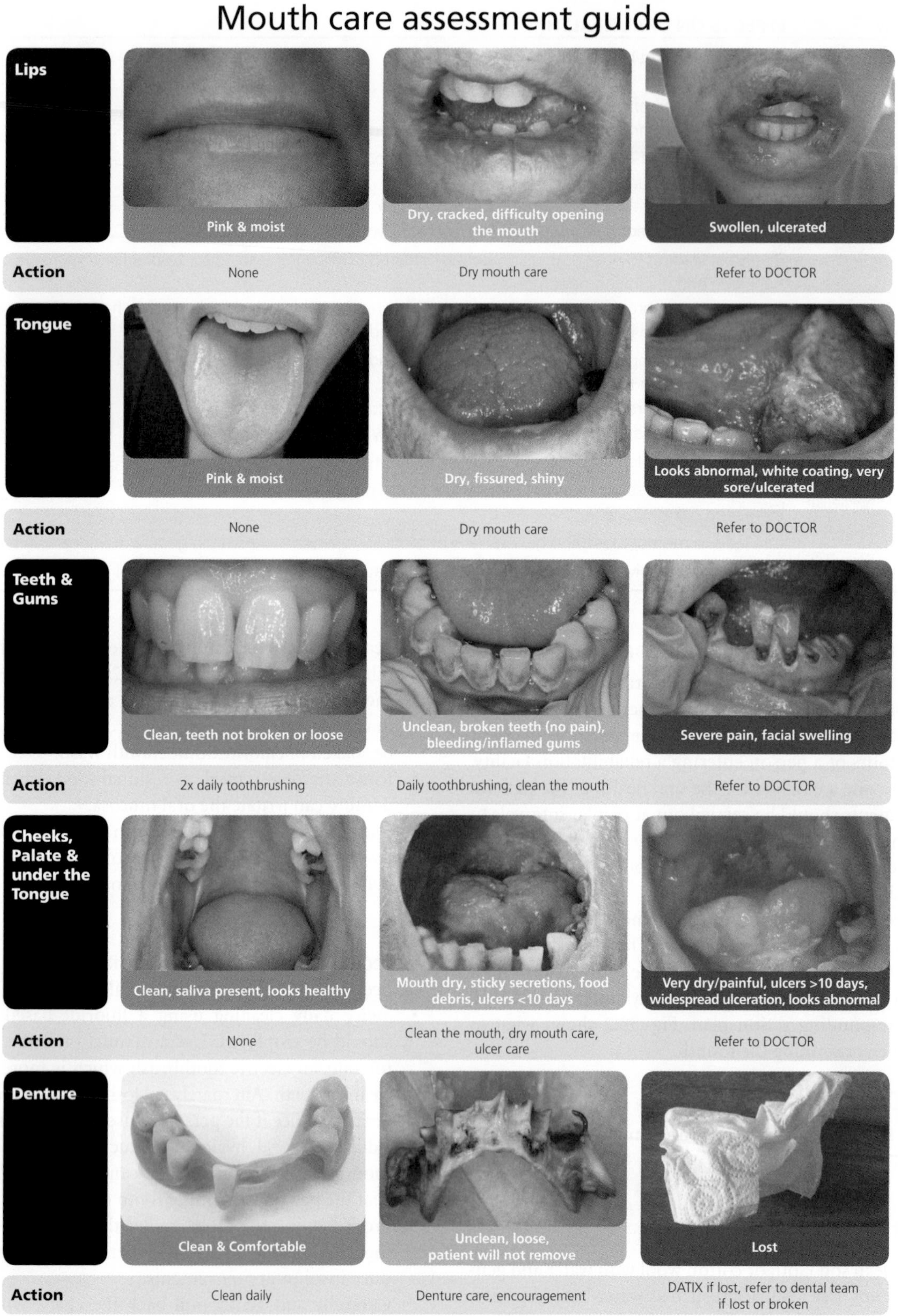

Mouth care assessment guide

Lips	Pink & moist	Dry, cracked, difficulty opening the mouth	Swollen, ulcerated
Action	None	Dry mouth care	Refer to DOCTOR
Tongue	Pink & moist	Dry, fissured, shiny	Looks abnormal, white coating, very sore/ulcerated
Action	None	Dry mouth care	Refer to DOCTOR
Teeth & Gums	Clean, teeth not broken or loose	Unclean, broken teeth (no pain), bleeding/inflamed gums	Severe pain, facial swelling
Action	2x daily toothbrushing	Daily toothbrushing, clean the mouth	Refer to DOCTOR
Cheeks, Palate & under the Tongue	Clean, saliva present, looks healthy	Mouth dry, sticky secretions, food debris, ulcers <10 days	Very dry/painful, ulcers >10 days, widespread ulceration, looks abnormal
Action	None	Clean the mouth, dry mouth care, ulcer care	Refer to DOCTOR
Denture	Clean & Comfortable	Unclean, loose, patient will not remove	Lost
Action	Clean daily	Denture care, encouragement	DATIX if lost, refer to dental team if lost or broken

FIG. 33.1 Sample data recording set. (Courtesy www.mouthcarematters.hee.nhs.uk) Available at http://www.mouthcarematters.hee.nhs.uk/wp-content/uploads/2019/06/MCAssessmentA3-Posterv3.pdf

What to look for?

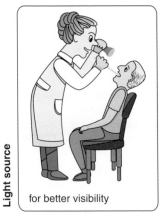
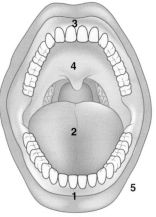

Light source for better visibility

1. Lips: Pink & moist
2. Tongue: Pink, moist & clean
3. Teeth & gums: Clean, teeth are not broken or loose. Gums are not bleeding / inflamed
4. Cheeks / palate / under tongue: Clean, saliva present & looks healthy
5. Dentures: Clean & comfortable It is important that both the dentures and the mouth are cleaned daily

FIG. 33.2 A visual guide to the appearance of the commonest oral health conditions that a patient, particularly an older person, may suffer from, with a corresponding action plan. (Courtesy www.mouthcarematters.hee.nhs.uk) Available at http://mouthcarematters.51.143.169.215.xip.io/wp-content/uploads/sites/6/2016/10/Mouthsinfoposter-v3.pdf

- When cooperation problems arise, such as limited opening or biting down of the toothbrush, you can utilise finger guards to prop one side of the mouth open while the other side is brushed.
- All staff should wear disposable latex-free gloves in order to maintain appropriate cross infection control.
- Keep the atmosphere comfortable. Playing a person's favourite music, especially if it is classical, can ensure the ambience is calm. Seating a person in their favourite armchair in an environment they are familiar with also helps.

Nutrition

Diet should be kept low in sugar as far as achievable. The higher the levels of sugar, the higher the dental decay risk. As a person's cooperation may deteriorate, especially in dementia, reducing or eliminating risk factors for dental decay is extremely important. Avoiding sugar in drinks and discouraging sweet treats is the place to start.

Education and Training

Oral healthcare training programmes need to be relevant and hands on with a strong evidence base. The central core should be the repeated emphasis of how detrimental to oral health age-related changes, impact of disease, and medications can be.

SUMMARY POINTS

- Dental pain and discomfort can affect general health, behaviour and well-being
- Long-term conditions, such as arthritis, Parkinson's disease and dementia, can make it harder to hold a toothbrush
- Reduced manual dexterity combined with certain medications that can reduce saliva production leading to a dry mouth will place patients in the high risk for poor oral health category
- Brushing natural teeth twice daily with fluoride toothpaste, cleaning and soaking dentures overnight, and limiting sugar in a high-risk patients' diet are all simple steps in maintaining a good standard of oral health

MCQs

Q.1 Which of the following is true about oral health problems?
  a. If dentures are not cleaned properly, food can trap around them, and settle on teeth, leading to dental decay.
  b. Toothache is the first sign of gum disease
  c. The most common cause of dry mouth is poor oral intake
  d. Denture sore mouth is caused by infection of the denture resting tissues
  e. People with Parkinson's disease should avoid brushing their teeth

Q.2 Which of the following is NOT good oral health practice?
  a. Mark dentures with owner's name
  b. Clean dentures with an individual toothbrush under cold water
  c. If a person can rinse, use a fluoride-based toothpaste; if they cannot, dampen the brush in fluoride mouthwash, for natural teeth
  d. When cooperation problems arise, use sedation to help with teeth cleaning
  e. Twice daily cleaning using a fluoride-based toothpaste should be employed for natural teeth

REFERENCES

Curzon, M., & Preston, A. (2004). Risk groups: nursing bottle caries/ caries in the elderly. *Caries Research, 38*(suppl 1), 24–33.

Department of Health. (2005). Meeting the challenges of oral health for older people: a strategic review. *Gerodontology, 22*(suppl 1), 3–48.

Griffiths, J., & Boyle, S. (2005). *Holistic oral care: a guide for health professionals* (2nd ed.). London: Stephen Hancocks.

Haumschild, M., & Haumschild, R. (2009). The importance of oral health in long-term care. *Journal of the Association of Physicians, 10,* 667–671.

Marcenes, W., Kassebaum, N., Bernabe, E., Flaxman, A., Naghavi, M., Lopez, A., & Murray, C. J. L. (2013). Global burden of oral conditions in 1990-2010: a systematic analysis. *Journal of Dental Research, 92,* 592–597.

Murray Thomson, W. (2014). Epidemiology of oral health conditions in older people. *Gerodontology, 31*(suppl 1), 9–16.

Porter, S., Scully, C., & Hegarty, A. M. (2004). An update of the etiology and management of xerostomia. *Oral Medicine, Oral Pathology, Oral Radiology and Endodontics, 97,* 28–46.

Puryer, J. (2016). Denture stomatitis–a clinical update. *Dental Update, 43,* 529–535.

Singh, S., & Hamdy, S. (2006). Dysphagia in stroke patients. *Postgraduate Medical Journal, 82,* 383–391.

Walls, A., & Steele, J. (2004). The relationship between oral health and nutrition in older people. *Mechanisms of Ageing and Development, 125,* 853–857.

White, D., Tsakos, G., Pitts, N., Fuller, E., Douglas, G. V. A., Murray, J. J., & Steele, J. G. (2012). Adult Dental Health Survey 2009: common oral health conditions and their impact on the population. *British Dental Journal, 213,* 567–572.

FURTHER READING

Promoting older people's oral health. Retrieved from: http://www.wales.nhs.uk/documents/Promoting-older-peoples-oral-health_NursingStandards.pdf.

Very useful guide that underpins a lot of the advice provided in this chapter.

Further reading and support material including Oral Health Needs Assessment. Retrieved from: www.mouthcarematters.hee.nhs.uk.

NHS Scotland. (2010). Caring for smiles: better oral care for dependent older people. Retrieved from: http://www.knowledge.scot.nhs.uk/media/7460397/caringforsmilescarehomes2013.pdf.

Relatives and Residents Association. *Keep smiling: dental care and oral health for older people in care homes.* Retrieved from: www.relres.org.

Making Sense of the Mouth – Training package including DVD and many images available from Petrina Sweeney, Glasgow Dental School, 378 Sauchiehall Street, Glasgow G2 3JZ.

British Dental Health Foundation. An independent charity working to improve standards of oral health care in the UK and around the world: www.dentalhealth.org.

34

Weight Loss and Overweight

Margot Gosney

LEARNING OBJECTIVES

- Identify the frequency of under- and overnutrition in older adults
- Describe measures of nutrition e.g. body mass index (BMI), skinfold thickness, biochemical measures and risk scoring systems such as the Mini Nutritional Assessment (MNA)

- Explain the effects of being either over- or underweight during rehabilitation and the underlying physiological and psychological causes
- Describe how to deal with weight outside the normal range during rehabilitation with particular reference to malnutrition

CASE

Marjorie is a 78-year-old lady who lives alone. She has osteoarthritis of both hips, and her hands are particularly affected. She falls in the kitchen while making lunch and fractures her right hip. Postoperatively it is noted that she has early cognitive impairment, a poor nutritional status as identified by a body mass index (BMI) of 18 kg/m² and a poor appetite. Her rehabilitation is slow to progress, and there are concerns about whether she will return home after this period of hospitalisation.

INTRODUCTION

Malnutrition can be defined as a state of nutrition in which a deficiency or excess of energy, protein and other nutrients cause measurable adverse effects on tissue/body, form and function and clinical outcome. What is poorly recognised is that malnutrition therefore refers to both obesity and undernutrition and whilst undernutrition is significantly more common, obesity also affects patients during rehabilitation.

BMI is a classification of body fatness, which is calculated from height and weight. Although this is problematic in older people who experience height loss due to osteoporosis, there are other surrogates that are described later. BMI is used by the World Health Organisation to classify body fatness (see Table 34.1).

Unfortunately, when BMI is used alone it probably underpredicts the prevalence of undernutrition, as many older people may have lost more than 10% of their body weight in the preceding 6 months and are at risk of undernutrition; however, they still have a BMI above 20 kg/m². The prevalence of undernutrition in patients undergoing rehabilitation has been reported as 30%–50% (Watterson et al., 2009).

Obesity as indicated by a high BMI is usually due to excess body fat. This in itself will cause increased health risks and mortality. Although cardiovascular risks and type 2 diabetes are more commonly seen in patients with obesity, the largest challenge in rehabilitation is the prevalence of osteoarthritis as a result of articular cartilage damage and the physical requirement of rehabilitating a large person rather than a small person. Obesity is associated with increased length of stay in rehabilitation (Padwal et al., 2012). In one study, the prevalence of obesity in older people was 38% and was associated with higher levels of functional limitation (Vasquez et al., 2014).

WHAT CAUSES UNDERNUTRITION?

In older individuals the majority of undernutrition is due to impaired intake. This can be caused by environmental situations such as poverty, homelessness, social isolation and difficulty with food preparation. It may also be due to psychological factors such as depression or dementia. Manual dexterity, difficulties with swallowing, poor dentition (see Chapter 33 Oral Health) or arthritis of the hands can also reduce oral intake. Many of the underlying conditions that have resulted in someone requiring rehabilitation (such as gastrointestinal surgery) may also cause impaired digestion or absorption. Any individual who has had illness or surgery will have increased nutrient requirements at a time when they are not keen to eat due to the hospital environment, postoperative pain, constipation, drugs causing nausea and vomiting as well as anxiety and depression.

HIP FRACTURE

Hip fracture gives us a model to illustrate cause and effect, assessment methodology, changing physiology, prognosis and advice.

Baseline dietary energy intake, serum albumin, weight/BMI and skin fold thickness are significantly and inversely related to subsequent hip fracture (Huang, Himes, & McGovern, 1996). In some series, over 80% of patients with hip fractures have protein malnutrition (Diaz de Bustamante et al., 2018). There

TABLE 34.1   Classification of body fatness based on body mass index according to the World Health Organisation.

BMI CLASSIFICATION (kg/m²)	
<18.5	Underweight
18.5–24.9	Healthy
25–29.9	Overweight
30–39.9	Obese
>40	Morbidly obese

is a significantly lower intake of energy in hip fracture patients when compared with age matched but frail older individuals attending day centres (Lumbers et al., 2001).

Prospective studies have shown that patients with a hip fracture and an abnormal albumin and low total lymphocyte count were 2.9 times more likely to have a length of stay greater than 2 weeks (P = 0.03), 3.9 times more likely to die within 1 year after surgery (P = 0.02) and 4.6 times less likely to recover their pre-fracture level of independence in basic activities of daily living (P < 0.01) (Koval et al., 1999). In a study of 20,278 patients, hypoalbuminaemia was predictive of readmission, re-intubation, mortality and length of stay (Ryan et al., 2018a) and when combined with the American Society of Anaesthesiologists (ASA) score provides enhanced risk stratification (Ryan et al., 2018b).

Both being underweight and having obesity are associated with increased mortality within the first 30 days following surgery (Woo et al., 2019).

The resting energy expenditure following hip fracture is particularly high on day 3 post-surgery although falling by day 8–9. There is a clear mismatch between energy requirement and calorific intake with spontaneous protein intake not meeting energy and protein requirements with calculations suggesting that an extra 200–300 kcal per day containing 20 g of protein are required (Jallut et al., 1990). Unfortunately, oral nutritional supplements (ONS) are poorly consumed, and therefore usually do not prevent weight loss after hip fracture (Bruce et al., 2003). Body composition is important for rehabilitation, and significant changes in body composition are usually seen between 10 days and 2 months, i.e., during some of the most prolonged rehabilitation periods during which time total body mass and hip bone mineral density all decrease. During the first 5 days after surgery the energy intake is only 56% of the preoperative value and probably accounts for poor rehabilitation.

In order to ensure that older people have optimum nutrition during a period of rehabilitation, it is important to explore some areas in greater detail.

ANTHROPOMETRIC MEASUREMENTS

To determine an individual's BMI, an accurate measurement of height and weight must be obtained. Even the frailest person can be weighed, but a variety of conditions common to older individuals result in difficulties in measuring height.

With age, height diminishes and this may be partly explained by change in posture as well as osteoporosis reducing vertebral height. It is important to always measure height at the same time, as vertebral height diminishes during the day. The most useful alternative to height is the measurement of arm span. There are validated equations for younger individuals, but adjustments must be made for older individuals and certain races. The equation from Weinbrenner et al. (2006) is the best validated in the copious literature published.

Knee height can be used to calculate height in somebody who is unable to rise from the bed (Muncie et al., 1987) and may be useful after stroke or when arm span is impossible to measure (Zhang, Hsu-Hage, & Wahlqvist, 1998). Where possible all measurements should be made with the patient out of bed as errors occur when individuals are supine (Beghetto et al., 2006).

DOES ANTHROPOMETRY PREDICT OR MATCH BIOCHEMICAL PARAMETERS?

There is much debate about the linkage of anthropometry to biochemistry. If one measurement could give an indication of nutritional status, life would be much easier.

Triceps skin fold thickness and upper arm circumference are frequently used to assess the nutritional status of patients. Triceps skinfold gives an indication of subcutaneous fat stores, and depletion of this compartment can reflect chronic inadequate intake or nutrient deprivation. Evidence of protein stores can be estimated by calculating the arm muscle circumference and arm muscle area using triceps skin fold and arm circumference measurements. Protein stores are commonly reduced during chronic protein depletion. They are easy to measure (but must be sitting or standing) and give an indication of gross changes (Jensen, Dudrick, & Johnston, 1981).

A calf circumference cut-off of 30.5 cm is also used to determine whether an individual is malnourished or not. It correlates well with triceps skin fold thickness, fat free mass, BMI and serum albumin, and is valid at this level for both men and women (Bonnefoy et al., 2002).

There has however been much debate about anthropometric thresholds particularly as populations are larger and taller, and therefore reference charts that were appropriate have ceased to be so. This is particularly the case for BMI where large numbers of individuals still have a normal BMI but have malnutrition on every other variable (Corish et al., 2000) or when the BMI is high but protein stores are low as occurs in some individuals with obesity. High BMI can also mask the presence of sarcopenia (loss of muscle mass); the concept of sarcopenic obesity has several important consequences as shown in Fig. 34.1.

BIOCHEMICAL MARKERS

Although frequently measured, albumin concentration is not a useful measure of nutritional state because it is affected by so many coincidental medical and surgical conditions. It is more useful for population surveys than for individuals (Forse & Shizgal, 1980). Although serum albumin is a non-specific

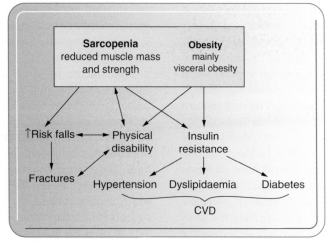

FIG. 34.1 Possible consequences of sarcopenic obesity in older people. (From Zamboni M, Mazzali G, Fantin F, et al. Sarcopenic obesity: a new category of obesity in the elderly. *Nutr Metab Cardiovasc Dis.* 2008;18(5):388–95, with permission).

marker, it is a strong predictor of death, length of stay and re-admission (Herrmann et al., 1992). During rehabilitation the most important measure of nutrition is a biomedical parameter that can show longitudinal changes as nutrition alters. There is an argument that plasma prealbumin (transthyretin) should become a routine screening blood test for protein status. Prealbumin is a sensitive measure of nutritional status but also reflects changes in nutrition during rehabilitation (Mears, 1996) as changes occur in both those over- and underweight.

Mini Nutritional Assessment

The Mini Nutritional Assessment (MNA) has been designed and validated to provide a rapid single assessment of nutritional status in older people that is appropriate for outpatient, hospital and nursing home use. It can be completed in approximately 10 minutes and will define patients as having adequate nutritional status (MNA >/= 24), protein calorie malnutrition (MNA < 17) and those who fall between 17 and 23.5 who are defined as being at risk of malnutrition (Vellas et al., 1999). The MNA correlates with better rehabilitation goal delivery, length of stay and mortality. Although the MNA takes 10 minutes, there is a short form (MNA-SF) that can be used as a screening version of the instrument (Rubenstein et al., 2001). The MNA can be used during rehabilitation to focus on those who are most at nutritional risk and should be used as part of a multidisciplinary comprehensive geriatric assessment.

ORAL INTAKE

The primary aim during rehabilitation is to increase oral intake, particularly protein containing foods. However, there are a number of physiological changes that occur particularly in older age that result in reduced appetite and interest in food. Xerostomia is the subjective feeling of a dry mouth and impacts on the quality of life of those affected. It increases with ageing, but is also seen in a number of autoimmune conditions, radiotherapy to the head and neck and more importantly with certain medications (Eliasson, Birkhed, & Carlen, 2009). Xerostomia

can cause decreased oral intake and food must be moist with plenty of sauce or gravy with patients encouraged to drink whilst eating their meals. Issues with a dry mouth may also complicate denture fixation, and individuals should consider the use of artificial saliva to help improve oral comfort prior to meals.

Part of our enjoyment of food is due to olfaction (sense of smell) but it deteriorates with age. Patients should be prompted as to what is being served and aroma increased by covering food until serving to help with recognition and overall oral intake.

Taste threshold deteriorates with age and underlying medical conditions. Therefore many older individuals need increased intensity of flavour to aid enjoyment. This is commonly seen in the addition of salt to foods. Alterations in taste are distressing and can lead to food aversions with a resultant reduction in food intake and nutritional deficits. Taste perceptions alter following mental or physical stress (Nakagawa, Mizuma, & Inui, 1996), and it is therefore important to provide a variety of foods. Of surprise to many relatives is that during rehabilitation, patients may make different food choices than at any other time.

Drugs alter taste perceptions and may cause abnormal taste, and therefore should be kept to a minimum during rehabilitation. Flavour enhancements of food can improve nutritional status and amplification of certain flavours, such as the addition of umami-rich naturally occurring ingredients, can result in increased oral intake as it compensates for chemosensory losses. A simple measure such as tongue cleaning also increases perceived intensity of various tastes and is a simple measure during oral hygiene (Seerangaiyan et al., 2018).

THE ROLE OF ORAL NUTRITIONAL SUPPLEMENTS

Whilst ONS provide calories and are particularly high in protein, their consumption is variable (Hubbard et al., 2012). Sweetness intensity correlates with the overall product dislike when considering chocolate, vanilla and strawberry ONS. If rejection of sweet ONS occurs during rehabilitation, savoury rather than sweet supplements should be considered (Kennedy et al., 2010). When consumption is high with increased calorie and protein intake, depression scores can improve when compared with placebo products, which should aid rehabilitation (Gariballa & Forster, 2007). Although there is concern that supplementation will result in reduced oral intake during meals, this is not confirmed (Turic et al., 1998). Most ONS are provided as a single serving with a straw to be inserted; however, individuals with cognitive impairment have increased intake when the ONS is served in a glass or beaker rather than with a straw (Allen, Methven, & Gosney, 2014). If sweetness intensity is a negative factor for patients, chilling the ONS reduces the perceived sweetness and therefore delivering the ONS directly from the fridge may encourage oral intake.

WHAT OTHER MEASURES MAY IMPROVE NUTRITION

There are varying feelings regarding protected mealtimes. It is important that mealtimes become an event and routine activities such as doctors' rounds, drug administration and rehabilitation do not distract from the consumption of a meal. However, the presence of family members to support at mealtimes and indeed using this time as an opportunity for rehabilitation such as learning to use an arm affected by trauma or stroke can be very useful. Generally, protected mealtimes do increase oral intake and therefore decisions should be flexible (Porter, Haines, & Truby, 2017). The role of trained volunteers to help support ward staff has been perceived by staff and patients to improve the quality of mealtime care (Robison et al., 2015) and mealtime assistance leads to statistically significant increases in energy and protein intake (Tassone et al., 2015). Mealtime is not just about calories consumed but also social interaction, which improves mood and therefore engagement and outcomes of rehabilitation. Whilst in hospital the role of social dining is part of nutrition action plans.

HOSPITAL FOOD SERVICE

In order to improve nutrition in hospital, a number of quality improvement projects have been undertaken. The first area is the discrepancy between what is planned and what is delivered and how this affects the outcome for the recipient (Collins et al., 2017). A number of barriers can be categorised into environmental, nutrition intervention, patients, implementation process and food service staff. Food should be as attractive as possible, and the beliefs and perceptions of the staff serving the food can provide positive reinforcement before eating commences. This must be backed up by knowledge and those who have the most work satisfaction will interact more with patients. The delivery of foods to the ward and the timing of meals are important. There is evidence that more frequent smaller meals are better consumed, and flexibility to implement this is important. Many hospitalised individuals have their last meal of the day between 1700 and 1800 hours

and then no breakfast until 0800 hours. The availability of snacks outside normal mealtimes, which are high in calories and protein, provides further opportunities for better nutritional input.

Many menus focus on low fat and calcium-rich foods, although rehabilitation patients may be better served by a higher fat, higher protein, higher calorie food being available and encouraged. Indeed snacks such as crisps, biscuits, cheese and cake are as important as the served meals. There is some evidence that cook-chill food services have menus that are more likely to meet nutritional recommendations although in contrast they are less likely to offer a choice of serving size, which may be difficult for both under- and overnourished patients (McClelland & Williams, 2003). Ensuring that a patient receives the food that they ordered, food that they like, at an appropriate time and at the correct food temperature is vital. The serving of a soup with a main course and a dessert on the same tray often reduces the appetite of the patient, and many will commence on the easier-to-eat dessert rather than the main course. The size of portion and indeed the size of the plate should be tailored to the needs of the individual.

When patients are asked about the presented meals, there are three recurring themes. The hot food being too cool, not receiving what was ordered and finally the satisfaction with the food service staff. When a patient is undergoing rehabilitation, food service staff should be aware that their role is equally important to that of the physiotherapist or the occupational therapist in ensuring that nutrition is adequate for maximal effect of rehabilitation input. They should be prepared to swap a poorly consumed meal for another requested item and provide snacks throughout the day. 'Shake and bake' where exercise is undertaken and then afternoon tea is served provides a focus for rehabilitation and improved nutrition. Presentation of a small portion or increased variety also increases patient satisfaction and overall consumption.

MEASURING ORAL INTAKE

As nutrition is so important in rehabilitation, it is vital that there is accurate recording of a patient's intake. Whilst in smaller units or in the patient's own home this is easy to undertake, it is more of a challenge in a large hospital ward. On the whole, patients who are undernourished overestimate their oral intake and there is underreporting by those subjects who are classified as obese (Moshfegh et al., 2008). In a community setting, a 24-hour dietary recall is more accurate when determined by a telephone call or when recorded directly onto a database. However, individuals with cognitive issues poorly reflect their oral intake. A 7-day food diary is more accurate than a food frequency questionnaire, and the recording of grams of intake by direct weighing is far superior to looking at serving size or number of servings. The gold standard for oral nutritional assessment is definitely the photographic method where pre- and post-ingestion photographs can be used to calculate calories and grams of protein consumed (Monacelli et al., 2017).

SUMMARY POINTS

- Both underweight and overweight have a negative impact on rehabilitation
- Many factors cause poor appetite during rehabilitation, and these should be systematically identified and managed
- Mealtimes should be an event; an opportunity to engage family members, to assist with rehabilitation and to socialise
- Smaller meals are better consumed; snacks should also be encouraged outside of mealtimes. Food service staff play a vital role in supporting rehabilitation
- Older people undergoing rehabilitation may need higher fat, higher protein, higher calorie food in contrast to those who are prioritising cardiovascular health

MCQs

Q.1 Which one of the following is correct?
- a. Malnutrition is a deficiency of energy or protein
- b. BMI used alone probably underpredicts the prevalence of undernutrition
- c. Obesity is due to excess body carbohydrate stores
- d. Height and weight can be accurately estimated from the end of the bed
- e. The Mini Nutritional Assessment is reserved for specialised assessment of nutrition

Q.2 Which of the following interventions should be considered to improve nutrition in hospital?
- a. Provision of extra snacks throughout the day
- b. Higher fat, higher protein, higher calorie food
- c. Providing assistance at mealtimes
- d. Adding umami-rich naturally occurring ingredients
- e. All of the above

REFERENCES

Allen, V. J., Methven, L., & Gosney, M. (2014). Impact of serving method on the consumption of nutritional supplement drinks: randomized trial in older adults with cognitive impairment. *Journal of Advanced Nursing, 70,* 1323–1333.

Beghetto, M. G., Fink, J., Luft, V. C., & de Mello, E. D. (2006). Estimates of body height in adult inpatients. *Clinical Nutrition, 25,* 438–443.

Bonnefoy, M., Jauffret, M., Kostka, T., & Jusot, J. F. (2002). Usefulness of calf circumference measurement in assessing the nutritional state of hospitalized elderly people. *Gerontology, 48,* 162–169.

Bruce, D., Laurance, I., McGuiness, M., Ridley, M., & Goldswain, P. (2003). Nutritional supplements after hip fracture: poor compliance limits effectiveness. *Clinical Nutrition, 22,* 497–500.

Collins, J., Huggins, C. E., Porter, J., & Palermo, C. (2017). Factors influencing hospital foodservice staff's capacity to deliver a nutrition intervention. *Nutrition & Dietetics, 74,* 129–137.

Corish, C. A., Flood, P., Mulligan, S., & Kennedy, N. P. (2000). Apparent low frequency of undernutrition in Dublin hospital in-patients: should we review the anthropometric thresholds for clinical practice? *British Journal of Nutrition, 84,* 325–335.

Diaz de Bustamante, M., Alarcon, T., Menendez-Colino, R., Ramirez-Martin, R., Otero, A., & Gonzalez-Montalvo, J. I. (2018). Prevalence of malnutrition in a cohort of 509 patients with acute hip fracture: the importance of a comprehensive assessment. *European Journal of Clinical Nutrition, 72,* 77–81.

Eliasson, L., Birkhed, D., & Carlen, A. (2009). Feeling of dry mouth in relation to whole and minor gland saliva secretion rate. *Archives of Oral Biology, 54,* 263–267.

Forse, R. A., & Shizgal, H. M. (1980). Serum albumin and nutritional status. *Journal of Parenteral and Enteral Nutrition, 4,* 450–454.

Gariballa, S., & Forster, S. (2007). Effects of dietary supplements on depressive symptoms in older patients: a randomised double-blind placebo-controlled trial. *Clinical Nutrition, 26,* 545–551.

Herrmann, F. R., Safran, C., Levkoff, S. E., & Minaker, K. L. (1992). Serum albumin level on admission as a predictor of death, length of stay, and readmission. *Archives of Internal Medicine, 152,* 125–130.

Huang, Z., Himes, J. H., & McGovern, P. G. (1996). Nutrition and subsequent hip fracture risk among a national cohort of white women. *American Journal of Epidemiology, 144,* 124–134.

Hubbard, G. P., Elia, M., Holdoway, A., & Stratton, R. J. (2012). A systematic review of compliance to oral nutritional supplements. *Clinical Nutrition, 31,* 293–312.

Jallut, D., Tappy, L., Kohut, M., Bloesch, D., Munger, R., Schutz, Y., …, & Jequier, E. (1990). Energy balance in elderly patients after surgery for a femoral neck fracture. *Journal of Parenteral and Enteral Nutrition, 14,* 563–568.

Jensen, T. G., Dudrick, S. J., & Johnston, D. A. (1981). A comparison of triceps skinfold and upper arm circumference measurements taken in standard and supine positions. *Journal of Parenteral and Enteral Nutrition, 5,* 519–521.

Kennedy, O., Law, C., Methven, L., Mottram, D., & Gosney, M. (2010). Investigating age-related changes in taste and affects on sensory perceptions of oral nutritional supplements. *Age Ageing, 39,* 733–738.

Koval, K. J., Maurer, S. G., Su, E. T., Aharonoff, G. B., & Zuckerman, J. D. (1999). The effects of nutritional status on outcome after hip fracture. *Journal of Orthopaedic Trauma, 13,* 164–169.

Lumbers, M., New, S. A., Gibson, S., & Murphy, M. C. (2001). Nutritional status in elderly female hip fracture patients: comparison with an age-matched home living group attending day centres. *British Journal of Nutrition, 85,* 733–740.

McClelland, A., & Williams, P. (2003). Trend to better nutrition on Australian hospital menus 1986-2001 and the impact of cook-chill food service systems. *Journal of Human Nutrition and Dietetics, 16,* 245–256.

Mears, E. (1996). Outcomes of continuous process improvement of a nutritional care program incorporating serum prealbumin measurements. *Nutrition, 12*, 479–484.

Monacelli, F., Sartini, M., Bassoli, V., Becchetti, D., Biagini, A. L., Nencioni, A., …, & Odetti, P. (2017). Validation of the photography method for nutritional intake assessment in hospitalized elderly subjects. *The Journal of Nutrition Health and Aging, 21*, 614–621.

Moshfegh, A. J., Rhodes, D. G., Baer, D. J., Murayi, T., Clemens, J. C., Rumpler, W. V., …, & Cleveland, L. E. (2008). The US Department of Agriculture Automated Multiple-Pass Method reduces bias in the collection of energy intakes. *American Journal of Clinical Nutrition, 88*, 324–332.

Muncie, H. L., Jr., Sobal, J., Hoopes, J. M., Tenney, J. H., & Warren, J. W. (1987). A practical method of estimating stature of bedridden female nursing home patients. *Journal of American Geriatrics Society, 35*, 285–289.

Nakagawa, M., Mizuma, K., & Inui, T. (1996). Changes in taste perception following mental or physical stress. *Chemical Senses, 21*, 195–200.

Padwal, R. S., Wang, X., Sharma, A. M., & Dyer, D. (2012). The impact of severe obesity on post-acute rehabilitation efficiency, length of stay, and hospital costs. *Journal of Obesity, 2012*, 972365.

Porter, J., Haines, T. P., & Truby, H. (2017). The efficacy of Protected Mealtimes in hospitalised patients: a stepped wedge cluster randomised controlled trial. *BMC Medicine, 15*, 25.

Robison, J., Pilgrim, A. L., Rood, G., Diaper, N., Elia, M., Jackson, A. A., …, & Roberts, H. C. (2015). Can trained volunteers make a difference at mealtimes for older people in hospital? A qualitative study of the views and experience of nurses, patients, relatives and volunteers in the Southampton Mealtime Assistance Study. *International Journal of Older People Nursing, 10*, 136–145.

Rubenstein, L. Z., Harker, J. O., Salva, A., Guigoz, Y., & Vellas, B. (2001). Screening for undernutrition in geriatric practice: developing the short-form mini-nutritional assessment (MNA-SF). *The Journals of Gerontology: Series A Biological Sciences and Medical Sciences, 56*, M366–M372.

Ryan, S., Politzer, C., Fletcher, A., Bolognesi, M., & Seyler, T. (2018a). Preoperative hypoalbuminemia predicts poor short-term outcomes for hip fracture surgery. *Orthopedics, 41*, e789–e796.

Ryan, S. P., Politzer, C., Green, C., Wellman, S., Bolognesi, M., & Seyler, T. (2018b). Albumin Versus American Society of Anesthesiologists Score: which is more predictive of complications following total joint arthroplasty? *Orthopedics, 41*, 354–362.

Seerangaiyan, K., Juch, F., Atefeh, F., & Winkel, E. G. (2018). Tongue cleaning increases the perceived intensity of salty taste. *Journal of Nutrition, Health, & Aging, 22*, 802–804.

Tassone, E. C., Tovey, J. A., Paciepnik, J. E., Keeton, I. M., Khoo, A. Y., Van Veenendaal, N. G., & Porter, J. (2015). Should we implement mealtime assistance in the hospital setting? A systematic literature review with meta-analyses. *Journal of Clinical Nursing, 24*, 2710–2721.

Turic, A., Gordon, K. L., Craig, L. D., Ataya, D. G., & Voss, A. C. (1998). Nutrition supplementation enables elderly residents of long-term-care facilities to meet or exceed RDAs without displacing energy or nutrient intakes from meals. *Journal of American Dietetic Association, 98*, 1457–1459.

Vasquez, E., Batsis, J. A., Germain, C. M., & Shaw, B. A. (2014). Impact of obesity and physical activity on functional outcomes in the elderly: data from NHANES 2005-2010. *Journal of Aging Health, 26*, 1032–1046.

Vellas, B., Guigoz, Y., Garry, P. J., Nourhashemi, F., Bennahum, D., Lauque, S., & Albarede, J. L. (1999). The Mini Nutritional Assessment (MNA) and its use in grading the nutritional state of elderly patients. *Nutrition, 15*, 116–122.

Watterson, C., Fraser, A., Banks, M., Isenring, E., Miller, M., Silvester, C., …, & Ferguson, M. (2009). Evidence based practice guidelines for the nutritional management of malnutrition in adult patients across the continuum of care. *Nutrition and Dietetics, 66*, S1–S34.

Weinbrenner, T., Vioque, J., Barber, X., & Asensio, L. (2006). Estimation of height and body mass index from demi-span in elderly individuals. *Gerontology, 52*, 275–281.

Woo, S. H., Cha, D. H., Park, E. C., & Kim, S. J. (2019). The association of under-weight and obesity with mortality after hip arthroplasty. *Age Ageing, 48*, 94–100.

Zhang, H., Hsu-Hage, B. H. -H., & Wahlqvist, M. L. (1998). The use of knee height to estimate maximum stature in elderly Chinese. *The Journal of Nutrition. Health & Aging, 2*, 84–87.

35

Continence and Elimination

Rebecca Lee, William Gibson & Adrian Wagg

LEARNING OBJECTIVES

- Describe common problems involving the bladder and bowels that may occur in older people
- Explain how to identify and manage urinary incontinence
- Describe the causes and management of faecal incontinence
- Explain how to effectively manage constipation

BLADDER

Urinary Incontinence in Older People

When considering urinary continence in older adults, it is important to remember that the maintenance of continence is not an automatic process, but rather is a learned skill. The awareness of the need to void (empty the bladder) and the ability to delay voiding requires the coordination of sensory information from the bladder being processed by numerous areas of the brain including the periaqueductal gray matter, the frontal and pre-frontal cortices, and the hypothalamus, which in turn activate the pontine micturition centre (PMC), which acts as a 'switch', to change the bladder from storage to voiding (Fowler, Griffiths, & de Groat, 2008). Additionally, continence relies on the ability to defer voiding in order to locate and walk to a suitable toileting facility, undress, void, redress, wash and return to normal previous activity. As such, the assessment of continence in older adults must include both assessing lower urinary tract symptoms (LUTS) as well as medical conditions, medications, cognitive and physical function. Incontinence therefore is a typical multifactorial geriatric syndrome akin to falls and cognitive impairment.

CASE

Lee, an 83-year-old man in rehabilitation following a fractured hip, reports a 3-year history of urinary incontinence. He describes a daytime frequency of 12, nocturia (nighttime voiding) of 3, with moderate to severe urinary urgency and urgency urinary incontinence most days. He reports some hesitancy but no slow stream and feels that he empties his bladder fully. He does not have any stress (exertional) incontinence. He passes a hard, lumpy stool twice weekly with straining. He drinks two cups of coffee per day and one to two glasses of water. His medical history includes type 2 diabetes, for which he takes gliclazide and canagliflozin, hypertension, for which he takes ramipril, and ischaemic heart disease, for which he takes atorvastatin and aspirin. Surgical history included an appendicectomy and inguinal herniorrhaphy. He currently uses a frame to aid walking and usually lives with his wife. There are no concerns about his memory or cognition. He was started on tamsulosin by the orthopaedic surgeons.

Examination revealed a normal abdomen. Digital rectal examination (DRE) found hard stool in the rectum and a smooth, golf-ball sized prostate. Urinalysis was positive for glucose ++++ and his post-void residual volume (PVR) was 120 ml. Neurological and musculoskeletal examination of the lower limbs was normal.

Lower Urinary Tract Symptoms

LUTS can be divided into *storage symptoms*, those experienced in the storage phase, *voiding symptoms* and *post-micturition symptoms* (Table 35.1). Fig. 35.1 shows the anatomy of the lower urinary tract.

Storage Symptoms

Storage symptoms include urgency, the sudden compelling desire to void which is difficult to defer (Abrams et al., 2009), which should be distinguished from urinary urge, the physiological sensation of a full bladder. Urgency can occur at any point in bladder filling. Patients who experience urgency will often tell you that 'when I've got to go, I've got to go'. A helpful measure to quantify urgency is the *holding or warning time*, a subjective measure of the time between urgency and incontinence or voiding. Clinically this can be explored with patients by asking whether they would interrupt an activity to go to the toilet if they were to experience their normal urgency.

Frequency is the complaint of voiding too often (Abrams et al., 2002); it is subjective and subject to wide variation. In general, more than 8 times per day is accepted as the upper limit of normal.

Nocturia, the complaint that an individual has to wake at night one or more times to void (Abrams et al., 2002), is bothersome to both the individual and their bedroom partner.

The most common cause of urinary incontinence in older adults is overactive bladder (OAB), the clinical syndrome comprising urgency, with or without urgency incontinence, usually with nocturia and frequency, in the absence of infection or

TABLE 35.1   Lower urinary tract symptoms.

STORAGE SYMPTOMS	VOIDING SYMPTOMS	POST-MICTURITION SYMPTOMS
Frequency	Hesitancy	Terminal dribble
Nocturia	Intermittency	Post-micturition dribble
Urgency	Slow stream	
Urgency incontinence	Straining	
Nocturnal enuresis	Spraying, splitting of stream	
Exertional (stress) incontinence	Sense of incomplete emptying	
Passive incontinence	Repositioning to void	

other causative urological pathology. The prevalence of OAB increases with age, and is strongly associated with cerebrovascular disease and cognitive impairment (Kuchel et al., 2009), and is a marker of frailty (Rolfson et al., 2006).

Stress urinary incontinence (SUI), also known as exertional incontinence, occurs when the pressure within the abdomen rises above the pressure generated by the pelvic floor, by actions such as coughing, laughing or sneezing. In women, the pelvic floor is often weakened by pregnancy and childbirth. In men, SUI is almost exclusively seen in those who have had prostate surgery.

Voiding Symptoms

Voiding symptoms are those experienced during urination. Hesitancy, where the onset of urination is delayed, and intermittency, a stop-start flow, are both common and often of little significance. Spraying and splitting of the stream can indicate urethral stricture. Needing to strain to void or a slow stream are symptoms which may result from failure of the detrusor muscle or bladder outflow tract obstruction.

Detrusor failure, in which the contractile function of the bladder is impaired, is associated with diabetes, neurological conditions such as multiple sclerosis, vascular disease and many medications, particularly those with anticholinergic effects. The failure of contractile function appears to be as a result of architectural change to the bladder wall, resulting in a dampening of conduction of contractile force, leading to ineffective emptying. Bladder outlet obstruction may be caused by prostatic obstruction in men, prolapse in women or as a result of surgery for stress incontinence. Constipation can also interfere with effective bladder emptying because of either a mass effect of a full rectum or secondary to nervous system cross talk between bladder and bowel.

Nocturia is commonly ascribed to prostatic obstruction in men but may also be due to excessive night-time urine production, from heart failure, a delayed diuresis to a fluid load, or to dependent oedema which is reabsorbed when lying flat. In addition, some older adults lose their circadian variation in antidiuretic hormone leading to an increase in nocturnal urine production (Ouslander et al., 1998). People with nocturia have higher levels of sodium in the urine at night than those without. The normal nocturnal production in people >65 years should be less than a third of the 24-hour total.

Factors Outside the Lower Urinary Tract

As well as LUTS, the assessment of continence in older people should include a comprehensive assessment of other conditions, prescribed medication and functional ability. Medical conditions can affect the bladder and its control directly, such as stroke or Parkinson's disease, or influence the volume and timing of urine production. Impaired mobility and cognition can also significantly affect people's ability to

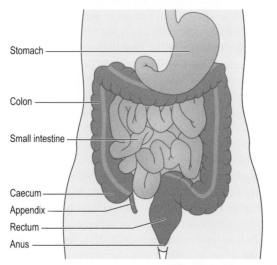
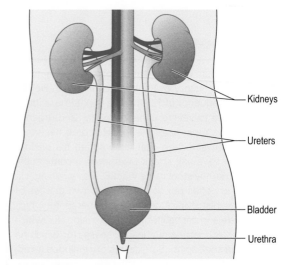

FIG. 35.1 The gastrointestinal and urinary tracts.

TABLE 35.2   Conditions affecting continence.

Diabetes	Microvascular and neurological changes in the bladder Osmotic diuresis
Osteoarthritis	Impaired mobility
Chronic obstructive pulmonary disease	Cough leading to SUI
Congestive cardiac failure	Increased urine production from oedema at night
Dementia	Impaired ability to suppress urgency Impaired ability to locate toileting facilities
Parkinson's disease	Impaired ability to suppress urgency
Obstructive sleep apnoea	Nocturia due to increased atrial natriuretic peptide at night

successfully toilet. People living with dementia may find it difficult to locate a toilet, particularly when in an unfamiliar environment such as in hospital. Poor mobility increases the time taken to reach a bathroom, exacerbating the reduction in holding time experienced by those with urinary urgency. There is evidence that general exercise interventions can improve continence in both community dwelling older people and nursing home residents (Danforth et al., 2007). Conditions which may affect continence are summarised in Table 35.2, and medications that can influence the function of the lower urinary tract are listed in Table 35.3. These are not comprehensive. Finally, an assessment of fluid intake should identify those who are over drinking, leading to polyuria (production of abnormally large volumes of dilute urine), and those who have excessively restricted fluid to reduce incontinence, paradoxically worsening the situation by inducing constipation and never fully filling the bladder.

TABLE 35.3   Medications affecting continence.

Alpha antagonists	Urethral sphincter relaxation
ACE inhibitors	Cough
Anticholinergic drugs	Impaired bladder emptying
Calcium-channel blockers	Oedema leading to nocturnal polyuria and constipation
Cholinesterase inhibitors	Induce urgency
Diuretics	Increased urine production
Lithium	Nephrogenic diabetes insipidus
Opioids, e.g. morphine	Constipation
Gabapentin	Impaired bladder emptying
SGLT2 inhibitors for diabetes	Glycosuria
Non-steroidal anti-inflammatory drugs	Oedema leading to nocturnal polyuria

Management of Urinary Incontinence in Older Adults

Active case finding is a crucial part of continence management. Over half of people with urinary or faecal incontinence (FI) will never seek help (Burgio et al., 1994), and as such asking at-risk populations, such as older people with frailty, is recommended (Wagg et al., 2015). Validated screening questionnaires such as the Bladder Control Symptom Assessment Questionnaire (BSAQ) are available (Basra et al., 2007).

Initial management should address remediable factors: treating underlying comorbidities such as improving diabetes, stopping culprit drugs where possible, and addressing constipation and fluid intake. People with incontinence will often severely limit fluid intake to avoid LUTS, and incontinence, which then worsens constipation, is ineffective and exposes them to the problems of dehydration. Persuading people with incontinence to increase fluid intake can be a challenge. There is much misinformation about adequate fluid intake but a minimum of a litre to a litre and a half daily plus that contained within foodstuffs meets most requirements.

Behavioural Interventions

Urgency suppression and bladder training. Urgency is, by definition, a compelling desire to void that is difficult to defer. However, the sensation of urgency can be reduced by rapid contraction of the pelvic floor, with 5 or 6 squeezes lasting 1 second each. Slow, deep breathing, or sitting on a hard surface, can also reduce the sensation of urgency. To retrain the bladder, patients are asked to suppress their urgency, then to count to 5 (or 3, or even 1), before going to the toilet. Once this is achievable, increase the count to 10, then 20, and so on. By so doing, people can increase their hold time and reduce their storage LUTS. Most published data suggest an interval of 3–4 hours between voids as being an indicator of success. Bladder retraining doesn't appear to be as successful in older people as in younger individuals. This may be due to increased central inability to suppress urgency in older people.

Pelvic floor muscle therapy. Pelvic floor muscle therapy forms the basis of conservative management, for different reasons, for all subtypes of incontinence. Evidence from high-quality trials supports its use and data from older people, albeit rarer, show a benefit, although of a lesser magnitude. As long as an older person can contract the pelvic floor, then this should be offered. Evidence supports supervised, rather than unsupervised, therapy, either in groups or individually, lasting for a minimum of four months.

Pharmacotherapy

Several drugs for the treatment of OAB and urgency incontinence have been developed. In broad terms, they comprise the antimuscarinics (oxybutynin, tolterodine, solifenacin, darifenacin, fesoterodine, propiverine and trospium) and beta-3 agonists (mirabegron and vibegron). The efficacy and rates of side effects for all the agents are broadly similar. Of the anticholinergics, oxybutynin has the highest discontinuation rates due to treatment emergent adverse events and has been shown to induce cognitive dysfunction in older adults. Solifenacin and fesoterodine both have data to support use in mild cognitive impairment and vulnerable elders, respectively. The rate of adverse cognitive events is low (approximately 1%) even in those >75 years of age, but long-term data are lacking. Use of the beta-3 agonists is associated with few anticholinergic side effects, which may be a consideration in those with concomitant neurological disease.

Interventions Beyond Medications

For older people without a successful response to either conservative or pharmacotherapy for urgency incontinence, evidence supports the use of intradetrusor onabotulinumtoxinA therapy, even in frail older persons. However, the results do not appear to reach the magnitude of effect seen in non-frail older people and the incidence of adverse effects is higher. Recipients should be advised of a potential risk of having to perform intermittent self-catheterisation (<3%) and urinary tract infection (up to 20%) following the procedure.

Prompted Voiding

Prompted voiding describes a process where patients are given positive reinforcement for successful toileting and are encouraged to toilet with verbal prompts in response to verbal and non-verbal clues from patients. It aims to recognise and respond to a person's voiding pattern and encourage successful toileting. A 3-day trial of prompted voiding should be used and if a 20% reduction in incontinence episodes or wet checks is not achieved, then the process should be abandoned, and the person managed with check and change. Timed voiding is where care staff will take people to the toilet at regular intervals with no reference to their voiding pattern. In those who are likely to require the assistance of two people to transfer in the long term, *check and change* using appropriate containment is often the only appropriate strategy.

Pads, Appliances and Catheters

A huge variety of hand-held urinals, bedpans and collection devices are available for those with urinary incontinence and for those whose incontinence is complicated by physical impairment. The International Consultation on Incontinence in collaboration with the International Continence Society hosts a comprehensive products directory for use by patients or their families which enables them to gain advice on the suitability of different products (http://www.continence-productadvisor.org/). The most expensive product is not necessarily the best and, likewise, neither is the cheapest the worst performing (Fader et al., 2008b; Fader, Cottenden, & Getliffe, 2007, 2008a). Attention should be paid to the type of pad, frequency of changing, ease of application and removal and overall, the personal preference of the intended user. The use of intermittent catheterisation for voiding inefficiency in older people should not be neglected. There are aids to assist with difficult catheterisation and, many home care services will perform this task on a twice or three times daily basis should the older person or willing and able caregiver be unable to perform this.

Lee is describing OAB, with urgency, frequency, nocturia and urgency incontinence. His risk factors for this include diabetes, and it is likely that his symptoms are exacerbated by constipation and glycosuria from his SGLT2 inhibitor. His poor mobility will also increase his risk of incontinence, as he takes longer to get to the toilet.

His initial management will include increasing his fluids, addressing his constipation and stopping his canagliflozin. He should be taught urgency suppression and bladder retraining, and he may benefit from physiotherapy to improve his gait and balance. If these measures are unsuccessful, he should be considered for treatment with one of the newer bladder antimuscarinic agents, such as solifenacin or fesoterodine, or a beta-3 agonist.

BOWELS

CASE

Aisha is a 76-year-old lady who was noted to have FI interfering with her physiotherapy sessions on most days and often with little to no warning. She is very distressed by this and has stopped attending recreation therapy and communal dining as a result.

She has a past medical history of hypertension, arthritis and diabetes, with her most recent HBA1C being 5.8%. She is currently taking ramipril, paracetamol and metformin. She had a prolonged labour with her first of two children and required a forceps delivery. She lives alone and hopes to return home with home care for bathing only. She mobilises slowly with a Zimmer frame. She is a non-smoker and a non-drinker.

On examination, her abdomen was soft and non-tender. Bowel sounds were active. Rectal examination revealed reduced anal tone, reduced rectal sensation and an absent anal reflex. There was evidence of chemical dermatitis. There was no evidence of any masses, faecal loading or impaction.

Faecal Incontinence

This lady presents with the socially debilitating issue of FI. The reported prevalence of FI is likely an underestimate as many patients do not mention it due to the associated perceived stigma (Brown et al., 2018). This has led to it being called the 'silent affliction' (Johanson & Lafferty, 1996). A recent systematic review reported a median prevalence of 7.7% (with a range of 2.0%–20.7%) increasing with age from 5.7% in 15–34 year olds to 15.9% in over 90 year olds and 42.3%–57.8% in institutionalised older persons (Ihnat et al., 2016; Jerez-Roig et al., 2015; Ng et al., 2015).

FI results in significant psychosocial consequences on patients, caregivers and society. Individual consequences include social isolation, depression, reduced sexual activity and increased dependence (Ihnat et al., 2016). It is a leading cause of caregiver stress and burnout (Wilson, 2007). From a societal perspective, it has been associated with higher rates of institutionalisation (Grover et al., 2010).

FI can be divided into four main categories. Passive FI is when incontinence occurs without any awareness of the need to defecate. Urge FI occurs when there is a strong urge to defecate and the patient is unable to retain the stool until they reach a toilet. Overflow incontinence occurs when there is leakage of liquid stool around impacted faeces. Functional incontinence occurs when the patient is unable to get to the toilet in time due for example to lack of access of toilets or reduced mobility. FI can also be mixed with a combination of two or more different types contributing. Fig. 35.1 shows the anatomy of the gastrointestinal tract.

Identifying FI is the first and most important step. A comprehensive history and examination is essential for differentiating the different types of FI. Ascertaining whether urgency is present or whether the loss is passive will help differentiate. It is important to clarify if the incontinence is gas, liquid or solid faeces and how often the incontinence occurs. Asking the patient to complete a stool chart can provide very useful information about the frequency and consistency of the stool (Lewis & Heaton, 1997). A detailed medical and obstetric history will help to identify risk factors. In our case history, the patient describes passive loss. Her risk factors for FI include poorly controlled diabetes, a prolonged labour with forceps delivery and reduced mobility. Other risk factors which can cause FI are shown in Table 35.4.

Examination should include a neurological exam looking for signs of underlying disease such as Parkinson's disease and stroke and an abdominal exam for evidence of masses or constipation. Anorectal examination should also be performed.

The next step in examination is to perform a DRE. This will detect any significant anal pathology such as faecal impaction or masses. During the DRE, the resting sphincter tone can be assessed. The patient can then be asked to 'squeeze' to assess their tone during contraction.

Finally, a vaginal examination should be completed to look for faeces in the vagina which would suggest the rare finding of a rectovaginal fistula. A vaginal exam will also allow assessment of any vaginal prolapse present.

Further investigations may be required if it is thought there is an underlying cause to the FI or importantly if there has been a recent change in bowel habit. Investigations could include sigmoidoscopy, colonoscopy, stool cultures and coeliac serology.

There are many conservative management strategies to try for patients with FI. The exact strategies will depend on what medications they are taking, any underlying medical conditions and the consistency of the stool. Table 35.5 outlines some potential approaches.

In our case example, Aisha required zinc oxide cream to act as a barrier. We stopped her metformin but, despite this, she continued to have low volume loose stool. We therefore started her on psyllium 3.4 g twice daily and advised her on a low residue diet. On her return to clinic 3 months later, she was passing a soft, formed stool every 2 days and had not had any FI for 2 months.

Should conservative measures fail, consideration should be given to referral for further investigations, such as anorectal

TABLE 35.4	Conditions affecting faecal incontinence.
Dementia Reduced mobility Delirium Depression	Functional impairment
Bile salt malabsorption Inflammatory bowel disease Coeliac disease Medications Microscopic colitis	Diarrhoea
Obstetric injury Surgery Diabetes Spinal cord injury Infiltrative process (e.g. systemic sclerosis)	Weakness of anal sphincter
Ulcerative colitis Radiation proctitis Proctectomy	Reduced rectal compliance Reduced reservoir capacity
Slow transit constipation Medications Dehydration Hypothyroidism Hypercalcaemia Parkinson's disease	Faecal impaction
Multiple sclerosis Spinal cord injury Diabetes Dementia Stroke	Rectal hyposensitivity

manometry and endoanal ultrasound. Subsequent management will then depend on findings from further investigations but could include biofeedback therapy and sacral nerve stimulation.

Constipation

Constipation is a common complaint of older people. There continues to be a widely held belief that 'once a day' is the normal bowel emptying frequency when in fact there is a wide variation between three times daily and three times weekly. The frequency of bowel emptying does not change in association with ageing in the absence of coexisting medical conditions, mobility impairment or medications. There is also a mismatch between older people's report of constipation and the medical definition (which in addition to bowel opening frequency includes the need to strain, the passage of hard or lumpy stool at least a quarter of the time, a sense of incomplete evacuation, hard or lumpy stools, prolonged time to stool or a need for manual manoeuvres to pass stool, which have been present for at least 3 of the prior 12 months). Needless to say, in older people with constipation there is usually more than one underlying cause (Gallegos-Orozco et al., 2012). The Bristol stool form chart (Fig. 35.2) is a useful tool that allows pictorial depiction of seven consistencies ranging from type 1 (hard lumps) to type 7 (watery diarrhoea).

TABLE 35.5	Approaches to management of faecal incontinence.
Supportive care	• Chemical irritation – barrier cream, e.g. zinc oxide; apply to affected areas as required • Reduce alcohol intake • Maintain adequate fluid intake • Use of moist wipe or tissue for wiping
Functional incontinence	• Improve signage to toilets – pictorial signs • Easy to remove clothing, e.g. jogging bottoms • Scheduled/timed/prompted toileting • Aids such as grab rails, raised toilet seats, mobility aids (Goodman et al., 2017)
Chronic constipation resulting in overflow	• Stop or reduce offending medications, e.g. opiates, tricyclic antidepressants, anticholinergics, calcium-channel blockers • Increase fluid intake • Increase fibre intake • Bulk forming laxatives, e.g. ispaghula husk, methylcellulose • Osmotic laxatives, e.g. lactulose, polyethylene glycol 3350 • Stimulant laxatives, e.g. senna, bisacodyl • Suppositories – glycerin, bisacodyl
Low-volume, loose stools	• Bulking agent, e.g. ispaghula husk, methylcellulose, psyllium (Markland et al., 2015) • Low residue diet
Chronic diarrhoea	• Treat underlying cause • Consider bile salt malabsorption – use cholestyramine • Stop offending drugs, e.g. metformin, antibiotics, magnesium salts, colchicine, cholinesterase inhibitors, proton pump inhibitors, laxative overuse • Antidiarrhoeal agent, e.g. loperamide (Omar & Alexander, 2013) • In some cases, loperamide to induce constipation with twice weekly suppositories/enemas to evacuate stool • Daily rectal washout (e.g. Peristeen) • Anal plug

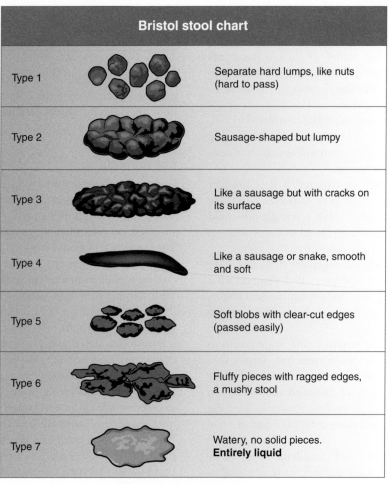

Bristol stool chart

Type 1	Separate hard lumps, like nuts (hard to pass)
Type 2	Sausage-shaped but lumpy
Type 3	Like a sausage but with cracks on its surface
Type 4	Like a sausage or snake, smooth and soft
Type 5	Soft blobs with clear-cut edges (passed easily)
Type 6	Fluffy pieces with ragged edges, a mushy stool
Type 7	Watery, no solid pieces. **Entirely liquid**

FIG. 35.2 Bristol stool chart.

Self-reported constipation is more common in women (26%) than men (16%) who are 65 years or older, rising to 34% and 26% among those 84 years or older (Talley et al., 1996). In patients undergoing rehabilitation, immobility, opiate analgesics (pain medication), anticholinergic medications and calcium supplements, for example, can exacerbate constipation as can having other coexisting conditions such as Parkinson's disease (Table 35.6).

Any acute change in bowel habit in older people, particularly if there is blood in the stool, should be taken seriously and screening for colon cancer should be undertaken. Examination should comprise a DRE and inspection for the presence of haemorrhoids or prolapse, masses, anal strictures, fissures or stool impaction. Treatment consists of establishing a regular bowel habit, taking advantage of the increase in bowel motility after breakfast and encouragement of mobility. Attention to position with the use of a footstool at the toilet is useful. Using prunes, prune juice (Hull et al., 2011), polyethylene glycol (Lyseng-Williamson, 2018) or insoluble fibre (Spinzi et al., 2009) to produce a type 4 stool which is easy to pass is the first target of treatment. Docusate should not be used as the evidence suggests little if any effect and it has been accordingly removed from many formularies. If then there is difficulty in achieving successful bowel emptying, a stimulant laxative such as senna or bisacodyl should be used. There are several newer drugs which successfully treat chronic constipation by improving the motility of the lower bowel (e.g. linaclotide), but these are best reserved for specialist practice. Glycerine suppositories are a useful aid to evacuation, and low-volume enemata sometimes have to be employed; large volume enemata should be avoided as they can cause problems with absorption of salts in those with heart conditions.

TABLE 35.6 Correlates of constipation.	
MEDICATION	
Analgesics (opiates, NSAIDs)	Calcium-channel blockers
Antacids containing calcium or aluminium	Calcium supplements
Anticonvulsants	Diuretics
Tricyclic antidepressants	Iron supplements
Antipsychotics	
Antihistamines	
Bile acid binders	
MEDICAL CONDITIONS	
Chronic kidney disease	Hypothyroidism
Diabetes mellitus	Hypercalcaemia
Hyperparathyroidism	Hypermagnesaemia
Autonomic neuropathy	Hypokalaemia
Dementia	Multiple sclerosis
Parkinson's disease	Scleroderma
Stroke	Spinal cord injury
Depression	Immobility
Dehydration	

SUMMARY POINTS

- Urinary and faecal incontinence are common conditions which result in significant impairment in well-being and quality of life for patients and their caregivers
- All patients presenting with urinary or faecal incontinence should have a thorough history and examination to determine the underlying contributing factors. All patients should be offered supportive treatment if required. Other management will vary depending on the underlying cause
- The majority of older patients with urinary or faecal incontinence can be successfully managed with a combination of conservative techniques in combination with suitable containment products
- Constipation is increasingly common in late life; maintenance of mobility and hydration and avoidance of precipitating medications are key interventions in management

MCQs

Q.1 The most common cause of urinary incontinence in older adults is
   a. Nocturia
   b. Stress urinary incontinence
   c. Overactive bladder
   d. Voiding dysfunction
   e. Functional incontinence

Q.2 Medications which can predispose to urinary incontinence include:
   a. Metformin
   b. Alpha adrenoreceptor antagonists

   c. Senna
   d. Dapagliflozin
   e. Potassium supplements

Q.3 Management of incontinence in older people can include:
   a. Easy to remove clothing
   b. Prompted voiding
   c. Pictorial toilet signs
   d. Maintenance of mobility
   e. All of the above

REFERENCES

Abrams, P., Artibani, W., Cardozo, L., Dmochowski, R., Van Kerrebroeck, P., & Sand, P. International Continence Society. (2009). Reviewing the ICS 2002 terminology report: the ongoing debate. *Neurourol Urodyn, 28*, 287.

Abrams, P., Cardozo, L., Fall, M., et al. Standardisation Subcommittee of the International Continence Society. (2002). The standardisation of terminology of lower urinary tract function: report from the Standardisation Sub-committee of the International Continence Society. *Neurourol Urodyn, 21*, 167–178.

Basra, R., Artibani, W., Cardozo, L., Castro-Diaz, D., et al. (2007). Design and validation of a new screening instrument for lower urinary tract dysfunction: the Bladder Control Self-Assessment Questionnaire (B-SAQ). *European Urology, 52*, 230–237.

Brown, H. W., Guan, W., Schmuhl, N. B., Smith, P. D., Whitehead, W. E., & Rogers, R. G. (2018). If we don't ask, they won't tell: screening for urinary and fecal incontinence by primary care providers. *Journal of the American Board of Family Medicine, 31*, 774–782.

Burgio, K. L., Ives, D. G., Locher, J. L., Arena, V. C., & Kuller, L. H. (1994). Treatment seeking for urinary incontinence in older adults. *Journal of American Geriatrics Society, 42*, 208–212.

Danforth, K. N., Shah, A. D., Townsend, M. K., Lifford, K. L., Curhan, G. C., Resnick, N. M., & Grodstein, F. (2007). Physical activity and urinary incontinence among healthy, older women. *Obstetrics and Gynecology, 109*, 721–727.

Fader, M., Cottenden, A. M., & Getliffe, K. (2007). Absorbent products for light urinary incontinence in women. *Cochrane Database of Systematic Reviews, 2*, CD001406.

Fader, M., Cottenden, A. M., & Getliffe, K. (2008a). Absorbent products for moderate-heavy urinary and/or faecal incontinence in women and men. *Cochrane Database of Systematic Reviews, 4*, CD007408.

Fader, M., Cottenden, A., Getliffe, K., et al. (2008b). Absorbent products for urinary/faecal incontinence: a comparative evaluation of key product designs. *Health Technology Assessment, 12*, iii–iv, ix–185.

Fowler, C. J., Griffiths, D., & de Groat, W. C. (2008). The neural control of micturition. *National Reviews Neuroscience, 9*, 453–466.

Gallegos-Orozco, J. F., Foxx-Orenstein, A. E., Sterler, S. M., & Stoa, J. M. (2012). Chronic constipation in the elderly. *The American Journal of Gastroenterology, 107*, 18–25, quiz 26.

Goodman, C., Norton, C., Buswell, M., et al. (2017). Managing Faecal INcontinence in people with advanced dementia resident in Care Homes (FINCH) study: a realist synthesis of the evidence. *Health Technology Assessment, 21*, 1–220.

Grover, M., Busby-Whitehead, J., Palmer, M. H., Heymen, S., Palsson, O. S., Goode, P. S., Turner, M., & Whitehead, W. E. (2010). Survey of geriatricians on the effect of fecal incontinence on nursing home referral. *Journal of the American Geriatrics Society, 58*, 1058–1062.

Hull, M. A., Mcintire, D. D., Atnip, S. D., Dreadin, J., Nihira, M. A., Drewes, P. G., Schaffer, J. I., & Wai, C. Y. (2011). Randomized trial comparing 2 fiber regimens for the reduction of symptoms of constipation. *Female Pelvic Medicine & Reconstructive Surgery, 17*, 128–133.

Ihnat, P., Kozakova, R., Rudinska, L. I., Peteja, M., Vavra, P., & Zonca, P. (2016). Fecal incontinence among nursing home residents: is it still a problem? *Archives of Gerontology & Geriatrics, 65*, 79–84.

Jerez-Roig, J., Souza, D. L., Amaral, F. L., & Lima, K. C. (2015). Prevalence of fecal incontinence (FI) and associated factors in institutionalized older adults. *Archives of Gerontology Geriatrics, 60*, 425–430.

Johanson, J. F., & Lafferty, J. (1996). Epidemiology of fecal incontinence: the silent affliction. *The American Journal of Gastroenterology, 91*, 33–36.

Kuchel, G. A., Moscufo, N., Guttmann, C. R., Zeevi, N., Wakefield, D., Schmidt, J., Dubeau, C. E., & Wolfson, L. (2009). Localization of brain white matter hyperintensities and urinary incontinence in community-dwelling older adults. *The Journals of Gerontology. Series A, Biological Sciences and Medical Sciences, 64*, 902–909.

Lewis, S. J., & Heaton, K. W. (1997). Stool form scale as a useful guide to intestinal transit time. *Scandinavian Journal of Gastroenterology, 32*, 920–924.

Lyseng-Williamson, K. A. (2018). Macrogol (polyethylene glycol) 4000 without electrolytes in the symptomatic treatment of chronic constipation: a profile of its use. *Drugs & Therapy Perspectives, 34*, 300–310.

Markland, A. D., Burgio, K. L., Whitehead, W. E., Richter, H. E., Wilcox, C. M., Redden, D. T., Beasley, T. M., & Goode, P. S. (2015). Loperamide versus psyllium fiber for treatment of fecal incontinence: the Fecal Incontinence Prescription (Rx) Management (FIRM) randomized clinical trial. *Diseases of the Colon and Rectum, 58*, 983–993.

Ng, K. S., Sivakumaran, Y., Nassar, N., & Gladman, M. A. (2015). Fecal incontinence: community prevalence and associated factors—a systematic review. *Diseases of the Colon and Rectum, 58*, 1194–1209.

Omar, M. I., & Alexander, C. E. (2013). Drug treatment for faecal incontinence in adults. *Cochrane Database of Systematic Review*, CD002116.

Ouslander, J. G., Nasr, S. Z., Miller, M., Withington, W., Lee, C. S., Wiltshire-Clement, M., Cruise, P., & Schnelle, J. F. (1998). Arginine vasopressin levels in nursing home residents with nighttime urinary incontinence. *Journal of the American Geriatrics Society, 46*, 1274–1279.

Rolfson, D. B., Majumdar, S. R., Tsuyuki, R. T., Tahir, A., & Rockwood, K. (2006). Validity and reliability of the Edmonton Frail Scale. *Age Ageing, 35*, 526–529.

Spinzi, G., Amato, A., Imperiali, G., Lenoci, N., Mandelli, G., Paggi, S., Radaelli, F., Terreni, N., & Terruzzi, V. (2009). Constipation in the elderly: management strategies. *Drugs Aging, 26*, 469–474.

Talley, N. J., Fleming, K. C., Evans, J. M., O'Keefe, E. A., Weaver, A. L., Zinsmeister, A. R., & Melton, L. J., III. (1996). Constipation in an elderly community: a study of prevalence and potential risk factors. *The American Journal of Gastroenterology, 91*, 19–25.

Wagg, A., Gibson, W., Ostaszkiewicz, J., Johnson, T., 3rd, Markland, A., Palmer, M. H., Kuchel, G., Szonyi, G., & Kirschner-Hermanns, R. (2015). Urinary incontinence in frail elderly persons: Report from the 5th International Consultation on Incontinence. *Neurourol Urodyn, 34*, 398–406.

Wilson, M. (2007). The impact of faecal incontinence on the quality of life. *British Journal of Nursing, 16*, 204–207.

36

Sexuality

Mary Ni Lochlainn

LEARNING OBJECTIVES

- Discuss sexuality in the context of older age
- Describe the ways sexuality can be influenced by ageing, age-related conditions and the treatment of these conditions
- Explain the different considerations for men and women
- Consider sexuality in the context of rehabilitation and cognitive impairment

CASE

Clark is an 80-year-old gentleman who was recently discharged from hospital. He spent 6 weeks on the ward. His elective admission for a cardiac procedure on his aortic valve was complicated by a heart attack and severe pneumonia. Before he went into hospital, he was living independently with his 74-year-old wife Lois. Both had been in good health and enjoyed an active sex life, albeit less often than when they were younger.

Now that he is back at home, he gets breathless after walking short distances, and has lost a few kilograms in weight. He takes several new medications. He is having erectile dysfunction and is not sure if this is related to his illness, his medications or his fear of having another heart attack while exerting himself.

INTRODUCTION

Sexuality is an important component of emotional and physical well-being that people experience throughout their lives. Studies showing that many men and women remain sexually active as they age refute the prevailing myth that ageing equates to celibacy. Age-related physiological changes do not render sexual relationships impossible, and many are modifiable. There are several therapeutic options available to improve sexual capacity in old age. An understanding of sexual changes that accompany ageing, as well as those that accompany certain illnesses and medications, may help healthcare practitioners to give practical advice on sexuality in the rehabilitation setting. Good awareness of this aspect of older people's lives could raise meaningful expectations and improve quality of life for ageing adults.

Studies have shown that many older adults remain sexually active well into their later years (Ni Lochlainn & Kenny, 2013). For example, one survey of 335 people aged 50–90 years in the UK found that 82% were currently involved in one or more sexual relationships (Gott, 2001). Research by the Irish Longitudinal Study on Ageing (TILDA) involved over 8000 adults over 50 years, and found that frequent sexual activity is the norm with 59% being sexually active and of those, 69% were sexually active weekly or monthly (Orr, McGarrigle, & Kenny, 2017). These results clearly counteract the stereotype of the 'asexual older person'.

Sexuality may include touching, caressing, fantasy, masturbation, physical closeness and the warmth created by emotionality. Intimacy and relationships are important quality of life issues from birth until death. Psychological well-being has been closely linked with sexuality, with a bidirectional relationship. Both physical and mental health have been linked with sexuality (Freak-Poli et al., 2017; Waite et al., 2017), and sustained sexual interest and sexual enjoyment are linked to successful ageing in both genders (Štulhofer et al., 2018). The frequency and importance of sexual behaviours have been positively correlated with quality of life (Flynn & Gow, 2015), and sexually active adults tend to be more positive in their perceptions of ageing (Orr et al., 2017). With such a close link to overall well-being, sexuality is clearly an important consideration in the rehabilitation process.

One must also consider lesbian, gay, bisexual, transgender and queer (LGBTQ+) older adults when contemplating sexual health. It has been estimated that the number of older LGBTQ+ adults in the US will exceed 5 million by 2060 and could be up to 20 million (~6% of US population) when accounting for those who don't publicly identify as LGBTQ+ but have engaged in same-sex attraction or sexual activity (Goldsen, 2018). Discrimination on the basis of sexual orientation has been reported in accessing sexual healthcare in older age and in retirement homes (Knochel et al., 2012; Westwood, 2019). Notably, LGBTQ+ older adults in the US have also shown higher rates of chronic health conditions including strokes and heart attacks (Goldsen, 2018). As the population continues to age, it is imperative that we provide inclusive rehabilitation options for all older adults.

INFLUENCE OF AGEING ON SEXUAL FUNCTION

It is not typically age that affects the importance placed on sex, but health problems experienced by an individual and/or their partner. Poor physical and mental health have been associated with lower levels of sexual activity and satisfaction, and higher prevalence of sexual dysfunction (any problem related to sexual activity) (Beckman et al., 2014; Lee et al., 2016; Orr et al., 2017). Physical illness can affect sexual function directly by interfering with endocrine, neural and vascular processes that mediate the sexual response, indirectly by causing weakness or pain and psychologically by provoking changes in body image or self-esteem.

Age-associated medical problems that have been linked to sexual dysfunction are listed in Table 36.1. This is not an exhaustive list and some people may have more than one of the conditions listed. In addition, drugs commonly affect sexual function (see Table 36.2).

In terms of the indirect effects of health conditions, changes in appearance caused by ageing itself or by illness may affect self-esteem, which can then influence sexual functioning. Fatigue caused by illness or medications may lead to reduced interest in sex. Alcohol and stress are other causes of sexual dysfunction, although this is not specific to older adults.

It is worth noting that it is not all negative. Retirement, with increased free time, as well as not having to worry about getting pregnant means that many older couples report increased satisfaction with their sex lives. Sexual activity is equivalent to mild-moderate physical activity, in the range of 3–5 metabolic equivalents (METs) (Levine et al., 2012). METs

TABLE 36.1 **Medical problems that have been linked to sexual dysfunction.**
Diabetes
High blood pressure
Lower urinary tract symptoms (bladder/prostate/ penis-related issues)
Heart disease including heart attack
Prostate cancer and its treatment
Pelvic surgery
Parkinson's disease
Epilepsy
Stroke
Multiple sclerosis (MS)
Kidney disease and dialysis
Lung disease
Disease of arteries/veins in the legs
Hysterectomy
Ovarian cancer
Disease of lumbar spine
Arthritis
Incontinence
Obesity

TABLE 36.2 **Drugs that can affect sexual function.**
Antidepressants
Other psychiatric medications, e.g. lithium, risperidone, chlorpromazine
Antihistamines
Parkinson's medications
Cardiac medications, e.g. digoxin, beta blockers, diuretics
Anti-inflammatories
Hormone treatments for some cancers, e.g., goserelin
HIV treatments, e.g. protease inhibitors
Steroids, e.g. prednisolone
Immunosuppressants
Recreational drugs and alcohol

are a way of estimating the energy expenditure for many common physical activities. An activity which is 4 METs (e.g. sexual activity) uses approximately 4 times as much oxygen than at rest. Running at approximately 7 mph is 11 METs. Therefore sexual activity can contribute to physical fitness and well-being.

SEXUAL CONSIDERATIONS FOR OLDER WOMEN

Female-specific surgery, such as mastectomy, hysterectomy and pelvic floor surgery, and pregnancy-related complications can affect the sexual function of older women. Women live on average 30 years after the menopause (Speroff & Fritz, 2005), indicating the importance of good post-menopausal health. Menopausal changes that arise from loss of oestrogen include decreased vaginal lubrication, vasomotor symptoms (hot flushes and night sweats), and changes including irritability, anorgasmia (inability to achieve orgasm), decreased libido, and impaired sexual performance (Speroff & Fritz, 2005). However these only affect some women and there are therapies available including dilators to improve dyspareunia (pain during sex), vaginal lubricants and topical or oral oestrogen, which may help with vaginal thinning and dryness (Amin, Kuhle, & Fitzpatrick, 2003). Vaginal dryness can affect other activities such as prolonged sitting or bike riding (Huang et al., 2009), and therefore can have a big impact on quality of life.

SEXUAL CONSIDERATIONS FOR OLDER MEN

Significant changes in penile structure occur with ageing. The concentration of elastic fibres, smooth muscle and collagen decreases with age. In addition, mechanical sensitivity of the penis is decreased (Seftel, 2003). These changes may contribute to the development of erectile dysfunction in older men. This indicates that for some men, the normal ageing process can be sufficient to produce erectile dysfunction, in the absence of disease. Other causes of erectile dysfunction include medications (see Table 36.2), disease (see Table 36.1),

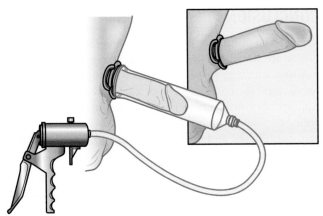

FIG. 36.1 Vacuum erection device. (From Creager M, Beckman J, Loscalzo J. *Vascular Medicine: A Companion to Braunwald's Heart Disease*, 3rd edn, Elsevier; 2020, with permission.)

particularly disease of the blood vessels (vascular), psychological or hormonal causes (Yafi et al., 2017). Vascular causes are the most common (Yafi et al., 2017): erectile dysfunction can be considered an early marker for cardiovascular risk and its development should prompt medical review (Billups, 2005).

In terms of medications, above-average prevalence for erectile dysfunction has been reported among men treated with vasodilators, cardiac drugs, antihyperglycaemic, antihypertensive agents and antidepressants (Ni Lochlainn & Kenny, 2013). In addition, behaviour including smoking, alcohol consumption, lack of physical activity and television viewing time have been associated with erectile dysfunction (Bacon et al., 2003).

Currently available therapies for erectile dysfunction include oral medication, e.g. sildenafil, penile self-injection therapy, hormone injections, vacuum constriction devices (see Fig. 36.1), arterial revascularisation, penile prostheses and psychological treatment (Seftel, 2003; Montorsi et al., 2010).

SEXUALLY TRANSMITTED DISEASE IN OLDER ADULTS

The number of new sexually transmitted infections (STIs) diagnosed among 50–70 year olds increased by 38% between 2010 and 2014 in the UK (Davies, 2015). It has also been reported that older adults are less likely to use condoms (Davies, 2015). Older adults may engage in riskier sexual behaviour as they no longer are concerned about pregnancy (post-menopause). It is important that people of all ages engage in safe sex practices and get annual testing for STIs if they have any new partners.

SEXUALITY AND COGNITIVE IMPAIRMENT

A large study in the US reported that approximately 50% of men and women with dementia reported being sexually active, refuting the idea that cognitive impairment equates to celibacy (Lindau et al., 2018). However, cognitive impairment has been associated with a decline in emotional intimacy, reduced sexual activity, reduced marital cohesion and increased feelings of 'separateness' (Holdsworth & McCabe, 2018). Sexuality in dementia is often discussed in terms of 'appropriateness'. The simplified binary labelling and classification of sexual behaviour in dementia as appropriate or inappropriate, often applied in institutional settings, fails to account for complex factors that may influence staff decisions on the ethical dilemmas raised by dementia. The prevalence of sexual behaviour which is distressing/disruptive to the person themselves and/or people around them ranges between 2% and 17% of patients with dementia and is more commonly seen in men (Black, Muralee, & Tampi, 2005; Stubbs, 2011).

Interestingly, a 2016 study found a significant association between sexual activity and number sequencing and recall in men, and between sexual activity and recall in women (Wright & Jenks, 2016), suggesting that maintaining a healthy sex life in later life could be beneficial for cognitive function.

ATTITUDES TOWARDS SEXUALITY OF OLDER ADULTS

Prejudice exists at all levels of society, finding its basis in overgeneralised, learned attitudes towards individuals who do not conform to what is perceived to be normal within that society. In a study of reactions of college students to various sexual scenarios, they were more surprised and more disgusted by incidents of sexuality in people who were 70–75 years than those who were 30–35 years (Waterman, 2012). They also found the scenarios less acceptable and less appropriate.

One suggested reason for the negative attitudes towards older persons could be the media's portrayal of the elderly as frail and asexual. When reporting on sexuality and health among older adults, 'NBC News' wrote 'many older people are surprisingly frisky' and described how 'sexed up seniors' take part in 'intimate acts that would make their grandchildren blush' (Sexed up seniors do it more than you'd think, 2007). On the same topic 'ABC News' reported 'grandma's still got it' with a similar air of surprise (Bord, 2007). Even the United Kingdom's NHS (National Health Service) website, in a piece which looked at the link between sex life and health in older age, remarked 'birds do it, bees do it, even OAPs do it (Sex life linked to elderly health, 2010).

SEXUAL ACTIVITY CONSIDERATIONS IN REHABILITATION

Current practice does not routinely include any consideration of sexual health in the rehabilitation setting. Typically, it is not mentioned unless a patient brings it up themselves and a number of studies have reported that older adults consider intimacy and sexual issues important, yet rarely addressed (Ni Lochlainn & Kenny, 2013). Other ways in which sexual well-being can be considered include simple measures such as allowing partners to stay overnight at rehabilitation facilities, with adequate privacy, or planning overnight visits to home.

The British Heart Foundation advises that sexual activity can be restarted as soon as one feels well enough after a heart attack, usually 4–6 weeks. They advise taking longer after cardiac surgery. As sex is a form of exercise, it is generally considered that if you can walk briskly, or climb two flights of stairs without discomfort, then you are ready to resume having sex. It is always worth taking things slowly and stopping if you experience any chest pain or dizziness. In terms of other surgery, injuries or medical problems, generally the advice is similar; once you feel well enough, sexual activity can be gradually reintroduced. Individual concerns should be discussed with a doctor before resuming sex.

Physical activity is usually a key component of rehabilitation, and luckily this can also be beneficial for sexual health in some contexts (Belardinelli et al., 2005). Physical activity is a strong predictor of normal erectile function for example (Pohjantähti-Maaroos, Palomäki, & Hartikainen, 2011). In this way, building up one's strength and exercise abilities is likely to also benefit sexual functioning.

CONCLUSION

Regular sexual activity is normal in older age. Many older people are sexually active despite the increase of sexual dysfunction with age. Notably, there is a strong link between a satisfactory sex life, good health and better quality of life. Appropriate consideration must be given to the needs of the ageing population in the planning and delivery of healthcare, and institutional and support services to help sustain their right to a sex life.

CASE CONCLUSION

For Clark and his partner Lois, several factors may be causing Clark's erectile dysfunction, and he should discuss this with his GP. There are therapeutic options available; his current medications could be changed, or he could trial medications specifically for erectile dysfunction. His anxiety can be addressed, for example, the exertion associated with sexual activity may actually be beneficial for his overall rehabilitation, and he can be reassured that he and Lois can reintroduce this gradually.

SUMMARY POINTS

- Sexuality continues to be an important aspect of life for many older adults
- Good sexual function is associated with good physical and psychological health, in a bidirectional relationship
- Sexual dysfunction for women can increase after the menopause; however, treatment options are available
- Erectile dysfunction and other male sexual dysfunction can increase with age and can be a marker of other disease such as cardiovascular disease – new-onset erectile dysfunction should prompt a medical review
- A balanced diet, regular exercise, avoiding or stopping smoking, reducing stress and getting enough sleep are all important factors for a healthy sex life

MCQs

Q.1 What is the probable cause of Clark's erectile dysfunction?
  a. Vascular disease
  b. Antihypertensive medications
  c. Anxiety/worry
  d. All the above

Q.2 Which of the following is a therapeutic option for post-menopausal vaginal dryness?
  a. St John's Wort
  b. Oestrogen cream
  c. Showering more often
  d. Steroids

REFERENCES

Amin, S. H., Kuhle, C. L., & Fitzpatrick, L. A. (2003). Comprehensive evaluation of the older woman. *Mayo Clinic Proceedings, 78*(9), 1157–1185.

Bacon, C. G., Mittleman, M. A., Kawachi, I., Giovannucci, E., Glasser, D. B., & Rimm, E. B. (2003). Sexual function in men older than 50 years of age: results from the health professionals follow-up study. *Annals of Internal Medicine.,139*(3), 161–168.

Beckman, N., Waern, M., Östling, S., Sundh, V., & Skoog, I. (2014). Determinants of sexual activity in four birth cohorts of Swedish 70-year-olds examined 1971-2001. *Journal of Sexual Medicine, 11*(2), 401–410.

Belardinelli, R., Lacalaprice, F., Faccenda, E., Purcaro, A., & Perna, G. (2005). Effects of short-term moderate exercise training on sexual function in male patients with chronic stable heart failure. *International Journal of Cardiology, 101*(1), 83–90.

Billups, K. L. (2005). Erectile dysfunction as a marker for vascular disease. *Current Urology Reports, 6*(6), 439–444.

Black, B., Muralee, S., & Tampi, R. R. (2005). Inappropriate sexual behaviors in dementia. *Journal of Geriatric Psychiatry and Neurology, 18*(3), 155–162.

Bord, S. (2007). Grandma's still got it: sex persists into the 80s. *ABC News*. Retrieved from: http://abcnews.go.com/Health/ActiveAging/story?id=3511604&page=1.

Davies, S.C. (2015). Annual Report of the Chief Medical Officer 2015. Retrieved from: https://assets.publishing.service.gov.uk/government/uploads/system/uploads/attachment_data/file/654806/CMO_baby_boomers_annual_report_2015.pdf [Accessed: 31 July 2019].

Flynn, T. -J., & Gow, A. J. (2015). Examining associations between sexual behaviours and quality of life in older adults. *Age and Ageing, 44*, 823–828.

Freak-Poli, R., Kirkman, M., De Castro Lima, G., Direk, N., Franco, O. H., & Tiemeier, H. (2017). Sexual activity and physical tenderness in older adults: cross-sectional prevalence and associated characteristics. *Journal of Sexual Medicine, 14*(7), 918–927.

Goldsen, K. F. (2018). Shifting social context in the lives of LGBTQ older adults. *Public Policy & Aging Report, 28*(1), 24–28.

Gott, C. M. (2001). Sexual activity and risk-taking in later life. *Health & Social Care in the Community, 9*(2), 72–78.

Holdsworth, K., & McCabe, M. (2018). The impact of younger-onset dementia on relationships, intimacy, and sexuality in midlife couples: a systematic review. *International Psychogeriatrics, 30*(1), 15–29.

Huang, A. J., Luft, J., Grady, D., & Kuppermann, M. (2009). The day-to-day impact of urogenital aging: perspectives from racially/ethnically diverse women. *Journal of General Internal Medicine, 25*(1), 45–51.

Knochel, K. A., Croghan, C. F., Moone, R. P., & Quam, J. K. (2012). Training, geography, and provision of aging services to lesbian, gay, bisexual, and transgender older adults. *Journal of Gerontological Social Work, 55*(5), 426–443.

Lee, D. M., Nazroo, J., O'Connor, D. B., Blake, M., & Pendleton, N. (2016). Sexual health and well-being among older men and women in England: findings from the English Longitudinal Study of Ageing. *Archives of Sexual Behavior, 45*(1), 133–144.

Levine, G. N., Steinke, E. E., Bakaeen, F. G., Bozkurt, B., Cheitlin, M. D., Conti, J. B., …, & Stewart, W. J. (2012). Sexual activity and cardiovascular disease: a scientific statement from the American Heart Association. *Circulation, 125*(8), 1058–1072.

Lindau, S. T., Dale, W., Feldmeth, G., Gavrilova, N., Langa, K. M., Makelarski, J. A., & Wroblewski, K. (2018). Sexuality and cognitive status: a U.S. nationally representative study of home-dwelling older adults. *Journal of the American Geriatrics Society, 66*(10), 1902–1910.

Montorsi, F., Adaikan, G., Becher, E., Giuliano, F., Khoury, S., Lue, T. F., …, & Wasserman, M. (2010). Summary of the recommendations on sexual dysfunctions in men. *Journal of Sexual Medicine, 7*(11), 3572–3588.

Ni Lochlainn, M., & Kenny, R. A. (2013). Sexual activity and aging. *Journal of the American Medical Directors Association, 14*(8), 565–572.

Orr, J., McGarrigle, C.A., & Kenny, R.A. (2017). Sexual activity in the over 50s population in Ireland. Retrieved from: https://tilda.tcd.ie/publications/reports/pdf/Report_SexualActivity.pdf.

Pohjantähti-Maaroos, H., Palomäki, A., & Hartikainen, J. (2011). Erectile dysfunction, physical activity and metabolic syndrome: differences in markers of atherosclerosis. *BMC Cardiovascular Disorders, 11*, 36.

Seftel, A. D. (2003). Erectile dysfunction in the elderly: epidemiology, etiology and approaches to treatment. *Journal of Urology, 169*(6), 1999–2007.

Sex life linked to elderly health. (2010). Retrieved from: http://www.nhs.uk/news/2010/03March/Pages/sexual-health-general-health-elderly.aspx.

Sexed up seniors do it more than you'd think. (2007). Retrieved from: https://www.nbcnews.com/healthmain/sexed-seniors-do-it-more-youd-think-1C9468751.

Speroff, L., & Fritz, M. A. (2005). *Clinical gynecologic endocrinology and infertility*. Philadelphia: Lippincott Williams & Wilkins. Retrieved from: http://stella.catalogue.tcd.ie/iii/encore/record/C__Rb12355457__SClinical+gynecologic+endocrinology+and+infertility__P0%2C1__Orightresult__X5;jsessionid=972CD5F9D080DB4F8E55EE45C6C68747?lang=eng&suite=cobalt.

Stubbs, B. (2011). Displays of inappropriate sexual behaviour by patients with progressive cognitive impairment: the forgotten form of challenging behaviour? *Journal of Psychiatric and Mental Health Nursing, 18*(7), 602–607.

Štulhofer, A., Hinchliff, S., Jurin, T., Hald, G. M., & Træen, B. (2018). Successful aging and changes in sexual interest and enjoyment among older european men and women. *Journal of Sexual Medicine, 15*(10), 1393–1402.

Waite, L. J., Iveniuk, J., Laumann, E. O., & McClintock, M. K. (2017). Sexuality in older couples: individual and dyadic characteristics. *Archives of Sexual Behavior, 46*(2), 605–618.

Waterman, E. (2012). Reactions of college students to the sexuality of older people. *Journal of Student Research, 2*, 46–50.

Westwood, S. (2019). *Ageing, diversity and equality: social justice perspectives*. Retrieved from: www.routledge.com/series/SE0511.

Wright, H., & Jenks, R. A. (2016). Sex on the brain! Associations between sexual activity and cognitive function in older age. *Age and Ageing, 45*(2), 313–317.

Yafi, F. A., Jenkins, L., Albersen, M., Corona, G., Isidori, A. M., Goldfarb, S., …, & Hellstrom, W. J. G. (2017). Erectile dysfunction. *Nature Review Disease Primers, 2*, 16003.

FURTHER READING

American Council on Exercise on METs: https://www.acefitness.org/education-and-resources/professional/expert-articles/6434/5-things-to-know-about-metabolic-equivalents.

British Heart Foundation advice on relationships and sex in the context of heart disease: https://www.bhf.org.uk/information-support/support/practical-support/sex-and-heart-conditions.

What happens to your penis as you age? https://metro.co.uk/2019/06/15/happens-penis-age-9967741/.

37

Optimising Pharmacotherapy

Donal Fitzpatrick & Paul Gallagher

LEARNING OBJECTIVES

- Describe how drugs work differently in older adults and how this influences prescribing decisions
- Explain what polypharmacy is and how drugs and drug interactions impact on mobility, cognition, functional status and rehabilitation
- Explain the value of deprescribing, reducing medication burden and medication reconciliation
- Describe the importance of putting the patient at the centre of medication management and using shared decision making in all prescribing decisions

CASE

Agatha is an 85-year-old woman with a history of gout, hypertension, type 2 diabetes and epilepsy. She fell at home and sustained a hip fracture. She is now day 7 postop and has been transferred for off-site rehabilitation. She reported frequent episodes of dizziness occurring in the morning shortly after getting out of bed and reported a similar episode causing the fall leading to her hip fracture. She is a widow who lives alone in a two-storey house and was independently mobile without any aid and did her own shopping and cooking.

List of medications, day 7 postop:

Bendroflumethiazide 2.5 mg once daily

Lisinopril 100 mg once daily

Atorvastatin 10 mg at night

Alprazolam 0.5 mg at night

Oxybutynin 10 mg once daily

Phenytoin 100 mg once daily

Added during her admission

Insulin glargine 10 units at night

Tramadol 50 mg three times daily

Ibuprofen 400 mg three times daily as needed

Questions to Consider

Which medications are likely to have contributed to her fall?

What potential drug interactions is the patient exposed to?

Which drugs would you stop (deprescribe)?

What medications would you consider starting?

Which medications may potentially be difficult for the patient to administer?

INTRODUCTION

Modern medicine provides more medications and treatment options for patients than ever before. This can have enormous benefits in prolonging and improving quality of life. Older adults are the largest per capita consumers of prescription and over-the counter drugs in most developed nations (Health and Social Care Information Centre, 2015; Qato et al., 2008). Many older people have multiple health conditions and hence take multiple medications, referred to as polypharmacy. Whilst many of these medications are necessary, they do carry the

risk of serious adverse effects. Frail older adults with polypharmacy are at the highest risk of these effects. Adverse drug events (ADEs) cause an estimated 6.5% of unplanned hospital admissions in the United Kingdom, accounting for 4% of hospital bed capacity (Pirmohamed et al., 2004).

Many older people requiring rehabilitation do so because of impairments acquired as the result of falls due to polypharmacy. This may not have been adequately addressed before they start rehabilitation, so needs to be considered as part of their management. Gait (the way a person walks) and cognitive disorders are highly associated with inappropriate polypharmacy. Some classes of medications deserve particular caution in the frail older person. These include certain antidepressants, opioids, sleeping tablets and medications with anticholinergic side effects (Ambrose, Paul, & Hausdorff, 2013; Clegg & Young, 2011; Langeard et al., 2016). There are also age-related changes in how medications affect the body (see Box 37.1 for more detail).

Older adults in rehabilitation settings are especially likely to have multiple health conditions and be prescribed multiple medications. A US study found that 39.2% were taking more than 10 medications (Runganga, Peel, & Hubbard, 2014). Careful review of an older person's medications is essential to preserving and maximising mobility, cognition and functional ability.

> *"A significant proportion of patients require rehabilitation because of adverse drug events related to inappropriate polypharmacy"*

INAPPROPRIATE PRESCRIBING AND POLYPHARMACY

Polypharmacy can be appropriate or inappropriate. Inappropriate polypharmacy refers to a patient being prescribed more medications than clinically necessary, putting the individual at risk of harm, through ADEs and drug interactions. The more medications a person takes, the greater the potential

BOX 37.1   Age-Related Changes in Drug Pharmacology

Age-related changes mean drugs can have very different effects in older adults even at much lower doses than in young and middle-aged adults. The way a drug moves through the body, i.e. is absorbed, distributed, metabolised and excreted, is referred to as pharmacokinetics. Pharmacodynamics refers to the physiologic effect of the drug including both therapeutic and adverse effects. Table 37.1 shows how these processes change with age.

Older people have proportionately higher levels of body fat and lower levels of muscle and bone (lean body mass). This can lead to delayed excretion of fat-soluble drugs, such as morphine, benzodiazepines and antipsychotics, and higher concentrations of water-soluble drugs, such as lithium, digoxin and gentamycin. In older patients, drugs should often be started at a low dose and titrated up cautiously: 'Start low, go slow'.

The liver and kidney are the two most important organs in metabolising and excreting drugs from the body. Most medications are excreted through the kidneys. In older adults, it is essential to be aware of kidney function and to adjust dosages as needed, e.g. metformin, dabigatran, apixaban, digoxin and alendronate. Some drugs should be avoided altogether in patients with severely impaired kidney function and prescribers should refer to standard formularies for guidance.

Similarly, older patients have reduced liver volume with a consequent decline in liver metabolism and clearance of drugs, such as propranolol and theophylline. Essential to drug metabolism in the liver is a group of proteins called the cytochrome p450 system (CYP450). Many drugs are broken down to inactive forms by CYP450, and many of the most common drug interactions are mediated by this system. Drugs such as clarithromycin and amiodarone inhibit the activity of CYP450 leading to accumulation of other drugs. Other drugs such as phenytoin and carbamazepine promote CYP450 leading to increased drug breakdown. For example, clarithromycin may impede the breakdown of warfarin (an anticlotting medication) thus increasing the risk of serious bleeding.

TABLE 37.1   Age-related changes in pharmacokinetics and pharmacodynamics.

PHARMACOKINETICS		
Pharmacokinetic Change	**Consequence**	**Examples of Drugs Affected**
Proportionately higher level of total body fat	Slower elimination of fat-soluble drugs	Morphine, benzodiazepines, antipsychotics and amitriptyline
Proportionately reduced lean body mass	Higher serum concentration of water-soluble drugs	Lithium, theophylline and gentamycin
Low albumin levels in acute and chronic disease	Higher proportion of drug unbound to albumin (active)	Benzodiazepines, antipsychotics, non-steroidal anti-inflammatory drugs (NSAIDs), warfarin and phenytoin
Reduced kidney function	Higher serum concentrations of drugs excreted by the kidney	Direct oral anticoagulants, lithium, paracetamol, metformin, allopurinol
Reduced liver function	Higher concentrations of drugs metabolised by the liver	Propranolol and theophylline
PHARMACODYNAMICS		
Drug	**Influence of Age on Effect of Drug**	**Potential Clinical Response**
Morphine	↑	Excessive sedation, confusion, constipation, respiratory depression
Dabigatran Warfarin Apixaban	↑	↑ Bleeding risk
Angiotensin-receptor blocker, e.g. enalapril	↑	Hypotension (↑ acute antihypertensive effect)
Frusemide	↓	↓ Diuretic effect and size of peak of diuretic response
Benzodiazepines	↑	Excessive sedation, confusion, postural sway, falls
Levodopa	↑	Dyskinesia, confusion, hallucinations

↑: Drug has more potent effect in older adults; ↓: reduced potency of drug in older adults.

for harmful drug interactions. People taking two concurrent medications have a 13% risk of an ADE which rises to 38% for four medications and 82% for greater than seven medications (Runganga et al., 2014). Older people are also more likely to have multiple chronic disorders that may be worsened by the drug or affect drug response. Approximately 10%–20% of hospital admissions of older patients are directly related to the adverse effects of inappropriately prescribed drugs (Gallagher & O'Mahony, 2008; Hamilton et al., 2011).

Inappropriate prescribing refers to the use of a drug where the risk of an adverse outcome outweighs the potential for clinical benefit. This includes overuse (no clinical indication,

TABLE 37.2	**Polypharmacy in older patients: clinical associations.**
1.	↑ Risk of adverse drug events including drug-drug and drug-disease interactions
2.	↑ Likelihood of inappropriate prescribing including use of drugs without clear clinical indication
3.	↑ Likelihood of prescribing cascades, i.e. where a drug is prescribed to treat a symptom attributable to an adverse effect of another drug
4.	↑ Incidence of geriatric syndromes, i.e. cognitive and functional decline, weight loss and falls
5.	↑ Risk of non-compliance and poor adherence with medication regimen
6.	↑ Healthcare costs (drug costs and resource utilisation to investigate and manage adverse outcomes)

duplication or excessive duration), misuse (increased risk of ADE including drug-drug and drug-disease interactions) and underuse of medications (omission). Polypharmacy is the principal risk for inappropriate prescribing (Maher, Hanlon, & Hajjar, 2014). Older patients attending multiple doctors and multiple pharmacies are at high risk (Frank et al., 2001). Polypharmacy and inappropriate prescribing are associated with unnecessary drug use and prescribing cascades (where a drug is prescribed to treat an adverse effect of another drug), ADE's and wasted healthcare resources (see Table 37.2).

It is important to remember that many medications are essential to older patients in rehabilitation programmes, for treating the underlying illnesses leading to functional impairment and to aid the rehabilitation process. For example, ACE (angiotensin-converting enzyme) inhibitors improve exercise tolerance in patients with heart failure (Hutcheon et al., 2002), inhalers can improve exercise tolerance in patients with COPD (chronic obstructive pulmonary disease) and adequate analgesia (pain medication) facilitates mobility in those with pain. Antidepressants can improve symptoms of low mood, apathy, poor concentration and poor appetite, thus enabling patients with depression to engage in rehabilitation.

MEDICATION RECONCILIATION

Older adults engaging in inpatient rehabilitation will have undergone multiple transitions of care, e.g. from home to the acute hospital, transitions within the hospital and from the acute hospital to a rehab facility. Each of these transitions represents an opportunity for medication errors to occur, e.g. drug omission or transcription errors pertaining to drug name, dose, duration and frequency (Wheeler et al., 2018). This is all the more likely in older patients who may be on many different medications and are not able to reliably discuss their medication regimens. Meticulous medication reconciliation is vital to eliminate these errors. Medication reconciliation, usually undertaken by a clinical pharmacist, is the process of creating and maintaining the most up-to-date and accurate medication list for a patient, checking for all potential discrepancies.

MEDICATION ADMINISTRATION AND ADHERENCE

Medication administration can be challenging for older people. They may have physical impairments such as poor vision and impaired manual dexterity. Cognitive impairment can make it difficult for older people to organise, understand and remember their medications.

Medication non-adherence is highly prevalent in the older population (approximately 40%; Mongkhon & Kongkaew, 2017). Blister packs (see Fig. 37.1) and assistance from carers can overcome some of these difficulties and improve adherence (Conn et al., 2015). The simplest medication regimen should be chosen wherever possible, e.g. once daily rather than four times daily administration, if possible.

Oropharyngeal dysphagia refers to impaired swallowing usually due to neurological disease such as stroke, dementia and Parkinson's disease. It is very common in older adults and is associated with pneumonia, malnutrition and weight loss (Baijens et al., 2016). Liquid or topical formulations may be available instead of tablets. It should not be assumed that all tablets can be crushed and given with a soft food such as yogurt. This is particularly relevant to extended release capsules which are not appropriate to crush. These tablets are designed to deliver the drug slowly to the bloodstream. If crushed, the drug will not be released slowly, may not be absorbed and can cause significant adverse effects (Royal Pharmaceutical Society, 2011). Advice should be sought from speech and language therapists and pharmacists in optimising medicine formulations in patients with dysphagia. If oral medications are particularly burdensome for a patient to take, a pragmatic approach should be adopted, and non-essential drugs deprescribed.

MEDICATIONS AND COMMON CONDITIONS SEEN IN OLDER REHABILITATING ADULTS

Falls, Mobility and Fractures

Polypharmacy is associated with falls in older people, with culprit medications being well recognised (see Table 37.3) (Ambrose et al., 2013; Fried et al., 2014). Antihypertensive (blood pressure lowering) medications frequently cause significant drops in blood pressure on standing (postural hypotension) leading to dizziness, falls and syncope (temporary loss of consciousness). Other drugs can cause sedation and cognitive impairment, increasing falls risk.

As people age, bone mineral density reduces. Osteoporosis is highly prevalent in older people and is associated with a much higher incidence of fractures after relatively low impact trauma (Compston et al., 2017). Medications, including corticosteroids, antiepileptic drugs, selective serotonin receptor inhibitors and proton pump inhibitors, can accelerate osteoporosis.

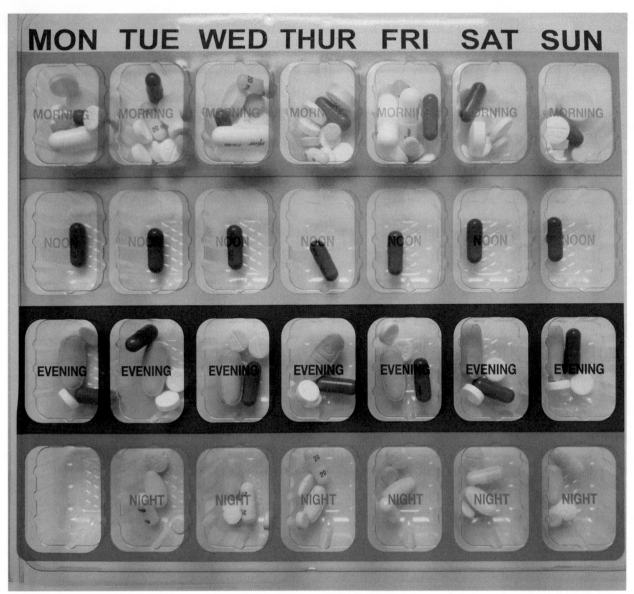

FIG. 37.1   Blister packed medications.

Medications, including vitamin D, bisphosphonates, denosumab and teriparatide, are effective treatments for osteoporosis. This is often neglected in the acute setting, but the rehabilitation team has the opportunity to review treatment options including non-pharmacological interventions to reduce the risk of further fractures.

Cognitive Impairment

Cognitive impairment can be acute and transient in the case of delirium, or chronic and progressive in the case of dementia. Cognition influences an individual's ability to engage with the rehabilitation team and to retain skills learned from one rehab session to the next ('carry over'). Multiple medications can impair cognition (see Table 37.3).

Anticholinergic drugs, which block acetylcholine, a neurotransmitter in the brain, should be avoided if possible (Fox et al., 2011). These drugs include common medications for urinary incontinence, antihistamines and antidepressants. Benzodiazepines and antipsychotics also cause cognitive impairment and should be avoided if possible (Drake, Nixon, & Crew, 1998). These drugs, especially benzodiazepines, often need to be weaned very gradually to avoid withdrawal reactions.

Incontinence

Incontinence may be urinary, faecal or both, and has a major impact on quality of life and independence. Many drugs are implicated in both urinary and faecal incontinence (see Chapter 35 Bladder and Bowel Problems) and, again, polypharmacy is a significant risk factor (Kashyap, Tu, & Tannenbaum, 2013). Several drugs interfere with bladder and bladder outlet muscular tone, e.g. alpha-adrenergic blockers and anticholinergics. Drugs which impair bladder contractility or increase bladder outlet tone are more likely to cause urinary retention in men because of prostate enlargement. Drugs such as benzodiazepines and opioids cause incontinence

TABLE 37.3 Potentially harmful medications in older patients engaged in rehabilitation.

Medication Class	Examples	Effect
Antipsychotics	*Typical:* Haloperidol, chlorpromazine, *Atypical:* quetiapine, risperidone, olanzapine	• Impaired mobility and balance, gait disorders, parkinsonism (tremor, rigidity, bradykinesia), dystonia and akathisia (more commonly with typical than atypical antipsychotics). • Postural hypotension • Sedation and cognitive impairment. • Weight gain • Anticholinergic side effects (listed below) • Increased risk of incontinence
Benzodiazepines, Z-drugs	Alprazolam, diazepam, flurazepam, zopiclone, zolpidem	• Sedation and cognitive impairment • Mobility and balance impairment with increased falls risk • Drug dependence • Impaired consciousness and respiratory depression in toxicity • Increased risk of incontinence
Opioids	Morphine, oxycodone, tramadol, codeine, buprenorphine, fentanyl	• Sedation, impaired cognition and hallucinations • Nausea, vomiting, constipation • Mobility and balance impairment with increased falls risk • Respiratory depression in toxicity • Drug dependence • Postural hypotension • Increased risk of incontinence
Vasodilators	Calcium-channel blockers, e.g. amlodipine, nitrates, e.g. isosorbide mononitrate, alpha blockers, e.g. doxazosin, tamsulosin	• Postural hypotension, generalised lethargy, increased falls risk
Diuretics	Furosemide, bendroflumethiazide, bumetanide	• Postural hypotension, dehydration, sodium and electrolyte disorders • Urinary incontinence
Corticosteroids	Prednisolone	• Proximal myopathy • Osteoporosis
Alpha-adrenergic antagonists	Doxazosin	• Reduces bladder outflow resistance (Ruby et al., 2010). Can increase the risk of incontinence fivefold • Potent vasodilator causing postural hypotension and falls
Tricyclic antidepressants	Amitriptyline, trimipramine, nortriptyline	**Anticholinergic side effects** • Cognitive impairment: associated with both delirium and dementia
Antipsychotics	Olanzapine, clozapine, trifluoperazine	• Dry mouth
Bladder antispasmodics	Oxybutynin	• Balance impairment and falls • Drowsiness
Antihistamines	Diphenhydramine, chlorpheniramine	• Blurred vision • Urinary retention and overflow incontinence Constipation

indirectly, through sedation and impaired mobility. Drugs causing diarrhoea (laxatives, metformin, antibiotics) and constipation (oral iron supplements, opioids, anticholinergics) can cause faecal incontinence (Drake et al., 1998).

DEPRESCRIBING

There are many guidelines detailing when to initiate drug treatments. However, identifying inappropriate polypharmacy and stopping potentially inappropriate medications can make a big difference to the life of an older person with frailty. There are several useful tools for systematically examining patients' medication regimens, such as the Beers criteria (American Geriatrics Society, 2019), and STOPP (Screening Tool of Older Persons' Prescriptions)/START (Screening Tool to Alert doctors to Right Treatment) (O'Mahony et al., 2015). STOPP contains recommendations relating to the most common, potentially harmful instances of inappropriate prescribing. START comprises recommendations identifying common instances of prescribing omission. For patients with frailty and reduced life expectancy, often encountered in the rehab setting, the STOPPFrail criteria are specifically focussed on this group (Lavan et al., 2017).

EDUCATION AND COMMUNICATION

Teaching people to overcome physical limitations is a key part of rehabilitation for older people. Empowering older adults and their carers by educating them about their medications should be a part of this teaching process. Medication education prevents drug errors and improves adherence (Esposito, 1995). It is essential that details of medication changes are communicated properly between transitions in care and, especially to the patient's primary care provider on discharge.

SUMMARY POINTS

- Shared decision making should be used when prescribing/deprescribing
- All medications must have a clear purpose to avoid inappropriate polypharmacy – otherwise consider stopping the medication; tools such as STOPP/START criteria can be used
- Medications should be started at the smallest dose and titrated up slowly according to response

- The simplest dosing regimen and the most appropriate formulation should be used, e.g. liquid in patients with swallowing difficulties
- Medication reconciliation should be performed with any transition in care
- Beware of medications that contribute to falls and cognitive impairment in older adults

ANSWERS TO CASE-BASED QUESTIONS

Which Medications Contributed to Her Fall?

Bendroflumethiazide and lisinopril are antihypertensive medications that can cause postural drops in blood pressure leading to falls and syncope. Bendroflumethiazide is a thiazide diuretic, associated with hyponatremia (low sodium levels) and hypokalaemia (low potassium levels), which also impair balance. Blood pressure should be checked to avoid excessive dosages. Kidney function and serum electrolyte levels should be monitored.

Alprazolam is a benzodiazepine which causes falls by impairing balance and causing sedation.

Oxybutynin is an anticholinergic drug used for urinary urgency. It causes cognitive impairment and poor balance which makes falls more likely. Phenytoin also has sedative side effects increasing falls risk.

What Potential Drug Interactions Is She Exposed to?

With this number of drugs, there is significant potential for drug interactions and consequent adverse events. Phenytoin is a cytochrome P450 inducer which can reduce the level of metformin, alprazolam, tramadol, atorvastatin and oxybutynin. The combination of an ACE inhibitor (lisinopril) and an nonsteroidal anti-inflammatory drug (NSAID) places an older patient at very high risk for acute kidney injury. Alprazolam and tramadol can synergistically increase sedation levels.

Which Drugs Would You Stop (Deprescribe)?

Oxybutynin, tramadol and alprazolam should be stopped because of the harmful effects of these drugs on balance and cognition. Alprazolam should be weaned slowly to avoid withdrawal symptoms, especially if she has been on the drug for a long time. Ibuprofen is an NSAID and likely to cause significant toxicity in older adults, renal impairment and increased risk of cardiovascular events. Alternative analgesics should be used. The thiazide diuretic should be stopped because it causes postural hypotension (the cause of her fall), low sodium levels and will exacerbate her gout. The lisinopril may also need to be stopped.

What Medications Would You Consider Starting?

The patient has had an osteoporotic fracture. DEXA scan is not necessary; the low-impact fracture is much more convincing evidence of the need for osteoporosis treatment. Vitamin D supplementation and a bone antiresorptive such as a bisphosphonate or denosumab (a six-monthly subcutaneous injection) will reduce the risk of further fractures, provided there are no contraindications.

Which Medications May Potentially Be Difficult for the Patient to Administer?

This lady lives alone. Insulin can be difficult for older patients to administer to themselves. In this case, another oral antidiabetic drug, such as metformin, would be preferable to discharging her home on insulin. However, in some cases, adequate blood sugar control cannot be achieved without insulin.

Final Prescription on Discharge

Atorvastatin 10 mg at night
Denosumab 60 mg subcutaneous injection every 6 months
Calcium/vitamin D3 (1 g/800 units) one tablet daily
Metformin 1 g twice daily
Paracetamol 1 g three times daily or as needed for pain

MCQs

Q.1 Which of the following medications can potentially worsen cognitive impairment in an older adult?
   a. Benzodiazepines
   b. Antihistamines
   c. Opioids
   d. Tricyclic antidepressants
   e. All of the above

Q.2 Which one of the following medications does not increase the risk of falls?
   a. Thiazide diuretic
   b. Apixaban (direct oral anticoagulant)
   c. Atypical antipsychotics
   d. Benzodiazepines
   e. Oxybutynin (anticholinergic for urinary urge incontinence)

REFERENCES

Ambrose, A. F., Paul, G., & Hausdorff, J. M. (2013). Risk factors for falls among older adults: a review of the literature. *Maturitas*, *75*(1), 51–61.

American Geriatrics Society. (2019). American Geriatrics Society 2019 Updated AGS Beers Criteria® for potentially inappropriate medication use in older adults. *Journal of the American Geriatrics Society*, *67*, 674–694.

Baijens, L. W., Clavé, P., Cras, P., et al. (2016). European Society for Swallowing Disorders - European Union Geriatric Medicine Society white paper: oropharyngeal dysphagia as a geriatric syndrome. *Clinical Interventions in Aging*, *11*, 1403–1428.

Clegg, A., & Young, J. B. (2011). Which medications to avoid in people at risk of delirium: a systematic review. *Age and Ageing*, *40*(1), 23–29.

Compston, J., Cooper, A., Cooper, C., et al. (2017). UK clinical guideline for the prevention and treatment of osteoporosis. *Archives of Osteoporosis*, *12*(1), 43.

Conn, V. S., Ruppar, T. M., Chan, K. C., Dunbar-Jacob, J., Pepper, G. A., & De Geest, S. (2015). Packaging interventions to increase medication adherence: systematic review and meta-analysis. *Current Medical Research and Opinion*, *31*(1), 145–160.

Drake, M. J., Nixon, P. M., & Crew, J. P. (1998). Drug-induced bladder and urinary disorders. *Drug Safety*, *19*(1), 45–55.

Esposito, L. (1995). The effects of medication education on adherence to medication regimens in an elderly population. *Journal of Advanced Nursing*, *21*(5), 935–943.

Fox, C., Richardson, K., Maidment, I. D., et al. (2011). Anticholinergic medication use and cognitive impairment in the older population: the Medical Research Council Cognitive Function and Ageing Study. *Journal of the American Geriatrics Society*, *59*(8), 1477–1483.

Frank, C., Godwin, M., Verma, S., Kelly, A., Birenbaum, A., Seguin, R., & Anderson, J. (2001). What drugs are our frail elderly patients taking? Do drugs they take or fail to take put them at increased risk of interactions and inappropriate medication use? *Canadian Family Physician*, *47*, 1198–1204.

Fried, T. R., O'Leary, J., Towle, V., Goldstein, M. K., Trentalange, M., & Martin, D. K. (2014). Health outcomes associated with polypharmacy in community-dwelling older adults: a systematic review. *Journal of the American Geriatrics Society*, *62*(12), 2261–2272.

Gallagher, P., & O'Mahony, D. (2008). STOPP (Screening Tool of Older Persons' potentially inappropriate Prescriptions): application to acutely ill elderly patients and comparison with Beers' criteria. *Age and Ageing*, *37*(6), 673–679.

Hamilton, H., Gallagher, P., Ryan, C., Byrne, S., & O'Mahony, D. (2011). Potentially inappropriate medications defined by STOPP criteria and the risk of adverse drug events in older hospitalized patients. *Archives of Internal Medicine*, *171*(11), 1013–1019.

Health and Social Care Information Centre. (2015). Prescriptions dispensed in the community - statistics for England, 2004-2014 - NHS Digital. Retrieved from: https://digital.nhs.uk/data-and-information/publications/statistical/prescriptions-dispensed-in-the-community/prescriptions-dispensed-in-the-community-statistics-for-england-2004-2014 (Accessed 2 April 2019).

Hutcheon, S. D., Gillespie, N. D., Crombie, I. K., Struthers, A. D., & McMurdo, M. E. T. (2002). Perindopril improves six minute walking distance in older patients with left ventricular systolic dysfunction: a randomised double blind placebo controlled trial. *Heart*, *88*(4), 373–377.

Kashyap, M., Tu, L. M., & Tannenbaum, C. (2013). Prevalence of commonly prescribed medications potentially contributing to urinary symptoms in a cohort of older patients seeking care for incontinence. *BMC Geriatrics*, *13*, 57.

Langeard, A., Pothier, K., Morello, R., et al. (2016). Polypharmacy cut-off for gait and cognitive impairments. *Frontiers in Pharmacology*, *7*, 296.

Lavan, A. H., Gallagher, P., Parsons, C., & O'Mahony, D. (2017). STOPPFrail (Screening Tool of Older Persons Prescriptions in Frail adults with limited life expectancy): consensus validation. *Age and Ageing*, *46*(4), 600–607.

Maher, R. L., Hanlon, J., & Hajjar, E. R. (2014). Clinical consequences of polypharmacy in elderly. *Expert Opinion on Drug Safety*, *13*(1), 57–65.

Mongkhon, P., & Kongkaew, C. (2017). Medication non-adherence identified at home: a systematic review and meta-analysis. *Quality in Primary Care*, *25*(2).

O'Mahony, D., O'Sullivan, D., Byrne, S., O'Connor, M. N., Ryan, C., & Gallagher, P. (2015). STOPP/START criteria for potentially inappropriate prescribing in older people: version 2. *Age and Ageing*, *44*(2), 213–218.

Pirmohamed, M., James, S., Meakin, S., et al. (2004). Adverse drug reactions as cause of admission to hospital: prospective analysis of 18 820 patients. *BMJ*, *329*(7456), 15–19.

Qato, D. M., Alexander, G. G., Conti, R. M., Johnson, M., Schumm, P., & Lindau, S. T. (2008). Use of prescription and over-the-counter medications and dietary supplements among older adults in the United States. *JAMA*, *300*(24), 2867.

Royal Pharmaceutical Society. (2011). Pharmaceutical issues when crushing, opening or splitting oral dosage forms. Retrieved from: https://www.rpharms.com/Portals/0/RPS%20document%20library/Open%20access/Support/toolkit/pharmaceuticalissuesdosageforms-%282%29.pdf (Accessed 24 August 2019).

Ruby, C. M., Hanlon, J. T., Boudreau, R. M., Newman, A. B., Simonsick, E. M., Shorr, R. I., Bauer, D. C., & Resnick, N. M. (2010). The effect of medication use on urinary incontinence in community-dwelling elderly women. *Journal of the American Geriatrics Society, 58*(9), 1715–1720.

Runganga, M., Peel, N. M., & Hubbard, R. E. (2014). Multiple medication use in older patients in post-acute transitional care: a prospective cohort study. *Clinical Interventions in Aging, 9*, 1453–1462.

Wheeler, A. J., Scahill, S., Hopcroft, D., & Stapleton, H. (2018). Reducing medication errors at transitions of care is everyone's business. *Australian Prescriber, 41*(3), 73.

38

Osteoporosis and Bone Health

Louise Statham, Gavin Snelson & Terry Aspray

LEARNING OBJECTIVES

- Describe the structure of normal bone and the changes seen in osteoporosis
- List common treatments for osteoporosis and their side effect profile
- Explain the benefits and harms of calcium and vitamin D supplements

CASE

Lisa is a 77-year-old female who presented with acute back pain; an x-ray confirms new vertebral fractures (VFs) at T4 and T9. Osteoporosis had previously been diagnosed following a wrist fracture 2 years before, when she had been seen by her local Fracture Liaison Service (FLS) and she had been treated with alendronic acid 70 mg tablets weekly. However, on questioning it became evident that she had stopped taking this prescription soon after it was initiated. Reasons for non-adherence were explored; adverse effects of nausea and severe heartburn were identified. A shared decision-making approach was used with the patient and her prescription was changed to annual intravenous zoledronic acid infusions. These were scheduled for 3 years, in the first instance, provided she experiences no problems with the medication prior to this time. Her back pain was managed with pain medication and exercises recommended by a physiotherapist.

INTRODUCTION

Bone

Bone is a dynamic tissue composed of a protein matrix of *osteoid*, which is mineralised by calcium hydroxyapatite to increase its strength, while remaining relatively lightweight. Two sorts of bone exist. Compact (or cortical) bone is dense and comprises layers of bone tissue which makes up the outer structure of long and flat bones such as the skull and the long bones, whereas cancellous (trabecular or spongy) bone is encased in cortical bone but has a much more porous network of interconnected bone tissue (called trabeculae), interspersed with blood vessels and with a large surface area, as shown diagrammatically in Fig. 38.1. The main types of bone cell (which are not all presented in the figure) comprise osteoblasts, responsible for bone formation; osteoclasts, responsible for bone resorption; and osteocytes, which are the commonest cells to be seen, offering some structural function but also now known to be important in cell signalling and coordination of bone turnover.

Bone Disorders

Osteoporosis

Osteoporosis is 'a skeletal disorder characterised by compromised **bone strength** predisposing a person to an **increased risk of fracture**' (NIH Consensus Development Panel on Osteoporosis Prevention, 2001). Under the microscope, osteoporotic bone has fewer trabeculae, with an overall reduction in trabecular bone volume and significant differences in microstructure when compared with normal bone. Bone mineral density (BMD) can be measured using dual-energy x-ray absorptiometry (DXA). This procedure, where a focused band of x-rays pass through the bone to estimate the mineral content of the tissue, has proven useful as a non-invasive way to estimate the quality of bone, as a lower BMD is associated with lower bone mineral content and osteoporosis. BMD increases from the day we are born up until around the age of 25–30 years, when we achieve our *peak bone mass*, which is higher in men than women (see Fig. 38.2). Thereafter, BMD decreases slowly until about the age of 50 years, in women, at which time there is a rather rapid decrease in BMD over 5–10 years. For men, the decrease is much more gradual.

Case Finding

Patients with a low BMD have **no symptoms whatsoever** and, while the risk of breaking bones may be increased with lower BMD, any two people with exactly the same BMD measured using DXA can have very different *fracture risk*. We therefore consider a number of other clinical risk factors in practice to help make decisions about diagnosis and treatment. Other risk factors include excessive alcohol intake, smoking cigarettes, previous low trauma fractures, body mass index, parental history of hip fracture, rheumatoid arthritis, medications and falls risk. There are also a number of conditions which are associated with an increased fracture risk, via a range of mechanisms, such as hyperthyroidism, hyperparathyroidism, type 1 diabetes, myeloma, chronic liver disease and cancer. Evidence-based assessment tools such

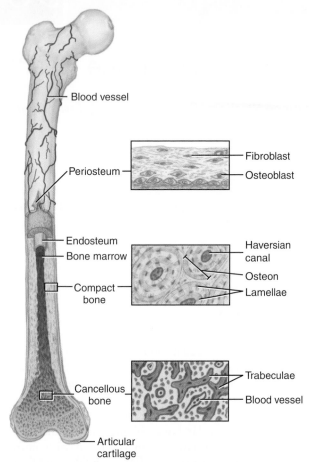

FIG. 38.1 A typical long bone, comprising mostly compact bone with cancellous bone also present, where there is a complex of trabeculae and blood vessels.

as FRAX and QFracture are useful in practice, allowing clinicians to translate the combined information given from clinical risk factors and BMD to estimate a 10-year risk of major osteoporotic fractures and hip fractures. Some element of clinical judgement is required as, for example, these tools do not take into account falls risk, spinal BMD or prescribed medications other than steroids. An important group to consider are those who sustain their first low trauma fracture, for whom FLS may be provided to evaluate their future fracture risk and advise on treatment options.

Common Misunderstandings

People can be confused by clinical terms used, including *osteopaenia*. This term is commonly applied to an appearance on routine x-rays, where the bones appear to be less mineralised. This can be seen in a local region, for example in rheumatoid arthritis, where *periarticular osteopaenia* is commonly seen. It can also be a more generalised feature possibly indicating an increased likelihood of underlying osteoporosis. However, it is most commonly used (rather unhelpfully in our opinion) as a term to represent a BMD which is low on DXA scanning (a T-score between –1.0 and –2.5) but not low enough to place it in the osteoporotic range (T-score less than –2.5). We would reiterate that there is no medical condition of *osteopaenia* and in clinical practice the consideration of fracture risk due to underlying osteoporosis is a much more useful concept. T-scores come from a statistical model which assumes that BMD is distributed *normally*. They use a normal young adult reference for BMD. Sometimes, we use Z-scores, which use the age of the patient as a reference point, and are very important in assessing BMD in children and young adults and when considering whether secondary osteoporosis is likely. Another confusing term is *osteoarthritis*, which is completely unrelated to osteoporosis, as it is a condition which affects joints, while *osteomalacia* (literally *soft bones*) is a metabolic bone condition, unrelated to osteoporosis, where the underlying protein matrix, or *osteoid,* is formed in the skeleton but there is a failure of mineralisation of the bone.

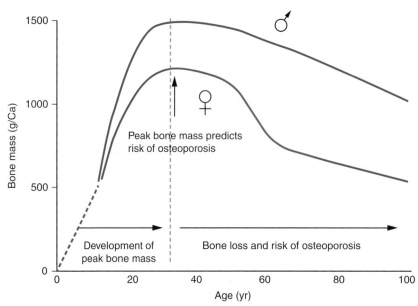

FIG. 38.2 Bone mass increases from birth to the third decade, when we achieve peak bone mass. Thereafter, there is a decrease, more rapid in women than in men.

BONE IN HEALTH AND DISEASE

Osteomalacia in Older People

Osteomalacia is associated with deformity of the bone leading to pain at specific sites, including the thigh, shoulder and pelvis as well as muscle weakness. It can be caused by a number of health issues, commonly vitamin D deficiency and less commonly dietary calcium deficiency or a combination of both. While there are other, much rarer, causes of osteomalacia, unrelated to calcium or vitamin D, they are beyond the remit of this book. The recommended nutritional intake in the UK is 700 mg of elemental calcium daily. This is relatively easily obtained from a balanced diet, even into old age. However, some people, particularly those who take little or no dairy food, may require calcium supplementation. The recommended intake for vitamin D is 400 IU (10 µg) daily, which is much more difficult to achieve from diet alone. Between May and October, virtually all of our vitamin D requirements can be met by sun exposure, as we synthesise vitamin D in our skin. However, this may not apply to many older people who get less exposure to the sun and whose skin may be less efficient at synthesising vitamin D under the influence of sunshine. Therefore, many older people will need to take supplements of vitamin D, with or without calcium, particularly in the winter and early spring months.

Bone and Muscle

Ageing is associated with a loss of muscle mass and strength. This decline starts at around 40 years of age and can be as much as 20% to 40% by age 70 years. In young adults bone responds to exercise stimulation by increasing osteogenesis (bone formation) and reducing reabsorption of bone. In people who do little physical activity, the converse happens and bone can be reabsorbed. Bones remodel over time, in response to the loading during exercise, and providing the appropriate bone strength required. Muscle mass and strength respond in a similar fashion to loading and both can be increased though progressive strength training or reduced through inactivity. In people of all ages exercise can help to maintain BMD at the hip and spine. Older people tend to have more sedentary lifestyles and so there is less stimulation for the muscles to strengthen. However, many factors can influence muscle mass and strength, which decrease with age, resulting in a condition termed *sarcopenia,* which is associated with functional consequences for older adults who are living with frailty and leading to increased falls risk due to muscle weakness and fatigue.

TREATMENT

Available Drug Therapies

Pharmacological therapy of osteoporosis affects the bone density and aims to reduce fracture risk. The mode of action of drugs generally falls into two categories: antiresorptive agents which decrease the resorption of bones (mediated by osteoclast cells) and anabolic agents which promote new bone formation (mediated by the action of osteoblasts). The choice of treatment may be influenced by the site of action of the drugs in question, specifically their effects on the balance between bone formation (anabolic effects) and bone loss/resorption (antiresorptive effects). These are summarised in Table 38.1.

It should be noted that, while medications can significantly reduce the risk of fracture, they do not eliminate that risk and there is always a chance that someone may fracture while on treatment. If this occurs, adherence and administration should be checked along with any other factors that may contribute to treatment failure. Particularly where multiple fractures on treatment occur, it may be necessary to consider alternative treatment options.

While osteoporosis has no symptoms, skeletal pain is common after a fracture and may be from other conditions such as damage or spasm in muscles and ligaments. As such, pain medications are often required following fractures or in patients with long-term back pain, after osteoporotic fractures. However, patients should be aware that osteoporosis treatment aiming to prevent fractures does not provide symptomatic pain relief, as misunderstanding around this can result in reduced adherence.

Bisphosphonates

The most commonly prescribed treatments are the bisphosphonates taken by mouth: alendronic acid and risedronate. If patients are unable to follow administration requirements (see Table 38.1), bisphosphonates given into the vein such as zoledronic acid may be considered, usually in a hospital setting. As it does not touch the gastrointestinal tract, unwanted gastrointestinal symptoms, which are common with oral bisphosphonates, are not usually seen, although transient 'flu-like' symptoms can occur. In addition, a once yearly infusion may be more convenient than taking daily, weekly or monthly tablets.

Denosumab

Denosumab is a monoclonal antibody which decreases bone resorption by a different mechanism. It is given as a six-monthly subcutaneous injection, increasing BMD and reducing the risk of vertebral and non-VFs, including hip fracture. In practice it can be given as a second-line agent if bisphosphonates are not suitable.

Other Medications

Less commonly prescribed drugs include hormone replacement therapy (HRT), raloxifene, strontium ranelate and teriparatide (see Table 38.1 for details). While HRT is licensed for the management of osteoporosis in postmenopausal women, its prescription beyond the sixth decade is not encouraged, as the balance of benefits is generally seen to be outweighed by the risks of treatment.

Adverse Effects: Hypocalcaemia, Atypical Fracture, Osteonecrosis

Any medication that reduces bone resorption can decrease blood calcium levels (hypocalcaemia), particularly when

TABLE 38.1   Characteristics of the drugs most commonly used in the treatment of osteoporosis.

DRUG	MECHANISM OF ACTION	FORMULATION & ADMINISTRATION	NOTABLE SIDE EFFECTS	NOTES
Alendronic acid	Bisphosphonates: reduce bone loss by inhibiting the cells that resorb bone (osteoclasts). They remain in the skeleton for many years	Once weekly tablets (most common)/ liquid/effervescent preparations Once daily tablets	Most commonly gastrointestinal discomfort, particularly heartburn with oral preparations Bone, joint or muscle pain (often transient), headache, eye inflammation	To facilitate absorption, tablets (and effervescent/liquid preparations) must be taken according to strict administration guidelines: first thing in the morning on an empty stomach, with a full glass of water and remaining in an upright position for at least 30 minutes after taking Gastrointestinal side effects *may* be less common with risedronate
Risedronate		Tablets: daily or weekly		
Ibandronic acid		Tablets: once monthly IV injection: three monthly		Similar oral administration requirements to above Lack of robust data to suggest that ibandronic acid reduces hip fracture
Zoledronic acid		Annual intravenous infusion, usually in a hospital setting	Low blood calcium (check vitamin D, serum calcium and kidney function before each dose) 'Flu-like' symptoms common especially with first dose Eye inflammation, possible increased risk of atrial fibrillation (unclear)	Useful when patients unable to follow administration requirements or have gastrointestinal side effects with oral bisphosphonates. Paracetamol can be advised to reduce flu-like symptoms around time of administration
Denosumab	Monoclonal antibody (RANK ligand inhibitor): reduce bone loss by inhibiting osteoclast cells that resorb bone. Not retained in the bone	Six monthly subcutaneous injection	Skin infection Low blood calcium (check vitamin D, serum calcium and kidney function before each infusion)	Can be used cautiously at lower levels of kidney function but this increases the risk of serious hypocalcaemia It is important that patients continue to take this medication once initiated, as evidence is emerging that the benefits of treatment can rapidly wear off and vertebral fractures may occur soon after stopping treatment in some patients
Strontium ranelate	Reduces bone loss through its effect on osteoclast cells, may also increase new bone formation	Daily sachet of granules to be mixed with water	Nausea, diarrhoea Increased risk of blood clots and heart attack Serious skin reactions (rare)	Administration instructions: take at night at least 2 hours after eating Cardiovascular risk must be regularly assessed during use. Withhold during periods of prolonged immobility

TABLE 38.1   Characteristics of the drugs most commonly used in the treatment of osteoporosis. (*Cont.*)

DRUG	MECHANISM OF ACTION	FORMULATION & ADMINISTRATION	NOTABLE SIDE EFFECTS	NOTES
Teriparatide	Recombinant human parathyroid hormone: stimulates bone formation through its action on bone building cells (osteoblasts) and other indirect effects	Daily subcutaneous injection for a maximum of 2 years	Dizziness, headache, joint pain High blood calcium	Antiresorptive medication should be given following the course so that benefits of bone gained can be maintained Lack of robust data to suggest teriparatide reduces hip fracture risk High cost
Raloxifene	Selective estrogen receptor modulator: mimics the positive action of oestrogen at the bone, while blocking its negative action elsewhere in the body	Daily tablet	Commonly causes menopause like symptoms including hot flushes, ankle swelling, flu-like symptoms, leg cramps. Associated with increased risk of blood clots.	May have a protective effect against breast cancer. Lack of robust data to suggest raloxifene reduces hip fracture risk
Romosuzumab	Monoclonal antibody (sclerostin inhibitor) reduces bone loss *and* increases bone formation	Subcutaneous injection		New drug awaiting approval at the time of writing

given by routes other than by mouth. Prior to treatment, serum calcium and vitamin D levels should be reviewed and any deficiency treated. Patients on these medications should also be advised how to identify symptoms associated with low serum calcium levels, such as muscle spasm, cramps or numbness or tingling of the fingers or around the mouth.

With longer term use of antiresorptive medication, there appears to be an increased risk of rare side effects such as atypical fracture and osteonecrosis of the jaw (see Fig. 38.3).

For this reason, the risks and benefits of treatments should be periodically reassessed.

Duration of Therapy

The optimal duration of treatment for bone protection is currently unknown. For oral bisphosphonates, treatment is typically reviewed at 5 years, though there is evidence for 10 years of use (Bone et al., 2004); those at high risk of fracture and particularly VF may benefit from use beyond 5 years. There is

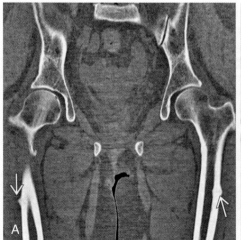
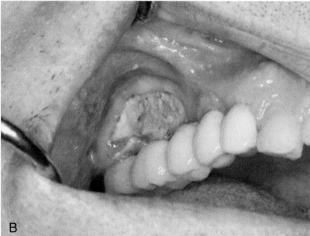

FIG. 38.3   (A) Bilateral non-traumatic subtrochanteric fractures and (B) osteonecrosis of the jaw in two separate cases, with prior exposure to bisphosphonate therapy.

also some evidence that, on stopping long-term bisphosphonates, the benefits of treatment are sustained, though one study found a slightly higher rate of VFs without pain on follow-up x-rays (Black et al., 2006). Bisphosphonates are retained in the bone for many years, and thus a residual benefit may be seen on stopping treatment. Some clinicians therefore recommend a 'drug holiday', where bisphosphonate therapy is suspended for a period of time, usually up to 2 years, to reduce the risk of atypical fracture, while remaining at a relatively reduced fracture risk. Before stopping or changing treatment, it is important to have confidence that the level of adherence has been good. When initiating a drug holiday, appropriate follow-up should be ensured as benefits of treatment are not sustained indefinitely and incorrect administration of a drug holiday without appropriate review may be associated with an increased risk of fracture. Zoledronic acid is longer acting than the oral bisphosphonates. Therefore, review and consideration of stopping treatment can typically occur after 3 years of therapy.

For denosumab therapy, drug holidays are not appropriate. Treatment with denosumab should therefore be continued indefinitely, or measures considered to try to reduce the rapid increase in bone turnover on cessation, such as use of bisphosphonates following treatment. This is still an area of emerging evidence.

Calcium and Vitamin D Supplements

Benefits

Calcium is a key constituent of bone and is important for good bone health, while vitamin D is important in facilitating the absorption of calcium. There are conflicting studies on the safety and efficacy of giving calcium and vitamin D through supplements. A small reduction in fracture risk has been shown with calcium and vitamin D supplements for patients living in nursing homes, but this effect has not been replicated in studies assessing patients in community settings. Of course, it is important to identify any untreated osteomalacia in this patient group. Even in the absence of osteomalacia, the effects of antiresorptive therapies are likely to be impaired if vitamin D deficiency is present. Vitamin D supplementation given alone does not reduce fracture risk, although there is some evidence that it may help prevent falls at commonly used maintenance doses.

Harms

Can supplementation cause harm? Suggested links between calcium supplementation and an increased risk of heart attack remain controversial. As calcium intakes are satisfactory for the majority of patients, blanket prescription of calcium supplements is not a logical stratagem. An assessment of dietary calcium intake should form part of routine patient care and, if dietary calcium intake of 700 mg per day is not possible for an individual, supplementation can be considered with an extra 500 mg of elemental calcium enough for most patients. As vitamin D deficiency is much more common, supplementation should be considered to ensure adequate levels in those at risk of osteomalacia. The routine coprescription of calcium and vitamin D with osteoporosis treatments is often unnecessary, particularly where dietary calcium intake and vitamin D status are adequate.

Rehabilitation

Physiotherapy aims to help people affected by injury such as fractures, illness or disability through exercise prescription, manual therapy, education and advice. It can also maintain health for people of all ages, helping patients to manage pain and prevent disease. Physiotherapists will tailor a combination of exercises, including those which promote range of movement such as those involved in posture, strengthening exercises that use resistance and balance exercises that involve challenge to maintain postural control. Things to consider include an individual's exercise capacity at the time of assessment and the rehabilitation goals that the patient would like to achieve. Manual therapy, including the use of hot and cold packs, taping to the skin to reinforce correct movement, bracing to restrict movement and passive stretches, may all be used as an adjunct to exercise.

Targeted rehabilitation to patients with osteoporotic fractures will be offered. For example, for patients with a wrist fracture, there will be initial immobilisation, typically for around 4 weeks. However, it is also essential that range of movement exercises are started at the elbow, shoulder and fingers, as pain allows, to optimise the range of movement around the wrist in the long term and this will continue, once the cast is removed. Once the patient is able to move through range, undertake strengthening and weight bear on the wrist, then any specific activities can be reintroduced slowly. This might include golf, cycling or racket sports.

Another particularly challenging scenario is VFs, which are often not discovered acutely (see Chapter 46 Vertebral and Lower Limb Fractures and Surgery). Physiotherapy will focus on early mobilisation and weight bearing as able with multidisciplinary team review of analgesia requirements often required. The *natural history* of VF is pain lasting from 6 to 8 weeks, as patients can then increase their activity. However, chronic and persistent pain is not uncommon and a clinical challenge, as the aetiology may be multifactorial. Recognition of frailty is increasingly relevant to rehabilitation in an ageing population at risk of fracture. It is estimated that frail older people make up 30% of medical inpatients and physiotherapists are well placed to measure known identifiers of frailty such as grip strength and gait speed in practice and to promote balance and strengthening exercise, which have been shown to reduce frailty, improve balance and reduce falls risk.

Healthcare practitioners are often unsure how to enable people with osteoporosis to exercise, so The Royal Osteoporosis Society exercise guidelines (Strong, Steady and Straight - An Expert Consensus Statement, National Osteoporosis Society, n.d.) are a valuable resource for clinicians and people with osteoporosis alike, since they help to clarify the role of exercise in bone strength, reducing falls and fractures. There is very limited evidence that exercise itself will cause either a VF or fragility fracture, and so exercises should be adapted to individual capability rather than bone density. Back strengthening should be complemented by balance exercise, particularly for fallers. Monitoring is crucial, as muscles take around 6 weeks to show measurable improvement, so physiotherapists may need to review progression at set intervals depending on the patient ability.

Overall the risks of inactivity are greater than those for exercise. Patients with osteoporosis, including those with VF should be encouraged to undertake exercises including strengthening, balance and weight bearing, and impact cardiovascular ones to promote a healthy lifestyle. These exercises need to be tailored (with VF it is recommended that this is done by a physiotherapist) to individuals based on their current impairment and capabilities.

SUMMARY POINTS

- Most drugs used to treat osteoporosis, including bisphosphonates such as alendronic acid, decrease bone resorption
- Older people are at particular risk of vitamin D deficiency, and many will need to take supplements of vitamin D, with or without calcium, particularly in the winter and early spring months
- Loss of muscle mass and strength occurs with age with the decline starting at around 40 years of age and can decrease by as much as 20% to 40% by age 70 years

- When deciding whether to treat for osteoporosis, it is most important to consider fracture risk, rather than just bone mineral density
- The benefits to the skeleton of exercise outweigh the risks of inactivity. Evidence supports weight-bearing exercise to increase muscle strength to improve the skeleton. To gain maximum benefit exercise should be tailored to individuals' capabilities

MCQs

Q.1 A 78-year-old male patient had a history of multiple vertebral fracture and left hip fracture, for which he had received annual zoledronic acid infusions for the previous 2 years. He was vitamin D replete (on a maintenance dose of 800 units colecalciferol daily), and he was tolerating the medication without any problems. In order to reduce the risk of longer-term adverse effects such as atypical fracture, his treatment was reviewed for consideration of a 'drug holiday'.
What is the most appropriate course of action?
  a. Commence denosumab, continue vitamin D
  b. Continue zoledronic acid, continue vitamin D
  c. Continue zoledronic acid, discontinue vitamin D
  d. Discontinue zoledronic acid, continue vitamin D
  e. Discontinue zoledronic acid, discontinue vitamin D

Q.2 A 70-year-old woman had been taking alendronic acid 70 mg once weekly for 3 years. A recent endoscopy confirms that she had a gastric ulcer. She has no significant kidney impairment and her past medical history includes osteoporosis, diabetes and rheumatoid arthritis.

What would be the most appropriate plan of action for her?
  a. Continue current regimen with an agent to protect stomach
  b. Switch to risedronate 35 mg weekly
  c. Switch to alendronic acid 10 mg daily
  d. Switch to strontium ranelate 2 g daily
  e. Switch to zoledronic acid 5 mg yearly

Q.3 An independent 76-year-old female patient with osteoporosis and a slight kyphosis presented, having lost her balance 6 weeks previously, whilst gardening and sustained a wrist fracture. She had been advised that the wrist fracture had fully healed and she was keen to become more active again.
What exercise advice do you think will give most benefit?
  a. Do not exercise due to the falls risk
  b. Get back to normal activities straight away
  c. Prioritise back strengthening and postural exercises
  d. Prioritise balance exercise, walking practice and leg muscle strengthening
  e. Prioritise muscle strengthening and impact exercise for bone health

REFERENCES

Black, D. M., Schwartz, A. V., Ensrud, K. E., Cauley, J. A., Levis, S., Quandt, S. A., …, & Cummings, S. R. (2006). Effects of continuing or stopping alendronate after 5 years of treatment: the Fracture Intervention Trial Long-term Extension (FLEX): a randomized trial. *JAMA, 296*, 2927–2938.

Bone, H. G., Hosking, D., Devogelaer, J. -P., Tucci, J. R., Emkey, R. D., Tonino, R. P., …, & Liberman, U. A. (2004). Ten years' experience with alendronate for osteoporosis in postmenopausal women. *New England Journal of Medicine, 350*, 1189–1199.

NIH Consensus Development Panel on Osteoporosis Prevention, Diagnosis, and Therapy. (2001). Osteoporosis prevention, diagnosis, and therapy. *JAMA, 285*, 785–795.

Strong, Steady and Straight: An Expert Consensus Statement | National Osteoporosis Society [WWW Document] (n.d.). Retrieved from: https://theros.org.uk/healthcare-professionals/tools-and-resources/clinical-guidance/documents/strong-steady-and-straight-an-expert-consensus-statement-on-physical-activity-and-exercise-for-osteoporosis-ros-2018/ (Accessed 7 April 2019).

39

Vision and Hearing

Joanna Preston & Kimberley Kok

LEARNING OBJECTIVES

- Explain the impact of visual and hearing sensory impairments on rehabilitation
- List common causes of visual and hearing deficits in older adults
- Describe how to adapt rehabilitation programmes to be inclusive for older adults
- Explain how to recognise when sensory impairments may be impacting on communication and engagement
- Describe how simple measures can be used to manage many causes of hearing loss

CASE

Cheng is a 92-year-old man who developed pneumonia requiring hospital admission. He has a background of mild cognitive impairment but had been living independently prior to admission with no concerns. He has macular degeneration and is registered partially sighted. He has hearing aids for presbycusis, and these were lost in the emergency department (ED). He develops a marked delirium a couple of days into admission even as his pneumonia is treated. For 3 weeks he is unable to follow commands, has little carry over between therapy sessions and remains distracted. A decision is made to refer for bed-based rehabilitation. While he is waiting, a replacement hearing aid is sourced. Within 2 days, his delirium has settled and he begins to make good progress and is able to be discharged with rehabilitation at home. In his familiar environment he returns to normal level of function within a week.

VISION

Undiagnosed visual impairments may become more apparent in unfamiliar environments or undertaking less familiar tasks. Age-related macular degeneration is the commonest cause of visual impairment in older adults. Other significant causes include cataracts and glaucoma. Referral to an ophthalmologist is usually necessary, both for diagnosis and access to support from low vision services.

Vision is an important and modifiable risk factor for falls. Good eye health contributes to a lower rate of falls, depression and isolation; and better quality of life (International Longevity Centre UK, 2012). 'Severely visually impaired' or 'partially visually impaired' are the preferred terms, over 'blind'.

The eye has many functions and seeing is more than just visual acuity. Other common problems encountered include visual field defects and double vision (Table 39.1). Each will have a particular contribution to overall vision and impact

rehabilitations. This chapter will explore the common conditions and their management as relevant to rehabilitation, followed by more rehabilitation specific strategies.

Epidemiology

Sight loss affects people of all ages, but as we get older we are increasingly likely to experience it.

- One in five people aged 75 years and over are living with sight loss.
- One in two people aged 90 years and over are living with sight loss.
- Nearly two-thirds of people living with sight loss are women.
- People from black and minority ethnic communities are at greater risk of some of the leading causes of sight loss.
- Adults with learning disabilities are 10 times more likely to be blind or partially sighted than the general population.

Types of Visual Impairment

Low Visual Acuity

There are many causes of low visual acuity as shown in Table 39.1. This section will focus on those pertinent to rehabilitation.

Cataracts. Cataracts are very common and cause gradual onset of a sensation of glare, particularly at night and when driving in low light. Cataracts are almost always operable. It is a short operation performed under local anaesthetic as a day case. It has a good result in being able to improve vision and as such is a modifiable risk factor for falls. The procedure itself requires the person to be able to lie still and flat for about 30 minutes. If both eyes are affected, they are usually operated on one eye at a time because of concerns regarding the risk of infection (1 in 1000), to minimise the risk of complication in both eyes at the same time.

Glaucoma. Glaucoma is raised pressure in the eye due to problems with circulation of fluid in the front of the eye (the aqueous humour), anterior chamber, in front of the iris.

TABLE 39.1	Types of visual impairment.		
	LOW VISUAL ACUITY	**VISUAL FIELD DEFECT**	**DOUBLE VISION**
Front of eye (anterior segment)	Cataracts Refractive error of lens Glaucoma		
Back of eye (posterior segment)	Hypertensive retinopathy Diabetic retinopathy Macular degeneration	Vascular occlusion Macular degeneration	
Neuro-ophthalmic & neurological causes	Cortical blindness	Stroke	Conditions causing weakness of eye muscles Stroke

It causes progressive peripheral visual field loss and is often otherwise asymptomatic.

First-degree relatives over 40 years old of someone with glaucoma are entitled to free eye tests in some countries including the UK.

Drops are the mainstay of treatment to improve drainage of the eye and maintenance of a stable pressure. It is therefore important to avoid missing doses of drops. For those undergoing rehabilitation with upper limb weakness or malcoordination, this may mean finding alternative ways for these to be administered. Options might include:

- OT (occupational therapist) review for aids for drops
- Teaching someone else to administer
- Consideration of need for a carer to help.

Refractive Errors (Lens Changes). Many older adults will need glasses for myopia (short sightedness), hypermetropia (long sightedness) or both. In some countries, e.g. the UK, free eye tests are available for older people. This is a simple way to improve someone's vision and reduce their falls risk. There is debate about whether varifocals contribute to an increased falls risk. Varifocals have the lens for reading at the bottom of the glasses, so that they can look down to read and up to see the rest of the world. This means that wearing varifocals whilst walking and looking downwards will cause the floor, or the stairs, etc. to be out of focus. Individuals need to learn to use varifocals so it is likely that the introduction of these as a new pair of glasses, particularly in those with some cognitive impairment, can potentially increase risks of falls, at least initially, until the person is able to adjust to them.

Macular Degeneration. Dry macular degeneration (also known as age-related macular degeneration or ARMD) has a gradual onset over many years. It causes a central loss of visual acuity (termed a central scotoma). People usually complain of worsening vision, thinking that they need new glasses, but it is not a refractive lens problem. There is no medical treatment available to slow the progression but fish oils and green vegetables may be beneficial.

Visual Field Defects

These are areas of the visual field that do not contain images (see Fig. 39.1). They can be caused by conditions affecting the retina, for example vascular occlusions or ARMD, or neurological conditions affecting the pathways between the eyes and the occipital cortex at the back of the brain. Stroke can cause different patterns of defects dependent on the area of the brain affected and similarly, will often be associated with other neurological deficits. Brain tumours may cause similar patterns for the same reason.

Double Vision

Double vision (diplopia) is when you can see two objects where there should be one. This can be caused by problems with the muscles, nerves or the brain (see Table 39.2). Treatment of diplopia depends on the cause and whether the double vision can be reversed. There are some non-surgical treatments that can be considered. These are:

- An eye patch
- Fresnel prism applied to glasses – the strength can be adjusted

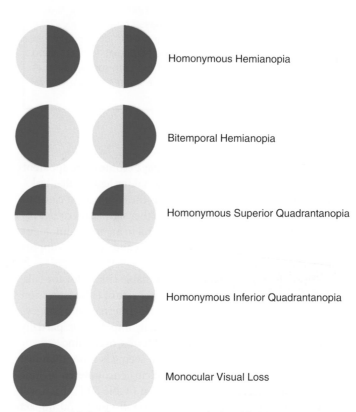

Homonymous Hemianopia

Bitemporal Hemianopia

Homonymous Superior Quadrantanopia

Homonymous Inferior Quadrantanopia

Monocular Visual Loss

FIG. 39.1 Common patterns of visual field loss.

TABLE 39.2 **Causes of double vision.**		
MUSCLES	**NERVES**	**BRAIN**
Nerves that control the muscles	Multiple sclerosis	Stroke (brainstem)
Autoimmune diseases, e.g. myasthenia gravis, Graves' disease	Guillain-Barré syndrome	Migraine headaches
	Diabetes	

- Occlusive lens applied to glasses, or as a contact lens
- Visual perceptual therapy – to overcome visual perception disorders following a stroke and to improve hand-eye coordination.

Management

- Consider referral to a community optometrist as they are able to undertake initial assessments in a care home or at home if the individual is unable to get to clinic
- Consider assessment by an optician who will have equipment to undertake a fuller assessment, e.g. check visual fields, check for cataracts, refractive errors, check prescription of glasses
- Inform GP so the individual can access additional services
- Referral to Low Visual Aid (LVA) Clinic (Ophthalmology clinic)
- Signpost towards charity groups such as the Royal National Institute for Blind People (RNIB) in the UK
- Ensure all available useful aids are offered, e.g. large font for letters, braille
- Explore local links to social services
- Adapt your communication to enhance non-visual components (Box 39.1).

Driving

In most countries, it is essential for individuals to wear glasses or contact lenses whenever they drive if they need them. Individuals have to inform the licencing agency (DVLA in the UK) if they have visual impairment that affects both eyes, or the remaining eye if they only have one eye (Gov.UK, 2019).

Legal Blindness

Individuals can choose to register as visually impaired. This is optional and registering as visually impaired can entitle the individual to benefits in some countries such as:

- Allowance or a tax-free benefit to help with any costs relating to your disability or illness

BOX 39.1   **Communication Tips – Visual Impairment**
- Talk as you approach - Introduce yourself and who else is with you - Explain where you are, e.g. I'm to your left - Consider tactile cues to demonstrate location - Ensure good lighting - Avoid being in their visual field defect - Use glasses - If no glasses: use other magnifiers, e.g. for reading

- Reduction in TV licence fee
- Discounted public transport
- Parking concessions.

HEARING

Hearing problems in rehabilitation are most likely to be due to pre-existing conditions such as age-related hearing loss (presbycusis) or wax.

Practically, hearing conditions cause problems with communication which thereby impacts on the effectiveness of rehabilitation. One study showed 43% of patients had misheard a healthcare professional in their recent attendance to hospital (Cudmore et al., 2017). The goal therefore is to identify and manage any hearing impairments early to optimise participation. Management is often easily accessible and very effective depending on the cause.

Epidemiology

Hearing loss is common in older adults. It is the fourth leading cause of disability globally. Prevalence doubles with every 10-year increase in age and is seen in half of 60 year olds, two thirds of over 70 year olds and 85% of over 85 year olds. An ageing population will lead to an ever-increasing absolute number of people with hearing loss because the commonest cause of hearing loss in older adults is age related, or presbycusis.

Hearing loss itself is usually benign in terms of its causes. It can however adversely affect communication if left untreated which leads to increased levels of social isolation, mood disorders and there is an association with increased rates of cognitive impairment which has a direct impact on both the need for and success of rehabilitation.

Causes

The ear itself anatomically is split into three parts: inner, middle and outer. All three parts need to be functioning well as does the nerve connecting the ear to the brain and the brain itself (Fig. 39.2).

There are two main categories of hearing loss: sensorineural and conductive. Sensorineural relates to any problem relating to the nerve impulses between the brain and the cochlear in the inner ear. Conductive is any problem between the middle and outer ear.

It is recommended that for those over 60 years, if the hearing impairment appears to be progressive, bilateral and sensorineural in origin – with normal ear examination; GPs and hospital clinicians should diagnose age-related hearing loss and make a direct referral to hospital audiology

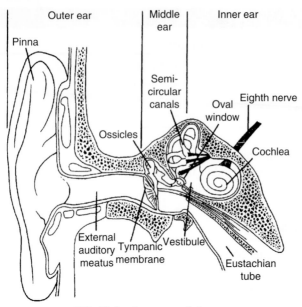

FIG. 39.2   Anatomy of the ear.

departments for management. Further investigation is rarely indicated unless another condition is suspected – a guide to this is below.

Sensorineural vs Conductive

The sensorineural element of hearing involves the inner ear. The cochlea is a small circular organ in the inner ear which collects sounds from the ear and converts them to electrical signals to send to the brain and the majority of sensorineural hearing loss is due to a problem here. It can be damaged by drugs, noise and the ageing process. Sensorineural hearing loss largely causes bilateral hearing loss with the exception of acoustic neuroma.

Conductive hearing loss involves the middle and outer ear. The commonest cause of conductive hearing loss is ear wax which will usually have a gradual onset but can have a sudden deterioration on top. Other conductive causes tend to be acute problems with the ear drum itself and either fluid or inflammation on either side of it.

Common Causes of Hearing Impairment
Presbycusis

The commonest cause of sensorineural hearing loss in older adults is presbycusis, or age-related hearing loss.

It is slowly progressive and usually bilateral, although often one side may be affected earlier. It is caused by degeneration of both the sensory hair cells in the cochlea and the nerve cells that send sensory inputs to the brain. There is also atrophy of the stria vascularis, a membrane of the cochlea that makes endolymph. There is a genetic predisposition.

Typically, higher pitched sounds are lost earlier so talking at a lower pitch may aid communication. Hearing aids amplify remaining hearing ability. Approximately 86% of patients benefited from hearing aid correction with age-related hearing loss; 14% of people with hearing loss reported wearing hearing aids (Cunningham & Tucci, 2017). One study showed that using a hearing aid slows the progression of cognitive decline (Maharani et al., 2018).

Wax

Initial treatment is with standard olive oil ear drops, 2 drops twice a day for a week, followed by ear irrigation and sometimes microsuction. Although it is common for people to use cotton buds to attempt to clear wax, this often leads to further impaction or accidental introduction of new foreign material into the ear and it is not advised.

Other Causes of Hearing Impairment

Other causes tend to be acute onset and require further assessment for diagnosis. Table 39.3 summarises other frequently encountered causes of hearing loss.

Management
Screening

Screening for hearing loss is not routine in the general population. This is because many people with mild hearing loss are not significantly affected and hearing aids may provide minimal benefit to them at an early stage. If someone is not ready to start wearing a hearing aid, then diagnosing the hearing loss has little utility. In the context of rehabilitation,

TABLE 39.3   Causes of hearing loss.

	PRESBYCUSIS	COCHLEAR STRESSORS	ACOUSTIC NEUROMA	WAX IMPACTION	PERFORATED EAR DRUM	OTITIS MEDIA
Type	Sensorineural	Sensorineural	Sensorineural	Conductive	Conductive	Conductive
Onset	Gradual	After insult	Gradual	Gradual	Sudden	Sudden
Bilateral	Yes	Can be	No	Can be	No	No
Pain	No	No	No	No	Yes	Yes
Associations	May run in families	Exposure to stressor	Facial weakness/ numbness Tinnitus Dysphagia Diplopia	None	Recent otitis media Trauma to area	Recent URTI

however, it is important to screen for hearing deficits in those with

- Communication deficits, e.g. not participating in conversations normally
- Suspected cognitive impairment, e.g. not able to follow instructions
- Social isolation, e.g. low mood as a consequence, difficulty hearing in busy places.

Assessment of hearing function is usually carried out at the local audiology department. Options are available for testing over the phone and online (links in resources). Some pharmacies and opticians offer free hearing tests. In the UK, the charity AgeUK may be able to help arrange domiciliary visits.

Hearing Amplification

Choice of hearing aid is largely related to aesthetics and ease of use, as well as cost. There is an increasing variety of hearing aid models available and a selection of these are supplied for free in the UK by the NHS, largely the behind the ear versions. Aftercare with batteries and repairs is also free. Privately it can cost £500 to £3500 per hearing aid. It takes at least 6 weeks for the hearing aid to work, due to reprogramming of neural pathways, so persistence is required during the acclimatisation period.

New hearing aids can take several months to organise. For those in whom rehabilitation is impacted by their hearing, it may be worth asking for an urgent appointment or trying to establish pathways for such people. In the meantime, or as an alternative, Communicaids can be used to amplify sound through an external microphone attached to headphones. Some people prefer this longer term.

It is sensible to involve speech and language therapists when discussing difficult decisions if communication may be impaired, in particular around capacity assessment.

Battery life for standard behind the ear (BTE) hearing aids is between 6 and 14 days, depending on usage. Battery compartments often need to be opened to 'turn off' the hearing aid and therefore save battery, e.g. overnight. As a general rule, the smaller the hearing aid, the smaller the battery, the shorter the battery life. Box 39.2 provides some help with common problems.

BOX 39.2 Hearing Aid Troubleshooting

Is It On?
- Normally switched on by pushing battery clip in
- Older versions have an on and off button

Using Loop Devices
- Buses, banks, theatres and some telephones may transmit a signal to be picked up by the hearing aid directly
- Set it to telecoil mode to use (T mode if available)

It's Whistling
Always abnormal: check for source of feedback
- Wax in external auditory canal
- Ill-fitting mould: can be re-made relatively easily and quickly (weeks)

No sound/muffled sound
Checklist
- Is it switched on?
- Turn the volume up
- Is it on the telecoil setting?
- Is the tubing patent?
- Is the battery in the right way round?
- Try a new battery

BOX 39.3 Communication Tips – Hearing Impairment

- Gain attention before starting to speak
- Gain eye contact
- Do not cover your mouth so that lip reading can be used
- Use gestures and body language for context including demonstrating exercises
- Speak to the 'better ear' if they have one
- Use a whiteboard/notepad to use writing
- Check understanding
- Ensure hearing aid on

Communication

It is worth thinking about how you can enhance the non-auditory elements of communication (Box 39.3) to improve the interaction.

SUMMARY POINTS

- Sensory impairment impacts function in a variety of ways through a reduction in visual and auditory feedback that we often take for granted
- This has a direct impact with regards to social isolation, low mood and delirium
- It is important to be aware of enhancing use of other sensory modalities instead. Many are modifiable
- Screening for deficits and referring/signposting for further assessment can have a big impact on optimising rehabilitation participation

---

MCQs

Q.1 Good eye health contributes to:
- **a.** Increased risk of depression
- **b.** Reduced risk of isolation
- **c.** Falls
- **d.** Lower quality of life
- **e.** Reduced risk of institutionalisation

Q.2 The following condition is the commonest cause of hearing impairment:
- **a.** Presbycusis
- **b.** Acoustic neuroma
- **c.** Physical head injury
- **d.** Otitis media
- **e.** Perforated ear drum

Q.3 A standard hearing aid battery has a life of:
- **a.** 1–2 days
- **b.** 3–4 days
- **c.** 6–14 days
- **d.** 14–21 days
- **e.** 21–28 days

REFERENCES

Cudmore, V., Henn, P., O'Tuathaigh, C. M. P., & Smith, S. (2017). Age-related hearing loss and communication breakdown in the clinical setting. *JAMA Otolaryngology Head Neck Surgery*, *143*(10), 1054–1055.

Cunningham, L. L., & Tucci, D. L. (2017). Hearing loss in adults. *New England Journal of Medicine*, *377*(25), 2465–2473.

Gov.UK. (2019). Check if a health condition affects your driving. Retrieved from: https://www.gov.uk/health-conditions-and-driving (Accessed 12 May 2019).

International Longevity Centre UK. (2012). Undetected sight loss in care homes: an evidence review. International Longevity Centre UK. Retrieved from: https://www.bl.uk/collection-items/undetected-sight-loss-in-care-homes-an-evidence-review (Accessed 11 August 2019).

Maharani, A., Dawes, P., Nazroo, J., Tampubolon, G., & Pendleton, N. SENSE-Cog WP1 Group. (2018). Longitudinal relationship between hearing aid use and cognitive function in older Americans. *Journal of the American Geriatrics Society*, *66*(6), 1130–1136.

FURTHER READING

Action on hearing loss. (2019). Hearing health. Retrieved from: https://www.actiononhearingloss.org.uk/hearing-health/ (Accessed 12 May 2019).

Age UK. (2019). Hearing loss. Retrieved from: https://www.ageuk.org.uk/information-advice/health-wellbeing/conditions-illnesses/hearing-loss/ (Accessed 12 May 2019).

MDTea Podcast. (2017). Episode 4.06 Vision. Retrieved from: https://thehearingaidpodcasts.org.uk/4-06-vision/ (Accessed 12 May 2019).

MDTea Podcast. (2018). Episode 5.08 Hearing. Retrieved from: http://thehearingaidpodcasts.org.uk/5-08-hearing/ (Accessed 12 May 2019).

NHS.UK. (2018). Blindness and vision loss. Retrieved from: https://www.nhs.uk/conditions/vision-loss/ (Accessed 12 May 2019).

Royal National Institute of Blind People (RNIB). (2019). Royal National Institute of Blind People. Retrieved from: https://www.rnib.org.uk (Accessed 12 May 2019).

40

Skin Care and Podiatry

Belinda Longhurst & Gill Gibson

LEARNING OBJECTIVES

- Explain why healthcare professionals, patients and their families should undertake regular skin inspections
- Identify skin and nail changes in the older person and the associated risk factors

- Describe the appropriate treatment and prevention of common skin disorders
- Explain how to incorporate a person-centred care package to include a regular skin-care regime

INTRODUCTION

Skin integrity is a common care need which requires integrated care and support to minimise the impact of risks and vulnerability in ageing skin (NICE CG22, 2015). Any breach of the skin increases the risk of developing healthcare-associated infection as microorganisms can penetrate the surface of the broken skin and cause anything from boils to bacteraemia (Bissett, 2010). Healthcare professionals (HCPs), patients and their families should be aware of the structural and functional skin changes that occur in the older person and recognise signs and symptoms of skin disease. This will assist implementation, monitoring and responding to person-centred skin care plans.

Skin care, in the form of treating dry skin conditions, preventing incontinence-associated dermatitis and superficial ulcerations, is 'regarded as a major strategy for maintaining the skin barrier, skin integrity and health' (Kottner, Lichterfeld, & Blume-Peytavi, 2013). This chapter briefly highlights the treatments and prevention of some common skin pathologies associated with older people and presents a case study to aid with learning outcomes.

CASE

Luca is an 89-year-old man, with well-managed diabetes mellitus (type 2) and was discharged from primary care following recovery from an acute episode of ulcerative lower limb cellulitis (infection of the deeper layers of skin) associated with meticillin-resistant Staphylococcus aureus (MRSA). The portal of entry for the bacterial infection was traced to an open wound between the fourth and fifth toes of his left foot, associated with chronic tinea pedis ('athletes foot'). The initial misdiagnosis of stasis eczema (impaired blood flow causing leakage of blood into body tissues, so the skin becomes red, dry and irritated) led to inappropriate management and a delay in receiving the right care at the right time, by the right health professionals. His family has since been advised on how to recognise the signs and symptoms of tinea pedis and secondary bacterial infection and has been issued a copy of

the British Association of Dermatologists' guidelines on preventing cellulitis (British Association of Dermatologists, 2018). With this case in mind, the following subheadings on changes in older persons' skin and the associated vulnerabilities should aid in the prevention of inappropriate hospital admissions and an overall improvement to the quality of life in an older person.

CHANGES IN OLDER PERSONS' SKIN

- Anhidrosis (dry skin): Sweat glands produce less sweat and sebaceous glands produce less sebum (oily secretion of the sebaceous glands). The result is dry and itchy skin. Sebum also contains antimicrobial peptides, which form part of the innate immune defence against pathogens such as bacteria and fungus. Thus, the reduction of sebum increases an older person's risk of infection, such as with Luca in our case study.
- Atrophy: The dermis (the layer of skin beneath the epidermis that consists of dense connective tissue to cushion the body from injury) becomes thinner and a slower rate of skin cell turnover in the epidermis (the outer layer of skin) renders the skin weaker and 'parchment' like, prone to damage and at risk of delayed wound healing.
- Pigment changes: The skin appears paler. There is a reduction in the number of melanocytes (skin cells responsible for skin colour), but the remaining melanocytes become larger, Solar lentigines (age spots) appear on sun exposed areas.
- Haemosiderosis: Venous insufficiency and increased venous pressure result in venule leakage and lead to iron deposits in skin, resulting in dark-coloured haemosiderin staining around the lower legs.
- Elastosis: Collagen (connective tissue) and elastin (protein in connective tissue which allows skin to resume its shape after stretching or contraction) fragment, reducing the skin's underlying strength and it thus becomes more fragile and wrinkled, which leads to a 'leathery' appearance.

• Dehydration: The intercellular glue (natural moisturising factors in the skin) that holds collagen and elastin in place reduces, so the stratum corneum (outer layer of the epidermis) becomes dehydrated.

ECZEMA

Eczema and dermatitis are interchangeable terms for a group of inflammatory skin conditions.

Asteatotic eczema (eczema cracquelée) is associated with dry, older skin and initially appears on the shins with a 'crazy paving' appearance. Uncomfortable, pruritic (itchy) fissures or grooves then manifest, but tend to only affect the epidermal layers of the skin. Other areas that can be affected are upper arms, thighs and lower back, but it more often manifests on the legs (Fig. 40.1).

Stasis eczema (gravitational dermatitis) is triggered by impaired circulation. Insufficient venous return causes pressure to build up as the blood tries to flow upward, but instead pools in the lower limbs. This pressure causes fluid to leak out of the veins and into the skin, which creates swelling, dark red/brown pigmented areas that are vulnerable to ulceration, secondary infection and cellulitis (Fig. 40.2). Elevating the legs whilst sitting, regular exercise and use of compression hosiery can reduce the swelling.

Both asteatotic and stasis eczema require frequent and generous applications of emollients to the legs. Occasional use of topical steroids can reduce the itch and assist in healing. If infection is suspected, then antibiotics may be prescribed.

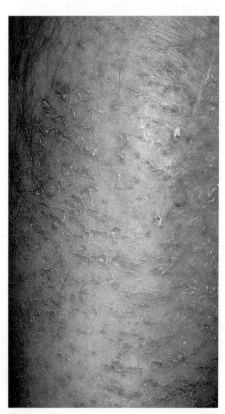

FIG. 40.1 Asteatotic eczema. (From James W, Elston D, Treat J, Rosenbach M, Neuhaus I. *Andrews' Diseases of the skin*, 13th edn, Elsevier; 2020, with permission.)

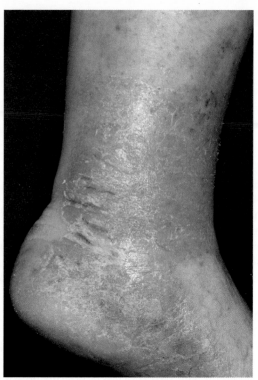

FIG. 40.2 Stasis eczema. (From Habif TP. *Clinical Dermatology: A Color Guide to Diagnosis and Therapy*, 6th en. Elsevier; 2016, with permission.)

TINEA PEDIS AND ONYCHOMYCOSIS

Tinea pedis (athlete's foot) and onychomycosis (fungal nail) are superficial fungal infections (Fig. 40.3) of the epidermis and nail bed, most often caused by the dermatophyte Trichophyton rubrum. These infections are among the most common diseases worldwide and cause serious chronic illness in the older person (Thomas et al., 2010).

Tinea pedis is divided into three types:

1) Interdigital tinea is the most common clinical manifestation and is characterised by maceration and fissuring of the skin mainly in the space between the toes.
2) Plantar (moccasin) tinea presents with hyperkeratotic and squamous plaques which cover the soles, heels and sides of the foot. This type is often misdiagnosed as eczema.
3) Vesiculobullous tinea produces clusters of pruritic blisters or pustules, which can ulcerate.

Tinea can cause fissuring and lead to bacterial infections, especially in people with impaired circulation. In our case study, Luca had a history of chronic interdigital tinea, which caused a breach in the epidermis and subsequent infection spreading to the lower leg. Unfortunately, the misdiagnosis of stasis eczema delayed the appropriate treatment. Thus, it is important that patients are assessed by the relevant HCP, at the right time. Older people, such as Luca, with diabetes mellitus are at increased risk of developing cellulitis, so should be assessed frequently by carers for any signs of tinea (or other skin infections) and then referred to a podiatrist for diagnosis and treatment. It is appropriate to treat any episode of tinea with topical antifungals and consider prophylactic

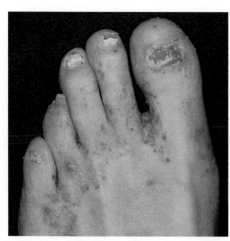

FIG. 40.3 Tinea pedis and onychomycosis. (From Habif TP, Dinulos JGH, Chapman MS, Zug K. *Skin Disease: Diagnosis and Treatment*, 4th edn. Elsevier; 2018, with permission.)

use of antifungals to prevent further complications (Bristow & Spruce, 2009).

Prevalence of onychomycosis is seen in nearly 20% of patients aged over 60 years (Loo, 2007). These have specific risk factors and poor response to therapy, including frequent nail dystrophy, slow growth of nails and increased prevalence of peripheral vascular disease and diabetes mellitus.

Treatment of onychomycosis and other nail changes, such as thickening, is person and pathology specific, so should be discussed with a podiatrist who can advise on the most appropriate course of evidence-based treatments (e.g. iea tree oil is not recommended). A podiatrist is also trained to assess, diagnose and treat many other dermatological conditions of the foot, such as corns, callus and HPV-associated lesions. They also advise on the importance of good-fitting footwear, which can prevent many hyperkeratotic lesions, and improve gait and quality of life by keeping people mobile.

SKIN TEARS

Rubbing or pulling on fragile skin can result in the separation of the skin at the dermo-epidermal junction. These tears can occur anywhere on the body although they are more common on the extremities. If mismanaged, the delayed healing can give rise to infection, so carers and family members should seek the help of a qualified health professional as soon as the wound appears.

Carers and patients can reduce the risk of skin tears by keeping finger and toenails short, padding bed rails and wheelchairs and taking care when transporting patients. A good skin care regimen, in the form of frequent applications of emollients, will also reduce the risk of skin tears in an older person by preserving the integrity of the epidermal barrier. The emollient can be self-applied or with the support of a family member or carer.

PRESSURE SORES

Restricted movement due to frailty, poor general health and decreased mobility are identified risks for developing pressure ulcers. Able-bodied patients will adjust their sitting or lying position to counteract pressure build-up, even whilst sleeping, but older patients may be incapable of doing so. A combination of pathological pressure (commonly from a hard surface such as a chair or a firm bed mattress) and compromised arterial supply to a focal area of skin deprives the epidermis and underlying tissues of oxygen and nutrients, leading to painful breakdown and ulceration. Other contributing factors such as increased body temperature, advanced age, poor nutritional status and reduced sensory feeling should be identified to reduce the risk of pressure sores (National Pressure Ulcer Advisory Panel, 2014).

HCPs can advise on suitable aids to redistribute pressure if the patient is permanently in bed or reliant on sitting for most of the day. Common areas for pressure sores are the sacral and lower leg areas. The latter requires protection in the form of properly fitting hosiery, shoes and slippers and monitoring.

Prevention is key, with a focus on frequent observation and assessment of the skin integrity. There are recognised assessment tools for identifying pressure problems. One such model is the Waterlow scale (Anthony et al., 2008) which explores risk factors including weight for height ratio, continence, skin condition, mobility, sex and age, nutrition and hydration, neurological function, major surgery or trauma and current medication. These assessment scales are not standalone screening tools. They are intended to complement other health assessments and identify risk factors enabling HCPs to offer and deliver person-centred care, which is tailored for individual health care needs (Chamang, 2010).

Another useful assessment tool for families and healthcare workers is the SSKIN Framework (NHS Framework, 2017) five-step approach to preventing pressure ulcers:

- **S**urface: make sure your patients have adequate support
- **S**kin inspection: early inspection means early detection
- **K**eep your patients moving
- **I**ncontinence/moisture: patients need to be clean and dry
- **N**utrition/hydration: a healthy diet is required and plenty of fluids.

The treatment of pressure ulcers is carried out by specialists within a multidisciplinary team, which includes tissue viability nurses and podiatrists who will assess the wound and, if necessary, swab the area to identify infection, remove any non-viable tissue and deflect pressure to promote healing (Fig. 40.4).

There are four recognised stages of pressure ulcers (Table 40.1). Knowing the appropriate stage assists in the prognosis and management of the ulcer. Each stage should be documented to include the surface area. If possible, use a validated measurement technique (for example, transparency tracing or a photograph).

A variety of wound dressings are available, with an equally wide range of uses according to the type and stage of ulceration. They vary in material, size, absorbency and whether they adhere to skin and conform to creases (NICE KTT14, 2015). Some are designed for wet wounds and are used in conjunction with other treatments, such as negative pressure therapy. Others may promote hydration and are manufactured as foams, gels and other compounds. An HCP can advise patients and their families on the most appropriate dressing.

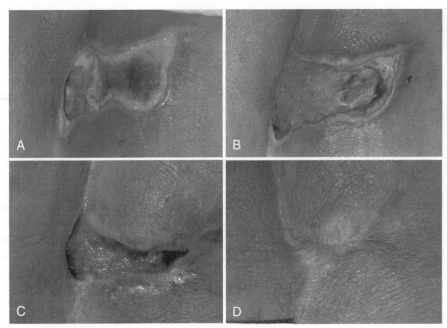

FIG. 40.4 Pressure ulcers. Pressure sore grading: A: Ungradable – depth unknown until slough removed. A/B: Deep Category – unclassified pressure ulcer progress to Grade 3. B/C: Superficial Category – Grade 2. D: Superficial Category – Grade 1. (From Cifu D. *Braddom's Physical Medicine and Rehabilitation*, 5th edn. Elsevier; 2016, with permission.)

INCONTINENCE ASSOCIATED DERMATITIS

Prolonged contact of urine with skin not only causes breakdown of the tissues, it also triggers an innate inflammatory response. Simultaneously, the enzyme urease hydrolyses urea forming ammonia, which then leads to an increase in skin pH. Bacteria will then multiply and potentially result in infection (Fig. 40.5).

Treatment consists of two key interventions: cleaning and protection. Soap is alkaline so can further raise the skin's pH and reduces natural moisturising factors and lipids, which increases dryness.

Ideally, a leave-on cleanser should be used. A barrier is then needed to protect the skin. This should not be a thick, occlusive layer as it will affect the absorbency of incontinence pads and lead to overhydration. Instead, carers and patients should use a proprietary film, which leaves a thin, semipermeable coating providing protection for recurrent episodes of incontinence.

Alternatively, a specialised barrier cream can be used, which does not have to be reapplied for every episode of incontinence. If bacterial infection is suspected, barrier creams or sprays should not be used, and a swab should be taken by the HCP so appropriate treatment can be given (Wilson, 2018).

It should be noted that:
- Incontinence is not an inevitable consequence of old age and should be treated whenever possible
- Skin should be kept clean, dry and well hydrated
- Patients should be encouraged to drink regularly to maintain hydration, reduce the risk of constipation and reduce the concentration of urine.

TABLE 40.1	**The four stages of pressure ulcers.**
STAGE	**EXAMPLES OF TREATMENT**
Stage 1: Non-blanching surface of intact skin. The skin may appear red and feel warm	Derma emollient and pressure relieving aids, such as air flow mattresses and heel elevators
Stage 2: Partial thickness wound which involves the epidermis and dermis (the first two layers) or both	Relieve pressure by repositioning, frequent moving and padding of hard surfaces
Stage 3: Full thickness wound which involves the epidermis and dermis and subcutaneous tissue (where all the nerves, sweat glands and hair follicles lie)	Turn the patient every 2 hours. Keep the skin clean and dry. Swab open sores for infection and subsequent antibiotic cover. Debride non-viable tissue and dressing of wound by HCP. Promote movement and proper nutrition and hydration
Stage 4: Full-thickness wound which involves the epidermis and dermis, subcutaneous tissue and the deep fascia (in the muscle)	As stage 3 and consider referral for surgical opinion

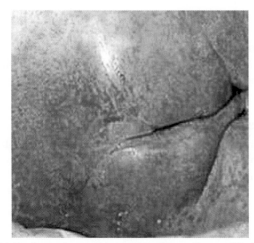

FIG. 40.5 Incontinence dermatitis. (From Bryant RA, Nix DP. *Acute & Chronic Wounds: Current Management Concepts*, 4th edn, Mosby; 2011, with permission)

COMPLETE EMOLLIENT THERAPY

Washing with soaps can cause irritation and strip the natural oils that keep our skin healthy. However, washing with an emollient will both clean and soothe fragile, vulnerable skin and forms part of the complete emollient therapy, recommended for people with dry skin (Penzer, 2005). Aqueous cream is not an emollient and should only be used as a soap substitute (rinsed off). It contains sodium lauryl sulphate, which is a sensitiser for contact dermatitis and increases transepidermal water loss (TEWL), thereby drying out the skin.

Maintaining and restoring the skin's natural barrier by increasing hydration and reducing TEWL, emollients also reduce itching, redness and inflammation. There are an array of emollients available, but generally they come under the following groups:

- Cleansing products which are formulated as bath additives and wash products (soap substitutes)
- Leave on products such as creams, ointments, gels, mousses and sprays
- Some emollients (such as creams and ointments) can be used as both a cleanser and a leave-on product.

In addition to being easy to apply, emollients should be used in a way that fits within the individual's lifestyle, which will promote concordance with treatment (Loden, 2003). It should be noted that many emollients/moisturisers are petroleum, or paraffin, based which can be a fire hazard when soaked into dressings and bedding. Whilst a moisturiser will hydrate the skin, an emollient has the added benefit of forming a barrier which retains natural moisture.

Bristow (2016) makes the following recommendations for emollient therapy:

- The best emollient is the one that the patient likes and therefore will use!
- Apply straight after a bath, wash or shower when the skin is warm and slightly damp to trap in moisture. Some preparations can be slippery so preferably should be applied at night to reduce the risk of falls

- Emollients should be applied daily and at least twice daily in cases of severe eczema and dry skin. The amount of emollient applied will vary from one part of the body to another. For example, an average pair of feet can use 4 g of emollients per day. As a guide, most emollients come with a convenient pump dispenser and one full 'press' on the pump equals to approximately 1 g
- Efficacy is improved when applied under occlusion (covering of skin to trap TEWL), which is useful for areas of hyperkeratosis, such as heels. This can be in the form of hydrocolloid dressings, socks or heel sleeves.

Emollients should not be applied between the toes, as this will increase the risk of developing tinea pedis. These interdigital areas should be washed and carefully dried every day. If the webspaces are still damp after towel drying, an astringent (such as surgical spirit) can be applied with a cotton bud to further dry the area.

While emollients are regarded as safe and with limited side effects, some individuals do report stinging or discomfort on application of those containing urea. This is usually transient; however, consideration of patient-specific treatment in use of emollients should be utilised, particularly for those with sensitive skin, such as eczema and psoriasis.

It does not necessarily equate that the emollient that is applied to a sacral area will be the same for the feet, as heels can be callused and require a thicker emollient with added keratolytic (break down the clumped-up skin cells) ingredients, whilst other areas would be too sensitive to tolerate a keratolytic.

PREVENTION OF LOWER LEG ULCERATION

Lower leg ulceration (LLU) is a common, debilitating and costly condition. It is estimated that the annual cost to the NHS of managing chronic wounds is between £4.5 and £5.1 billion. Over one third of these wounds affect the lower limb, such as leg and foot ulcers (Guest et al., 2015).

In addition to the recommended regular use of emollients, as part of the routine foot and leg care regime in older people for prevention of LLU, a structured wound assessment tool such as TIME (Fletcher, 2007) can aid diagnosis and subsequent treatment of any LLU:

- Tissue: assess tissue quality. Is there evidence of slough and necrosis?
- Infection: colonisation is common in leg ulcers. Assess for signs of surrounding cellulitis indicating infection
- Moisture imbalance: exudate should be assessed in terms of colour, viscosity and volume
- Edge of wound: assess for signs of over-granulation, 'rolled' edges, shallowness, depth and colour, i.e. a purple edge (Todhunter, 2019).

The Legs Matter campaign (Adderly, 2018) is a public health drive, supported by an online website and aims to increase awareness of conditions that affect the lower leg and foot. It is designed to help patients across all ages, from young pregnant women to the older person, their families and carers. Crucially, the campaign aims to outline the importance of seeking the right treatment at the right time, as well as educating people as to the type of care they can expect from HCPs.

Luca is an example of an older person who encountered several HCPs along his journey from correct diagnosis to treatment, including the pharmacist, the community nurse, his GP and other hospital staff. This patient-centred approach of care by a multidisciplinary team assists in critical sharing of communication, in addition to improving coordination of care and results in positive outcomes for older people with skin conditions.

SUMMARY POINTS

- Skin disorders, infection and ulceration are recognised risks as people undergo biological changes along with other health conditions associated with an older person
- Healthcare professionals, patients and their families can perform an assessment of skin and nails, identify and treat various conditions
- Complications of skin conditions can be reduced by implementing person-centred skin-care plans to maintain the integrity of the skin

MCQs

Q.1 What is the five-step approach to preventing and treating pressure ulcers?
  a. Increase moisture, keep moving, promote a healthy diet, surface support and inspect skin
  b. Restrict mobility, increase fluids, use incontinence pads, surface support and inspect skin
  c. Surface support, skin inspection, keep moving, reduce moisture, promote a healthy diet including plenty of fluids
  d. Inspect skin, use incontinence pads, sit the patient up, promote a healthy diet including plenty of fluids, keep moving

Q.2 Tinea pedis and onychomycosis is:
  a. A bacterial infection of skin and nails
  b. Only a cosmetic problem, so requires no treatment
  c. A common complaint and can lead to complications and chronic morbidity
  d. Treated with tea tree oil

REFERENCES

Adderly, U. (2018). Legs matter. *Journal Community Nursing, 32*(4), 32–36.

Anthony, D., Parboteeah, S., Saleh, M., & Papanikolaou, P. (2008). Norton, Waterlow and Braden scores: a review of the literature and a comparison between the scores and clinical judgement. *Journal of Clinical Nursing, 17*(5), 646–653.

Bissett, L. (2010). Skin care as a tool in the prevention of health care-associated infection. *British Journal Community Nursing, 15*(5), 226 228, 231.

Bristow, I. (2016). The podiatric dermatology blog. Emollients – what's best practice? Retrieved from: https://www.foot.expert/single-post/2016/05/05/Emollients---Whats-best-practice (Accessed 15 April 2019).

Bristow, I., & Spruce, M. (2009). Fungal foot infection, cellulitis and diabetes: a review. *Diabetic Medicine, 26*, 548–551.

British Association of Dermatologists. (2018). Patient information leaflet on cellulitis and erysipelas. Retrieved from: http://www.bad.org.uk/shared/get-file.ashx?id=156&itemtype=document (Accessed 30 April 2019).

Chamang, E. T. (2010). A critical review of the Waterlow Tool. *Journal of Community Nursing, 24*(3), 26–32.

Fletcher, J. (2007). Wound assessment and the TIME framework. *British Journal Nursing, 16*(8), 462–466.

Guest, J. F., Ayoub, N., McIlwraith, T., Uchegbu, I., Gerrish, A., Weidlich, D., Vowden, K., & Vowden, P. (2015). Health economic burden that wounds impose on the National Health Service in the UK. *BMJ Open*. Retrieved from: https://bmjopen.bmj.com/content/5/12/e009283 (Accessed 20 May 2018).

Kottner, J., Lichterfeld, A., & Blume-Peytavi, U. (2013). Maintaining skin integrity in the aged: a systematic review. *British Journal of Dermatology, 169*(3), 528–542.

Loden, M. (2003). The skin barrier and use of moisturisers in atopic dermatitis. *Clinical Dermatology, 21*(2), 145–157.

Loo, D. (2007). Onychomycosis in the elderly: drug treatment options. *Drugs and Aging, 24*(4), 293–302.

National Institute of Health and Care Excellence. (2015). Older people with social care needs and multiple long-term conditions. Clinical guideline [CG22]. Retrieved from: https://www.nice.org.uk/guidance/ng22 (Accessed 15 April 2019).

National Institute of Health and Care Excellence. (2015). Wound Care Products. Key therapeutic topic [KTT14]. Retrieved from: https://www.nice.org.uk/advice/ktt14 (Accessed 17 July 2019).

National Pressure Ulcer Advisory Panel. (2014). Prevention and treatment of pressure ulcers – a quick reference guide. Retrieved from: http://www.epuap.org/wp-content/uploads/2016/10/quick-reference-guide-digital-npuap-epuap-pppia-jan2016.pdf (Accessed 16 July 2019).

Penzer, R. (2005). Emollients: selection and application. *Podiatry Now, 9*, S1–S8.

SSKIN Framework. NHS National Stop the Pressure programme Improvement date November 2017 Publication code: IG 24/17.

Thomas, J., Jacobson, G., Narkowicz, C., Peterson, G., Burnet, H., & Sharpe, C. (2010). Toenail onychomycosis: an important global disease burden. *Journal of Clinical Pharmacy and Therapeutics, 35*(5), 497.

Todhunter, J. (2019). Understanding the differential diagnosis of leg ulcers: focus on atypical ulcers. *Wound Care Today, 1*(3), 1–19.

Wilson, M. (2018). Incontinence-associated dermatitis from a urinary incontinence perspective. *British Journal of Nursing, 27*(9), 4–12.

Specialised Rehabilitation

41

Rehabilitation in the Acute Setting

Kenneth Rockwood

LEARNING OBJECTIVES

- Explain how an understanding of baseline function can allow individualised goals of care to be set that emphasise prevention of deconditioning, and a plan for rehabilitation, as part of treating acute illness in older people with frailty who are admitted to hospital
- Demonstrate that goals of care should be informed by the baseline state, established where possible by veri-

fied history (usually with an informant) of cognition, mobility, balance, continence and social engagement
- Describe the importance of understanding early changes in how a patient mobilises, including how they improve in bed
- Illustrate that mobilisation, a key aspect of rehabilitation, should be early, aggressive and documented

CASE

Ada, an 84-year-old woman, presents to hospital after a fall. She was alone and on her floor for 4 hours before her daughter found her, at which point she was unable to get up, and so an ambulance was called. At the emergency department, no fracture was demonstrated, but Ada was found to have a mild low level of serum sodium (recorded as Na+ 129; the lower limit of normal was 135); mild acute kidney injury – urea elevated to 16 (from a baseline of 7.2, with an upper limit of normal of 8.0, and creatinine 101, from a baseline of 60); an elevated creatinine kinase (1322, upper limit 215) and a 'positive urinalysis'. Her investigations also revealed evidence of a prior heart attack not present on an ECG from 4 years before. Her past history was recorded to include hypertension, dyslipidaemia, transient ischaemic attack, peripheral vascular disease, abdominal aortic aneurysm last visualised 2 years ago at a maximum diameter of 3.3 cm, hypothyroidism, vitiligo, osteoporosis, Colles fracture 2 years ago, chronic (20+ years) daily headache and anxiety. No comment is made about her current or prior ability to walk, or of prior falls, although it is noted that 'she did not lose consciousness'. On this basis, her fall is adjudged 'mechanical' (a common term that commonly betrays a lack of understanding of the approach to falls in frail older adults).

Her daughter, who lives in an apartment in the same building, came with her and said she felt that her mother was not safe to be sent home and would need hospital admission as she could no longer 'check on her all the time'. Just why she feels so stressed is not clear.

On the basis of a urinary tract infection (UTI) and being 'unable to cope', Ada was admitted to hospital late the same evening. Her goals of care were indicated as: 'No code, no ICU, but will accept escalation on the ward'. The pre-admission medications were re-ordered, although the indapamide and perindopril were held in view of her acute kidney injury. A 3-day course of a fluoroquinolone was initiated for the UTI. She was given 'cautious fluid replacement with IV normal

saline' with the serum sodium measured every 4 hours. Two days later, after a repeat ultrasound showed the aneurysm to be 'essentially unchanged', physiotherapy was consulted for mobilisation. The physiotherapist further suggested a consultation to geriatric medicine 'for rehabilitation'.

COMMENT ON THE CASE

Let's start with the obvious. Although what has been done for Ada is not wrong in and of itself, there are multiple errors of omission. As a consequence, her care falls well short of what might be accomplished. To begin, it is not at all clear that she has a UTI, and the record has insufficient information about whether symptoms referable to the lower urinary tract were present, without which antibiotics are not recommended (Nicolle et al., 2019). No attention has been paid to what might have caused the fall, and the label 'mechanical' is unhelpful. Apart from stopping a diuretic (and with it her ACE inhibitor), there has been no discussion of medication changes. The examination does not record whether her blood pressure falls when she stands, making her lightheaded ('symptomatic orthostatic hypotension'), or whether there is evidence of impaired vision, deconditioning, parkinsonism or impaired proprioception. No information has been gathered on the source of the carer daughter's stress, what might be done to mitigate it and how either the stress or its possible mitigation might impact Ada's ability to return home.

Perhaps a shade less obvious is the reasoning behind the note about the 'cautious IV fluid replacement' reflecting an apparent tension between an undocumented but apparently considered need for fluid replacement and the need not to correct the serum sodium level too quickly. It is not clear from the note whether the patient is considered to have had a normal fluid status (i.e. to be 'euvolemic', or for her to be relatively dry or 'hypovolemic') and how this might affect fluid management. (Usually it is of limited relevance in the setting of a patient chronically taking a diuretic, who can have low absolute body sodium but still appear not to be dry, having largely consumed hypotonic fluids (Miller, Tennankore, & Rockwood, 2017).)

Two other points stand out. First, an ultrasound of the aorta has been carried out. It can be argued that the meaning of this is that the team really does not know how to tackle the issues in front of them – that is why essential items in relation to the presentation have not been documented – so instead they default to doing what they know how to do. What they appear not to know is how to have a plan for mobilisation, beyond the desultory 'consult physio' after 2 days. This is important because what happens in the first 2 days can have a determining influence on the patient's course in hospital.

Briefly, people whose mobility improves in the first 48 hours of hospital admission have a low chance of dying within the first 30 days. In one patient series death occurred only in about one in 20 older adults admitted to acute medicine. In contrast, those whose mobility worsened – especially including their ability to move in bed – show a much higher risk of death, about three in four (Hubbard et al., 2011). Early worsening in mobility was more often seen in patients with greater baseline frailty (Hatheway, Mitnitski, & Rockwood, 2017). This pattern did not extend to patients admitted to a cardiovascular intensive care unit (Goldfarb et al., 2018). In the setting of critical illness, early mobilisation is safe (Nydahl et al., 2017) and some evidence supports it lessening cognitive and functional decline (Rengel et al., 2019). However well early mobilisation might work, and it appears to work best as part of a more comprehensive program (Inouye et al., 2000) – failure to observe changes in the first 48 hours can mean the loss of a great deal of useful information. This can include information vital to medical management, such as worsening shortness of breath during aided mobilisation. The false dichotomy between what must be done 'acutely' and what can wait 'for rehab' is as dangerous as it is invidious.

Also to be highlighted is that the goals of care discussion revolved around 'code status'. There is no mention of goals of care that might impact on what the patient needs to get home, save a despairing note from the first day about Ada's daughter being overwhelmed and unable to cope. There is no care plan in the record, beyond observing the effects of the treatments initiated in the emergency department.

The extent to which useful information has not been gathered is revealed in Fig. 41.1, which is the information that can be inferred from the recorded history and physical examination that would inform a Comprehensive Geriatric Assessment. This can be contrasted with Fig. 41.2, which records the results of that assessment. Although it might seem daunting, the information needed in a CGA is essential to designing a care plan that can allow more patients to be alive and in their homes 1 year after treatment (Ellis et al., 2017). Key to this

is incorporating interventions that also are essential in rehabilitation, further illustrating how for patients who are frail, change in function must be interpreted in a way that is alert to it potentially being a sign of illness.

THE CARE PLAN

Fundamentally the goals in healthcare are to avoid premature death, relieve pain and suffering, and improve function. A common take on this in the care of older adults living with frailty is further to 'prevent the preventable, treat the treatable and care for the carer'. This is the point of a care plan, which needs to be the result of an interprofessional collaborative evaluation, done in consultation with the patient and family. That whole process, including its implementation, is known, admittedly somewhat ambiguously, as 'Comprehensive Geriatric Assessment' (see Chapter 2).

The key to a care plan that can actually help an older person living with frailty who is judged likely to be able to recover from their current acute illness is to understand their baseline state. This is a contemporary take on the old joke 'Doctor, will I be able to play the violin after the operation?' – to which the answer is 'That depends, can you play it now?' It appears that the baseline state can be best estimated – including by corroboration – by understanding their cognition, affect, nutrition, mobility, balance, continence and function 2 weeks prior to the acute illness (Jarrett et al., 1995). This is not just a matter of taking at face value what people say, but by cross-classifying their account with what seems clinically plausible. For example, a patient with a right hip flexion contracture who claims to have been walking 2 weeks ago, or a functionally blind patient who says that they were driving (to quote two actual examples), is unlikely to be giving a justifiably true account, no matter what anyone else might say. The point is that arriving at a care plan requires judgement.

Judgement, like any attribute, is normally distributed – reasonable in most cases, gifted in some others and reliably prone to error in others still. As a consequence, the care planning process requires some processes that can accommodate variable judgement. An important source of disagreement can be over the practicality of having the patient 'return to baseline' – a goal that can be either too optimistic or, at times, not nearly optimistic enough. Much to be guarded against is the narrow view that the duty to care is met once the patient has recovered to a baseline that might well be itself remediable (Bergl, 2019).

Most teams have experience which validates the need for an adjudication process when judgements are at odds – otherwise the default is for the loudest or most passive-aggressive person to win out. As such, it is best to be clear about the need for differences in judgements to be resolved at the outset. The real world of developing a care plan must also acknowledge that negotiation is necessary. The menu of what a team can offer to do is not unlimited. In addition to variation in what patients can desire, there is variation in the resources to which teams have access.

Figure 1

Capital Health
Comprehensive Geriatric Assessment Form

Mrs. AC
Age 82

WNL = Within Normal Limits   ASST = Assisted   IND = Independent   DEP = Dependent

○ **Cognition** ☒ WNL   ☐ CIND   ☐ MCI   ☐ Dementia   ☐ Delirium   MMSE: _____   FAST: _____

    Chief lifelong occupation: _____   Education (years): _____

● **Action Required**	
○ **Monitor**	

○ **Emotional**   ☐ WNL   ☐ ↓ Mood   ☐ Depression   ☒ Anxiety   ☐ Fatigue   ☐ Halluncination   ☐ Delusion   ☐ Other

○ **Motivation**   ☐ High   ☐ Usual   ☐ Low   **Health Attitude**   ☐ Excellent   ☐ Good   ☐ Fair   ☐ Poor   ☐ Couldn't say

○ **Communication**   **Speech** ☒ WNL   ☐ Impaired   **Hearing** ☒ WNL   ☐ Impaired   **Vision** ☒ WNL   ☐ Impaired

○ **Strength**   ☐ WNL   ☐ Weak   Upper: PROXIMAL   DISTAL   Lower: PROXIMAL   DISTAL

○ **Exercise**   ☐ Frequent   ☐ Occassional   ☒ Not

Patient contact:
☒ Inpatient
☐ Clinic
☐ GDH
☐ NH
☐ Outreach
☐ Home
☐ Assisted Living
☒ ER
☐ Other

PT = PATIENT
CG = CAREGIVER

		BASELINE (two weeks ago)				CURRENT (today)				NOTES
○ **Balance**	Balance	WNL	Impaired			WNL	(Impaired)			
	Falls	N	Y	Number ____		N	(Y)	Number ____		
○ **Mobility**	Walk Outside	IND		ASST	Can't	IND		ASST	Can't	
	Walking	IND	SLOW	ASST	DEP	IND	SLOW	ASST	DEP	
	Transfers	IND	Stand by	ASST	DEP	IND	Stand by	ASST	DEP	
	Bed	IND	PULL	ASST	DEP	IND	PULL	ASST	DEP	
	Aid	None	Cane	Walker	Chair	None	Cane	Walker	Chair	
○ **Nutrition**	Weight	GOOD	UNDER	OVER	OBESE	STABLE	LOSS	GAIN		
	Appetite	WNL	FAIR	POOR		WNL	FAIR	POOR		
○ **Elimination**	Bowel	CONT	CONSTIP	INCONT		CONT	CONSTIP	INCONT		
	Bladder	CONT	CATHETER	INCONT		CONT	CATHETER	INCONT		
○ **ADLs**	Feeding	IND	ASST	DEP		IND	ASST	DEP		
	Bathing	IND	ASST	DEP		IND	ASST	DEP		
	Dressing	IND	ASST	DEP		IND	ASST	DEP		
	Toileting	IND	ASST	DEP		IND	ASST	DEP		
○ **IADLs**	Cooking	IND	ASST	DEP		IND	ASST	DEP		
	Cleaning	IND	ASST	DEP		IND	ASST	DEP		
	Shopping	IND	ASST	DEP		IND	ASST	DEP		
	Medications	IND	ASST	DEP		IND	ASST	DEP		
	Driving	IND	ASST	DEP		IND	ASST	DEP		
	Banking	IND	ASST	DEP		IND	ASST	DEP		

Current Frailty Score:

Scale	PT	CG
1. Very fit		
2. Well		
3. Well with Rx'd co-morbid disease		
4. Apparently vulnerable		
5. Mildly frail		
6. Moderately frail		
7. Severely frail		
8. Very severely frail		
9a. Terminally ill - walker		
9b. Terminally ill - bed		

○ **Sleep**   ☐ Normal   ☒ Disrupted   ☐ Daytime drowsiness   **Socially Engaged** ☐ Frequent   ☐ Occasional   ☐ Not

○ **Social**

	Lives	**Home**	**Supports**	**Caregiver Relationship**	**Caregiver Stress**
☐ Married					
☐ Divorced	☒ Alone	☐ House (Levels___)	☐ Informal	☐ Spouse	☐ None
☐ Widowed	☐ Spouse	☐ Steps (Number ___)	☐ HCNS	☐ Sibling	☐ Low
☐ Single	☐ Other	☒ Apartment	☐ Other	☒ Offspring daughter	☒ Moderate
		☐ Assisted Living	☐ Req. more support	☐ Other	☐ High
○ **Advance directive**		☐ Nursing home	☐ None		
in place? ☐ Yes ☐ No		☐ Other	○ **Code Status** ☐ Do not resuscitate ☐ Rescuscitate		Caregiver occupation (CG): _____

ACTION REQUIRED (check appropriate circles)

Problems: Med adjust req.   Associated Medication: (*mark meds started in hospital with an asterisk)

#	Problem		Medication
1.	Urinary tract infection	○	IV N Saline 50ml/h
2.	Fall with long lie (CK 122)	○	Norfloxacin
3.	Acute kidney injury	○	Atorvastatin
4.	Hyponatremia 129	○	Metoprolol 25mg BID
5.	Dyslipidemia	○	ASA [Hold]
6.	Ischemic heart disease [Prior MI]	○	Indapamide perindopril [Hold]
7.	Abdominal aortic aneurysm	○	Alendronate once weekly
8.	Peripheral vascular disease	○	Levothyroxine
9.	Anziety	○	
10.	Hypertension	○	
11.	Osteoporosis	○	
12.	Hypothryoidism	○	

Assessor/Physician: _Signature_____   Date: ___Date___

                                                     (YYYY/MM/DD)

FIG. 41.1 Comprehensive Geriatric Assessment Template information available from a medical history and physical examination. The standard 'history and physical exam' pays scant attention to baseline function, but records prior diagnoses, translates 'typical' current symptoms into new diagnoses, including the dubious one of 'urinary tract infection', and lists current medications.

Figure 2

Capital Health
Comprehensive Geriatric Assessment Form

Mrs. AC
Age 82

WNL = Within Normal Limits   ASST = Assisted   IND = Independent   DEP = Dependent

○ **Cognition** ☒ WNL   ☐ CIND   ☐ MCI   ☐ Dementia   ☐ Delirium   MMSE: __27__   FAST: __2__

● Action Required
○ Monitor

Chief lifelong occupation: __Nurse__   Education (years): __14__

● **Emotional**   ☐ WNL   ☐ ↓ Mood   ☐ Depression   ☒ Anxiety   ☐ Fatigue   ☐ Halluncination   ☐ Delusion   ☐ Other

Patient contact:
☒ Inpatient
☐ Clinic
☐ GDH
☐ NH
☐ Outreach
☐ Home
☐ Assisted Living
☐ ER
☐ Other
PT = PATIENT
CG = CAREGIVER

○ **Motivation**   ☐ High   ☒ Usual   ☐ Low   **Health Attitude**   ☐ Excellent   ☒ Good   ☐ Fair   ☐ Poor   ☐ Couldn't say

○ **Communication**   **Speech** ☒ WNL   ☐ Impaired   **Hearing** ☒ WNL   ☐ Impaired   **Vision** ☐ WNL   ☒ Impaired

○ **Strength**   ☐ WNL   ☒ Weak   Upper: PROXIMAL DISTAL   Lower: (PROXIMAL) DISTAL

● **Exercise**   ☐ Frequent   ☐ Occasional   ☒ Not

Current Frailty Score:

Scale	PT	CG
1. Very fit		
2. Well		×
3. Well with Rx'd co-morbid disease		
4. Apparently vulnerable		
5. Mildly frail	×	
6. Moderately frail		
7. Severely frail		
8. Very severely frail		
9a. Terminally ill - walker		
9b. Terminally ill - bed		

BASELINE (two weeks ago) / CURRENT (today) / NOTES

		BASELINE (two weeks ago)				CURRENT (today)				
● **Balance**	Balance	WNL	(Impaired)			WNL	(Impaired)			
	Falls	(N) Y	Number ___			N (Y)	Number 1			
● **Mobility**	Walk Outside	(IND)	ASST	Can't		IND	ASST	(Can't)		Asst x 2 10 meters
	Walking	(IND)	(SLOW) ASST	DEP		IND	SLOW (ASST)	DEP		
	Transfers	(IND)	Stand by ASST	DEP		IND	Stand by (ASST)	DEP		
	Bed	(IND)	PULL ASST	DEP		IND	PULL (ASST)	DEP		
	Aid	None	Cane (Walker)	Chair		None	Cane (Walker)	Chair		
● **Nutrition**	Weight	(GOOD)	UNDER OVER	OBESE		(STABLE)	LOSS	GAIN		
	Appetite	(WNL)	FAIR	POOR		WNL	FAIR	(POOR)		
● **Elimination**	Bowel	CONT	(CONSTIP)	INCONT		CONT	(CONSTIP)	INCONT		
	Bladder	(CONT)	CATHETER	INCONT		CONT	(CATHETER)	INCONT		
● **ADLs**	Feeding	(IND)	ASST	DEP		(IND)	ASST	DEP		
	Bathing	IND	(ASST)	DEP		IND	ASST	(DEP)		
	Dressing	(IND)	ASST	DEP		IND	ASST	(DEP)		
	Toileting	(IND)	ASST	DEP		IND	ASST	(DEP)		
● **IADLs**	Cooking	IND	(ASST)	DEP		IND	ASST	(DEP)		
	Cleaning	IND	(ASST)	DEP		IND	ASST	(DEP)		
	Shopping	IND	ASST	(DEP)		IND	ASST	(DEP)		
	Medications	(IND)	ASST	DEP		IND	ASST	(DEP)		
	Driving	IND	ASST	(DEP)		IND	ASST	(DEP)		
	Banking	IND	ASST	(DEP)		IND	ASST	(DEP)		

● **Sleep**   ☐ Normal   ☒ Disrupted   ☐ Daytime drowsiness   **Socially Engaged** ☒ Frequent   ☐ Occassional   ☐ Not

○ **Social**   ☐ Married   ☐ Divorced   ☒ Widowed   ☐ Single

Lives   ☒ Alone   ☐ Spouse   ☐ Other

Home   ☐ House (Levels ___)   ☐ Steps (Number ___)   ☒ Apartment   ☐ Assisted Living   ☐ Nursing home   ☐ Other

Supports   ☒ Informal   ☐ HCNS   ☐ Other   ☒ Req. more support   ☐ None

Caregiver Relationship   ☐ Spouse   ☐ Sibling   ☒ Offspring daughter   ☐ Other

Caregiver Stress   ☐ None   ☐ Low   ☒ Moderate   ☐ High

○ **Advance directive in place?**   ☐ Yes   ☒ No

○ **Code Status**   ☒ Do not resuscitate   ☐ Rescuscitate

Caregiver occupation (CG): Nurse (also cares for disabled adult daughter)

ACTION REQUIRED (check appropriate circles)

Problems:

Med adjust req. / Associated Medication: (*mark meds started in hospital with an asterisk)

	Problems	Med adjust	Associated Medication
1.	Acute kidney injury Urea 16/Cr101	●	IV N Saline 100ml/h
2.	Hyponatremia (sodium 129)	●	Norfloxacin
3.	Metabolic alkalosis	●	Indapamide perindopril [Hold]
4.	Fall with long lie (CK 1322)	●	Atorvastatin 20mg/day
5.	? UTI	●	Metoprolol 25mg BID [Hold]
6.	Hypertension	●	ASA [Hold]
7.	Symptomatic orthostatic hypotension	●	Alendronate x15 years; once weekly
8.	Dyslipidemia	●	Levothyroxine
9.	Ischemic heart disease (Old MI)	●	Zopiclone 15 mg
10.	Abdominal aortic aneurysm (3.3cm)	●	Lorazepam 1 mg
11.	Peripheral vascular disease	○	
12.	osteoporosis/remote colles	○	
13.	Hypothyroidism	○	
14.	Insomnia	○	
15.	Anxiety	○	
16.	Mild Parkinsonism	○	
17.	Polypharmacy	○	
18.	Cataract	○	

Assessor/Physician: __Signature__   Date: __Date__ (YYYY/MM/DD)

Assessment Forms
CD0184MR_06_09

Page 1 of 1

FIG. 41.2 Comprehensive Geriatric Assessment, now with the information added by the CGA. The latter records information about baseline and current cognition, mental status, motivation and health attitude; specifically assesses special senses and motor functions; and screens for nutrition (asking about baseline and protective factors and current appetite and weight loss), exercise and prior social engagement. New diagnoses have been revealed (parkinsonism, deconditioning with isolated hip flexion weakness, polypharmacy) and a rational approach to the hyponatraemia (despite being clinically euvolemic, the patient's low serum sodium represents an absolute sodium deficit). There is no evidence for a urinary tract infection, so that is no longer a diagnosis and the antibiotic has been stopped. The carer assessment reveals the extent and sources of the daughter's stress, allowing these to be targeted as part of the care plan.

ACTIONABLE INFORMATION ADDED BY A COMPREHENSIVE GERIATRIC ASSESSMENT

With these caveats in mind, it is worth turning again to Fig. 41.2, to explore some examples of how rehabilitation considerations can be built into the initial care plan. Let's be clear: this is in the setting of acute illness and the uncertainty associated with prognosis in older people who are frail.

First, a geriatric assessment reveals a great deal of additional information that will inform a proactive approach to rehabilitation. To begin, the patient's fall is no longer a curiosity, but a matter of inquiry. We should expect – and thereby look for – multiple causes. One, recognised at a glance by several team members, is that Ada has several signs of parkinsonism. This diagnosis, which is new, makes Ada's unsteady gait and postural instability important contributors to her falls, and to her worsening disability. As part of the Comprehensive Geriatric Assessment, lying and standing blood pressures were assessed –'we put the "C" in CGA' is a team refrain). Those measurements revealed that the blood pressure fell 26 points on standing, with symptoms, and without a compensatory increase in the heart rate. Whether this impaired autonomic reflex comes from the metoprolol (which slows the heart rate response), or together with the constipation is part of the newly diagnosed parkinsonism, or both, is not yet clear. The orthostatic hypotension (fall in blood pressure upon standing) itself could also reflect a parkinsonism-related dysautonomia, or be another adverse medication effect – here chronic diuretic use (indapamide) which depletes the patient's fluid status. Although the chronic diuretic use with inadequate fluid replacement could account for the orthostatic hypotension, the hyponatraemia suggests that however fluid was replaced was inadequate. Here, the indapamide and perindopril are each put on hold in the face of the acute kidney injury, and the metoprolol is initially reduced by half. Fluid replacement remains cautious, but the extent of the volume depletion is now better understood; in any case the serum sodium is being checked frequently to guard against overcorrection.

The new diagnosis of parkinsonism helps to explain the predisposition to falls (as does the volume depletion and blunted heart rate response. So too does deconditioning, evidenced here by hip flexor weakness (and arguably the hyponatraemia, reflecting impaired mobility).

In this context, the impetus for rehabilitation includes fixing what has been broken. This patient is not 'naturally' unsteady due to age. Instead, many factors are implicated, including iatrogenic (due to medications) illness. Early mobilisation is now not just part of 'rehab' but part of treatment. Early mobilisation now has a greater chance of success, due to the revelation of parkinsonism impairing gait and movement (here, it will prove to be responsive to dopamine).

Likewise, better mobility and balance offer the prospect of better function including being able to return to greater independence in cooking and cleaning. Knowing that local practice means that a care package is easier to arrange and more comprehensive if it requires weekly assistance with bathing, the team will act accordingly in suggesting goals.

On the basis of some realistic hope of her mother becoming less dependent, the daughter's sense of burden can be addressed. This inquiry reveals that Ada's daughter herself has an adult daughter who has lifelong intellectual disability. Whereas for most of her granddaughter's life Ada had helped provide care, this is no longer the case. With this information, the social worker is also able to explore options for socially engaging activities for Ada's dependent granddaughter. Means of engaging both her mother and her disabled daughter – sometimes together – can offer needed relief.

REHABILITATION ON THE ACUTE CARE WARD AND THE NEED FOR FURTHER INPATIENT REHABILITATION

Given this more optimistic sense of what is achievable, more can be achieved. Even so, there are important issues to be addressed. The daughter's sense of burden will not be alleviated by the hope that things will be better. Some demonstration of this is needed, as is follow-up. Here, the response to dopamine therapy will prove to be persuasive – the daughter will see her mother walk better than she has done in a couple of years. At this point, however, she is still unable to supervise exercise in the home, so admission to a rehabilitation ward is needed. That cannot happen until the fluids are better sorted, which will take a few days.

Those hospital days are risky ones. The same lack of understanding of why the patient fell here is not rare. It translates into hospital routines that increase risk – e.g. deconditioning from failure to mobilise, *Clostridium difficile* diarrhoea from promiscuous prescribing and delirium from inadequate sleep added to everything else. 'Everything else' can include, for example, not routinely checking that a meal tray once delivered is accessible, or food has been eaten. There is no communal dining. The patient is expecting to stay in their pyjamas. 'Ambulation' is felt to be the responsibility of physiotherapy, and 'too risky' for her daughter to help with, even were she available.

Advocacy by the geriatric medicine team is only a partial remedy, so early transfer to a 'restorative care' ward where routine care is less hazardous is arranged. In the interval, the consult team will take responsibility for ongoing management of fluids and electrolytes and medication adjustments. Their calculation is that being on a ward that gives more priority to function, mobility, nutrition and sleep in a patient who is reasonably stable tips the balance in favour of transfer, even if there are ongoing medical issues.

The reality is that functional impairment in older adults who live with frailty reflects not just the need for rehabilitation but the manifestation of acute illness. Here the consulting team and the rehab team are able to accommodate that request, even if the acute care team is not yet there. This circumstance, though far from ideal, is not rare. Further, a pragmatic challenge is that the attitude of acute care teams, which do not understand how to care for acutely ill older people who are functionally impaired as a result of their acute illness, is rarely to reform care. Instead, it can manifest simply as the idea that such patients 'don't belong here'. It is rare to find that the attitude instead is 'we must learn how to provide better care for the full range of people who are acutely ill, including this very common group of older adults with frailty'.

CONCLUSION

How to achieve a responsible attitude to patient mobilisation, cognition, function, nutrition and comfort is a particular challenge for healthcare leadership in the early part of the 21st century. It must be faced. These days are what we soon are likely to refer to as 'the good old days' when it is not the parents of the baby boomers who so challenged healthcare, but the boomers themselves (Statistics Canada, 2011). Making rehabilitation practices part of routine care in which all team members can engage will be an essential part of facing up to frailty. Knowing how to do it, and to do it well, will be an important part of delivering care. Given that there will not be enough geriatricians and specialised interprofessional care teams to provide all such care directly, it is essential that we all act as catalysts in spreading the joy of geriatrics.

SUMMARY POINTS

- Acute decline in function, mobility and balance are not just indications of 'old age', or even 'need for rehabilitation', but of illness
- To know that decline is acute means establishing baseline function as part of routine history taking
- A sensible physical examination of acutely ill older patients must include the evaluation of signs that are associated with acute decline in function, mobility and balance, but that are neglected in the traditional exam. These include assessment of vision and hearing, or orthostatic blood pressure and heart rate change, mobility – gait and for patients who cannot walk, the degree of mobility in bed – balance, muscle tone and lower limb function, especially including the feet
- Especially in patients who cannot get out of bed on their own, how they move in bed offers powerful prognostic information especially in the first 48 hours, or if it changes during the hospital stay
- A patient whose mobility improves in the first 48 hours has a low risk of death within 30 days. For someone whose mobility worsens in the first 48 hours of hospital admission, the risk of dying is much higher

MCQs

Q.1 Regarding mobilisation during acute illness, which one of the following is correct?
  a. Patients should be encouraged to remain in bed until 48 hours have passed
  b. As family members know the patient best, they should decide when mobilisation begins
  c. Early mobilisation is safe and should be encouraged
  d. Family members should not help their relative to mobilise
  e. Patients should not sit out of bed until a physiotherapist has seen them

Q.2 Regarding a patient's baseline level of function, which one of the following is correct:
  a. Information provided by the patient should be corroborated by family or carers where possible
  b. It may be possible to improve beyond that level with adequate diagnosis and rehabilitation
  c. It is best estimated by understanding their cognition, affect, nutrition, mobility, balance, continence and function 2 weeks prior to the acute illness
  d. Acute illness can lead to a rapid and dramatic change from their baseline level of function
  e. All of the above

REFERENCES

Bergl, P. A. (2019). At baseline. *The New England Journal of Medicine, 380*(19), 1792–1793.

Ellis, G., Gardner, M., Tsiachristas, A., Langhorne, P., Burke, O., Harwood, R. H., …, & Shepperd, S. (2017). Comprehensive geriatric assessment for older adults admitted to hospital. *Cochrane Database of Systematic Reviews, 9*, CD006211.

Goldfarb, M., Afilalo, J., Chan, A., Herscovici, R., & Cercek, B. (2018). Early mobility in frail and non-frail older adults admitted to the cardiovascular intensive care unit. *Journal of Critical Care, 47*, 9–14.

Hatheway, O. L., Mitnitski, A., & Rockwood, K. (2017). Frailty affects the initial treatment response and time to recovery of mobility in acutely ill older adults admitted to hospital. *Age Ageing, 46*(6), 920–925.

Hubbard, R. E., Eeles, E. M., Rockwood, M. R., Fallah, N., Ross, E., Mitnitski, A., & Rockwood, K. (2011). Assessing balance and mobility to track illness and recovery in older inpatients. *Journal of General Internal Medicine, 26*(12), 1471–1478.

Inouye, S. K., Bogardus, S. T., Jr., Baker, D. I., Leo-Summers, L., & Cooney, L. M. (2000). The Hospital Elder Life Program: a model of care to prevent cognitive and functional decline in older

hospitalized patients. *Journal of the American Geriatrics Society,*
48(12), 1697–1706.

Jarrett, P. G., Rockwood, K., Carver, D., Stolee, P., & Cosway, S.
(1995). Illness presentation in elderly patients. *Archives of*
Internal Medicine, 155(10), 1060–1064.

Miller, A., Tennankore, K., & Rockwood, K. (2017). Disorders of
water and electrolyte metabolism. In H. Fillit, K. Rockwood, & J.
Young (Eds.), *Brocklehurst's textbook of geriatric medicine & ger-*
ontology, Ch. 82 (8th edn, pp. 681–688). Philadelphia: Elsevier.

Nicolle, L. E., Gupta, K., Bradley, S. F., Colgan, R., DeMuri, G. P.,
Drekonja, D., ..., & Siemieniuk, R. (2019). Clinical practice
guideline for the management of asymptomatic bacteriuria:
2019 update by the Infectious Diseases Society of America.
Clinical Infectious Diseases, 68(10), e83–e110.

Nydahl, P., Sricharoenchai, T., Chandra, S., Kundt, F. S., Huang, M.,
Fischill, M., & Needham, D. M. (2017). Safety of patient mobilization and rehabilitation in the intensive care unit. Systematic
review with meta-analysis. *Annals of the American Thoracic*
Society, 14(5), 766–777.

Rengel, K. F., Hayhurst, C. J., Pandharipande, P. P., & Hughes, C. G.
(2019). Long-term cognitive and functional impairments after
critical illness. *Anesthesia & Analgesia, 128*(4), 772–780.

Statistics Canada. (2011). Generations in Canada. Retrieved from:
https://www12.statcan.gc.ca/census-recensement/2011/as-sa/98-
311-x/98-311-x2011003_2-eng.cfm.

42

Stroke Rehabilitation

Daniel Oh & Joel Stein

LEARNING OBJECTIVES

- Define stroke and the different types of strokes
- List the risk factors for both ischaemic and haemorrhagic strokes
- Discuss factors that affect prognosis in the older person in the setting of a recent stroke
- Explain different interventions used in stroke rehab
- Discuss after-effects of stroke and treatments

CASE

Ahmed is a 75-year-old right-handed man with a history of hypertension, diabetes, paroxysmal atrial fibrillation and current smoking, who presents to the hospital after 2 hours of right arm and leg weakness, right facial droop and slurred speech. On arrival to the hospital, a computed tomography (CT) scan shows no evidence of intracranial bleeding. CT angiography shows an occlusion of the proximal left middle cerebral artery (MCA). He is taken to the endovascular suite where he undergoes mechanical thrombectomy. Several days later, he begins his rehabilitation course using task-oriented training in physical and occupational therapy. Over time, he develops spasticity of his right arm, which does not respond to oral baclofen, but is successfully managed with botulinum toxin injection. He is depressed which initially interferes with his rehabilitation but improves over several weeks after the initiation of a selective serotonin reuptake inhibitor (SSRI) antidepressant. Occupational therapy works with him on his activities of daily living. Speech and language therapists treat the patient for his aphasia. He experiences dysphagia, requiring thickened liquids initially, but resumes a regular diet within several weeks post-stroke.

Three weeks later, he returns home, where he receives physiotherapy, occupational therapy and speech therapy, as well as assistance from a home carer. After several weeks, he begins travelling to a rehabilitation centre where he receives ongoing rehabilitation therapies. Ultimately, he is able to walk independently with a walking stick and ankle-foot orthosis (AFO) but has limited recovery of right arm function. His speech is somewhat halting, but easily understood by others. He is able to live independently in the community with some assistance for shopping, cleaning and cooking.

INTRODUCTION

A stroke is a condition in which blockage of a blood vessel or bleeding within the brain causes damage to the brain with persistent neurological deficits. Ischaemic strokes are the most common, accounting for 88% of strokes and are primarily due to clot formation in an artery that supplies a part of the brain (thrombotic) or clot that travels through the bloodstream to the brain (embolic) (WHO, 2006). Haemorrhagic strokes come in two varieties: intracerebral or subarachnoid. Intracerebral haemorrhages occur within the brain tissue, while subarachnoid haemorrhages are caused by arterial bleeds into the area between two layers covering the brain tissue, called the arachnoid and pia mater. Common causes of haemorrhagic strokes are trauma, abnormalities with blood vessels (vascular) and high blood pressure (hypertension).

There are an estimated 12.6 million individuals living with the after-effects of stroke throughout the world and currently, it is the second leading cause of death (Hachinski et al., 2010; WHO, 2011). The prevalence is particularly high among older individuals with over 66% of hospitalised cases over the age of 65 years. While mortality due to stroke is expected to decline in developed countries, the burden of disability is expected to increase; already, 25% of stroke survivors are left with minor disabilities while 40% experience moderate-to-severe disabilities. This indicates an increasing need for quality stroke rehabilitation and a global effort to prevent strokes.

RISK FACTORS

Some risk factors for stroke are non-modifiable and are shared between ischaemic and haemorrhagic strokes (see Fig. 42.1). These include age, gender, race, family history and personal history of prior stroke. Stroke risk doubles for every decade beyond age 55 years and is more common in men than in women as well as in African Americans and Hispanics than in Caucasians. Additionally, an individual's risk of stroke increases if an immediate family member has had a stroke (Goodman & Fuller, 2009).

Among the modifiable risk factors, hypertension is the most important for both ischaemic and haemorrhagic strokes, with about 30% of adults having hypertension, doubling the

	Ischaemic	Both	Haemorrhagic
Non-modifiable	Genetics Systemic diseases (sickle cell anaemia, cancer, etc.)	> Age 55 years (increases with every decade of life) Male gender African-Americans/Hispanics Immediate family member with stroke	Asian Chronic kidney disease Cerebral amyloid angiopathy
Modifiable	Heart disease (atrial fibrillation, atrial cardiopathy, heart failure, etc.) Diabetes Carotid stenosis Dyslipidaemia Smoking Smoking with oral contraceptives Diet/nutrition Obesity Sedentary behavior Metabolic syndrome Sleep apnea Drugs (cocaine, heroin, amphetamines, MDMA) Inflammation/infection	Hypertension	Smoking Excessive alcohol consumption Aneurysm Anticoagulation Antiplatelet agent Sympathomimetic drugs (cocaine, heroin, amphetamine, PPA, ephedrine)

(Data from An et al., 2017; Boehme et al., 2018)

FIG. 42.1   Risk factors for stroke.

risk of stroke (Mackay & Mensah, 2004). Hypertension accounts for up to 54% of all strokes (Lawes, Vander Hoorn, & Rodgers, 2008). Other risk factors for ischaemic strokes include smoking, diet, sedentary lifestyle, hyperlipidaemia, diabetes, alcohol consumption and cardiac disease (Boehme, Esenwa, & Elkind, 2017). Other risk factors for haemorrhagic strokes are smoking, excessive alcohol consumption, certain drugs, presence of aneurysm (an abnormal outpouching of an arterial wall) and cerebral amyloid angiopathy where amyloid protein is deposited in medium-sized blood vessels in the brain, causing the blood vessels to become fragile and at increased risk for brain bleeds (An, Kim, & Yoon, 2017). Cardiac disease may include congestive heart failure and coronary artery disease, which increase the risk of ischaemic stroke twofold. Valvular heart diseases, such as valvular atrial fibrillation, increase the risk of ischaemic stroke fivefold. There are many other risk factors for ischaemic strokes, including diabetes, carotid artery stenosis (narrowing), combination of smoking and oral contraceptive use, sleep apnoea and systemic diseases that are associated with a propensity to form blood clots (sickle cell anaemia, cancer, etc.).

It is important to keep in mind that many of these risk factors are more common in older people. These include hypertension, cerebral amyloid angiopathy, heart failure, coronary artery disease and atrial fibrillation, helping to account for the increased prevalence of strokes in this population.

SIGNS AND SYMPTOMS

Signs and symptoms of a stroke include weakness or altered sensation of the face, arm and/or leg, headache, vision changes (visual field loss, blurriness), confusion, dizziness and slurred speech (Sullivan et al., 2004; WHO, 2006). Other notable symptoms include aphasia, which is the inability to understand and/or produce speech, as well as dysphagia or difficulty with swallowing. In right-sided strokes, patients can develop hemineglect syndrome in which they are unaware of items to their left side. Development of these signs or symptoms requires immediate medical attention. Other symptoms may include headache, vertigo or seizure.

INITIAL MANAGEMENT

If the stroke is ischaemic, blood supply may be restored through a thrombolytic agent (i.e. 'clot-busting' treatment) such as tissue plasminogen activator (tPA); however, this treatment has only been demonstrated to improve outcomes if administered within the first 4.5 hours of the event. Only a small percentage of patients actually receive tPA (generally 10% or less), due to certain criteria that must be met. Notably, tPA cannot be given in patients with a propensity for or presence of body or brain haemorrhage; if there has been recent neurosurgery, trauma or stroke; when there is uncontrolled hypertension; in the presence of brain tumours or aneurysm; and abnormal blood glucose. There are other precautionary factors as well, which are not covered here. If a patient has an acute ischaemic stroke caused by an occlusion of a large artery and has symptom onset within 24 hours, they may be a candidate for mechanical thrombectomy, regardless of whether they received a thrombolytic agent. Mechanical thrombectomy is an interventional procedure that is performed by a specialist to carefully remove the clot blocking the blood vessel via a catheter threaded through the blood vessels, thus restoring blood flow. The time window for thrombectomy is longer than for tPA, and the upper time limit has not been clearly defined. The presence of brain tissue that is at risk for death, but remains alive and salvageable, is the most important criteria for deciding whether this therapy may be appropriate. For those with an ischaemic stroke who do not receive thrombolysis or thrombectomy, aspirin (sometimes combined with clopidogrel) is the main initial medical treatment.

DIAGNOSIS

In most developed countries, definitive diagnosis of stroke is often made with CT or magnetic resonance imaging (MRI) scan. CT is used more commonly than MRI, as CT is generally more available, faster to acquire and less expensive than MRI (Calautti & Jean-Claude, 2003). Both CT and MRI can provide information about areas of infarction or haemorrhage (Kidwell et al., 2004). Echocardiography may be used to identify the cardiac origin of a blood clot responsible for an ischaemic event (Gunaratne, 2012). Carotid duplex scans can evaluate for carotid stenosis or occlusion, and angiography (typically CT or MRI) can delineate the vascular structure and reasons for a stroke or cerebral haemorrhage.

PROGNOSIS

Functional recovery is largely dependent on the severity of the stroke. Patients with mild strokes, such as someone with mild clumsiness of the hand as their only symptom, may have minimal permanent damage to the brain, and may essentially fully recover. Conversely, larger strokes, such as from a blockage of the left MCA, may cause complete paralysis of the right side, and often the inability to speak or understand speech. These more severe strokes tend to have a less positive prognosis overall, and a particularly poor prognosis for return of full use of the affected upper extremity. The chance of recovery declines if it takes longer for the patient to make functional gains, or to regain active hand motion (Kwakkel, van Dijk, & Wagenaar, 2000). Post-stroke recovery is dependent on intact areas of the brain that control related functions and may take over the lost function to some degree.

Impaired motor function after a stroke may lead to long-term disability. Early return of motor function is a good prognostic indicator of future functional improvement. Regaining voluntary shoulder and finger movements within 7 days of a stroke is associated with a good return of arm function (Nijland et al., 2010). Return of leg strength within 1 week is a good predictor of return to independent walking (Stinear, 2010). A study conducted in the Netherlands (Kwakkel et al., 2000) found that at 5 weeks post stroke, physiotherapists and occupational therapists are able to accurately predict a patient's walking ability and manual dexterity at 6 months post stroke.

There are many other factors that will affect a patient's outcome after stroke, including the presence of conditions such as hypertension, diabetes and obesity. The presence of cognitive or perceptual deficits may limit understanding of directions, negatively affecting a patient's motivation or insight into the deficits of the stroke. None of these factors preclude a good outcome, but they may increase the time it takes a patient to demonstrate functional improvement during rehabilitation.

Another factor that greatly affects prognosis is whether or not the patient will be given the opportunity to participate in a high-quality rehabilitation programme. The World Health Organization (WHO) and the World Stroke Organization both recommend rehabilitation services at a centre that specialises in the treatment of stroke (Hachinski et al., 2010; WHO, 2006). The interventions that may be used to promote recovery are discussed below.

In addition to the above, there are several considerations when an older person sustains a stroke. Muscle mass decreases with age, and this progressive decline in muscle size and strength is known as sarcopenia. Strokes resulting in weakness can further predispose patients to exacerbation of sarcopenia through a combination of factors, especially hemiparesis (weakness of one side of the body) and sedentary behaviour (Scherbakov & Doehner, 2011). Similarly, bone density decreases as people age, and can lead to osteopenia and osteoporosis. Hemiparetic strokes may cause or exacerbate osteoporosis. A further complication is that patients with strokes are at increased risk of falls due to motor, sensory and visual/perceptual deficits, ultimately leading to increased prevalence of hip fractures in this population (Poole, Reeve, & Warburton, 2002). As one ages, there are structural and functional changes in the brain that correlate with age-related cognitive changes; however, age-associated diseases, such as stroke, may further accelerate this process, contributing to cognitive decline.

There are also non-physical/non-cognitive implications of stroke that are not necessarily unique to the older person, but are accentuated in this population. For example, older people are already predisposed to social isolation and depression, while sustaining a stroke may leave a patient with even less social contact given physical/cognitive limitations thus increasing the risk for depression.

IMPAIRMENTS

Several impairments and functional limitations may occur after a stroke. Weakness involving the upper or lower extremity, or both, is one of the most common impairments that may need to be addressed by occupational therapists and physiotherapists. Patients may also experience sensory loss or altered sensation in the area of the body affected by the stroke. Other common impairments include decreased balance, visual and perceptual deficits, impaired cognition, impaired communication, decreased coordination, increased tone and spasticity (a condition characterised by involuntary muscle activation and stiffness), decreased motor control and impaired swallowing. These problems often lead to functional limitations such as difficulty moving in bed, transfers (change in position, such as rising to the standing position from sitting), walking and performing activities of daily living (ADLs) or self-care activities, especially those that require the use of both arms (e.g. dressing and bathing). Improving physical function plays an important role in quality of life after a stroke. Duncan et al. (2003) found that decreased physical abilities have the greatest effect on quality of life after stroke. Loss of hand function is reported as the most disabling.

The large spectrum of possible impairments in body structure or function, activity limitations and participation restrictions is the reason an interdisciplinary team approach that includes physiotherapists and occupational therapists, speech therapists, physicians, nurses and other health professions is crucial to the rehabilitation approach.

INTERVENTIONS

Historically, one of the more commonly used physiotherapy treatment approaches for post-stroke rehabilitation was the Bobath approach, also known as neurodevelopmental technique (NDT). This approach focuses on encouraging or facilitating normal movements and preventing abnormal movements. Other stroke physiotherapy methods have included proprioceptive neuromuscular facilitation, a stretching technique that relies on intact reflexes to improve muscle stretch, as well as approaches developed by Brunnstrom, Rood, Johnstone, and Ayres (O'Sullivan & Schmitz, 2007). Little empiric evidence supports the efficacy of any of these traditional physiotherapy techniques, however, and more contemporary therapy has focused more on practicing the functional tasks needed for the patient to regain independence.

Stroke rehabilitation can be broadly divided into two fundamental strategies: compensation and recovery. Compensation focuses on using existing motor abilities to accomplish mobility and ADL tasks in order to achieve independence. Examples include one-handed dressing techniques, or the use of a walking stick (see Fig. 42.2) or leg brace such as an AFO (see Fig. 42.3) to enhance walking. Conversely, recovery is the restoration or partial restoration of the underlying neurological disabilities. Considerable recovery occurs spontaneously after stroke. Contemporary stroke rehabilitation endeavours to maximise recovery by harnessing neuroplasticity (the ability of the brain to form and reorganise neural connections), as well as addressing functional deficits through compensatory techniques.

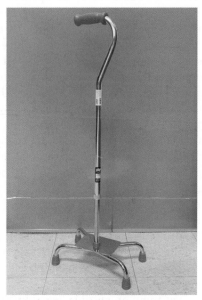

FIG. 42.2 Four-pronged walking stick. This is commonly used in those who suffer a stroke and have difficulty with ambulation.

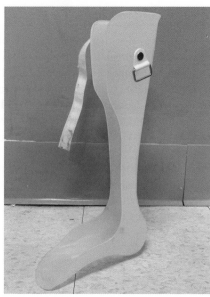

FIG. 42.3 Custom plastic solid ankle-foot orthosis (AFO). This is the most commonly prescribed AFO for foot drop.

One important factor in promoting neuroplasticity and recovery is making the rehabilitation activities salient, specific and functional. The activities need to have enough intensity and repetition to promote learning (Kleim & Jones, 2008). One such approach is the task-oriented approach which is based on the concept that learning is goal-oriented (Gordon, 2000). This typically involves real-life tasks (such as walking) with the intention of acquiring or reacquiring a skill. The tasks should be challenging, progressively adaptive and involve active participation. It differs from repetitive training in that the end goal is acquiring a skill, and not dividing a task into component parts.

While the primary motor deficit after stroke is typically decreased motor control, reduced strength also contributes to disability. Strength training has been shown to be a useful component of post-stroke rehabilitation (Canning et al., 2004; Forrester, Wheaton, & Luft, 2008; Morris, Dodd, & Morris, 2004; Patten, Lexell, & Brown, 2004). Several studies have demonstrated functional improvements in patients who participated in both strength training and task-oriented functional training (Jørgensen et al., 2010; Morris et al., 2004; Patten et al., 2006). There is no evidence that strength training adversely affects spasticity (Patten et al., 2004).

Electrical Stimulation

Modalities that are frequently used in stroke rehabilitation include neuromuscular electrical stimulation (NMES). NMES can be used to enhance the recovery of motor function, or to partially replace a lost functional ability (a neuroprosthesis). For example, a stroke survivor may experience persistent weakness when dorsiflexing the ankle (raising the foot upwards), often known as 'foot drop'. This can cause the foot to drag when walking, risking tripping and falls. An NMES system (such as the Bioness L300, or the Walkaide device) may be used to stimulate the nerve that supplies the muscles that lift up the ankle and improve walking as an alternative to an AFO. A multicentre randomised controlled trial showed similar improvement in gait speed and other functional outcomes when comparing NMES to AFO (Kluding et al., 2013), with some patients preferring the NMES devices.

NMES is also used for the arms, with the Bioness H300 as one example. These are primarily intended to enhance recovery of motor function. Additionally, there is strong evidence to support the use of NMES to decrease inferior subluxation (partial dislocation) of the glenohumeral joint in the shoulder and to increase shoulder external rotation passive range of motion (Van Peppen, Kwakkel, & Wood-Dauphinee, 2004).

Constraint-Induced Therapy

Achieving motor recovery of a weakened upper limb is challenging in many individuals after stroke. Constraint-induced therapy (CIT), also known as constraint-induced movement therapy or forced use, has been shown to be helpful in this goal. A constraining device such as a sling or mitt is applied to the other (non-paretic) arm to promote increased use of the weak arm (Mark & Taub, 2002). This is paired with 'massed practice' of functional activities and other exercises with the paretic arm, and restraint of the non-paretic arm for a target of 90% of waking hours (Mark & Taub, 2002). CIT has been most successful with patients who have some ability to extend the affected wrist and fingers (Lin et al., 2010; Mark & Taub, 2002), and has even been found beneficial in patients who are in the chronic phase of post-stroke (Wolf et al., 2006).

Locomotor Training

Despite some encouraging preliminary studies, bodyweight-supported treadmill training (also called locomotor training) was not found useful for improving gait in a large randomised trial (Duncan et al., 2011). Other techniques being explored include the use of robotic training to improve gait and upper extremity motor control (Frick & Alberts, 2006; Lum et al., 2002; Stein et al., 2004)(see Fig. 42.4) and virtual reality. Some interventions, such as mirror therapy (Yavuzer et al., 2008) and aquatic therapy (Chon, Oh, & Shim, 2009), require less technology and have recent research supporting

their use. These are promising approaches but are not yet standard of care for stroke rehabilitation.

Spasticity and Pain

Another common complication of stroke is spasticity, an abnormal increase in muscle activity and stiffness. Spasticity can interfere with positioning, use of a brace, mobility, ADLs, and hygiene, as well as cause discomfort. Oral medications, such as baclofen or tizanidine, are of limited value in stroke survivors, as the sedating side effects of these medications often limit the ability to achieve an effective dose. Local muscle injections with botulinum toxins can be quite effective, but typically need to be repeated every few months. Despite the widespread use of splinting, there is limited evidence to support the effectiveness of this approach. Stretching and passive range of motion exercises should be a component of management in most cases.

Shoulder pain is common after stroke, and often associated with shoulder subluxation. Treatment includes positioning of the upper limb, including the use of slings when necessary, as well as NMES or injections in selected cases.

Communication and Swallowing

Speech therapists will also work with a patient who suffered a stroke when there are impairments of speech, language, cognition, communication and/or swallowing. Aphasia therapy is an important component for affected patients and should include caregiver training to support practice outside of formal therapy sessions. Dysphagia is commonly managed with alterations in diet consistency initially, and often gradually resolves. In more severe cases of dysphagia, feeding tubes may be needed temporarily, or in rare cases, for the long term. Both topics are covered in more detail in the next chapter.

CONCLUSION

Stroke is a global problem that can result in a multitude of impairments and functional limitations. Improvement of healthcare and public awareness of the importance of reducing risk factors may help to decrease the incidence and severity of

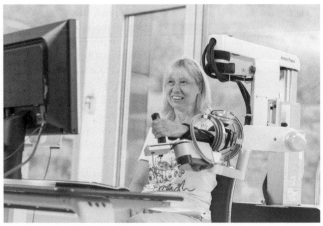

FIG. 42.4   Armeo®Power robotic upper limb device. Picture: Hocoma, Switzerland. Reprinted from Hocoma's website. Permission obtained on April 28, 2019.

this condition and decrease the global burden of this non-communicable disease. There are currently many types of physiotherapy interventions used to improve the functional abilities of patients after a stroke. More randomised, controlled clinical research is needed in this area to help therapists make informed decisions about which interventions are most appropriate for each patient.

SUMMARY POINTS

- Stroke can be ischaemic or haemorrhagic and is characterised by sudden neurological impairment (weakness, sensory loss, facial droop, etc.) lasting more than 24 hours
- Hypertension is the most important modifiable risk factor for both types of strokes
- An older person who sustains a stroke is more predisposed to sarcopenia, osteopenia/osteoporosis, cognitive decline, social isolation and depression than a younger person
- Stroke rehabilitation can be divided into two fundamental strategies: compensation and recovery
- There are many modalities that can aid with post-stroke recovery (i.e. NMES, CIT, task-oriented approach) and with management of after-effects (i.e. AFO, cane, walker, NMES, medications/injections)

MCQs

Q.1 A 75-year-old man had a stroke and is now with left arm and leg weakness. Which intervention is the least likely to be useful in improving functionality?
  a. Constraint-induced therapy
  b. Bodyweight-supported treadmill training
  c. Mirror therapy
  d. Strength training

Q.2 An 83-year-old man with hypertension, diabetes, excessive alcohol consumption, smoking and sedentary lifestyle sustained an acute ischaemic stroke. What modifiable risk factor is most strongly associated with increased risk of ischaemic stroke?
  a. Smoking
  b. Diabetes
  c. Age
  d. Hypertension

Q.3 A 73-year-old woman sustained a stroke a year ago and presents in clinic with spasticity of her left leg, including her foot. Which one of the following is least likely to aid with this patient's spasticity management?
  a. Stretching
  b. Passive range of motion
  c. Oral baclofen
  d. Botox injection

REFERENCES

An, S. J., Kim, T. J., & Yoon, B. W. (2017). Epidemiology, risk factors, and clinical features of intracerebral hemorrhage: an update. *Journal of Stroke, 19*, 3–10.

Boehme, A., Esenwa, C., & Elkind, M. (2017). Stroke risk factors, genetics, and prevention. *Circulation Research, 120*, 472–495.

Calautti, C., & Jean-Claude, B. (2003). Functional recovery after stroke in adults. *Stroke, 34*, 1553–1575.

Canning, C. G., Ada, L., Adams, R., & O'Dwyer, N. J. (2004). Loss of strength contributes more to physical disability after a stroke than loss of dexterity. *Clinical Rehabilitation, 18*, 300–308.

Chon, S. C., Oh, D. W., & Shim, J. H. (2009). Watsu approach for improving spasticity and ambulatory function in hemiparetic patients with stroke. *Physiotherapy Research International, 14*(2), 128–136.

Duncan, P. W., Bode, R. K., Min Lai, S., & Perera, S. (2003). Rasch analysis of a new stroke-specific outcome scale: the Stroke Impact Scale. *Archives of Physical Medicine and Rehabilitation, 84*(7), 950–963.

Duncan, P. W., Sullivan, K., Behrman, A., Azen, S., Wu, S., Nadeau, S., …, & Hayden, S. (2011). Body-weight-supported treadmill rehabilitation after stroke. *New England Journal of Medicine, 364*, 2026–2036.

Forrester, L. W., Wheaton, L. A., & Luft, A. R. (2008). Exercise-mediated locomotor recovery and lower-limb neuroplasticity after stroke. *The Journal of Rehabilitation Research and Development, 45*(2), 205–220.

Frick, E. M., & Alberts, J. L. (2006). Combined use of repetitive task practice and an assistive robotic device in a patient with subacute stroke. *Physical Therapy, 86*(10), 1378–1386.

Goodman, C. C., & Fuller, K. (2009). *Pathology: implications for the physical therapist* (3rd edn.). St Louis, MO: WB Saunders.

Gordon, J. (2000). *Assumptions underlying physical therapy intervention: theoretical and historical perspectives*. New York: Aspen Publishers Inc.

Gunaratne, P. S. (2012). *Stroke care*. Colombo, Sri Lanka: S Godage & Brothers (Pvt) Ltd.

Hachinski, V., Donnan, G. A., Gorelick, P. B., Hacke, W., Cramer, S. C., Kaste, M., …, & Tuomilehto, J. (2010). Stroke: working toward a prioritized world agenda. *International Journal of Stroke, 5*(4), 238–256.

Jørgensen, J. R., Bech-Pedersen, D. T., Zeeman, P., Sørensen, J., Andersen, L. L., & Schönberger, M. (2010). Effect of intensive outpatient physical training on gait performance and cardiovascular health in people with hemiparesis after stroke. *Physical Therapy, 90*, 527–537.

Kidwell, C. S., Chalela, J. A., Saver, J. L., Starkman, S., Hill, M. D., Demchuk, A. M., …, & Warach, S. (2004). Comparison of MRI and CT for detection of acute intracerebral hemorrhage. *JAMA, 292*(15), 1823–1830.

Kleim, J. A., & Jones, T. A. (2008). Principles of experience-dependent neural plasticity: implications for rehabilitation after brain damage. *Journal of Speech Language and Hearing Research, 51*, S225–S239.

Kluding, P., Dunning, K., O'Dell, M., Wu, S., Ginosian, J., Feld, J., & McBride, K. (2013). Foot drop stimulation versus ankle foot orthosis after stroke: 30-week outcomes. *Stroke, 44*, 1660–1669.

Kwakkel, G., van Dijk, G. M., & Wagenaar, R. C. (2000). Accuracy of physical and occupational therapists' early predictions of recovery after severe middle cerebral artery stroke. *Clinical Rehabilitation, 14*, 28–41.

Lawes, C. M. M., Vander Hoorn, S., & Rodgers, A. (2008). Global burden of blood-pressure-related disease, 2001. *Lancet, 371*, 1513–1516.

Lin, K. C., Chung, H. Y., Wu, C. Y., Liu, H. L., Hsieh, Y. W., Chen, I. H., …, & Wai, Y. Y. (2010). Constraint-induced therapy versus control intervention in patients with stroke: a functional magnetic resonance imaging study. *American Journal of Physical Medicine and Rehabilitation, 89*, 177–185.

Lum, P. S., Burgar, C. G., Shor, P. C., Majmundar, M., & Van der Loos, M. (2002). Robot-assisted movement training compared with conventional therapy techniques for the rehabilitation of upper-limb motor function after stroke. *Archives of Physical Medicine and Rehabilitation, 83*(7), 952–959.

Mackay, J., & Mensah, G. (2004). *The atlas of heart disease and stroke*. Geneva, Switzerland: WHO Press.

Mark, V. W., & Taub, E. (2002). Constraint-induced movement therapy for chronic stroke hemiparesis and other disabilities. *Restorative Neurology and Neuroscience, 22*, 317–336.

Morris, S. L., Dodd, K. J., & Morris, M. E. (2004). Outcomes of progressive resistance strength training following stroke: a systematic review. *Clinical Rehabilitation, 18*, 27–39.

Nijland, R. H., van Wegen, E. E., Harmeling-van der Wel, B. C., & Kwakkel, G. (2010). Presence of finger extension and shoulder abduction with 72 hours after stroke predicts functional recovery: early prediction of functional outcome after stroke: the EPOS cohort study. *Stroke, 41*, 745–750.

O'Sullivan, S. B., & Schmitz, T. J. (2007). Stroke. In *Physical rehabilitation* (5th edn.). Philadelphia, PA: FA Davis Company.

Patten, C., Dozono, J., Schmidt, S. G., Jue, M., & Lum, P. (2006). Combined functional task practice and dynamic high intensity resistance training promotes recovery of upper extremity motor function in post-stroke hemiparesis: a case study. *Journal of Neurologic Physical Therapy, 30*(3), 99–115.

Patten, C., Lexell, J., & Brown, H. E. (2004). Weakness and strength training in persons with poststroke hemiplegia: rationale, method and efficacy. *The Journal of Rehabilitation Research and Development, 41*, 293–312.

Poole, K., Reeve, J., & Warburton, E. (2002). Falls, fractures, and osteoporosis after stroke: time to think about protection? *Stroke, 33*, 1432–1436.

Scherbakov, N., & Doehner, W. (2011). Sarcopenia in stroke – facts and numbers on muscle loss accounting for disability after stroke. *Journal of Cachexia, Sarcopenia and Muscle, 2*, 5–8.

Stein, J., Krebs, H. I., Frontera, W. R., Fasoli, S. E., Hughes, R., & Hogan, N. (2004). Comparison of two techniques of robot-aided upper limb exercise training. *American Journal of Physical Medicine & Rehabilitation, 83*(9), 720–728.

Stinear, C. (2010). Prediction of motor recovery after stroke. *Lancet Neurology, 9*, 1228–1232.

Sullivan, K. J., Hershberg, J., Howard, R., & Fisher, B. (2004). Neurologic differential diagnosis for physical therapy. *Journal of Neurologic Physical Therapy, 28*(4), 162–168.

Van Peppen, R. P. S., Kwakkel, G., Wood-Dauphinee, S., Hendriks, H. J. M., Van der Wees, P. J., & Dekker, J. (2004). The impact of physical therapy on functional outcomes after stroke: what's the evidence? *Clinical Rehabilitation, 18*, 833–862.

WHO (World Health Organization). (2006). *WHO STEPS stroke manual: the WHO STEPwise approach to stroke surveillance*. Geneva, Switzerland.

WHO (World Health Organization) Media Centre. (2011). *The 10 leading causes of death by broad income group*. Geneva, Switzerland.

Wolf, S. L., Winstein, C. J., Miller, J. P., Taub, E., Uswatte, G., Morris, D., Giuliani, C., Light, K. E., & Nichols-Larsen, D. (2006). Effect of constraint-induced movement therapy on upper extremity function 3 to 9 months after stroke. *JAMA, 296*(17), 2095–2104.

Yavuzer, G., Selles, R., Sezer, N., Sütbeyaz, S., Bussmann, J. B., Köseoğlu, F., Atay, M. B., & Stam, H. J. (2008). Mirror therapy improves hand function in subacute stroke: a randomized controlled trial. *Archives of Physical Medicine and Rehabilitation, 89*, 393–398.

43

Speech and Swallow Rehabilitation After Stroke

Fiona Craven

LEARNING OBJECTIVES

- Describe communication and swallowing difficulties that can result from a stroke
- Describe some common treatment approaches for working with impairments of communication and swallowing following a stroke
- Identify specific communication support strategies to use with a person following a stroke

INTRODUCTION

About one third of people will experience communication difficulty after a stroke. Swallow impairments can occur in up to 80% of patients, most commonly in the initial phases of stroke recovery (Martino et al., 2005). Both communication and swallowing difficulties can resolve or reduce in severity with spontaneous recovery as well as with access to specialised speech and language therapy.

The type of communication and/or swallow difficulties that a person may experience following a stroke can be influenced by a variety of factors. The largest determinants are the type of stroke (i.e. haemorrhagic versus infarct), the location of the stroke and the extent of the damage. Other factors such as age, the person's overall health and their prior level of functioning will also impact.

COMMUNICATION IMPAIRMENTS FOLLOWING STROKE

Aphasia

Aphasia (also referred to as dysphasia) is the term given to language difficulties following damage to the brain. In the majority of the population, language is controlled by the brain's left hemisphere; therefore a stroke in this part of the brain frequently results in aphasia (Teasell & Hussan, 2013).

Aphasia can affect some or all of the components of language: receptive language (comprehension/understanding), expression (word finding and the ability to create sentences), reading, writing and the use of gestures. Difficulties can range from mild to severe. These difficulties can impact everyday activities and functioning in a variety of ways (see Fig. 43.1). The severity of the impairment and the impact it may have

on the person's functioning and well-being are not always directly correlated. For example, a person may have mild word-finding difficulties. This may present barriers to conversations at work or with their family and impact on how they participate in everyday life. In another person, these same mild word finding difficulties may be less of a barrier to communicating.

CASE 1

Tom is an 80-year-old man who had a left hemisphere stroke 2 weeks ago, resulting in difficulty talking and forming sentences. Assessment with the speech and language therapist (SLT) indicated a moderate to severe receptive and expressive aphasia. Tom can follow single commands but has difficulty understanding longer pieces of information. He can make some sounds and say 'hello' but he cannot say other functional words. Tom can read and understand single written words. He can write his name and copy words. He appears frustrated and is withdrawing from conversations with his family and the medical team.

The International Classification of Functioning, Disability and Health: ICF (WHO, 2001) is a useful framework to use when working with a person with aphasia. This is discussed in Chapter 15 and has been adapted specifically for working with people with aphasia as outlined below.

It is important to recognise that the impact of a language difficulty extends beyond the disruption of language alone. It impacts on how we communicate with the world around us, how we participate in life and how we feel and express ourselves on a day-to-day basis.

Therapy aims to address issues at all levels of the ICF framework. Therapy may target the underlying language

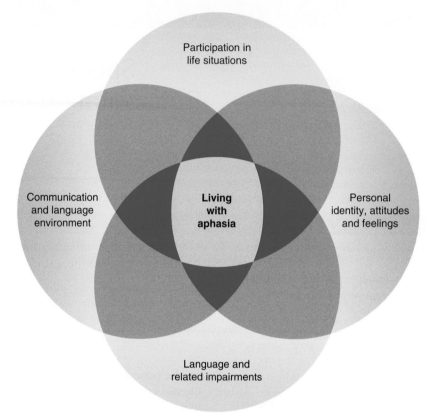

FIG. 43.1 Living with aphasia. (Adapted from Kagan et al., 2008, C. Aphasia Institute, with permission.)

difficulty, and/or aim to maximise participation in everyday conversations and interactions. It may also focus on supporting the person to express themselves and their emotions in the context of reduced language abilities. It is likely that therapy goals will straddle all these levels. Rehabilitation will require different intervention approaches depending on the communication impairment and the specific goals of the individual. For example, the person may want to communicate clearly on the phone, write a shopping list, ask their doctor about their medications or express their opinion about a news item.

Aphasia therapy focuses on:
- Helping the person to use remaining communication abilities
- Restoring language abilities as much as possible
- Compensating for language difficulties and using strategies
- Using other methods apart from speech to communicate
- Educating and coaching others (family and team members) to use strategies that support the person in understanding and communicating within conversations.

Table 43.1 details the different treatment approaches. Strategies to support someone with aphasia or communication difficulties after a stroke are outlined in Appendix 1.

CASE 1 Continued

The SLT meets with Tom and his family to set the goals for therapy.

Impairment-based exercises help Tom improve his reading, writing and understanding of words and sentences. Speech drills help Tom say functional words. A picture communication aid is provided for Tom to use when he needs to ask for something; for example, when asking for a family member or when requesting the toilet.

The SLT advises and works with Tom's family and the medical team to identify strategies that support Tom to communicate. For example, by writing down single words for Tom to read and point to he can indicate his choices and discuss issues related to his care needs. Rating scales help him to indicate his mood and levels of pain.

With this support, Tom becomes more engaged in conversations and social interactions with his family and members of the multidisciplinary team (MDT). He can take an active role in decision making and engaging with his overall rehab plan.

Cognitive Communication Deficits

Cognitive and social skills play an important role in effective communication. Attention, memory, problem solving, reasoning and organisation all impact communication. A stroke can interfere with these skills (see Table 43.2). The person may be able to use words and sentences; however, the way they communicate can be different. For example, they may talk lots but have trouble sticking to the topic or knowing when to stop talking. They may have difficulty with abstract language such as understanding jokes or metaphors. These difficulties can cause frustration and/or

TABLE 43.1 Treatment approaches for aphasia.

TREATMENT APPROACH	EXAMPLES
Impairment-based language therapy	- **Word-finding and word retrieval therapy**, e.g. helping the person name things by describing it or by giving them the starting letter - **Therapy that focuses on syntax** (grammar) and constructing grammatically accurate sentences - Therapy tasks that work on **improving the person's reading and/or writing abilities**
Functional communication therapy	- **Total communication** where the person with aphasia is encouraged to use gesture, facial expression and/or drawing to aid their verbal communication - In some cases **using a communication aid** can be helpful. This can be a picture or alphabet chart, or a computer-based system. This is known as augmentative and alternative communication (AAC) - **Script training** where the person with aphasia regularly practises and relearns vocabulary and sentences related to a topic of their interest, e.g. related to their favourite hobby
Psychosocial therapy	- Therapy that addresses the **psychosocial impact of aphasia** on the person, e.g. exploring how the person sees and expresses themselves in the context of language difficulties as well as supporting the person to explore and express their identity. This may be done in conjunction with a counsellor or psychologist. It may be carried out individually or with input from family or close friends
Family education	- **Conversation partner training** where key conversation partners (e.g. family members) are trained in strategies to help facilitate communication. This may involve verbal and non-verbal strategies, e.g. talking slowly and paying attention to the person's gesture and/or body language

TABLE 43.2 Cognitive communication difficulties.

AREA OF DIFFICULTY	EFFECT
Attention	Difficulties attending to and concentrating in conversation. They may be easily distracted or not able to follow conversation, especially where there is more than one person talking
Memory	Difficulties recalling information or events, especially recent events
Organisation	Difficulties putting information together or telling a story in a logical, well-sequenced manner
Perception	Difficulties reading words on one side of the page
Reasoning and problem solving	Difficulties solving a problem or discussing appropriate solutions
Social communication	Difficulties knowing when to take turns in the conversation, e.g. talking too much or continually talking about the same topics
Humour and sarcasm	Difficulty interpreting jokes or judging when someone is being sarcastic. They might be very literal in their interpretations and struggle with abstract language
Prosody	Their speech may sound unnatural and may be faster or slower than usual or lack natural intonation
Insight	The person may have difficulties recognising changes with their communication
Fatigue	This is extremely common after a stroke and can have a major impact on the person's ability to engage in conversations

embarrassment for the person and their communication partners.

Dysarthria

Dysarthria is a speech impairment resulting from weakness in the muscles involved in speech. It can affect any of the five subsystems used to control speech: respiration, phonation, articulation, resonance and prosody. It can range in severity (mild to moderate). A person with dysarthria may present with:
- Difficulty moving the muscles for speech in their jaw, lips, tongue, soft palate or vocal cords
- Slurred or mumbled speech

- Low volume or running out of breath when speaking
- Monotone speech
- Changes in voice (e.g. hoarse, breathy or strained)
- Nasal sounding speech
- Choppy or poorly coordinated speech
- Changes in rate of speech: slow or fast.

Someone with dysarthria can have difficulty being understood or may feel that they don't sound like themselves. This can result in frustration and/or embarrassment for the person themselves and/or for the person they are communicating with. When speech is effortful the person may start to withdraw from communicating and avoid certain situations; for example, using the phone or speaking with strangers.

TABLE 43.3 Treatment approaches for dysarthria.

TREATMENT APPROACH	EXAMPLES
Restorative treatments	Learning how to **breathe** in a way that best supports speech Using **voice exercises** to improve volume and vocal strength **Overarticulation** to emphasise placement and articulation of sounds in words **Rate modification** using audio feedback or finger tapping to help slow down speech Improving **intonation** by practising sentences with different stress, loudness and pitch
Compensatory treatments	Using **shorter sentences** or signalling the topic of the conversation Educating the listener to provide **feedback** when they don't understand or to ask questions to help get the correct message **Environmental modification**, e.g. sitting face to face in well lit room and reducing background noise and distractions Using augmentative and alternative communication (**AAC**) to support or replace speech, e.g. writing things down or using a speech generating device

Dysarthria treatment generally falls into two categories: restorative and compensatory. A restorative approach aims to improve the intelligibility and naturalness of speech by working directly on the muscles and subsystems of speech that have been affected. A compensatory approach identifies and addresses factors that make it difficult for the person to be understood. Table 43.3 lists some common treatments for dysarthria.

Apraxia of Speech

Unlike dysarthria that is caused by weakness of the muscles used for speech, apraxia of speech (AOS) results from difficulty planning, programming and coordinating these muscles. The person may be able to say words or phrases in automatic speech but not under volitional control, e.g. they can say goodbye when someone is leaving but not at other times. AOS can vary in severity and can co-occur with dysarthria, aphasia or other forms of apraxia (e.g. oral/limb). Mild AOS may be characterised by occasional mispronunciations of words or mild changes in the prosody of speech. For example, someone may have difficulty pronouncing longer words with multiple syllables, or their speech might lack typical intonation. In severe AOS the person may be unable to make any sounds or words. In some cases AOS can resolve quickly in the acute period after a stroke but in many cases it persists. Research shows mixed evidence for interventions working with AOS (West et al., 2005). Table 43.4 lists some common treatments for AOS.

SETTING GOALS IN THERAPY

The goals of therapy can change over time and vary depending on the person's communication needs and wants at that time. For example, a goal in the hospital setting may be to communicate basic needs with ward staff. A goal at home may be to re-engage with pastimes, e.g. read the newspaper, follow a favourite TV programme, or communicate with grandchildren.

TABLE 43.4 Treatment approaches for apraxia of speech.

TREATMENT APPROACH	EXAMPLES
Impairment-based approaches	Through **guided, repetitive practice** the person relearns how to produce sounds and words, e.g. use of a mirror to relearn how to shape sounds, or regular practice of functional words
Compensatory	**Strategies** to improve the ability to be understood, e.g. use of a pacing board to slow speech down Using augmentative and alternative communication (**AAC**) to support or replace speech, e.g. writing or using a computer/phone app

The person will identify their priorities or aspirations for the future, and the SLT will use clinical judgement based on the best available research evidence to shape these goals into therapy activities. Effective goals are relevant to the person and will take into account their individual strengths and needs. Factors such as fatigue, mood, insight and social supports will impact on goals and participation in therapy.

DYSPHAGIA DUE TO STROKE

Difficulty swallowing (dysphagia) is common following a stroke, especially in the acute phase. It results from muscle weakness, incoordination, reduced sensation and/or cognitive changes. As discussed in Chapter 15 dysphagia can impact on:

- Ability to eat, drink and take medicine safely
- Hydration and nutrition
- Respiratory status (aspiration pneumonia)
- Quality of life and mealtime enjoyment.

CASE 2

Sally is an 82-year-old woman who was admitted to hospital with a stroke. The medical team referred her to SLT for an assessment of her swallow. The team was concerned about the safety of giving her food and drink and her ability to take medications.

Dysphagia in the initial days following a stroke can result in aspiration pneumonia and is an important indicator of overall prognosis (Wang et al., 2001). It must be carefully managed by the SLT and members of the MDT. Initially, the person may not be safe to take food or drink by mouth. In this case they may receive food through a nasogastric tube, inserted through their nose into the stomach. This is always a short-term solution to ensure adequate hydration, nutrition and access to medications. Longer term tube feeding may involve inserting a tube into the stomach, called a percutaneous endoscopic gastrostomy (PEG) or a radiologically inserted gastrostomy (RIG).

Dysphagia therapy following stroke can be both compensatory and rehabilitative. Compensatory approaches aim to reduce the symptoms and risks associated with dysphagia, but do not change the underlying cause. Rehabilitative approaches aim to change the underlying cause with a positive impact on

swallow function and safety. Different approaches and combinations will be utilised by the SLT, depending on the time since the stroke (e.g. initial few days or one year later), which phase of the swallow has been affected (e.g. oral or pharyngeal) and the person's individual goals. Strategies to support someone with dysphagia after a stroke are outlined in Appendix 1.

CASE 2 Continued

The SLT completed a swallow assessment with Sally. She had fluctuating levels of alertness and difficulty sitting upright. She had facial weakness resulting in difficulty chewing food, and drinks spilled from the side of her mouth. She coughed drinking fluids.

The SLT recommended small teaspoons of level 4 pureed food and sips of level 3 moderately thick fluids and educated Sally's family to adequately thicken her drinks for her. The SLT liaised with the physiotherapist and occupational therapist to support Sally's sitting posture. Nurses were advised to feed Sally only when she was fully awake and to regularly clean Sally's mouth. Pharmacy recommended which tablets could be crushed to make them easier and safer to swallow.

A swallow rehabilitation programme was commenced, and Sally carried out exercises every day with the SLT and her family. Over the next few weeks, Sally's swallow improved gradually and 4 weeks later, she was eating and drinking normally.

SUMMARY POINTS

- Communication difficulties are common after a stroke. A person can present with language difficulties (aphasia, or cognitive communication difficulties) or speech difficulties (dysarthria and apraxia of speech)
- Assessment and intervention by an SLT is essential to promote recovery and optimise the person's engagement in communication. Therapy addresses the underlying impairment and explores factors influencing well-being and communication participation in everyday life

- Swallow difficulties (dysphagia) are also common following a stroke. Early detection and management is essential to reduce risks that can negatively impact on the person's recovery
- Dysphagia intervention can involve diet modification, use of adaptive equipment, behaviour changes and swallow exercises

MCQs

Q.1 The goal of communication therapy following a stroke is:
  a. To work with the patient to achieve goals of their choosing
  b. To support the patient to communicate to the best of their ability
  c. To educate the family in how best to communicate with the patient
  d. All of the above

Q.2 Dysphagia after a stroke can lead to:
  a. Aspiration pneumonia
  b. Difficulties taking essential medications
  c. Weight loss and dehydration
  d. Reduced quality of life
  e. All of the above

REFERENCES

Kagan, A., Simmons-Mackie, N., Rowland, A., Huijbregts, M., Shumway, E., McEwen, S., Threats, T., & Sharp, S. (2008). Counting what counts: a framework for capturing real-life outcomes of aphasia intervention. *Aphasiology*, 22(3), 258–280.

Martino, R., Foley, N., Bhogal, S., Diamant, N., Speechley, M., & Teasell, R. (2005). Dysphagia after stroke: incidence, diagnosis and pulmonary complications. *Stroke, 36*, 2756–2763.

Teasell, R., & Hussein, N. (2013). Clinical consequences of stroke. Evidence based review of stroke rehabilitation. Retrieved from http://www.ebrsr.com/evidence-review/2-clinical-conse-quences-stroke.

Wang, Y., Lim, L. L., Levi, C., Heller, R. F., & Fischer, J. (2001). A prognostic index for 30-day mortality after stroke. *Journal of Clinical Epidemiology, 54*(8), 766–773.

West, C., Hesketh, A., Vail, A., & Bowen, A. (2005). Interventions for apraxia of speech following stroke. *Cochrane Database of Systematic Reviews*, CD004298.

World Health Organisation (2001). *International classification of functioning, disability and health.* Geneva: ICF.

44

Swallow Rehabilitation in Frailty

Gill Main

LEARNING OBJECTIVES

- Describe the factors influencing eating and drinking for older people living with frailty
- Describe the role of the speech and language therapist (SLT) in dysphagia management
- Describe strategies that support someone with a swallowing difficulty

INTRODUCTION

Frailty is another way of talking about how our body responds and changes as we become older. Frailty results in the loss of in-built reserves, and sudden change in our abilities can be triggered by a seemingly minor or unrelated illness. Our ability to swallow can be affected in this way and result in dysphagia. Dysphagia, the term used to describe swallowing difficulties, is known to be both a consequence of frailty and a contributing factor (Hathaway et al., 2014). However, identifying changes to swallowing as specifically related to ageing can be challenging when several medical conditions occur simultaneously (Cichero, 2018).

This chapter will help you understand the changes to swallowing that occur as part of the ageing process, the impact of frailty on swallowing, and how SLTs work as part of the healthcare team to manage dysphagia. You will also learn about how to help promote recovery and, where possible, prevent deterioration. Finally, we will discuss what is meant by person-centred management, and the impact on prognosis.

CASE

Jim is an 89-year-old gentleman who was transferred to an inpatient rehabilitation unit to maximise his mobility following a fall. Jim had not made gains in physiotherapy, was losing weight and inconsistently showed non-specific signs of infection. Jim did not have a history of swallowing difficulties, but the consultant geriatrician referred him to the SLT team suspecting undiagnosed dysphagia.

We will follow Jim's story through this chapter to help illustrate the relationship between frailty and dysphagia.

THE NORMALLY AGEING SWALLOW

Changes to swallowing occur as a part of the normal ageing process and are the consequence of gradual muscle loss (sarcopenia). These changes include:
- variable initiation and duration of key mechanisms (Namasivayam-MacDonald, Barbon, & Steele, 2018)
- reduced tongue strength and higher incidence of pharyngeal residue (Tracy et al., 1989)
- altered activity patterns in the suprahyoid muscles and increased fatigue (Wakabayashi, Sashika, & Matsushima, 2015).

Older adults are often able to tolerate these changes while maintaining adequate swallowing and airway protection (Mulheren et al., 2018).

Patterns of eating and drinking also change as people become older. The range of foods people consume can become less varied due to reduced mobility, difficulties with food preparation or reduction of income. Changes to taste and smell, experiencing less hunger before meals, eating more slowly, feeling full rapidly during meals and eating less between meals are frequently reported. Missing or broken teeth, and ill-fitting, damaged or loose dentures can also significantly influence the type and amount of food a person eats, in addition to posing an increased risk of pneumonia (Müller, 2015). Older people can experience up to a 30% reduction of daily intake, increasing the risk of malnutrition and dehydration.

THE IMPACT OF FRAILTY ON SWALLOWING

Studies have found it is common for healthy older adults to describe changes in swallowing that clinicians anticipate to cause swallowing difficulties. However, the evidence also suggests that when older people are living well, these changes alone may have no perceived health impact (Checklin & Pizzari, 2018; González-Fernández et al., 2014; Serra-Prat et al., 2011). While stronger individuals may compensate without consequence, frailty may lead to an increased vulnerability to dysphagia (Maeda & Akagi, 2016; Wakabayashi, Takahashi, & Murakami, 2019). As one of the major risk factors for poor nutrition and hydration, sarcopenia and pneumonia, early diagnosis and management of dysphagia is key.

Of all the features of frailty, nutrition is central to the ability to recover. Swallowing difficulties and maintaining adequate oral intake can be so closely linked that it is often difficult to determine if the dysphagia is causal or symptomatic. Certainly, people on modified diet textures to manage dysphagia are at high risk of poor nutrition (Pezzana et al., 2015) and sarcopenia (Shimizu et al., 2018). In this context, does poor nutrition ultimately lead to progressive deterioration that reveals dysphagia, or does dysphagia lead to difficulties with maintaining adequate nutrition resulting in weight loss and decline? Regardless of cause, poor nutrition will often be the most significant limiting factor when considering prognosis or rehabilitation potential.

CASE Continued

Jim had been referred to the dietitian, but remained too fatigued to participate in active therapy and was beginning to show signs of further physical deterioration. No overt signs of dysphagia were reported and the nursing team routinely encouraged good positioning for eating and drinking (see Fig. 44.1). Although Jim was noted to occasionally throat clear, the team did not feel that this was in direct response to food or fluid and suspected his medication for a known heart condition was a more likely cause.

There are a number of reasons why someone may not display obvious signs of dysphagia. Slow and insidious change can gradually reduce sensation with common signs of dysphagia being significantly dulled or entirely absent. Signs of dysphagia can also easily be missed, or interpreted only as part of a larger picture. For example, delirium and undiagnosed dysphagia will have some commonality in symptoms, such as:
- apathy and reduced interaction
- losses in cognitive capacity
- rapid weight loss and further deconditioning.

THE DIAGNOSIS AND MANAGEMENT OF DYSPHAGIA IN THE CONTEXT OF FRAILTY

When dysphagia is suspected, an SLT should be asked to carry out a Clinical Swallow Examination (a description can be found in Chapter 15 Speech Therapy). Understanding the potential for undiagnosed dysphagia in this content hinges on understanding the relationship between events across time and spotting precursors to dysphagia. Depression, dementia and delirium can be described as both symptomatic and causal factors associated with nutrition and swallowing problems. Polypharmacy, diabetes, poor oral health, alcoholism, chronic lung disease, heart failure, changes to neurology, falls and recurrent infection are all examples of exacerbating factors.

Using the International Dysphagia Diet Standardisation Initiative (IDDSI) to describe the texture or consistency of food and fluids (Cichero et al., 2017), Jim was observed drinking thin fluids (IDDSI Level 0), and self-selecting soft and bite-sized food (Level 6) due to difficulties chewing harder food items. Jim reported he preferred to stay in bed and would often drink in a reclined position. Clinical assessment from SLT revealed signs of dysphagia when drinking, likely due to a combination of poor positioning and sarcopenia. Recommendations that minimised impact were agreed in discussion with Jim, and a referral for an instrumental assessment was made with his consent. In this case, the assessment would be a moving x-ray of Jim's swallowing, called a videofluoroscopy (VFS). For further information on IDDSI categorisation or VFS, refer to Chapter 15.

Following a clinical assessment, modification to consistency of food or drinks may be recommended. SLTs are highly skilled at making decisions based on both the bedside assessment and the individual's wider circumstance on a case-by-case basis.

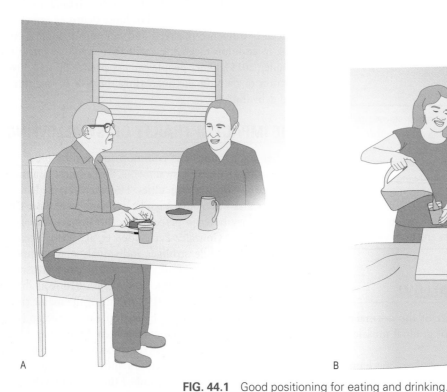
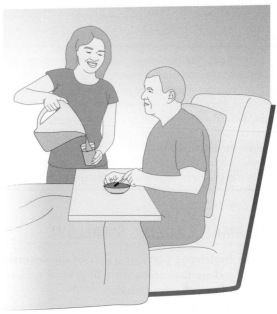

A   B

FIG. 44.1   Good positioning for eating and drinking.

However, it is recognised that the evidence base for modifying textures and consistencies is not robust (O'Keeffe, 2018). For this reason, best practice decisions regarding food or drink consistency, incorporating compensatory posture, strategy or rehabilitation prescription should be collaborative, informed by objective instrumental assessment measure where possible and informed by evidence. Decisions based on an undefined perceived level of 'risk' are inappropriate and have the potential to cause harm. Instrumental assessment supports management in the context of impairment, situation and consequence.

Prescription of targeted strength training exercises made by an SLT should be evidence based and in response to identification of specific deficit in order to avoid unnecessary harm. For example, the commonly used 'effortful swallow' strategy may result in reduced rather than improved swallow performance for some older people (Molfenter et al., 2018). Reviews of strength training exercises in dysphagia rehabilitation show improvements in generation of force, increased motor recruitment, and generally promote extended participation. However, strength-based rehabilitation often requires a high level of intensity, may be prolonged and have a significant impact on quality of life. Rehabilitation outcomes are also dependent on the slow and often lengthy process of restoring muscle mass. As this process is dependent on good nutrition, the relationship between dysphagia and nutrition often determines whether rehabilitation of this nature is successful. Where it is not possible to maintain adequate nutrition, it is unlikely that strength-based exercises will result in regained function.

Jim's VFS revealed he had difficulty with controlling fluid in his mouth until ready to swallow, poor coordination and strength of the elements that create a downward pressure, and reduced airway protection before and during the swallow. The consequence of this was fluid entering deep into the airway before he swallowed thin drinks (Level 0), and shallow penetration of the airway when swallowing slightly thick drinks (Level 1). Jim did not spontaneously cough in response to this. When prompted to cough, Jim was only successful in ejecting slightly thick drinks (Level 1) from the airway. Mildly thick drinks (Level 2) did not enter the airway initially, but residue remaining after the swallow slowly entered the airway despite multiple clearing swallows. The diet consistencies preferred by Jim (Level 6) were swallowed without concern.

Recommendations were for Jim to continue with IDDSI Level 6 diet, and to review the 'cost' versus 'benefit' of drink options with the treating therapist and medical team. Jim was also supported to consider rehabilitation targeting tongue strength and hyolaryngeal movement.

HOW CAN THE TEAM, RELATIVES AND CARERS HELP?

Targeted rehabilitation of a specific physiological impairment is only one of a range of tools in dysphagia management. Often, simple person-centred changes make the biggest difference for older people with dysphagia (Keller et al., 2017). The wider multidisciplinary team, relatives and carers play an important role in supporting a person with dysphagia. Examples of ways to support eating and drinking can be found in the Resources section at the end of the book.

Person-Centred Management Plans

Following joint discussion with the medical team and the SLT, Jim chose not to undertake a programme of rehabilitation, preferring a combination of strategy and modification. Jim chose to drink small, single sips of slightly thickened drinks (Level 1) most of the time, self-prompting a cough every third sip. He understood the 'cost' of drinking thin drinks was the possibility of developing a potentially devastating pneumonia, but felt having a 'normal cup of tea' with visitors, or enjoying a glass of sherry on occasion was important to him. Jim was aware of the strategies he could use to maximise his swallow and his family received training on how to best support him. For Jim this was, on balance, the greatest 'benefit' for the least accepted and agreed level of 'cost'.

Open discussion and collaborative decision making in relation to the 'cost' and 'benefit' of all available options are vital and require a whole team approach to be a truly person-centred management plan. Some more traditional models may talk about 'risk feeding' and focus more on perceived safety. Not even the most skilled dysphagia practitioner can make every swallow safe for every person in every situation. A high number of interacting variables may lead to a decision to work with the 'best' if not 'safest' option requiring a whole team approach to balance personal preferences, overall health, swallowing difficulties and long-term nutrition needs.

SUMMARY POINTS

- The ageing process results in changes to the mechanisms of swallowing that are normal and often without consequence
- In the presence of frailty, these changes may become more significant and impact on nutrition and overall health

- Early diagnosis and management that is evidence-based, informed and collaborative can positively influence rehabilitation outcomes

MCQs

Q.1 Swallowing difficulties in older people
  a. only occur when a person has been given a diagnosis of a progressive neurological condition
  b. are usually short lived and can be ignored
  c. can be the result of a combination of health needs and conditions that result in loss of strength and reduced swallow function in the long term
  d. mean all food and drink should be avoided

Q.2 Where dysphagia is suspected, the role of the SLT is to

   a. assess, diagnose, inform and support the person and their family to make an informed decision on management with the help of the whole team

   b. work collaboratively with the person and those around them to ensure the best possible environment and support for all eating and drinking

   c. offer a programme of rehabilitation exercises, strategies, prompts and support tips, as indicated

   d. all of the above

REFERENCES

Checklin, M., & Pizzari, T. (2018). Impaired tongue function as an indicator of laryngeal aspiration in adults with acquired oropharyngeal dysphagia: a systematic review. *Dysphagia, 33*, 778–788.

Cichero, J. A. Y. (2018). Age-related changes to eating and swallowing impact frailty: aspiration, choking risk, modified food texture and autonomy of choice. *Geriatrics, 3*, 69.

Cichero, J. A. Y., Lam, P., Steele, C. M., Hanson, B., Chen, J., Dantas, R. O., & Stanschus, S. (2017). Development of international terminology and definitions for texture-modified foods and thickened fluids used in dysphagia management: the IDDSI framework. *Dysphagia, 32*, 293–314.

González-Fernández, M., Humbert, I., Winegrad, H., Cappola, A. R., & Fried, L. P. (2014). Dysphagia in old-old women: prevalence as determined by self-report and the 3 oz. water swallowing test. *Journal of the American Geriatrics Society, 62*, 716–720.

Hathaway, B., Vaezi, A., Egloff, A. M., Smith, L., Wasserman-Wincko, T., & Johnson, J. T. (2014). Frailty measurements and dysphagia in the outpatient setting. *Annals of Otology, Rhinology & Laryngology, 123*, 629–634.

Keller, H. H., Carrier, N., Slaughter, S. E., Lengyel, C., Steele, C. M., Duizer, L., & Villalon, L. (2017). Prevalence and determinants of poor food intake of residents living in long-term care. *Journal of the American Medical Directors Association, 18*, 941–947.

Maeda, K., & Akagi, J. (2016). Sarcopenia is an independent risk factor of dysphagia in hospitalized older people. *Geriatrics & Gerontology International, 16*, 515–521.

Molfenter, S. M., Hsu, C. -Y., Lu, Y., & Lazarus, C. L. (2018). Alterations to swallowing physiology as the result of effortful swallowing in healthy seniors. *Dysphagia, 33*, 380–388.

Mulheren, R. W., Azola, A. M., Kwiatkowski, S., Karagiorgos, E., Humbert, I., Palmer, J. B., & González-Fernández, M. (2018). Swallowing changes in community-dwelling older adults. *Dysphagia, 33*, 848–856.

Müller, F. (2015). Oral hygiene reduces the mortality from aspiration pneumonia in frail elders. *Journal of Dental Research, 94*, 14S–16S.

Namasivayam-Macdonald, A. M., Barbon, C. E. A., & Steele, C. M. (2018). A review of swallow timing in the elderly. *Physiology & Behavior, 184*, 12–26.

O'Keeffe, S. T. (2018). Use of modified diets to prevent aspiration in oropharyngeal dysphagia: is current practice justified? *BMC Geriatrics, 18*, 167.

Pezzana, A., Cereda, E., Avagnina, P., Malfi, G., Paiola, E., Frighi, Z., Capizzi, I., Sgnaolin, E., & Amerio, M. L. (2015). Nutritional care needs in elderly residents of long-term care institutions: potential implications for policies. *Journal of Nutrition Health and Aging, 19*, 947–954.

Serra-Prat, M., Hinojosa, G., López, D., Juan, M., Fabré, E., Voss, D. S., & Clavé, P. (2011). Prevalence of oropharyngeal dysphagia and impaired safety and efficacy of swallow in independently living older persons. *Journal of the American Geriatrics Society, 59*, 186–187.

Shimizu, A., Maeda, K., Tanaka, K., Ogawa, M., & Kayashita, J. (2018). Texture-modified diets are associated with decreased muscle mass in older adults admitted to a rehabilitation ward. *Geriatrics & Gerontology International, 18*, 698–704.

Tracy, J. F., Logemann, J. A., Kahrilas, P. J., Jacob, P., Kobara, M., & Krugler, C. (1989). Preliminary observations on the effects of age on oropharyngeal deglutition. *Dysphagia, 4*, 90–94.

Wakabayashi, H., Sashika, H., & Matsushima, M. (2015). Head lifting strength is associated with dysphagia and malnutrition in frail older adults. *Geriatrics & Gerontology International, 15*, 410–416.

Wakabayashi, H., Takahashi, R., & Murakami, T. (2019). The prevalence and prognosis of sarcopenic dysphagia in patients who require dysphagia rehabilitation. *The Journal of Nutrition, Health & Aging, 23*, 84–88.

FURTHER READING

British Dietetic Association. (2018). Guiding food principles. [Online]. Retrieved from: https://www.bda.uk.com/uploads/assets/a1fb38ae-2dfd-46f0-888ad6278055b6e9/olderpeoplesgroupprinciples.pdf (Accessed 5 September 2019).

Campbell, N. (2018). ROC (Reliance On a Carer) Hydration Care Assessment Tool. [Online]. Retrieved from: https://www.hydrationcareconsultancy.co.uk/ (Accessed 7 May 2019).

45

Spasticity

Jacinta McElligott, Lesley Corcoran & Catherine Cornell

LEARNING OBJECTIVES

- Explain spasticity (involuntary muscle overactivity) in the context of impairments of weakness, coordination difficulties, hypertonicity and hyperactive reflexes (upper motor neuron syndrome) associated with injury to the brain or spinal cord

- Describe the stepwise approach to medical and physical therapeutic interventions that are effective in the multidisciplinary management of spasticity
- Explain the goal and outcome-oriented multidisciplinary assessment and management of spasticity

SPASTICITY

Spasticity refers to the abnormal, excessive increase in muscle tone (hypertonicity) in a muscle, or group of muscles, which may occur following injury to the brain or spinal cord where there is injury to motor tracts that control automatic adjustment to tone, posture, balance and dynamic stability of the body.

Upper motor neuron syndrome (UMNS) is the term used to describe the clinical presentation of injury to the brain or spinal cord involving upper motor neuron tracts that control purposeful (pyramidal) and automatic (extrapyramidal) movements respectively (see Table 45.1). Clinically patients with UMNS present with varying degrees of impairment related to weakness, coordination difficulties and excessive tone/spasticity related to abnormality in automatic adjustments to muscle tone, posture, balance and dynamic stability.

Spastic movement disorder presents differently in different conditions; for example, flexor spasms may be seen more commonly in spinal cord injury, whereas extensor posturing may be seen in severe brainstem injury. Spasticity is a dynamic condition which may change along the time course of different conditions (Bennett, 2008). The excessive tone or hypertonicity in spasticity is thought to be caused by lack of inhibition from extrapyramidal motor tracts that are responsible for automatic adjustments to muscle tone, posture and dynamic stability (see Figs. 45.1 and 45.2).

Spasticity is considered to be a disorder of spinal proprioceptive reflexes as noxious systemic or focal stimuli from the body (fever, anxiety, pain, skin conditions) can aggravate spasticity. Mild to moderate spasticity can be beneficial. It helps maintain muscle strength, prevent atrophy and can augment function. Spasticity may also prevent deep venous thrombosis (clots in a vein) and osteoporosis (bone thinning) (RCP, 2018). However, spasticity can have serious consequences in relation to comfort and function. Spasticity can disturb sleep and produce discomfort in posture and body alignment. It may contribute to difficulties in maintaining hygiene and to the development of pressure sores.

TABLE 45.1 Upper motor neuron syndrome (UMNS).	
IMPAIRMENTS ASSOCIATED WITH INJURY RELATED TO (Extrapyramidal Tracts) (AUTOMATIC) MOVEMENT	**IMPAIRMENTS ASSOCIATED WITH INJURY RELATED TO (Pyramidal Tracts) (PURPOSEFUL) MOVEMENT**
Spasticity	Weakness
Hypertonia	Reduced dexterity
Spastic dystonia	Decreased coordination
Co-contraction	Fatigue
Associated reactions	
Hyperreflexia/clonus	
Positive support reaction	
Spasms	
Positive Babinski sign	

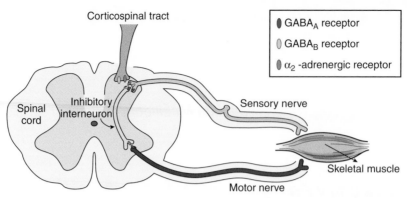

FIG. 45.1 The factors that contribute to spasticity in UMNS. Lack of inhibition from motor pathways from the brain is thought to contribute to hypertonicity. In addition, there is a heightened sensitivity to muscle stretch from spinal reflex pathways and sensory input. (From Wecker L. *Brody's Human Pharmacology*, 6th edn. Elsevier; 2019, with permission.)

Spasticity can inhibit function, particularly activity limitation associated with hygiene and dressing. Tonic contraction of muscles may result in biomechanical changes to muscle, tendons and soft tissue structures within and around joints that may result in shortening of the muscle or muscle tendon combination or contracture (Gracies, 2005a,b; Pingel, Bartels, & Nielsen, 2017) (see Fig. 45.3).

MANAGEMENT

The management of spasticity is a stepwise team approach with the use of a combination of physical and medical therapeutic interventions (RCP, 2018).
- Factors such as tight-fitting clothes or uncomfortable orthotics, inflamed or broken skin, ingrown toenails, pressure sores

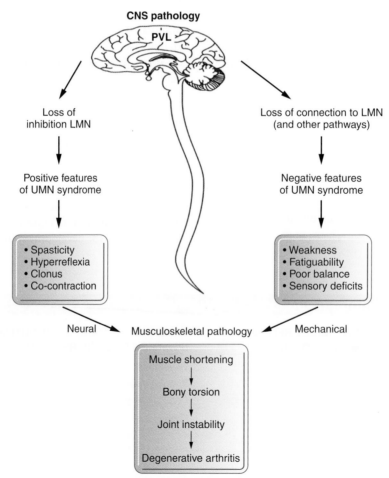

FIG. 45.2 Some of the consequences of spasticity, in the context of UMNS. (From Deon LL, Gaebler-Spira D. Assessment and treatment of movement disorders in children with cerebral palsy. *Orthop Clin North Am.* 2010;41(4):507–17, with permission.)

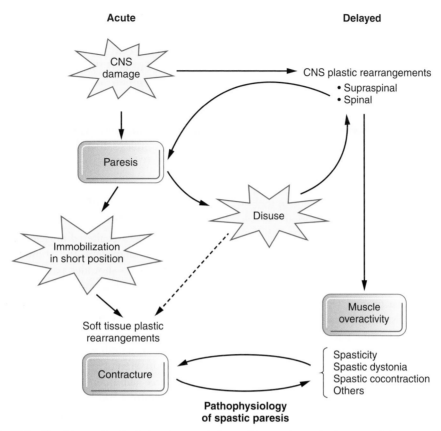

Acute   Delayed

FIG. 45.3 The biomechanical changes and disruption to the soft tissues of the body from spasticity, tonic contraction and development of contractures. (From Wissel J, Verrier M, Simpson DM. Post-stroke spasticity: predictors of early development and considerations for therapeutic intervention. *PM R*. 2015;7(1):60–7, with permission.)

or systemic medical issues can aggravate spasticity. Treating underlying factors that may be contributing to spasticity is the first step in reducing and managing spasticity.

• Preserving and/or improving range of movement (ROM), maintaining length in muscles and soft tissues, reducing pain and prevention of contractures are the cornerstones of effective multidisciplinary team (MDT) management and are incorporated into treatments that aim to increase function.

• Careful clinical reasoning guides the use of splints/casts for the treatment and correction of the biomechanical aspects of spasticity and contracture (Kilbride, 2015).

• Medications such as baclofen, tizanidine and dantrolene have been shown to be effective in reducing spasticity as shown in Fig. 45.4. These medications are most effective when used in conjunction with the MDT management plan (RCP, 2018).

• Botulinum toxin injected into muscles is effective in inhibiting the release of acetylcholine at the neuromuscular junction, thus reducing hypertonicity in targeted muscles or muscle groups. The use of phenol nerve block on peripheral nerves is also effective; however, it carries the risk of potential side effects, neurogenic pain and excessive weakness.

• Intrathecal baclofen therapy (ITB) is effective in the management of severe intractable spasticity of spinal or cerebral origin. ITB requires the insertion of a programmable implantable pump in the abdomen from which a catheter leads to the intrathecal space within the spinal cord. The pump is programmed to deliver a fixed or variable rate of baclofen directly into the intrathecal space. Patients with severe intractable spasticity, which is refractory to conservative multidisciplinary interventions, should be referred to specialist rehabilitation, neurology or anaesthesiology/pain management centre for assessment to benefit from ITB.

CASE

Maura is a 72-year-old widow, mother and grandmother, who had a right middle cerebral artery stroke 2 months prior to admission to the stroke rehabilitation unit. Maura lives in a bungalow and her daughter and grandson live close by.

Maura's rehabilitation team includes the following professionals: medical, nursing, healthcare assistants, physiotherapist, occupational therapist, speech and language therapist, psychologist and medical social worker. The team has access to splinting and orthotic services.

Maura presents with primary impairment related to UMNS with weakness and sensory deficits in the left arm and left leg. She has some mild cognitive deficits and inattention to her left side.

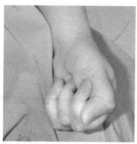

FIG. 45.4 Maura has spasticity and tonic contraction of her arm which has led to abnormal position and contractures of the long finger and thumb flexors as well as intrinsic muscles of the hand. Botulinum toxin was injected to reduce tone in targeted muscle groups in Maura's arm and hand. (From Cifu D. *Braddom's Physical Medicine and Rehabilitation*, 5th edn. Elsevier; 2016, with permission.)

GOAL SETTING

Goal setting is a collaborative process with the individual and/or family/carers, and substantial literature supports the usefulness of goal setting as a routine part of rehabilitation. Goal setting encourages communication, collaboration and effectiveness of the MDT team, and involvement of the patient and family is key to education and self-management. There is emerging evidence that goals are more likely to be achieved if patients are involved in setting them.

The literature encompasses a range of different approaches to goal setting and measurement of outcome related to specific interventions. We have used the Goal Attainment Scale (GAS) adapted from that used in the context of upper limb spasticity by Turner-Stokes (2009) to illustrate one method of capturing individual and person-centred goals.

Whilst not an outcome measure itself, the GAS is one tool that may be particularly helpful, incorporating and aligning patient, family, and team aims and expectations towards a goal-oriented multidisciplinary plan of care which addresses not only the specific therapeutic interventions for spasticity, but also the holistic rehabilitation interventions addressing impairments, activity limitations and participation restrictions.

An example has been used in Table 45.2 to express Maura's goals. The short-term GAS goals and outcome measures are merely examples rather than an exhaustive list.

Spasticity As Contributing to Impairment, and Barriers to Goals

- In Maura's case, altered muscle tone and soft tissue length influence alignment and shoulder joint movement and contribute to shoulder pain (Pain et al., 2019) which is associated with a poorer prognosis for recovery of movement, low mood, poor sleep and limits everyday activities (Tyson & Chissim, 2002).
- Overactivity, cocontraction, dysynergic patterns of activity, loss of length within muscles and joint & soft tissues result in stereotypical movement patterns which limit pain-free shoulder ROM and affect Maura's ability to dress/undress and cuddle with her grandson.
- Loss of ankle ROM secondary to spasticity and immobility, reduced power in the legs and trunk, and the arm's resting posture interfere with moving between sitting and standing from the sofa.
- Leg contractures are associated with reduced balance, higher risk of falls and increased dependency on walking aids (Hoang et al., 2013). The change in walking pattern limits Maura's ability to walk to her daughter's and participate in social activities.

TABLE 45.2   Example of goals for Maura.

	MAURA'S GOALS	BASELINE FUNCTION	GAS GOAL	OUTCOME MEASURES
1	To sleep through the night	Waking every 2 hours due to shoulder pain	To sleep for 3 consecutive hours in 1 week	• Visual Analogue Scale • Numeric Graphic Rating Scale • Observational sleep log
2	To dress by myself	Requires help of one person	a) To dress top half with setup b) To pull up trousers in standing with minimal assistance for fastening in 2 weeks	• Arm activity measure (Arm-A) • Leg activity measure (Leg-A) • Canadian Measure of Occupational Performance – Extended
3	To walk to my daughter's house (600 m)	Walking 240 m in 10 minutes	To walk 280 m in 10 minutes in 10 days	• 10-m walk test • 6-minute walk test • Video analysis
4	To read stories with my grandson on the sofa	Sits next to grandson at kitchen table with grandson holding the book	To sit with arm resting comfortably on the sofa armrest in 3 weeks	• The Spasticity Related Quality of Life Questionnaire

SPECIFIC MDT TEAM INTERVENTIONS

- Medical and nursing review identified no underlying medical factors contributing to or aggravating spasticity.
- Botulinum toxin was injected into targeted muscle groups in Maura's left arm and leg to reduce spasticity in the forearm, wrist and finger flexors and in the plantar flexors of the foot.
- A postural management plan across the 24-hour continuum is used to support Maura in attaining a comfortable position day and night. At night Maura's arm and body is supported in a comfortable position to reduce pain and sleep disturbance. Therapeutic positioning throughout the day aimed to place the limb in different positions to assist in maintaining ROM and soft tissue length.
- Providing support at the shoulder joint rather than further down the arm has been shown to give a greater pain-free ROM (Tyson & Chissim, 2002); therefore appropriate and effective handling of Maura's arm during transfers, positioning and repositioning by all staff is necessary to ensure consistency day and night.
- Self-management included tailored physical strategies to prevent biomechanical changes. Maura's may include self-stretches, positioning, strengthening, tasks to enhance the hand's sensory experience, task-specific practice and wearing a hand splint.
- Opportunities for practice are supported by all team members in all settings. Incidental practice, e.g. placing Maura's hand on the washbasin when brushing teeth in standing, all contribute to positive sensory information and meaningful experiences.
- Teaching Maura's family about postural management, effective supporting and moving of her arm and administering a sensory programme will ensure consistency within the hospital and at home.

- Stability of the pelvis and trunk, on which to base arm and leg movement, is vital as weakness and reduced stability can have a considerable effect on spasticity (Stevenson & Jarrett, 2016).
- Addressing impairments of weak trunk, poorly aligned shoulder blades/shoulder joint through physiotherapy and occupational therapy will strengthen the kinetic chain upwards from the pelvis to the arm. Improved passive ROM following shoulder girdle mobilisation results in reduced pain during sleep (Pain et al., 2019).
- Postural control affects both sides of the body following stroke (Silva et al., 2017). Strengthening antigravity leg and trunk muscles on both sides of the body is key in improving postural control which in turn will reduce the associated reactions in Maura's arm.
- Sit-to-stand and walking demand high levels of postural control. Improvements in sit-to-stand translate to improvements in walking (Chou et al., 2003). Repetitive task-specific training, e.g. sit-to-stand practice, has been shown to improve functional abilities in those people with activity (Veerbeek et al., 2014). Dose and intensity of practice is significant in improving functional outcome (Lohse, Lang, & Boyd, 2014; Teasell et al., 2005).
- To accommodate Maura's decreased ankle range and reduce its impact on walking, Maura required a custom-made ankle-foot orthosis. This stable alignment enabled activation and strengthening of appropriate muscle groups through an effective walking pattern and was designed to prevent potential vicarious knee joint trauma and pain from repeated hyperextension over time.
- Prior to discharge Maura's team will review management plan in the context of MDT discharge plan and follow up with outpatient and community services.

SUMMARY POINTS

- Interdisciplinary team interventions providing therapeutic goal-oriented physical interventions are the mainstay of evidence-based best practice management of complex spasticity
- Effective spasticity management relies on timely cohesive teamwork which demonstrates interlacing roles, consistent communication and a person-centred approach which respects the individual, their impairments and their functional environment
- Supporting patients and families in self-management is an integral part of managing spasticity in the long term

MCQs

Q.1 Upper motor neuron syndrome presents clinically with which of the following combinations of symptoms or signs?
- **a.** Weakness, coordination difficulties and hypotonia (reduced muscle tone tone)
- **b.** Weakness, coordination difficulties and hypertonia (increased muscle tone)
- **c.** Coordination difficulties and hypertonia (increased muscle tone)
- **d.** Coordination difficulties and hypotonia (reduced muscle tone)

Q.2 Which of the following management approaches is not used to treat spasticity?
- **a.** Treat underlying factors that may be contributing
- **b.** Force the limb back into the open position
- **c.** Maintain length in muscles and soft tissues
- **d.** Inject botulinum toxin into muscles
- **e.** Insert an abdominal pump for baclofen

REFERENCES

Bennett, D. J. (2008). Demystifying spasticity: reply to Dietz. *Journal of Neurophysiology, 99*(2), 1041–1043.

Chou, S. W., Wong, A. M., Leong, C. P., Hong, W. S., Tang, F. T., & Lin, T. H. (2003). Postural control during sit-to stand and gait in stroke patients. *American Journal of Physical Medicine & Rehabilitation, 82*(1), 42–47.

Gracies, J. -M. (2005a). Pathophysiology of spastic paresis. I: Paresis and soft tissue changes. *Muscle & Nerve, 31*(5), 535–551.

Gracies, J. -M. (2005b). Pathophysiology of spastic paresis. II: Emergence of muscle overactivity. *Muscle & Nerve, 31*(5), 552–571.

Hoang, P. D., Gandevia, S. C., Herbert, R. D. (2014). Prevalence of joint contractures and muscle weakness in people with multiple sclerosis. *Disability and Rehabilitation, 36*(19), 1588–1593.

Kilbride, C. (2015). *Splinting for the prevention and correction of contractures in adults with neurological dysfunction: practice guideline for occupational therapists and physiotherapists.* College of Occupational Therapists and Association of Chartered Physiotherapists in Neurology.

Lohse, K. R., Lang, C. E., & Boyd, L. A. (2014). Is more better? Using metadata to explore dose-response relationships in stroke rehabilitation. *Stroke, 45*(7), 2053–2058.

Pain, L. A. M., Baker, R., Sohail, Q. Z., Herbert, D., Zabjek, K., Richardson, D., & Agur, A. M. R. (2019). The three-dimensional shoulder pain alignment (3D-SPA) mobilization improves pain-free shoulder range, functional reach and sleep following stroke: a pilot randomized control trial. *Disability and Rehabilitation,* 1–12.

Pingel, J., Bartels, E. M., & Nielsen, J. B. (2017). New perspectives on the development of muscle contractures following central motor lesions. *Journal of Physiology, 595*(4), 1027–1038.

Royal College of Physicians National Guidelines. (2018). *Spasticity in adults: management using botulinum toxin.* London.

Silva, A., Sousa, A. S. P., Silva, C. C., Santos, R., Tavares, J. M. R. S., & Sousa, F. (2017). The role of the ipsilesional side in the rehabilitation of post-stroke subjects. *Somatosensory & Motor Research, 34*(3), 185–188.

Stevenson, V. L., & Jarrett, L. (2016). *Spasticity management. A practical multidisciplinary guide* (2nd edn). Boca Raton: CRC Press.

Teasell, R., Bitensky, J., Salter, K., & Bayona, N. A. (2005). The role of timing and intensity of rehabilitation therapies. *Topics in Stroke Rehabilitation, 12*(3), 46–57.

Turner-Stokes, L. (2009). Goal attainment scaling (GAS) in rehabilitation: a practical guide. *Clinical Rehabilitation, 23*(4), 362–370.

Tyson, S. F., & Chissim, C. (2002). The immediate effect of handling technique on range of movement in the hemiplegic shoulder. *Clinical Rehabilitation, 16*(2), 137–140.

Veerbeek, J. M., Van Wegen, E., Van Peppen, R. V., Van der Wees, P. J., Hendriks, E., Rietberg, M., & Kwakkel, G. (2014). What is the evidence for physical therapy poststroke? A systematic review and meta-analysis. *PLoS One, 9*(2), e87987.

FURTHER READING

Law, M., Baptiste, S., McColl, M., Opzoomer, A., Polatajko, H., & Pollock, N. (1990). The Canadian Occupational Performance Measure: an outcome measure for occupational therapy. *Canadian Journal of Occupational Therapy, 57*(2), 82–87.

National Institute for Care and Health Excellence Clinical Guideline. (2013). Stroke rehabilitation in adults. https://www.nice.org.uk/guidance/cg162.

Royal College of Physicians. (2016). *National clinical guideline for stroke,* 5th edn.

46

Vertebral and Lower Limb Fractures and Surgery

Rachael Doyle & Cliona Small

LEARNING OBJECTIVES

- Describe the management of vertebral fractures
- List types of lower limb fractures and outline their management

- Explain the role of the orthogeriatrician and the multidisciplinary team in rehabilitation of patients with vertebral and lower limb fractures or after joint surgery
- Outline the long-term consequences of hip fractures

CASE

Tariq is a 90-year-old man who was transferred to the emergency department (ED) after a fall at home. He stumbled and fell onto his right side while going to the bathroom. He activated his personal pendant alarm to call for help. On arrival to the ED, his right leg was shortened and externally rotated. X-ray revealed a right hip fracture. He was admitted under the orthopaedic team and reviewed by the orthogeriatrician. A collateral history from his daughter revealed that he was living alone and had a diagnosis of dementia. His family had noticed a decline in his memory and mobility over the preceding months.

He underwent surgery the following morning. That evening he was noted to be confused. On day 1 postoperatively, he was seen by the physiotherapist. Due to his delirium, he was slow to follow instructions and required a hoist transfer to sit out in a chair. On day 2, he was brighter and began to practise standing with the therapists and taking steps using a frame with the assistance of two people.

His postoperative course was complicated by fluctuating delirium. He required extensive multidisciplinary input including a home visit and referral to community services. He received intravenous zoledronic acid for osteoporosis treatment and was discharged home 4 weeks later with a home care package.

INTRODUCTION

As the population continues to age, fragility fractures are becoming more common. A fragility fracture is a fracture that results from 'low-impact' trauma, usually a fall from standing height. Fragility fractures occur most commonly in the spine, hip and wrist, and less often in the pelvis, ribs and other bones (Hertz & Santy-Tomlinson, 2018). These fractures result in pain and loss of function, which can affect quality of life and lead to increased dependency levels. For some, they can result in the inability to return home.

ORTHOPAEDIC SURGERY AND THE OLDER PATIENT

The number of older patients undergoing orthopaedic surgery is steadily increasing. Older people with fragility fractures are more likely to have multiple conditions, including dementia or polypharmacy, and are at increased risk of perioperative complications and mortality (Bachmann et al., 2010). Pre-fracture function, depression, nutrition and social support impact post-fracture recovery. Performing a comprehensive geriatric assessment (see Chapter 2, Comprehensive Assessment of Older People) allows for early identification of issues, such as cognitive impairment and frailty, that can adversely impact a patient's rehabilitation potential. Early communication with family members helps address potential concerns and barriers to discharge planning.

The orthogeriatric model of care is the standard of care for older orthopaedic patients. This uses a shared care approach where a geriatrician works closely with orthopaedic surgeons and the specialist multidisciplinary team (MDT) and encompasses the following:

- Optimising patients in the perioperative period to prevent complications
- Performing a falls assessment to look for possible causes including gait and balance problems, cardiac disease and neurological causes
- Early MDT engagement and early inpatient rehabilitation
- Assessment of bone health and treatment of osteoporosis if required
- Discharge planning.

VERTEBRAL FRACTURES

A vertebra is one of the bones of the spine. Ageing of the spine is characterised by two processes: the reduction of bone mineral density (BMD) and the development of degenerative changes (Papadakis et al., 2011). Alterations to the form and composition of the individual structures of the spine with increasing age can increase the risk of injury or fracture (Ferguson & Steffen, 2005). Vertebral fractures can be acute or chronic. Osteoporosis, trauma and malignancy are all potential causes. There is increased mortality risk associated with vertebral fractures (Cauley et al., 2000).

Clinical Presentation

Osteoporotic vertebral fractures can often occur without any symptoms. Some present with back pain, others with increasing kyphosis (stooped posture) and loss of height that can affect breathing as there is less room for the lungs to expand. Radiation of pain to the legs is rare with compression fractures but may signify spinal cord or nerve root compression from bone fragments. Acute urinary retention can also be a warning sign of spinal cord compression, as can bowel incontinence.

Diagnosis

Patients with a suspected vertebral fracture should have a full neurological exam followed by plain radiographs of the spine (see Fig. 46.1). A CT scan gives more information on the fracture pattern. An MRI is used to look at the posterior ligamentous complex and may be required especially if surgical management is being considered (Campbell et al., 1995) or if there are neurological symptoms. Stable fractures are those where the stability of the spinal column remains intact and there is no neurological compromise. Patients in whom an underlying malignancy is suspected will need further evaluation.

Management

Treatment strategies depend on patient fitness, the location of the fracture and whether it is stable or unstable. Several studies suggest that stable fractures can be treated successfully without surgical intervention (Spiegl et al., 2018). Initial management includes pain medication and activity modification. Bed rest poses a risk of further bone loss and deconditioning.

Surgery is typically required for unstable fractures where there is significant displacement, multiple bone fragments and where there is nerve injury due to parts of the vertebral body disrupting or pinching the spinal cord. Use of a back brace is not commonly recommended for the management of pain in the older person. If a brace is used, it should be for a short amount of time for pain control, but prolonged use poses risk of atrophy (wasting) of the core musculature (Kim et al., 2014). In addition adherence with bracing is low as it can be uncomfortable and restrict activity.

Physiotherapy is essential to prevent deformity and to promote strengthening of the spinal muscles and promote postural retraining. In addition, breathing exercises encourage thoracic expansion and reduce the risk of atelectasis (collapsed lung) and hospital-acquired pneumonia.

Lifestyle modification includes smoking cessation and reduced alcohol consumption.

A bone health assessment is required and osteoporosis treatment initiated where appropriate (see Chapter 38 Bone Health). Approximately 19% of patients who have a vertebral compression fracture will have another one in the next year (Lindsay et al., 2001). A vertebral fracture indicates an increased risk of hip fracture in future, so treatment of osteoporosis can help to reduce the likelihood of recurrence.

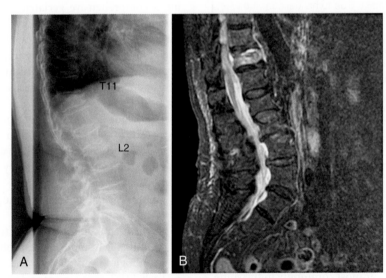

FIG. 46.1 (A) Lateral radiograph demonstrates fractures of T11 and L2 in an older woman with acute onset of thoracolumbar pain. (B) T2 sequence magnetic resonance imaging (MRI) shows increased signal in T11, while the L2 body has no increased signal compared with the surrounding vertebral bodies. This signifies the T11 fracture is acute and the L2 fracture is chronic and healed. (From Devlin D. *Spine Secrets Plus*, 2nd edn. Elsevier; 2012, with permission.)

LOWER LIMB FRACTURES AND TYPES OF SURGERY

Pelvic Fractures

The pelvis is a ring-like structure so more than one fracture may occur on the same side. Pelvic fractures may be classified as stable or unstable depending on whether the bones are misaligned. If the fracture is stable, then weight-bearing as tolerated is the treatment of choice. If the fracture is unstable, then surgery may be required. The acetabulum can occasionally be involved which may require extensive surgery.

The pubic rami make up a portion of the pelvis at the front. Pubic ramus fractures are usually due to a fall and may present with leg or groin pain on the affected side. Pubic ramus fractures do not require surgical intervention and will heal over time. Rehabilitation involves early mobilisation and adequate pain relief. Some patients may require a walking aid to help with mobility. The physiotherapist can provide a home exercise programme.

Hip Fractures

The hip is a ball and socket joint. Hip fractures are classified based on what area of the upper thigh bone (femur) is broken (see Fig. 46.2) and depending on whether the blood supply is affected.

- **Intracapsular:** occur at the level of the head and neck of the femur and within the joint capsule. Blood supply is commonly affected. Surgical treatment is a hemiarthroplasty (half a hip). A bipolar hemiarthroplasty is a ball within a ball to allow more movement and decrease wear and tear of the acetabulum.
- **Extracapsular:** Blood supply is not usually affected. Extracapsular fractures are further divided into intertrochanteric or subtrochanteric. Internal fixation with either a dynamic hip screw or an intramedullary nail (short or long) is the treatment. A cephalomedullary nail, which is a combination of sliding screw with the intramedullary nail, is sometimes used.
  - **Intertrochanteric:** Occurs between the neck of the femur and a lower bony prominence known as the lesser trochanter.

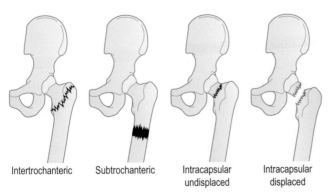

| Intertrochanteric | Subtrochanteric | Intracapsular undisplaced | Intracapsular displaced |

FIG. 46.2 Hip fracture subtypes/anatomical distribution. (https://www.bigstockphoto.com/image-221041627/stock-vector-types-of-hip-fracture-non-displaced-intracapsular%2C-extracapsular-trochanteric-and-subtrochanteric-f)

- **Subtrochanteric:** Occurs below the lesser trochanter.
- **Displaced Intracapsular:** Treatment is a hemiarthroplasty. A total hip replacement (THR) replaces the ball (head of femur) and the socket (acetabulum) and is used in more active patients.

Pain tends to resolve quicker after a hemiarthroplasty or a THR as the fracture has been removed compared to fixation of the fracture with screws or nails.

Surgery

Hip fracture surgery aims to restore mobility as well as optimising pain control and personal care. With all hip fractures, the aim is to have the patient able to fully weight-bear as tolerated in order to minimise complications. Surgery should be performed as soon as possible; ideally within 36 hours: 'The sun should never set twice on a hip fracture'. Patients often require preoperative orthogeriatric and anaesthetic assessment. The type of surgery (see Fig. 46.3) depends on the location of the fracture, whether the fracture is displaced (not aligned) and on the activity levels and independence of the person. In rare cases, a hip fracture may be treated conservatively without surgery.

Periprosthetic Hip Fractures

A periprosthetic hip fracture is a fracture that occurs around the implants of a previous THR. These fractures usually occur years after a THR and often result from a fall. Most patients are managed with surgery; however, some are managed conservatively (without surgery) with a period of non-weight-bearing and pain medication. These patients will require extensive MDT input as they will be less mobile and at high risk of developing complications.

Recovery After a Hip Fracture

Hip fracture recovery requires a multidisciplinary approach, and various aspects improve over different time frames. Recovery evolves first at the level of bone and muscle followed by recovery in function including gait and balance, cognition and strength followed by recovery in lower-extremity activities of daily living (ADLs) (Magaziner, Chiles, & Orwig, 2015).

The loss of femoral neck BMD in hip fracture patients is more than 12 times greater than expected compared to age-matched controls. Sarcopenia, a condition of muscle loss and muscle wasting, is present in about 35% of females within 1 week of their hip fracture and up to 60% at 1 year (Chiles et al., 2011).

The following factors are also important in recovery:

- **Comorbidities**

  Patients with more medical conditions at time of fracture have poorer outcomes in the year following hip fracture (Penrod et al., 2008).
- **Frailty**

  This is an increased state of vulnerability and is associated with adverse outcomes in older patients post-surgery, including prolonged length of stay, complications and postoperative mortality (Lin et al., 2016).

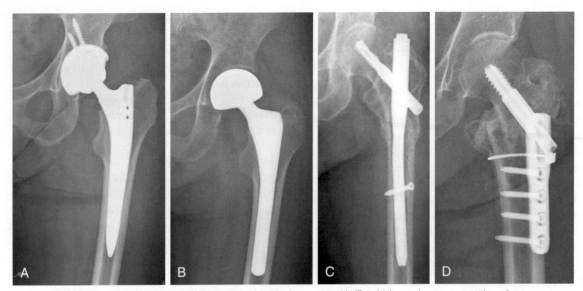

FIG. 46.3 Various surgical treatments for hip fractures. (A) Total hip replacement arthroplasty, (B) bipolar hemiarthroplasty, (C) proximal femoral nail antirotation, and (D) compression screw fixation. (From Cifu D, Lew HL, Oh-Park M. *Geriatric Rehabilitation*, 1st edition; Chapter 3; Osteoporosis and Fragility Fracture. Elsevier; 2018, with permission.)

- **Functional level**

    ADLs recover between 2 and 12 months after hip fracture. A lower functional level before the fracture has an adverse effect on recovery and the person is more likely to be more dependent at 6 months.

- **Cognition**

    Acute confusion (delirium) can occur in 50% of patients after a hip fracture. Approximately 25% of people still have cognitive deficits 2 months post-fracture. The degree of cognitive impairment has a large negative impact on regaining independence in the months after surgery. Approximately 50% of people with cognitive impairment require assistance of another person to walk 1 year after hip fracture surgery (Morghen et al., 2011).

- **Mood**

    Depression can make underlying cognitive frailty worse and affect the ability to participate in rehabilitation.

- **Nutritional status**

    Poor nutritional status is associated with poor functional outcome and increased mortality. Nutritional supplements are prescribed for a period of time after surgery. Patients with weight loss or who are malnourished should be seen by a dietician.

- **Social support**

    Patients with good social support are more likely to return to independent living than those with poor social support.

    Apart from pelvic and hip fractures, other common lower limb fractures are described in Table 46.1.

Weight-Bearing Status After a Fracture

The orthopaedic surgeon will prescribe the type of weight-bearing that is permissible following a lower limb fracture. This can be full weight-bearing or weight-bearing as tolerated, partial weight-bearing, toe touch weight-bearing or non-weight-bearing. While non-weight-bearing, it is important

that patients sit out as much as possible to prevent pressure ulcers, chest infections, blood clots, constipation and loss of muscle strength.

Some patients are non-weight-bearing for the first few days or weeks postoperatively. If well enough they can 'hop' and weight-bear on the non-injured limb with the aid of a frame or for ankle fractures they can use a scooter. Older people find non-weight-bearing more challenging. Using elbow crutches and ordinary crutches is more difficult due to muscle weakness and reduced balance. As a result, an older person may need to be cared for in a nursing home until they can weight-bear. Some patients can go home if they are living with someone and in a bungalow or on the flat with toilet/washing facilities downstairs as stairs mobility would not be recommended. Open chain exercises (a type of movement that allows the foot or the hand to move freely) are prescribed by the physiotherapist to cut down on loss of muscle strength. Once fracture recovery allows for weight-bearing, it can take several weeks to rehabilitate and this generally requires readmission for extensive MDT input.

Postoperative Period

The patient's goals and expectations after surgery will depend on what their function was prior to their fracture. Early mobilisation and adequate pain relief are priorities. Ideally the patient should be seen on the day of surgery or the next day by the physiotherapist, who will assess the patient and assist them to mobilise with a walking frame if they are safe and able to do so. Even transferring to a chair for a short amount of time can help minimise complications. The patient may feel unwell immediately postoperatively and unable to engage. Patients can have low blood pressure or blood pressure that drops when they stand. In these cases a review of blood pressure medication is

TABLE 46.1 Other lower limb fractures.

FRACTURE LOCATION	MANAGEMENT
Femoral shaft	• Almost always surgical fixation (plate or intramedullary [IM] nail) • Long leg cast if multiple comorbidities • Weight-bearing status determined by procedure/surgeon's preference • High risk of postoperative complications including blood loss, DVT and PE
Distal femur: supracondylar and intercondylar	• Surgery is generally using a plate or nail • Conservative (rare): above knee cast or a hinged brace at full range of movement (ROM) and non-weight-bearing for 6 weeks • Generally non-weight-bearing postop • Poor tolerance/pressure sores with above knee cast
Patella (kneecap)	• Minimally or undisplaced fracture often manageable in brace or cylinder cast and weight-bear as tolerated • Displaced fracture often needs surgery
Tibial plateau	• Usually plate and screws in a physically fit patient • Complex cases may need an external fixator • High risk of developing osteoarthritis in knee joint
Tibial shaft	• Usually an IM nail or plate and screws • Above knee cast if poor mobility or multiple comorbidities • Complex fractures may need an external frame • Usually non-weight-bearing postop • High risk for a potentially limb-threatening compartment syndrome (increased pressure in the muscles which can impede the blood supply)
Ankle	• Cast or surgery depending on fracture pattern and patient factors such as mobility and circulation • Below knee cast • Surgical wound, high risk of non-healing/infection • High DVT/PE risk
Mid- and hindfoot	• Often unstable or intra-articular fractures require surgery with a plate, screws or wires • Occasionally fusion may be needed • High risk of wound infection
Forefoot	• Minimally or non-displaced fractures usually don't need surgical fixation • Surgery is generally with small plates, screws or wires

required. Other causes include blood loss or dehydration. These factors and other complications can delay the rehabilitation process.

Interventions that help speed up recovery include:

- Sitting out of the bed for as long as tolerated during the day; having all meals sitting out.

Once the patient has been out of bed for the first time, the nurses and or healthcare assistants can assist with transfers to and from the bed.

- Walking to the toilet with assistance.
- Regularly walking on the ward with assistance.
- Washing and dressing: family and friends should bring in flat, supportive footwear, comfortable clothing, toiletries, and hearing aids or glasses (if required).
- Applying 'End PJ paralysis' and 'Get Up, Get Dressed, Get Moving' interventions (see Chapter 21 Avoiding Deconditioning).

Physiotherapy

A physiotherapist will concentrate on increasing walking distance daily (if able), leg exercises and ultimately stair/step practice if required. Moving around initially will cause some discomfort and the injured limb may feel heavy which is perfectly normal and should not stop people becoming active again.

Physiotherapists will prescribe exercises based on individual patient needs. Rehabilitation will involve muscle strengthening exercises and progressive mobilisation, aiming to increase a patient's mobility to pre-injury function (Petterson et al., 2009).

Exercises often include those specific to the area injured, for example strengthening muscles around the hip joint. They also include task-based exercises to promote a patient's return to function, for example sit to stand practice.

Example of exercises post-hip surgery

- Bridging: The patient lies on their back with knees bent and feet flat on the bed. The tummy muscles are tensed and the buttocks are squeezed together, lifting the bottom off the bed and holding for 5 seconds before returning to the starting position.
- Knee extension: Sitting in a chair, the leg is straightened and this is held for 5 seconds before being slowly lowered to the floor.
- Hip extension: Standing and holding on to a firm support, the affected leg is taken out behind with the foot facing

forward and the knee straight. This will be a very small movement. The patient should be able to stand tall and not bend at the waist or knee.

- Hip abduction: Same position as above, the buttocks are squeezed and the affected leg is lifted out to the side with the knee straight.
- Mini squats: Same starting position as above, the knees are slowly bent and then straightened. The knees should not move in front of the feet and the hip should not be bent more than 90 degrees.

Stairs Practice

The physiotherapist commences stairs practice if required once they feel it is safe to do so. As a general rule it is 'up for Heaven and down for Hell', i.e, the good leg goes up first when ascending and the bad leg goes first when descending.

Occupational Therapy

Initial assessment by an occupational therapist (OT) will focus on simple tasks such as getting out of bed and assessing seating needs. This is followed by a review of how patients manage ADLs such as washing, dressing, mobility indoors/outdoors and meal preparation.

The OT can then give the staff and families information to facilitate practice of the above activities with technical aids and prompting where required. Their goal is to assist patients to be as independent as possible after leaving hospital and to enable a safe discharge.

Postoperative Complications

Common complications after surgery are listed in Table 46.2.

PROMOTING HEALTHY BONES

A bone density (DEXA) scan cannot be carried out for 3 months after a hip fracture as it will not be possible to position the joint correctly. Patients should also be encouraged to carry out an exercise programme and participate in community exercises if appropriate. Fragility fractures should prompt assessment for osteoporosis treatment. See Chapter 38 Bone Health for more information.

PLANNED (ELECTIVE) JOINT REPLACEMENTS

THR and total knee replacements (TKR) are among the most successful and cost-effective operations for reducing pain and improving function (Culliford et al., 2015). Indications for an elective THR include:

- Pain that does not respond to pain relief and keeps the patient awake at night.
- Functional limitation, i.e., reduced mobility and difficulty carrying out ADLs. Stairs climbing and putting on shoes may become almost impossible.

Patients who undergo elective THR generally report Better health, emotional well-being, improved motivation and socialisation along with reduced levels of pain (Jones et al., 2007; Nilsdotter et al., 2003).

The THR operation replaces the worn head of the femur with a ball mounted on a stem and the socket (acetabulum) with a cup. Arthritic pain is relieved as early as 1 week after surgery (Aarons et al., 1996). There will be temporary pain after most operations. Chronic pain occurs in 2%–5% of patients after THR and 15%–20% after TKR. Even with a normal examination and good x-ray appearance, this can occur. Risk factors for chronic pain after TKR include younger

TABLE 46.2   Common postoperative complications.

COMPLICATION	PRESENTATION	MANAGEMENT
Delirium	Confusion, agitation, personality change, sleep disturbance	Treat potential causes, well lit and quiet room, sedation is occasionally required
Venous thromboembolism (DVT/PE)	A leg clot/DVT (swollen leg) that may travel to lung (PE) and presents with low oxygen levels, breathlessness or coughing up blood	Prevention includes early mobility, hydration, stockings and a blood thinning injection. Treatment is full dose anticoagulation
Pressure ulcer	Often occur over bony prominences. Skin colour change or blisters are early signs	Skin should be kept clean and dry. Incontinence managed. Dressings. Use of pressure relieving mattresses
Wound infection	Occurs if bacteria enter the incision. Can be superficial or deep (more serious)	Prevention is key. Management involves wound dressings and antibiotics may be required. Occasionally re-operation may be needed
Urinary retention	Decreased urine output, distended abdomen and abdominal discomfort	Catheter insertion for as short a period as possible and treatment of underlying constipation
Acute kidney injury	Reduced urine output can be a sign of a decline in kidney function	Stop contributing medications. Adequate hydration
Anaemia	Pallor, breathlessness, low energy	Transfusion where appropriate
Hospital-acquired infection	Pneumonia, urinary tract infection, gastroenteritis	Antibiotics may be required

patients who are highly active, females and those with a high body mass index (Beswick et al., 2012).

There is a large early postoperative loss of knee-extension strength with up to 30% post-THR and 80% post-TKR (Kehlet, 2013). This can lead to abnormal gait and the feeling of instability. Rehabilitation should address quadriceps strength to enhance recovery.

Complications after surgery can be reduced if the patient has an experienced surgeon in an experienced hospital. However, complications can still occur and include dislocation, deep venous thrombosis (DVT), pulmonary embolism (PE) and deep infection. These complications are highest in the immediate postoperative period and remain elevated in the first 3 months (De Vries et al., 2011). Occasionally the surgery can result in one leg being longer than the other. Longer term complications include loosening and breakage.

Prehabilitation

Prehabilitation is a strategy to enhance functional capacity and enable patients to withstand the stresses of surgery and associated inactivity (Ditmyer, Topp, & Pifer, 2002; Lemanu et al., 2013) by initiating the recovery process preoperatively. It helps to identify frailty or sarcopenia, for which nutritional supplements and an exercise programme can be prescribed preoperatively. Home assessments carried out by an OT can assist the patient in preparing for surgery and familiarising themselves with aids and adaptations as well as services that may be required on discharge home. Other interventions can include medication review, smoking cessation and weight loss.

Rehabilitation Following THR

Exercise-based rehabilitation is superior to minimal rehabilitation after THR or TKR. No one exercise programme has been found to be superior to another (Bandholm, Wainwright, & Kehlet, 2018). For the first few weeks after surgery, muscles around the joint are at their weakest, and therefore there is a higher risk of dislocating the new hip joint. In order to prevent dislocation after a THR, there are four basic movements that must be avoided for 12 weeks. These precautions apply in all situations including sitting and whilst moving in and out of bed or chair:

1. Avoid crossing of the legs.
2. Avoid bending the operated hip excessively.
3. Avoid twisting the operated leg in or out.
4. It is not advisable to lie on either side in the early stages of recovery. Patients are usually nursed on their back with the abduction pillow between their legs.

Driving

Normally, driving should be avoided for the first 6 weeks and travelling as a passenger for the first 3 weeks (except for essential journeys), as getting in and out of a car can risk straining the hip and stretching the healing tissues. Abstinence from driving for 8 weeks is recommended for knee replacements.

Flying After a Lower Limb Fracture

All hip and lower limb fractures increase a patient's risk of venous thromboembolism (clots) (Govilkar et al., 2018). This is compounded by air travel, especially a long-haul flight. All but essential travel should be avoided up to 6 weeks post-injury. If necessary the surgeon will prescribe anticoagulants and possibly consult haematology specialists in complex cases. During the flight, patients should wear TED (thromboembolic deterrent) stockings, mobilise both limbs as much as possible and drink plenty of water. Casts may need to be 'bi-valved', i.e. cut in half and fixed with straps to allow easy removal in emergency.

SUMMARY POINTS

- There is an association between frailty, falls, fractures and osteoporosis
- Vertebral fracture management depends on whether the fracture is stable or unstable
- Hip fractures almost always require surgical intervention but several fragility fractures involving spine and pelvis can be managed using conservative measures
- Pre-fracture function, cognitive status, comorbidities, depression, nutrition and social status impact recovery and possibly post-fracture outcome
- The orthogeriatric model of care is the standard of care to be provided to patients with a hip fracture and places a strong emphasis on MDT engagement

MCQs

Q.1 The following are all subtypes of hip fractures except which one?
 a. Intracapsular displaced
 b. Intracapsular undisplaced
 c. Distal femur
 d. Subtrochanteric
Q.2 Which of the following are possible complications post hip fracture surgery?
 a. Delirium
 b. Pressure ulcer

 c. Urinary retention
 d. All of the above
Q.3 Which of the following statements is true regarding vertebral fractures?
 a. Osteoporosis, trauma and malignancy are all potential causes of vertebral fractures
 b. Fractures may result in significant back pain, limited physical functioning and low mood
 c. Stable fractures are generally treated conservatively
 d. All of the above

REFERENCES

Aarons, H., Hall, G., Hughes, S., & Salmon, P. (1996). Short-term recovery from hip and knee arthroplasty. *Journal of Bone and Joint Surgery, 78*, 555–558.

Bachmann, S., Finger, C., Huss, A., Egger, M., Stuck, A. E., & Clough-Gorr, K. M. (2010). Inpatient rehabilitation specifically designed for geriatric patients: systematic review and meta-analysis of randomised controlled trials. *BMJ, 340*, c1718.

Bandholm, T., Wainwright, T., & Kehlet, H. (2018). Rehabilitation strategies for optimisation of functional recovery after joint replacement. *Journal of Experimental Orthopaedics, 5*, 44.

Beswick, A. D., Wylde, V., Gooberman-Hill, R., Blom, A., & Dieppe, P. (2012). What proportion of patients report long-term pain after total hip or knee replacement for osteoarthritis? A systematic review of prospective studies in unselected patients. *BMJ Open, 2*, e000435.

Campbell, S. E., Phillips, C. D., Dubovsky, E., Cail, W. S., & Omary, R. A. (1995). The value of CT in determining potential instability of simple wedge-compression fractures of the lumbar spine. *American Journal of Neuroradiology, 16*, 1385.

Cauley, J. A., Thompson, D. E., Ensrud, K. C., Scott, J. C., & Black, D. (2000). Risk of mortality following clinical fractures. *Osteoporosis International, 11*, 556–561.

Chiles, N., Alley, D., Hawkes, W., & Orwig, D. (2011). Sarcopenia and functional recovery after a hip fracture. *Gerontologist, 54*, 343.

Culliford, D., Maskell, J., Judge, A., Cooper, C., Prieto-Alhambra, D., & Arden, N. K. (2015). Future projections of total hip and knee arthroplasty in the UK: results from the UK Clinical Practice Research Datalink. *Osteoarthritis and Cartilage, 23*(4), 594–600.

De Vries, L. M., Sturkenboom, M. C. J. M., Verhaar, J. A. N., Kingma, J. H., & Stricker, B. H. C. (2011). Complications after hip arthroplasty and the association with hospital procedure volume. A nationwide retrospective cohort study on 50,080 total hip replacements with a follow-up of 3 months after surgery. *Acta Orthopaedica, 82*(5), 545–552.

Ditmyer, M., Topp, R., & Pifer, M. (2002). Prehabilitation in preparation for orthopaedic surgery. *Orthopaedic Nursing, 21*(5), 43–54.

Ferguson, S.J., & Steffen, T. (2005). Biomechanics of the aging spine. In *The aging spine*. Berlin, Heidelberg: Springer.

Govilkar, S., Patel, M., Bolt, A., & Hay, S. (2018). To fly or not to fly?—a review of the pertinent literature. *Orthopaedic & Muscular System, 7*, 2.

Hertz, K., & Santy-Tomlinson, J. (2018). *Fragility fracture nursing, holistic care and management of the orthogeriatric patient.* Springer.

Jones, C. A., Beaupre, L. A., Johnston, D. W., & Suarez-Almazor, M. E. (2007). Total joint arthroplasties: current concepts of patient outcomes after surgery. *Rheumatic Disease Clinics of North America, 33*, 71–86.

Kehlet, H. (2013). Fast-track hip and knee arthroplasty. *Lancet, 381*(9878), 1600–1602.

Kim, H. J., Yi, J. M., Cho, H. G., Chang, B. S., Lee, C. K., Kim, J. H., & Yeom, J. S. (2014). Comparative study of treatment outcomes of osteoporotic compression fractures without neurologic injury using a rigid brace, a soft brace and no brace: a prospective randomized controlled non inferiority trial. *The Journal of Bone and Joint Surgery American Volume, 96*, 1959.

Lemanu, D., Singh, P., MacCormick, A., Arroll, B., & Hill, A. (2013). Effect of preoperative exercise on cardiorespiratory function and recovery after surgery: a systematic review. *World Journal of Surgery, 37*(4), 711–720.

Lin, H. S., Watts, J. N., Peel, N. M., & Hubbard, R. E. (2016). Frailty and post-operative outcomes in older surgical patients: a systematic review. *BMC Geriatrics, 16*, 157.

Lindsay, R., Silverman, S. L., Cooper, C., Hanley, D. A., Barton, I., Broy, S., …, B., & Seeman, E. (2001). Risk of new vertebral fracture in the year following a fracture. *JAMA, 285*, 320.

Magaziner, J., Chiles, N., & Orwig, D. (2015). Recovery after hip fracture: interventions and their timing to address deficits and desired outcomes—evidence from Baltimore hip studies. *Nestlé Nutrition Institute Workshop Series, 83*, 71–81.

Morghen, S., Gentile, S., Ricci, E., Guerini, F., Bellilli, G., & Trabucchi, M. (2011). Rehabilitation of older adults with hip fracture: cognitive function and walking abilities. *Journal of the American Geriatrics Society, 59*(8), 1497–1502.

Nilsdotter, A. K., Petersson, I. F., Roos, E. M., & Lohmander, L. S. (2003). Predictors of patient relevant outcome after total hip replacement for osteoarthritis: a prospective study. *Annals of the Rheumatic Diseases, 62*, 923–930.

Papadakis, M., Sapkas, G., Papadopoulos, E. C., & Katonis, P. (2011). Pathophysiology and biomechanics of the aging spine. *The Open Orthopaedics Journal, 5*, 335–342.

Penrod, J. D., Litke, A., Hawkes, W. G., Magaziner, J., Doucette, J. T., Koval, K. J., & Siu, A. L. (2008). The association of race, gender, and co-morbidity with mortality and function after hip fracture. *The Journals of Gerontology Series A Biological Sciences and Medical Sciences, 63*, 867–872.

Petterson, S. C., Mizner, R. L., Stevens, J. E., Raisis, L., Bodenstab, A., Newcomb, W., & Snyder-Mackler, L. (2009). Improved function from progressive strengthening interventions after total knee arthroplasty. *A randomised clinical trial with an imbedded prospective cohort. Arthritis and Rheumatism, 61*(2), 174–183.

Spiegl, U. J., Fischer, K., Schmidt, J., Schnoor, J., Delank, S., Josten, C., Schulte, T., & Heyde, C. E. (2018). The conservative treatment of traumatic thoracolumbar vertebral fractures. *Deutsches Arzteblatt international, 115*(42), 697–704.

47

Upper Limb Fractures

Iain Wilkinson & Ibrahim Roushdi

LEARNING OBJECTIVES

- Explain the principles of management of upper limb fractures
- Describe the multidisciplinary approach to rehabilitation and delivering person-centred care in upper limb trauma

CASE

Shirley is an 88-year-old lady who lives at home with her husband. She is his primary carer. She presents to hospital following a fall at home, of which she has little recollection. She is identified in the emergency department (ED) to have a distal radius (wrist) fracture and an abnormal ECG with a postural blood pressure drop. Her fracture is immobilised in a back slab. She is taken to a medical ward for investigation and management of her fall. On the ward she has ongoing pain in her wrist, and does not walk for a number of days due to concerns about the stability of the fracture and looseness of her cast. When she can mobilise she is not able to use her usual walking stick. She has a prolonged admission requiring inpatient rehabilitation and short-term nursing home placement for her husband.

INTRODUCTION

One in three women over age 50 years will experience osteoporotic fractures, as will one in five men over age 50 years; one third of these will affect the upper limb. The most common sites of injury in older people are the distal radius (see Fig. 47.1) and proximal humerus (Fig. 47.2), both of which can lead to significant long-term problems. Less common but still frequently encountered injuries are fractures to the midshaft of the humerus, fractures around the elbow and fingers.

The incidence of upper limb fractures in older people appears to be increasing, most likely due to the changing demographic whereby we have increasing numbers of more active older people. However, as patients become increasingly frail, we see a progression in the pattern of injury from distal radial fractures to proximal humeral fractures and then onto proximal femoral fractures. This is felt to be related to a reduction in the protective reflex speed with age (Clement et al., 2011).

Injuries to the upper limb cause significant issues for older people and may lead onto a long-lasting disability. These injuries often affect ability to deliver key elements of personal care and perform activities of daily living (ADLs). Younger patients may be able to adapt to this, but often with older people it leads to new or increased care needs. The accurate assessment, management and rehabilitation of these patients requires thought and the expertise of a multidisciplinary team (MDT) to deliver a comprehensive geriatric assessment in tandem with the specific management of the injury.

PRINCIPLES OF INJURY MANAGEMENT

A good functional outcome after upper limb fracture starts with the initial management of both the bony and associated soft tissue injuries which may be operative or non-operative. Many upper limb injuries in older people are most appropriately managed non-operatively. There is a role for both internal fixation and primary arthroplasty in some cases. The use of external fixation (devices that hold bone in position from outside of the body) is limited to exceptional circumstances.

The aim of any management approach is to maximally restore function and minimise the risk of complications. With many upper limb injuries in older people, the balance of this may be unclear and a patient-centred approach should be taken, including discussion with the patient and/or carers.

During normal mobility the upper limb has little role in walking, but in polytrauma where patients have injuries to both upper and lower limbs the upper limbs often bear weight (around 25% of body weight with a walking stick, 45% with a standard crutch and 80% with an axillary crutch). This can significantly affect rehabilitation potential so the option which would soonest allow weight-bearing may well be the most appropriate. Simple adaptations may also be of great functional benefit, for example the use of a gutter crutch or frame in the context of a distal radius fracture allows immediate upper limb weight-bearing (see Chapter 11 Rehabilitation Equipment).

Principles of Specific Fracture Management

- Finger
  - The vast majority of finger fractures can be managed functionally with early active movement. If there is uncertainty, the hand can be placed in a position of

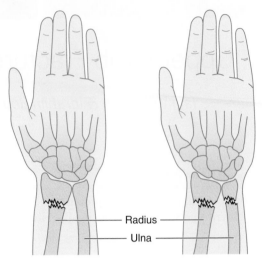

FIG. 47.1 A Colles fracture of the wrist, where the radius is broken near the wrist joint. On the right, the ulna has also fractured.

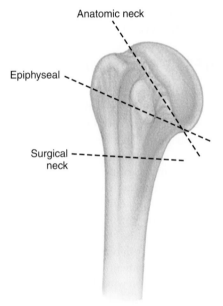

FIG. 47.2 Types of fracture of the proximal humerus. (From Matsen F, et al. *Rockwood and Matsen's Shoulder*, 5th edn, Elsevier; 2017, with permission.)

safe immobilisation with the wrist in slight extension, MCPs (metacarpophalangeal joints – knuckles) flexed and PIPJs (proximal interphalangeal joints – innermost finger joints) extended. A timely evaluation should occur in a hand trauma clinic as delays to treatment can compromise outcomes.
- Wrist
  - The recent BOAST (British Orthopaedic Association Standards for Trauma) guidelines suggest that the majority of distal radial fractures in older people can be managed non-operatively with 4 weeks of immobilisation. Stable fractures should be considered for a removable splint rather than a cast as this can allow significantly more independence.

- Proximal Humeral
  - Most proximal humeral fractures can be managed non-operatively with early physiotherapy and mobilisation. Prolonged immobilisation is associated with poor functional outcome. The role of reverse polarity arthroplasty is promising but remains to be fully defined.

PRINCIPLES OF REHABILITATION

Following injury and initial management (operative or non-operative), an appropriate rehabilitation regimen is key to obtaining a satisfactory outcome. Around one in three patients will require ongoing hospital admission for inpatient rehabilitation and their length of stay can be significant. This model of care is usually required for patients who are frail and do not have significant adaptability to be able to manage at home, either alone or with additional support, and attend key outpatient therapy sessions. The increased length of stay in this group of patients is specifically associated with older patients (over 80 years), patients from their own home and with two or more upper limb fractures where surgery is needed (Lübbeke et al., 2005). Within rehabilitation the goals are generally focused on gaining greater independence in personal care, grooming and other ADLs.

Due to the weight-bearing status of many of the upper limb bones during activities, these goals may need the full time of the fracture healing to be achieved. Patients from care homes often have a shorter length of stay due to their pre-existing additional care. Their increased care needs due to limb immobilisation can often be met in the residential care setting.

It is not uncommon for upper limb injuries to be neglected either in the context of a polytrauma or in the medically unwell patient as in the case above. Inappropriate splinting or delayed rehabilitation of these injuries can both delay the patient's general rehabilitation and lead to poor outcomes from the specific injury. For example, a poorly fitting splint or cast for a distal radial fracture which blocks the MCP joint (knuckle) can severely impede hand function, whereas in a well-fitted splint the hand can be used for most ADLs immediately.

Even a small delay in receiving treatment (Menendez & Ring, 2014) or therapy can lead to significant long-term complications and functional loss. Immediate physiotherapy after a minimally displaced proximal humeral fracture results in faster recovery, with maximal functional benefit being achieved at 1 year. A delay in rehabilitation by 3 weeks with shoulder immobilisation during this time produces a slower recovery, which continues for at least 2 years after the time of injury (Hodgson et al., 2007). This difference is likely the effect of immobilisation of the joint and tightening of the associated connective and muscular tissues. There is also emerging evidence that the amount of exercise currently prescribed across different health services worldwide may not be as effective as possible in reducing impairment and improving activity following an upper limb fracture. There is good rationale for starting exercise earlier after the injury with a much shorter immobilisation period. This is likely to be more effective in terms of pain (Hodgson et al., 2007) and function than starting exercise after a longer immobilisation period (Bruder et al., 2017).

There is evidence to support the role of specific exercise regimens in reducing impairments and improving upper limb function following specific upper limb fractures (Bruder et al., 2011). These exercise regimens often are progressive in nature starting with passive movement of the affected area and leading up to targeted weight training. In order to fulfil pre-injury strength and function, a guided exercise programme, with progressive intensity increases, will be needed.

Even minor upper limb fractures can be painful, and regular assessment of pain is an important part of rehabilitation. While simple pain relief with paracetamol may suffice, sometimes it can be necessary to use opioid pain medication such as codeine or morphine for a short period of time.

MULTIDISCIPLINARY WORKING

When the focus of management is on function, MDT working is needed for maximal benefit. This starts from surgical planning and runs through to discharge. For example, with Shirley's case above, early referral to the occupational therapy team would have resulted in a better, earlier functional assessment of her ADLs. Early physiotherapy and nursing assessments may have led to less functional decline, and earlier senior orthopaedic input would have resulted in a well-fitted cast with ultimately a better functional outcome.

Rehabilitation of this type usually does not need to be conducted whist the patient is an inpatient and there are a large number of patients who have home-based exercise programmes run through a virtual fracture clinic (McKirdy & Imbuldeniya, 2017) or similar service. In order for the patient to achieve their goals, they need to be motivated, informed and monitored during their rehabilitation period. Early assessment for this type of patient pathway is needed to see maximal benefits.

There is also evidence that for simple, uncomplicated injuries, home-based patient led exercise programmes are effective with no additional physiotherapy input (Wakefield & McQueen, 2000). Where patients need some additional guidance specialist videos, virtual reality and telehealth solutions may also be possible (Tousignant et al., 2014).

As with other types of fracture, investigation and management for osteoporosis should be a routine part of the plan. Starting bone protection medication if appropriate may reduce the risk of more serious fractures in future.

SUMMARY POINTS

- Upper limb fractures are a common presentation after a fall in an older person
- Many fractures can be managed non-operatively and without admission to hospital
- Upper limb trauma can result in significant loss of function and increased care needs
- An individualised approach to rehabilitation should be taken

MCQs

Q.1 Regarding upper limb fractures, which one of the following is true?
   a. Physiotherapy should not start until the fracture has healed
   b. The most common site is the proximal radius (elbow)
   c. It is not uncommon for them to be missed in the context of a polytrauma, or multiple injuries
   d. Most patients will require admission for management
   e. The use of external fixation is limited to exceptional circumstances

Q.2 Which of the following is true regarding rehabilitation of upper limb fractures?
   a. Multidisciplinary management is generally not needed
   b. A virtual fracture clinic is a reasonable approach for diagnosis
   c. Even a small delay in receiving therapy can lead to significant long-term complications and functional loss
   d. A well-fitted splint will impair hand function to avoid further injury
   e. Patients from care homes usually have a longer length of stay

REFERENCES

Bruder, A. M., Shields, N., Dodd, K. J., & Taylor, N. F. (2017). Prescribed exercise programs may not be effective in reducing impairments and improving activity during upper limb fracture rehabilitation: a systematic review. *Journal of Physiotherapy, 63*(4), 205–220.

Bruder, A., Taylor, N. F., Dodd, K. J., & Shields, N. (2011). Exercise reduces impairment and improves activity in people after some upper limb fractures: a systematic review. *Journal of Physiotherapy, 57*(2), 71–82.

Clement, N. D., Aitken, S. A., Duckworth, A. D., McQueen, M. M., & Court-Brown, C. M. (2011). The outcome of fractures in very elderly patients. *The Journal of Bone and Joint Surgery British Volume, 93*(6), 806–810.

Hodgson, S. A., Mawson, S. J., Saxton, J. M., & Stanley, D. (2007). Rehabilitation of two-part fractures of the neck of the humerus (two-year follow-up). *Journal of Shoulder and Elbow Surgery, 16*(2), 143–145.

Lübbeke, A., Stern, R., Grab, B., Herrmann, F., Michel, J. P., & Hoffmeyer, P. (2005). Upper extremity fractures in the elderly:

consequences on utilization of rehabilitation care. *Aging Clinical and Experimental Research, 17*(4), 276–280.

McKirdy, A., & Imbuldeniya, A. M. (2017). The clinical and cost effectiveness of a virtual fracture clinic service: an interrupted time series analysis and before-and-after comparison. *Bone & Joint Research, 6*(5), 259–269.

Menendez, M. E., & Ring, D. (2014). Does the timing of surgery for proximal humeral fracture affect inpatient outcomes? *Journal of Shoulder and Elbow Surgery, 23*(9), 1257–1262.

Tousignant, M., Giguère, A. M., Morin, M., Pelletier, J., Sheehy, A., & Cabana, F. (2014). In-home telerehabilitation for proximal humerus fractures: a pilot study. *International Journal of Telerehabilitation, 6*(2), 31.

Wakefield, A. E., & McQueen, M. M. (2000). The role of physiotherapy and clinical predictors of outcome after fracture of the distal radius. *The Journal of Bone and Joint Surgery British Volume, 82*(7), 972–976.

48

Rehabilitation After Surgery

Angeline Price & Arturo Vilches-Moraga

LEARNING OBJECTIVES

- Describe key issues that influence the approach to rehabilitation in older people after surgery
- Identify the key members of the multiprofessional team that are essential in the rehabilitation pathway of patients with frailty undergoing surgery
- Describe the common barriers to functional recovery after surgery
- Explain the importance of delirium screening, diagnosis and management in surgical patients with frailty

CASE

Maureen is a 76-year-old independent lady admitted to hospital with a history of abdominal pain and vomiting. A CT scan showed that she had a small bowel obstruction, and she had an emergency operation (emergency laparotomy and adhesiolysis) to resolve this. The surgery was successful, though as Maureen struggled to use the patient-controlled analgesia (PCA, pain medication) and found this ineffective, her postoperative pain was poorly controlled. She was unable to undertake deep breathing exercises, and was reluctant to sit out of bed or attempt to walk because of the pain. She developed constipation and nausea, and was unable to manage without a urinary catheter due to her restricted movement. Maureen became confused (delirium), and this impeded her ability to undertake personal care activities, or practise walking. Her sleep became disturbed, and she was drowsy throughout the daytime. Her hospital stay was prolonged whilst these issues were addressed, and as she lost a lot of strength throughout the admission, Maureen required a period of rehabilitation before she was able to return home. The problems Maureen faced are not uncommon in older people undergoing surgery, though measures can and should be taken to reduce the frequency and impact of these.

SURGERY IN OLDER PEOPLE

With changing demographics (ONS, 2018) and advances in surgical and anaesthetic techniques, the number of older people undergoing surgery has increased and will continue to do so (Partridge, Sbai, & Dhesi, 2018). Changes associated with normal ageing and with medical conditions translate into impaired physiological reserve and resilience to stress (frailty, see Chapter 4). Postoperative medical and functional complications are consequently higher in this group compared with their younger counterparts. Rates of peri-operative medical problems and even death are higher, length of stay is increased and the need for additional support at home or a transition into 24-hour care more likely (Carter et al., 2020; Desserud, Veen, & Soreide, 2016; Torrance, Powell, & Griffiths, 2015).

Surgical procedures in people over 75 years of age account for 23% of all surgical activity (Chana et al., 2017), with oesophageal, gastric and colon cancers being common reasons for older adults undergoing elective surgery. The enhanced recovery after surgery (ERAS) programme is a well-established component of perioperative care, and has been shown to reduce complications by up to 50%, even in older cohorts (Ljungqvist & Hubner, 2018). This multidisciplinary approach to care is built around evidence-based protocols aimed at reducing bodily stress reactions caused by injury during surgery, ensuring continuity across all stages of the perioperative period via designated ERAS teams and addressing important components of preoperative, intraoperative and postoperative care.

Unfortunately, older people are more likely to present in the emergency setting (Pearce et al., 2016), and surgery in this population conveys increased risk of complications and death. Biliary disease, hernias and bowel obstruction are the main diagnoses in this group. Emergency presentation reduces the time to effectively prepare for and carefully plan the surgical journey, hence the need for established multiprofessional acute abdominal pain care pathways adapted to local need and resources.

Rehabilitation extends from the time of diagnosis, through investigation and treatment of surgical illnesses. It facilitates a timely return to functional baseline through exercises and practice, along with psychological encouragement and support. Fig. 48.1 shows a flowchart of a patient's journey through rehabilitation: pre, during and after hospital admission.

ADDRESSING BARRIERS TO SUCCESSFUL REHABILITATION

The older surgical patient often has a background of multiple medical problems (comorbidity), takes a large number of long-term medications (polypharmacy), and has a degree

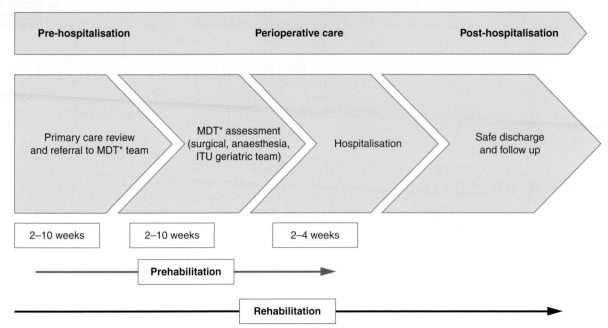

FIG. 48.1   Rehabilitation flowchart.

of functional or cognitive impairment and social isolation. Whilst 60% of those over the age of 60 years have a diagnosed long-term condition, this amount rises sharply to 85% of people in their 70s, and 93.5% of those in their 90s. Similarly, the number of individuals experiencing difficulties with activities of daily living increases with age, from 16.4% at 65 years to over half of those aged 85 years and older (Age UK, 2017).

Comprehensive geriatric assessment (CGA, see Chapter 2) will facilitate realistic goal setting, enable patient empowerment and provide targeted interventions aimed at regaining the highest possible functional status (sometimes even surpassing preoperative function). Patients identified as frail, cognitively impaired, functionally dependent or with impaired mobility should be considered for referral to appropriate multidisciplinary teams at the earliest opportunity. Fig. 48.2 shows the different members of the multidisciplinary team, working collaboratively to enhance patients' return to health.

Immediate and delayed surgical or medical complications may inhibit the person's ability to engage in rehabilitation. Complications should be managed promptly, including correction of significant or symptomatic anaemia, close fluid monitoring to ensure adequate rehydration, assessment for any signs of postoperative infection and timely treatment. Common medical complications encountered in the postoperative phase include heart failure, atrial fibrillation, acute coronary syndrome, infection (pneumonia, urinary tract, surgical site) and acute kidney injury, along with others more prevalent in the older person (delirium, constipation, gait instability and falls).

Delirium

Delirium is common in patients undergoing surgery. Unfortunately this condition impacts detrimentally on the rehabilitation process and should be prevented where possible and identified early to enable measures to be put in place to reduce its impact (Needham, Webb, & Bryden, 2017).

Delirium is defined as a disturbance of consciousness, with new-onset confusion and/or behavioural symptoms that develops over a short period of time and is fluctuating in nature (see Chapter 30 Cognitive Problems). Those with any pre-existing cognitive impairment are particularly at risk. Simple tools, such as the 4AT delirium assessment tool (MacLullich, Ryan, & Cash, 2014; Shenkin et al., 2017), can be used to identify delirium and the sooner it is identified, the easier it is to manage (Pryor & Clarke, 2017). Surgery is a significant risk factor in the development of delirium in older adults, with an incidence in this group of up to 50%, a result of a combination of factors including the use of perioperative medications (anaesthetic agents, opioids), reduced mobility, changing environments and disturbance to fluid status.

Patients experiencing delirium are likely to be inattentive, anxious and unable to comprehend or remember instructions relating to their ongoing rehabilitation. It is important to minimise the impact of this to facilitate the most effective recovery after surgery. In order to proactively reduce the risk and impact of delirium in the older surgical patient, regular assessment for common underlying precipitants to delirium should be undertaken routinely throughout the perioperative phase, and strategies implemented to prevent its development. The pneumonic PINCH ME is easy to remember, and allows for the assessment of the most common risk factors associated with delirium (see Resources section).

A holistic person-centred plan should be developed to optimise the person's ability to engage in rehabilitation activities, and with delirium prevention an overarching theme should take into account the following aspects.

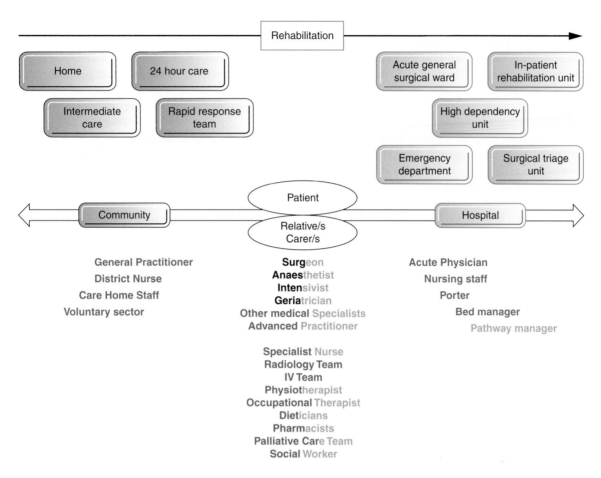

FIG. 48.2   Members of the surgical multidisciplinary team.

Communication

In an older population it is more likely that barriers to communication such as visual, auditory or those due to underlying medical conditions such as stroke or dementia-related dysphasia (communication difficulty) will exist.

Simple measures, such as ensuring functional hearing aids and access to spectacles, will enable clearer communication between patients, relatives and health professionals, ensuring information around goals of rehabilitation to be agreed as a partnership. Alternative methods of communication, including written instructions and picture cards, may be necessary in some cases, and the involvement of family is often vital in enabling older people to relay, recall and better understand any information relating to their rehabilitation.

In patients with delirium, cognition may fluctuate throughout the day, and it is important to take this into account in order to undertake mobility practice at a time when this will be best received. Planning rehabilitation interventions around patient behaviour and activity is important in optimising the likelihood of these being effective.

Pain

Pain and associated anxiety can be a significant deterrent for patients undertaking any meaningful rehabilitation activity

(see Chapter 25 Pain), and should be pre-empted and managed efficiently. Pain in the older person may present atypically, particularly in those with cognitive impairment or communication difficulty. The use of a simple pain scoring chart such as the Abbey Pain Scale may be of benefit in enabling a more accurate assessment and prompt intervention.

PCA is often used in the immediate period postoperatively, though any intravenous pain medication should be stepped down to oral, subcutaneous or topical, or a combination, at the earliest opportunity. Simple medication in the form of paracetamol should be given regularly, with the addition of short-acting opiates as required. The use of non-steroidal anti-inflammatory drugs (NSAIDs) should be avoided in the older population due to the increased risk of adverse effects. Fast-acting opiate preparations can be administered prior to any planned interventions or exercise-based activities to facilitate a more positive experience, which in turn will encourage further attempts at mobility practice.

Patients experiencing pain that is identified as complex or problematic should be referred to the local Acute Pain Service promptly, for specialist input (Faculty of Pain Medicine, 2015).

Nutrition

Poor nutrition in older adults impacts negatively on outcomes such as short- and long-term recovery, length of hospital stay and quality of life (Carli & Ferreira, 2018). In people who were unwell prior to the surgery, their nutritional status may have been inadequate for a long period of time, reducing their preoperative functional reserve. This is then further impacted by the stress of surgery.

Depending on the type of surgery, a period of tube feeding either as a replacement or supplement to normal eating may be needed. In accordance with advice from the surgical team on what food types can be taken, patients should be offered the widest variety of options available and relatives encouraged to bring any particular favourites from home, in order to increase the likelihood of nutritional requirements being successfully met. All patients should be screened in accordance with local policy, most commonly using the Malnutrition Universal Screening Tool (MUST) (BAPEN, 2003) and referred to the dietetics team for advice on optimisation of nutritional intake.

Hydration

Changes from usual oral intake, higher incidence of dehydration in the older population and the effects of surgery can all affect fluid status, and will affect the ability to engage with rehabilitation. It is imperative to ensure accurate fluid balance monitoring in order to pre-empt disturbance to fluid status, and manage any complications associated with this. All fluid losses should be documented, including drains, urinary output, stoma output and vomiting.

- Fluid depletion, due to inadequate hydration or excessive fluid loss, can lead to increased fatigue, low blood pressure and postural dizziness.
- Fluid overload as a consequence of large volumes of intravenous fluids, reduction or cessation of diuretics and/or pre-existing heart disease can result in symptoms of breathlessness, fatigue and significant peripheral oedema (causing heaviness of the legs, slowing progress with mobility and causing difficulty with functional activities such as washing and dressing).

Vigilance in observing for signs of fluid imbalance is important: reviewing consecutive daily fluid balance, observing for signs of peripheral oedema and daily weight fluctuation.

Mobility

Loss of muscle mass (sarcopenia) due to immobility occurs much more quickly in older patients with frailty, and prolonged bed rest is likely to lead to a downward spiral of deconditioning (see Chapter 21 Avoiding Deconditioning). This increases the risk of falls, pressure ulcers and continence issues, contributing to low mood and anorexia; all are likely to impede attempts at rehabilitation (Torrance, Powell, & Griffiths, 2015).

Traditionally, postoperative mobility was restricted in order to promote wound healing and reduction in rates of bleeding. More recently, with the implementation of ERAS pathways, earlier mobilisation is encouraged, with the aim of being out of bed as early as the day after abdominal surgery (sooner in some other types) where appropriate. Despite this, older people are still more likely to remain on bed rest for longer (McComb et al., 2018), and both encouragement and bed-based exercises should be given to those who remain in bed for any prolonged period.

Patients and relatives should be encouraged to bring in any familiar walking aids, which will enable them to begin to mobilise more confidently as their rehabilitation progresses, and allows for a more accurate assessment of their ability to manage normal routine. Assistance may be required in managing attachments including drips, drains and catheters, and forward planning of who will carry and adjust these is important in facilitating mobility practice.

Washing and Dressing

Taking into account the usual level of function of the individual, it is likely they will experience a degree of deconditioning postoperatively due to a combination of factors: pain, attachments, dressing sites and stomas.

Encouragement should be given to the patient to do as much activity as they feel able to, be this washing their hands and face initially or attending to their own oral hygiene. Attachments (drips, drains, catheters) should be removed at the earliest opportunity, and assistance given with these whilst maintaining as much independence as possible for the individual until they are removed. The early involvement of an occupational therapist should be sought if there are any issues relating to functional activity, or if equipment may be of benefit in maximising the patient's ability to manage.

Sleep

The postoperative period is often associated with higher levels of fatigue, weakness and lack of sleep (Carli & Ferreira, 2018), making any attempt at rehabilitation more challenging.

Measures should be in place to reduce excessive night-time noise and other disturbances, and ward moves should be avoided unless essential during normal sleeping hours (very important when also considering the prevention of delirium). Medications used long term to aid sleep, such as benzodiazepines, should not be withheld or withdrawn abruptly, though it is advisable to avoid any new use of these unless deemed essential, due to their association with the risk of delirium in older adults.

Death and Dying

Although the aim of surgical intervention is to improve life expectancy and quality of life, it is important to recognise that this may not always be the reality. Older patients undergoing emergency major gastrointestinal surgery face 12-month mortality rates of up to 50% (Desserud et al., 2016), and the number of older adults undergoing surgery in their final year of life, not just as a curative measure, but with palliative intent is increasing (Dunn, 2016). It is important to consider the long-term goals in each individual case, and whether prolonged and intensive rehabilitation is in their best interest. Maintaining quality of life is vital to older people (Holmes, Crome, & Arora, 2018), and this may mean an earlier return home below their previous baseline with equipment and/or ongoing therapy is preferable to a prolonged period undergoing rehabilitation in a designated facility. Only through discussion and shared decision making can these individualised goals be identified.

PREHABILITATION

Prehabilitation is an aspect of perioperative care that is growing in interest, and is pertinent to older people who undergo surgery. Through a programme of structured exercises and optimisation of nutritional status, functional reserve can be optimised in preparation for the surgery, reducing the impact of the postoperative stress response and aiming to reduce the likelihood of deconditioning (Carli & Ferreira, 2018; Ljungqvist & Hubner, 2018).

Those with the poorest physiological reserve are anticipated to benefit the most from even a modest improvement in overall functional status. Though the optimum time to begin any prehabilitation would be in the preoperative outpatient setting, any opportunity to continue and improve upon this during the hospital admission should be taken. This includes provision of and encouragement to maintain strengthening exercises and review of nutritional status, with subsequent advice/supplementation where required.

CONCLUSION

The care of older patients undergoing both emergency and elective surgery, and subsequent rehabilitation, can be complex and challenging. It is essential that clinicians are aware of the most common factors that will impact upon successful rehabilitation in this group, in order to deliver safe, effective and high-quality individualised care.

SUMMARY POINTS

- The number of older patients undergoing both emergency and elective surgery is steadily increasing
- Older patients undergoing surgery are more likely to have frailty, with reduced baseline function and mobility, and several long-term health diseases, making management particularly complex and challenging
- Rehabilitation of the older person following surgery requires a multidisciplinary, individualised and person-centred approach to care, and the ability to deliver this in the acute surgical setting is growing in significance for nursing and therapy teams
- Complications in the older surgical patient cohort are frequent, and it is important to pre-empt and reduce the impact of these in order to facilitate a speedier rehabilitation process
- Delirium is a major risk for the older person undergoing surgery, and preventative measures should be a routine aspect of their perioperative care

MCQs

Q.1 Which one of the following is true regarding surgery in older people?
   a. Delirium is common and cannot be prevented
   b. Pain medication should be used less often in people with cognitive impairment
   c. Patients should be screened for malnutrition
   d. Dehydration is less common in older people
   e. Patients should not get out of bed for a few days after surgery

Q.2 Which one of the following is NOT true about rehabilitation of the older adult after surgery?
   a. Relatives should be encouraged to bring in mobility aids
   b. Patients who take long-term night sedation should have it stopped during rehab
   c. Deconditioning is common, especially if pain is not well controlled
   d. Patients should be encouraged to be as independent as possible
   e. Catheters, intravenous lines and drains should be removed as soon as feasible

REFERENCES

Age UK. (2017). *Briefing: health and care of older people in England 2017*. Retrieved from https://www.ageuk.org.uk/Documents/EN-GB/For-professionals/Research/The_Health_and_Care_of_Older_People_in_England_2016.pdf?dtrk=true.

British Association of Parenteral and Enteral Nutrition (BAPEN). (2003). *Malnutrition Universal Screening Tool (MUST)*. Retrieved from http://www.bapen.org.uk/pdfs/must/must_full.pdf.

Carli, F., & Ferreira, V. (2018). Prehabilitation: a new area of integration between geriatricians, anesthesiologists, and exercise therapists. *Aging Clinical and Experimental Research, 30,* 241–244.

Carter, B., Law, J., Hewitt, J., Parmar, K. L., Boyle, J. M., Casey, P., …, & ELF Study Group. (2020). Association between preadmission frailty and care level at discharge in older adults undergoing emergency laparotomy. *British Journal of Surgery, 107*(3), 218–226.

Chana, P., Joy, M., Casey, N., Change, D., Burns, E. M., Arora, S., …, & Peden, C. J. (2017). Cohort analysis of outcomes in 69 490 emergency general surgical admissions across an international benchmarking collaborative. *BMJ Open, 7,* e014484.

Desserud, K. F., Veen, T., & Søreide, K. (2016). Emergency general surgery in the geriatric patient. *British Journal of Surgery, 103*(2), 52–61.

Dunn, G. (2016). Shared decision-making for the elderly patient with a surgical condition. *British Journal of Surgery, 103,* e19–e20.

Faculty of Pain Medicine. (2015). *Core standards for pain management services in the UK.* Retrieved from https://fpm.ac.uk/sites/fpm/files/documents/2019-07/Core%20Standards%20for%20Pain%20Management%20Services.pdf.

Holmes, E., Crome, P., & Arora, A. (2018). Patients' preferences and existential perspective: what to consider and how should patient's expectations be guided? *Aging Clinical and Experimental Research, 30,* 271–275.

Ljungqvist, O., & Hubner, M. (2018). Enhanced recovery after surgery—ERAS—principles, practice and feasibility in the elderly. *Aging Clinical and Experimental Research, 30,* 249–252.

MacLullich, A., Ryan, T., & Cash, H. (2014). *4AT: Rapid Clinical Test for Delirium. Version 1.2.* Retrieved from http://www.the4at.com.

McComb, A., Warkentin, L., McNeely, M., & Khadaroo, R. (2018). Development of a reconditioning program for elderly abdominal surgery patients: the Elder-friendly Approaches to the Surgical Environment–BEdside reconditioning for Functional ImprovemenTs (EASE-BE FIT) pilot study. *World Journal of Emergency Surgery, 13,* 21.

Needham, M. J., Webb, C. E., & Bryden, D. C. (2017). Postoperative cognitive dysfunction and dementia: what we need to know and do. *BJA: British Journal of Anaesthesia, 119*(suppl 1), i115–i125.

Office for National Statistics. (2018). *National population projections: 2018-based statistical bulletin.* London. Retrieved from https://www.ons.gov.uk/peoplepopulationandcommunity/populationandmigration/populationprojections/bulletins/nationalpopulationprojections/2018based.

Partridge, J., Sbai, M., & Dhesi, J. (2018). Proactive care of older people undergoing surgery. *Aging Clinical and Experimental Research, 30,* 253–257.

Pearce, L., Bunni, J., McCarthy, K., & Hewitt, J. (2016). Surgery in the older person: training needs for the provision of multidisciplinary care. *Annals for the Royal College of Surgeons England, 98,* 367–370.

Pryor, C., & Clarke, A. (2017). Nursing care for people with delirium superimposed on dementia. *Nursing Older People, 29*(3), 18–21.

Shenkin, S., Fox, C., Godfrey, M., Siddiqi, N., Goodacre, S., Young, J., & MacLullich, A. (2017). Protocol for validation of the 4AT, a rapid screening tool for delirium: a multicentre prospective diagnostic test accuracy study. *British Medical Journal Open, 8*(2), e015572.

Torrance, A., Powell, S., & Griffiths, E. (2015). Emergency surgery in the elderly: challenges and solutions. *Open Access Emergency Medicine, 7,* 55–68.

49

Rehabilitation in and After the Intensive Care Unit

Virginia Golightly & Rita Bakhru

LEARNING OBJECTIVES

- Name risk factors for ICU-acquired weakness
- Describe the levels of physiotherapy for ICU patients
- Explain how caregivers can assist at each level of mobility
- List contraindications for therapy

CASE

Filipe is a 70-year-old man who started feeling short of breath and having generalised weakness one week after going on a cruise. He has a past medical history of emphysema, coronary artery disease and type 2 diabetes. On initial presentation, he was found to have acute kidney injury, acute liver injury and heart failure. He was transferred to the intensive care unit (ICU) due to his altered mental status, tachycardia and low oxygen levels requiring intubation and ventilation (breathing machine). On day 4 of his hospitalisation, he was found to have an acute left MCA (middle cerebral artery) stroke. Physiotherapy was consulted on day 5 of his hospitalisation.

INTRODUCTION TO THE ICU

The ICU is the highest level of care in a hospital. Typically, a patient will be in the ICU because they require closer monitoring of vital signs, lab values and/or mental status, and/or require life-sustaining therapies/devices.

While in the ICU, patients commonly develop ICU-acquired weakness. This is a condition where weakness can be clinically detected and there is no other cause than critical illness. It is estimated that over half of the patients admitted to the ICU are over the age of 65 years and develop some form of weakness during their stay (Fossat et al., 2018; Verceles et al., 2018). Risk factors include age, bed rest, sepsis, multiorgan failure and duration of mechanical ventilation (Batt et al., 2013). This weakness is associated with longer hospital stays, prolonged time on the breathing machine and increased ICU mortality (Batt et al., 2013). ICU-acquired weakness can prevent patients from returning home at hospital discharge (Verceles et al., 2018; Zorowitz, 2016). In fact, it can persist several years after the hospital stay and may impact long-term quality of life (Zorowitz, 2016).

Delirium is also commonly found in patients in the ICU. It can manifest as hyperactive delirium with periods of restlessness and agitation, hypoactive delirium with periods of lethargy, slower processing or reasoning and decreased movement, or it can manifest as mixed delirium where the patient varies between both (Herling et al., 2018). Delirium is also associated with longer hospital stays, prolonged time on the ventilator, increased mortality and impaired quality of life after discharge (Herling et al., 2018).

Early mobility in the ICU is important to reduce the impact of ICU-acquired weakness, reduce delirium, decrease hospital length of stay and increase patients' level of independence at discharge (Fossat et al., 2018; Neufeld, 2017; Verceles et al., 2018). It has been shown to be effective and safe in the critically ill population (Fossat et al., 2018). Factors influencing implementation of early rehabilitation are shown in Fig. 49.1.

PROGRESSION OF REHABILITATION

In broad terms, exercise progresses from bed to chair to standing. Components of each stage are pictured in Fig. 49.2. In order to break down the progression of rehabilitation into more detail, it has been divided into five levels. We will start with evaluating our patient, Filipe, at the first level and work through rehabilitation at each level. See Table 49.1 for a summary of the progression of mobility (Morris et al., 2008).

Level 1

During this stage, the patient may be unconscious and is unable to actively participate in physiotherapy. This level is focused on preventative measures to ensure the patient has the best outcomes despite a sedated state. Rehabilitation during this time revolves around passive range of motion. It also involves positioning to reduce bed sores, oedema and contractures, including any splinting needs. During Filipe's evaluation, he is at this stage. The ICU team will ask his family members to provide background information about his prior level of function, his social history and his home

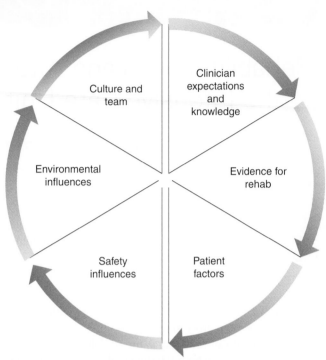

FIG. 49.1 Factors influencing implementation of early rehabilitation in the ICU. (From Parry SM, Remedios L, Denehy L, et al. What factors affect implementation of early rehabilitation into intensive care unit practice? A qualitative study with clinicians. *J Crit Care*. 2017;38:137–43, with permission.)

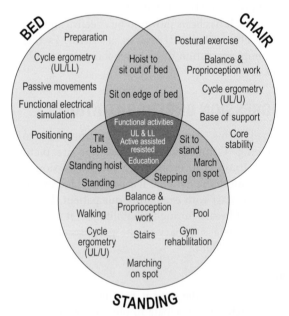

FIG. 49.2 Aspects of rehabilitation in the ICU in bed, in a chair and standing. (From Bersten AD, Handy J. *Oh's Intensive Care Manual*, 8th edn. Elsevier; 2018, with permission.)

arrangements. This can be a very hard time for family members because their loved one is very sick and unable to interact with them. Interested caregivers will be taught passive range of motion exercises as well as stretching and positioning.

Level 2

During this stage, the patient is conscious and will be able to actively participate in physiotherapy, at least intermittently. The patient will still be very weak during this stage and will be limited to activities in the bed. Regarding functional mobility, the focus will be on rolling and scooting in the bed. For strengthening, the patient will progress from passive range of motion (level 1) to active or active-assisted range of motion. Active-assisted range of motion means that the patient actively performs the motion, but needs assistance to complete the movement. Active range of motion means that the patient can perform the movement without assistance. For balance, the patient will work on improving upright tolerance of the trunk and ability to hold the head in midline. This can occur with increasing the head of bed height or long sitting in the bed. For coordination, the patient will work on reaching for targets, grasping objects and finger opposition while lying supine with the head of the bed elevated. Because the patient may be coming out of a sedated state, he/she will often need extra time or cues for motor planning tasks. The patient's endurance will be easily challenged at this stage, both mentally and physically, due to the limited activity in level 1.

During this stage, Filipe will be able to progress to active range of motion exercises on the left side of his body but still needs assistance for the right side of his body. He will roll in bed with minimal assistance to the right and with moderate assistance to the left side due to his weakness from this stroke. He may have trouble reaching for the handrail and for objects with his right hand despite being right handed, and this could make him quite frustrated. He will need rest breaks between each exercise and after bed mobility.

Caregivers can assist at this stage with exercise programmes, reminding patients to conserve their energy, providing hand-over-hand assistance with reaching tasks and feeding, increasing time with the head of bed elevated and engaging the patient mentally with conversation/re-orientation. Hand-over-hand assistance is when a caregiver places their hand over the patient's to help them complete the activity.

Level 3

The patient will be conscious and consistently able to participate in physiotherapy. In this stage, the patient progresses out of the bed.

Level 3a

The patient will be able to progress to sitting at the edge of the bed. For functional mobility, the patient will be working on bed mobility, supine to sit and sit to supine transfers. The patient will improve their sitting balance at the edge of the bed. Strengthening can transition to exercises performed while sitting at the edge of the bed. The patient will need to work on motor planning with these new activities and may need more cues initially. Due to these increased demands on the patient, he/she may develop fatigue due to a lack of endurance as well as mental status decline.

TABLE 49.1 Progression of mobility.

	PATIENT LEVEL OF INTERACTION	FUNCTIONAL MOBILITY
Level 1	Sedated, not following commands	• Passive range of motion • Positioning and splinting to prevent contractures and bed sores
Level 2	Intermittently alert and starting to follow commands	• Active-assisted range of motion and active range of motion • Dependent transfers to a chair • Rolling and scooting in bed • Long sitting in bed for balance and head control
Level 3a	Consistently alert and following commands	• Transfers to and from sitting at the edge of the bed • Sitting balance at edge of bed • Dependent transfers to a chair • Exercises while sitting edge of bed • Bed mobility
Level 3b	Consistently alert and following commands	• Transfers from bed to chair • Increasing endurance for out of bed • Sitting and standing balance at side of the bed • Exercises while weight bearing and seated in a chair • Bed mobility
Level 4	Consistently alert and following commands	• Walking with assistance • All active transfers and bed mobility • Balance in sitting and standing away from the side of the bed • Increasing endurance for standing
Level 5	Consistently alert and following commands	• Walking without assistance • All active transfers and bed mobility • Stairs • Dual task activities • Advanced balance tasks while walking • Increasing endurance for walking

During this stage, Filipe will be able to perform supine to sit transfers with minimal assistance by rolling onto his side, then pushing up into a seated position. He will sit at the edge of the bed with supervision using both arms for support. He will need external support of his trunk with dynamic sitting activities. He may be unable to clear his sacrum from the edge of the bed with attempts to stand.

Caregivers can assist at this stage by becoming involved in therapy sessions. They can provide encouragement and challenge the patient's sitting balance. They can encourage the patient to perform strengthening exercises outside of therapy sessions. Patients often tend to be discouraged at this level because they are now more aware and are often not used to being physically impaired.

Level 3b

The patient will be able to progress to sitting in a chair. For functional mobility, the patient will add sit to stand, stand to sit, bed to chair and chair to bed transfers. The patient will progress their sitting and standing balance by the side of the bed. Strengthening and coordination exercises are mostly still done while sitting, but one can use transfers as strengthening exercises. The patient's endurance will be challenged with more weight-bearing activities and sitting up for extended time in a chair. Typically, patients will start with only 1–2 hours sitting up and extending the time as able.

Filipe will work on sit to stand transfers with a focus on putting more weight on his right leg to strengthen it during physiotherapy sessions. He will have the chair on the right side of the bed so when he becomes fatigued from sitting for 3 hours he will be going toward his strong side to return to bed. He will work on self-feeding with his right hand.

Caregivers can assist by encouraging patients to increase their time out of bed, promoting self-feeding and performing exercises. They can bring in cards or games that challenge the patient's coordination and remind them of home.

Level 4

The patient will be conscious and will be able to progress to taking steps. Functional mobility will add walking to the previous transfers and bed mobility. These initial steps will likely need assistance from one or more staff members and use of an assistive device, like a rolling walker. Motor planning can be impaired, and the patient may need the therapist to break down walking into steps such as weight shift, lifting foot, advancing foot, shifting weight and repeating on other leg. Balance will be challenged while standing with static and dynamic activities. Strengthening and coordination exercises progress to standing if balance is sufficient. Endurance will be challenged with increased time spent standing.

During this stage, Filipe will have a physiotherapist and an assistant flanking him while working on walking laterally along the edge of the bed. He will continue to need frequent seated rest breaks due to shortness of breath and fatigue. He will need cues to pick up the toes on his right foot while walking when he becomes fatigued.

Caregivers can assist in this stage by promoting the patient to be as independent as possible with daily activities and providing less hand-over-hand assistance for feeding, brushing hair/teeth and washing face.

Level 5

The patient will be able to walk without external assistance but may use an assistive device. Functional mobility will focus on walking longer distances and stairs. Balance and coordination activities will involve challenges while walking, changes in surfaces or inclines. Endurance will be challenged with longer distances walked, increased walking speed and climbing stairs. Mental status will be challenged with finding objects while walking or delayed recall with giving directions prior to leaving the patient's room.

During this stage, Filipe will progress to walking with a single point cane with supervision in the hallways and minimal assistance for ascending four steps with use of one handrail. He will work towards becoming modified independent with stairs with a reciprocal pattern.

Caregivers can assist by helping walk with the patient each day and starting to take over assistance given by staff for mobility in order to prepare for home.

CHALLENGES IN THE ICU

While in the ICU, therapy sessions can be challenging due to unstable vital signs, severe weakness, delirium, injuries to multiple organ systems and the sheer number of devices connected to the patients (Malone et al., 2015). Fig. 49.3 shows a patient undergoing physiotherapy while on mechanical ventilation. Vital signs may need to be monitored during therapy sessions to assess how the patient is responding to the treatment. Therapy sessions can require extra staff to monitor equipment and provide physical assistance. Additionally, patients can have injuries to multiple organ systems that therapy needs to address. Because of the unstable nature of these patients, the therapist needs to have a contingency plan in place if a patient does not tolerate a therapy session. This can be as simple as returning the patient to supine, having a lift sheet in a chair to dependently return the patient to bed, or having a wheelchair following while walking.

While patients are in the ICU, they will have 'good days' and 'bad days' or even have both in the course of an hour. The therapist needs to know when to progress or regress the treatment for that day. This involves regular communication with the treatment team to see how the patient is doing. The goals for each session should always be in flux depending on the patient's clinical status. It is good practice to have a plan for possible regression, static level of activity and progression of activity for each session. Standardised outcome measures can also be used during the sessions to monitor if the patient is ready to progress to the next level of mobility. For example, manual muscle testing can be used during level

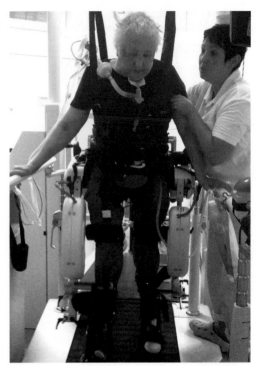

FIG. 49.3 A patient undergoing physiotherapy while on mechanical ventilation. (From Eifert B, Maurer-Karattup P, Schorl M. Integration of intensive care treatment and neurorehabilitation in patients with disorders of consciousness: a program description and case report. *Arch Phys Med Rehabil.* 2013;94(10):1924–33, with permission.)

2 to determine a patient's ability to progress to sitting at the side of the bed (Morris et al., 2008). The Function In Sitting Test can be used during level 3 to assess a patient's balance in sitting. This may be helpful because patients will have a hard time standing if they cannot maintain their balance in sitting. The Egress test can be used to assess a patient's ability to transfer safely to a chair.

There are times when physiotherapy needs to be suspended for patients in the ICU. Reasons may include specific ventilator settings, elevated intracranial pressure, arrhythmias, unstable heart rate or blood pressure, significant vasopressor dose, severe anaemia, seizures, severe dizziness or syncope symptoms (Dickinson, Taylor, & Anton, 2018). Patients can have more restrictive limitations placed by the medical team for specific disorders. Detailed suggestions for mobility with specific ICU devices and contraindications for physiotherapy are available (Hodgson et al., 2014).

PROGRESSION TO THE GENERAL WARD FROM THE ICU

As the patient progresses medically, they gradually need less close monitoring. This means fewer connected devices and more freedom for mobility. Transferring to the general ward is based on the patient's medical stability, not their mobility. The patient will continue to progress through the same levels of mobility whether they are in the ICU, a stepdown unit or in the general ward. The biggest difference in the type of unit is the reduction of lines/leads and frequency of monitoring. In the general ward, patients may have their own room where they can move around independently if given clearance to do so. They also may walk the halls or even go to certain outside areas if safe to do so. Patients typically will continue to progress through the levels of mobility on the general ward while preparing for discharge.

In Filipe's case, the physiotherapist would continue through the levels of mobility when he moves to a new unit.

All sessions should be well documented to ensure continuity of care between the ICU and the wards. A sample session on the general ward could include the physiotherapist demonstrating to the daughter how to provide assistance to Filipe as he climbs up stairs. As the patient progresses medically, they are getting closer to discharge from the hospital. Following discharge, it is possible that the patient may continue to receive physiotherapy for some time at home or at an outpatient clinic.

SUMMARY POINTS

- Early mobility in the ICU is a safe and effective way to decrease ICU-acquired weakness and delirium
- The goals for each physiotherapy session should always be in flux depending on the patient's status
- The physiotherapist needs to be in regular communication with the medical team to provide the best care for each patient

MCQs

Q.1 Filipe is able to sit up in a chair for the first time today; he is nervous and wants to know how long he should stay sitting up before returning to bed.
   a. 1–2 hours
   b. All day
   c. Until shift change
   d. 5 hours

Q.2 What test can be performed to see if Filipe is ready to get to a chair?
   a. Functional Gait Assessment
   b. Egress Test
   c. Function in Sitting Test
   d. Finger-to-Nose Coordination Test

REFERENCES

Batt, J., dos Santos, C., Cameron, J., & Herridge, M. (2013). Intensive care unit-acquired weakness. *American Journal of Respiratory and Critical Care Medicine, 187*(3), 238–246.

Dickinson, S., Taylor, S., & Anton, P. (2018). Integrating a standardized mobility program and safe patient handling. *Critical Care Nursing Quarterly, 41*(3), 240–252.

Fossat, G., Baudin, F., Courtes, L., Bobet, S., Dupont, A., Bretagnol, A., …, & Boulain, T. (2018). Effect of in-bed leg cycling and electrical stimulation of the quadriceps on global muscle strength in critically ill adults. *JAMA, 320*(4), 368.

Herling, S., Greve, I., Vasilevskis, E., Egerod, I., Bekker Mortensen, C., Møller, A., Svenningsen, H., & Thomsen, T. (2018). Interventions for preventing intensive care unit delirium in adults. *Cochrane Database of Systematic Reviews, 11,* CD009783.

Hodgson, C., Stiller, K., Needham, D., Tipping, C., Harrold, M., Baldwin, C., …, & Webb, S. (2014). Expert consensus and recommendations on safety criteria for active mobilization of mechanically ventilated critically ill adults. *Critical Care, 18*(6), 658.

Malone, D., Ridgeway, K., Nordon-Craft, A., Moss, P., Schenkman, M., & Moss, M. (2015). Physical therapist practice in the intensive care unit: results of a national survey. *Physical Therapy, 95*(10), 1335–1344.

Morris, P., Goad, A., Thompson, C., Taylor, K., Harry, B., Passmore, L., …, & Haponik, E. (2008). Early intensive care unit mobility therapy in the treatment of acute respiratory failure. *Critical Care Medicine, 36*(8), 2238–2243.

Neufeld, K. (2017). Interventions for ICU delirium—effect of physical therapy on attention in critically ill patients. *Innovation in Aging, 1*(suppl_1), 271–272.

Verceles, A., Wells, C., Sorkin, J., Terrin, M., Beans, J., Jenkins, T., & Goldberg, A. (2018). A multimodal rehabilitation program for patients with ICU acquired weakness improves ventilator weaning and discharge home. *Journal of Critical Care, 47,* 204–210.

Zorowitz, R. (2016). ICU–acquired weakness: a rehabilitation perspective of diagnosis, treatment, and functional management. *Chest, 150*(4), 966–971.

50

Rehabilitation in Cancer

Hannah Leach & Jo Jethwa

LEARNING OBJECTIVES

- Describe the significance of cancer to the older population
- Explain the benefits of rehabilitation in people with cancer
- Outline the unique side effects of cancer and anti-cancer treatment and how this can influence rehabilitation

CASE

Gina is a 75-year-old lady who was diagnosed with a gastro-oesophageal junction tumour after difficulty swallowing and unintentional weight loss. Due to a history of osteoarthritis and a period of poor nutrition before her cancer diagnosis, she was underweight and deconditioned. It was decided she would be treated with chemotherapy followed by surgery.

Outcome measures taken before and after chemotherapy showed a reduction in her fitness and function. Following treatment, she was referred for a period of prehabilitation to optimise her condition before surgery. Prehabilitation involved multidisciplinary input, including exercise interventions, dietary and lifestyle advice and psychological support.

She was admitted to hospital for an oesophagogastrectomy (surgery to remove part of the oesophagus and stomach). After her operation, she developed loose stools and was found to have chemotherapy-induced colitis which was treated with high-dose steroids. She then developed steroid-induced myopathy (muscle weakness) meaning daily activities became very difficult. For this reason, she was unable to be discharged home and had a prolonged inpatient stay. While her steroids were weaned, she received daily input from physiotherapy and occupational therapy to promote strength and independence, allowing her to eventually return home with ongoing community support.

CANCER AND THE OLDER POPULATION

Cancer continues to be a key international public health issue, affecting people of all backgrounds and ages. The United Nations, Department of Economic and Social Affairs (2015) estimated that there were over 17 million people with a new cancer diagnosis in 2018 worldwide. This number is expected to grow to 27.5 million by 2040. Poor diet, inactivity, genetics, obesity and smoking are recognised factors that can account for the increasing prevalence of cancer globally. Improved life expectancy however is considered to be the main factor influencing growing cancer rates.

As advances in cancer treatments continue to improve survival, a predicted 7% of the UK population will be living with cancer by 2040; of this number, an estimated 77% will be aged 65 years and over (Macmillan, 2019c). The most commonly diagnosed cancers in UK adults aged over 50 years are shown in Fig. 50.1.

CANCER AND ITS TREATMENT

Cancer care can be delivered at four levels:
- Acute treatment of the cancer
- Observation and follow-up care for disease recurrence
- Palliative care for advanced cancer
- End-of-life care (Aziz & Bellizzi, 2008).

Each person will follow a different treatment pathway, planned according to their disease, pre-existing medical conditions and functional status. When deciding on the appropriate treatment pathway, a person's general well-being and activity levels are measured using the World Health Organisation (WHO) Performance Status (also known as Zubrod scale) and Karnofsky score (see Fig. 50.2). Assessments and outcome measures such as incremental shuttle walk test (ISWT) or cardiopulmonary exercise testing (CPET) may also be used to assess fitness.

Treatments may be delivered alone or as a combination of surgery, chemotherapy, immunotherapy, targeted therapy, radiotherapy and hormone therapies. For this reason, each person requires a patient-centred rehabilitation plan to address their unique symptoms.

Despite accounting for the largest percentage of the cancer population, older people receive less intensive anti-cancer treatment than younger people, irrespective of fitness. However, the Cancer Reform Strategy clearly states that age should not be a barrier to treatment (Department of Health, 2007).

SYMPTOMS AND SIDE EFFECTS OF CANCER AND ITS TREATMENT

As cancer can develop anywhere in the body, the way in which it may affect people will vary greatly. The possible symptoms of cancer and side effects of treatment are numerous, but all have the potential to affect independence and function (see Table 50.1). In this chapter, non-tumour specific symptoms

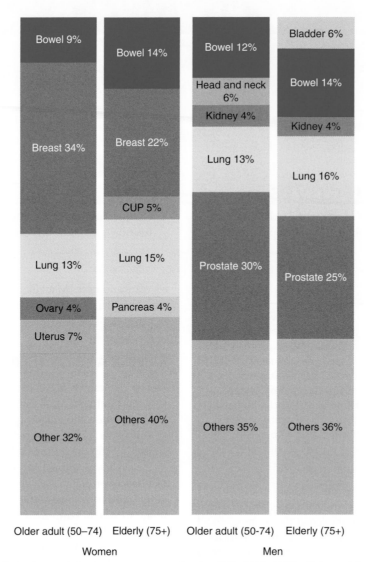

FIG. 50.1 The five most common cancers in the UK: 2013-2015. (Adapted from Cancer Research UK, 2015a, 2015b, with permission.) *CUP*, Cancer of unknown primary.

which require specialist rehabilitation are discussed in detail. Other symptoms that are also common to life-limiting diseases, such as breathlessness, are discussed in Chapter 64 Palliative Rehabilitation. Where cancer requires highly specialist treatment, for example, a lower limb amputation for a sarcoma tumour, equivalently specialist rehabilitation input will be required.

Weakness and Deconditioning

Older people will often be affected by normal age-related muscle deconditioning which can significantly impact their strength; this is known as sarcopenia. Older people may also be found to have frailty: 'a state of low energy, slow walking speed and poor strength' (British Geriatrics Society, 2018). Healthcare professionals should assess and offer support to those patients who are found to have frailty (NICE, 2016).

Research shows that people with cancer have significantly weaker muscles compared to healthy people of a similar age (Christensen et al., 2014). Reduced muscle strength is an independent predictor of cancer mortality and is correlated with slower postoperative recovery, poorer tolerance of anticancer treatment and reduced quality of life. Therefore older people with cancer are more at risk of weakness and deconditioning. Prehabilitation is made up of input from multidisciplinary professions in order to optimise these at-risk people before and during treatment.

Steroid-Induced Proximal Myopathy

Corticosteroids are used in oncology for several reasons, from curative treatment to symptom management. Despite their clinical effectiveness, corticosteroids may cause debilitating side effects. Steroid-induced proximal myopathy – a condition causing skeletal muscle weakness and atrophy in the muscles closest to the centre of the body – can affect up to 60% of users, irrelevant of dose or duration of use (Owczarek, Jasińska, & Orszulak-Michalak, 2005). Steroid myopathy can limit functional tasks such as stair climbing, sit to stand, and in more severe cases walking and moving in bed (Roth, Happold, & Weller, 2015).

Performance status scales

Zubrod scale	Karnofsky scale
0 Normal activity	100 Normal; no evidence of disease
	90 Able to perform normal activities with only minor symptoms
1 Symptomatic and ambulatory; care for self	80 Normal activity with effort; some symptoms
	70 Able to care for self but unable to do normal activities
2 Ambulatory >50% of time; occasional assistance	60 Requires occasional assistance; care for most needs
3 Ambulatory ≤50% of time; nursing care needed	50 Requires considerable assistance
	40 Disabled; requires special assistance
	30 Severely disabled
4 Bedridden	20 Very sick; requires active supportive treatment
	10 Moribund

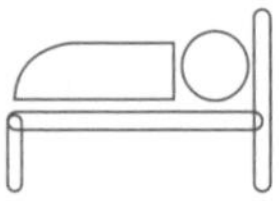

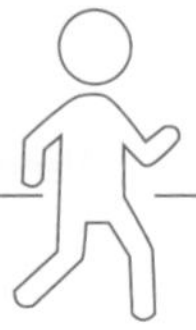

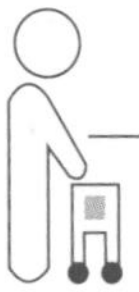

FIG. 50.2 Performance status scales.

TABLE 50.1 Symptoms and side effects of cancer and its treatment that will impact rehabilitation (Data adapted from Macmillan 2013, 2019b).

CANCER	ANTI-CANCER TREATMENT	SYMPTOM-MANAGEMENT MEDICATIONS
• Anxiety and depression • Ascites • Balance issues • Body image • Bone pain or fractures • Breathlessness • Fatigue • Incontinence • Nausea/vomiting • Pain • Paralysis • Visual changes • Weakness and deconditioning • Weight changes	• Anxiety and depression • Amputation • Balance issues • Body image issues • Bowel changes • Cardiac dysfunction • Cognitive changes • Memory issues • Fatigue • Infection • Lymphoedema • Malnutrition • Nausea/vomiting • Osteoporosis (bone weakness) and fractures • Pain • Peripheral neuropathy • Poor healing • Respiratory changes • Skin changes • Swelling • Visual changes • Weakness and deconditioning	• Balance issues • Bowel changes • Confusion/delirium • Dizziness • Drowsiness • Hallucinations • Muscle pain • Nausea/vomiting • Sleep disturbance • Steroid-induced myopathy

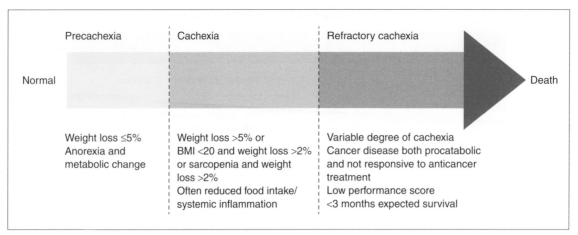

FIG. 50.3 Stages of cancer cachexia. (Data from Fearon et al., 2011.)

Medical management of steroid myopathy involves reduction or discontinuation of steroids, but muscle recovery itself can take months (Owczarek et al. 2005). Moderate exercise can be useful in preventing and treating steroid myopathy (Gupta & Gupta, 2013).

Malnutrition

Malnutrition is when the body does not receive the nutrients it requires. Malnutrition is more common with increased age and in advanced disease, particularly in gastrointestinal, head and neck, liver and lung cancers. Cancer-related malnutrition can develop into a more serious condition called cachexia.

The European Society for Clinical Nutrition and Metabolism (ESPEN) estimates that 10%-20% of deaths in the cancer population are due to malnutrition rather than the cancer itself. Despite this, only 30%-60% of patients at risk of malnutrition receive nutritional support. ESPEN recommends nutritional support, physical activity and anti-inflammatory medication as potential interventions (Arends et al., 2017).

Cachexia

Cachexia is an adverse effect of cancer which involves ongoing malnutrition, anaemia, systemic inflammation, altered immune function and skeletal muscle wasting that cannot be fully reversed with conventional nutritional support. This presents as reduced functional ability, fatigue, poor quality of life and reduced tolerance of anti-cancer treatments, and impacts survival (Christensen et al., 2014; Fearon et al., 2011; Milgrom et al., 2017).

Cachexia can be considered a three-stage continuum as described in Fig. 50.3. Carefully considered rehabilitation plans are needed for this group of patients, as placing further metabolic demands on the body may have negative effects (Fearon et al., 2011).

Fatigue

Fatigue is a debilitating symptom of cancer and a side effect of cancer treatment. It is a persistent sense of tiredness that interferes with usual activities which can have a profound impact on function and quality of life, even curtailing anti-cancer treatment (Chamberlain, 2010). However, evidence shows that fatigue can improve with exercise interventions delivered both during and after anti-cancer treatment (Cramp & Byron-Daniel, 2012; Lipsett et al., 2017; Loughney et al., 2018; Velthuis et al., 2010). Fatigue management, including pacing and sleep advice, is an important part of rehabilitation.

Chemotherapy-Induced Peripheral Neuropathy

Peripheral neuropathy (nerve damage) is a common complication of chemotherapy with approximately 38% of cancer patients on multi-agent chemotherapy experiencing chemotherapy-induced peripheral neuropathy (CIPN) (Hershman et al., 2014). CIPN may be sensory (nerves carrying feeling messages from the body back to the brain), motor (affecting the nerves carrying movement messages from the brain to the muscles) or autonomic (affecting the nerves that supply the organs).

Symptoms of CIPN and the effect it may have on quality of life will depend on the type of nerves affected. Motor nerve damage can cause weakness, cramping or poor coordination, whereas sensory nerve damage can cause pain, numbness or tingling. Motor or sensory deficits can affect a person's ability to balance, walk or carry out normal daily activities. Autonomic nerve damage can cause diarrhoea or constipation, irregular heartbeat or a drop in blood pressure on standing.

There is a higher risk of developing CIPN if you are taking or have previously taken multiple neurotoxic chemotherapy drugs, have a pre-existing peripheral neuropathy (e.g. diabetic neuropathy) or have low levels of vitamin E and B (Macmillan, 2019a).

Commonly neurotoxic drugs associated with CIPN are:
- Vinca alkaloids (vinblastine, vincristine, vinorelbine and vindesine)
- Platinum-based agents (cisplatin, oxaliplatin and carboplatin)
- Taxanes (docetaxel and paclitaxel)
- Thalidomide, bortezomib and interferon alpha (Macmillan, 2019a).

There is no treatment to reverse CIPN and while recovery is possible, it is usually very slow. For some people the damage can be permanent. For this reason, identifying CIPN may result in reduction or discontinuation of chemotherapy.

Good pain control is essential in the management of CIPN. Transcutaneous electrical nerve stimulation (TENS), acupuncture and psychological support are also useful adjuncts for pain management. People may also require splints, orthoses, walking aids or adaptive equipment to compensate (Macmillan, 2019a). There is evidence that exercise can be an important intervention both during and after treatment (McCrary et al., 2019).

Bone Disease

Bone disease in cancer can be attributed to cancer in the bones (primary or metastatic), development of osteoporosis or bone necrosis from treatment. Bone disease reduces the quality of the bone, putting a patient at risk of pathological fracture, pain, hypercalcaemia and spinal cord compression. The cancers that most commonly metastasise to the bone are prostate, breast and lung – some of the most prevalent cancers in older people (Singh, Haseeb, & Alkubaisi, 2014). It should also be considered that older patients, particularly women who are post-menopausal, are more likely to have age-related osteoporosis.

Macmillan (2018b) advises that people with bone disease remain active, with the following recommendations (see Table 50.2). Orthopaedic advice should be taken into consideration when developing a rehabilitation or exercise programme for this patient group; interventions should be considered holistically and led by specialist therapists.

THE CHANGING FACE OF REHABILITATION IN CANCER

The diversity in cancer can pose complex and multifaceted challenges for health practitioners and requires a holistic approach to rehabilitation. NICE (2004) states that 'Rehabilitation attempts to maximise patients' ability to function, to promote their independence and to help them adapt to their condition. It offers a major route to improving their quality of life, no matter how long or short a patient's prognosis may be. It aims to maximise dignity and reduce the extent to which cancer interferes with an individual's physical, psychosocial and economic functioning.'

People are now living an average of 10 years following cancer diagnosis, compared with 1 year in the 1970s (Quaresma, Coleman, & Rachet, 2015). Multidisciplinary rehabilitation in oncology, focusing on living with and beyond cancer, is becoming a more recognised and evidence-based aspect of the cancer care pathway. Dietz (1969) first classified cancer rehabilitation into the following categories: preventive, restorative, supportive and palliative. These remain relevant in current practice as seen in Fig. 50.4.

Preventative

Exercise has been shown to reduce the risk of cancer recurrence across 13 different cancer types (Moore et al., 2016), including bowel, breast and lung cancers which are common types of cancer amongst older persons. It has been hypothesised that activity reduces the risk of cancer due to improved immune system function, reduced inflammation, preventing obesity and lowering levels of hormones that are linked to cancer (Winzer et al., 2011). Lifestyle changes such as smoking cessation, weight loss and healthy eating can reduce the risk of cancer, even when such habits are long standing.

Restorative

Older people with frailty are known to have poorer outcomes from anti-cancer treatment (McIsaac et al., 2018). Prehabilitation (a period of multidisciplinary input prior to anti-cancer treatment) is becoming an increasingly well-evidenced area of the oncology pathway, showing improved outcomes of surgery, chemotherapy and radiotherapy (Macmillan, 2018b). The aim of prehabilitation is to maximise physical and psychological well-being to reduce the incidence and severity of future impairment (Silver & Baima, 2013). If prehabilitation was universally available for older people, they may be considered for more intensive treatment.

TABLE 50.2 Exercise recommendations for people with bone metastases (Data from Macmillan 2018a).

SITE AFFECTED BY METASTASES	EXERCISE MODE					
	Resistance Upper	Trunk	Lower	Aerobic WB	NWB	Flexibility Static
Pelvis	•	•	•**		•	•
Axial skeleton (lumbar)	•		•		•	•***
Axial skeleton (thoracic/ribs)	•*		•	•	•	•***
Proximal femur	•		•**		•	•
All regions	•*		•**		•	•***

Note that the efficacy and safety of this modular multimodal exercise programme is currently being determined, and this table should not act as an absolute guide.

*Exercise should exclude shoulder flexion/extension/abduction/adduction but can include elbow flexion/extension.
**Exercise should exclude hip extension/flexion but can include knee extension/flexion.
***Exercise should exclude spine/flexion/extension/rotation.
A dot indicates that a region of the body can be targeted for exercise. WB, weight bearing (e.g. walking); NWB, non-weight-bearing (e.g. cycling).

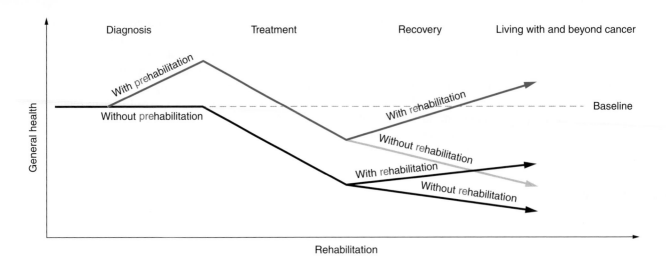

Diagnosis　　Treatment　　Recovery　　Living with and beyond cancer

With prehabilitation

Without prehabilitation

With rehabilitation

Without rehabilitation

With rehabilitation

Without rehabilitation

Baseline

General health

Rehabilitation

Preventative

Prehabilitation includes screening, assessment and, where appropriate, the development of a Personalised Prehabilitation Care Plan (PPCP) as part of an overall care plan.

This includes exercise, nutrition and psychological support interventions based on need, with continual monitoring and evaluation. The patient may go through this stage several times in preparation for different treatments.

Restorative

Prehabilitation can significantly improve the patient's ability to cope with effects of treatment of all kinds, including surgery, chemotherapy, radiotherapy, immunotherapy and treatment for palliative care.

People with treatable but not curable cancer may also benefit. It can help reduce the amount of time spent in hospital and to better quality of life.

Following treatment, the focus is restorative. Ideally, the patient will have an outcome assessment and will continue smoothly into rehabilitation and beyond.

By giving all patients, including people with treatable but not curable cancer a head-start, we can optimise their recovery from the effects of treatment.

Supportive and/or palliative

At this stage, we continue to reinforce the core principles of the programme, with health and wellbeing activities and cancer care reviews.

The patient can enjoy lifelong benefits from behaviours learned earlier. if there is further treatment, the patient goes through the cycle again.

FIG. 50.4 Classification of cancer rehabilitation. (From Macmillan 2018b, with permission.)

Supportive and/or Palliative

People with cancer have the same benefits from exercise as the general population, such as improving fitness, stamina and strength. In addition, exercise can help manage side effects of treatment and have a positive influence on quality of life (Segal et al., 2017). Exercise interventions for this population have been shown to be more effective in a group or supervised setting, compared with provision of a home exercise programme (Kramer Mikkelsen et al., 2019; Segal et al., 2017).

Exercise is considered safe during and after anti-cancer treatment. The risks of exercising in cancer are no greater than those in the general population, with the exception of those with bone metastases due to a higher risk of fracture and which require modified exercise advice from a specialist physiotherapist (Macmillan, 2018a). Although there is a positive

attitude towards exercise in older patients with cancer, fatigue and pre-existing comorbidities appear to be the biggest limitations (Kramer Mikkelsen et al., 2019). Exercise programmes that are adaptable to individual circumstances and abilities will be most beneficial (Kramer Mikkelsen et al., 2019).

It is equally important to address psychosocial concerns as part of holistic rehabilitation. The World Health Organisation (2017) reports that over 20% of adults aged 60 years or over have a mental health diagnosis. As the culture and stigma surrounding both cancer and mental health improves, public willingness to discuss such topics is increasingly acceptable (Fialka-Moser et al., 2003). It is therefore important to allow open conversations between patients and healthcare professionals, in order to improve care, rehabilitation and quality of life for our older patients.

SUMMARY POINTS

- Older people with cancer benefit from rehabilitation at all points of their journey, from diagnosis to palliative care, irrespective of their age
- Exercise can reduce the risk of cancer development or recurrence. It is a safe and important intervention in the management of cancer symptoms and the side effects of treatment

- The number of older people living with cancer continues to grow. Joined up, multidisciplinary rehabilitation, addressing both physical and mental health, is essential to allow them to maintain independence and quality of life despite their diagnosis

MCQs

Q.1 What is prehabilitation?
   a. A period of exercise to optimise a cancer patient prior to surgery
   b. A period of multidisciplinary input to optimise a cancer patient prior to surgery
   c. A period of multidisciplinary input to optimise a cancer patient prior to any anti-cancer treatment
   d. A period of exercise to optimise a cancer patient prior to any anti-cancer treatment

Q.2 When should a person with cancer not undertake exercise?
   a. When they are experiencing fatigue
   b. When they have uncontrolled pain
   c. When they have osteoporosis from treatment
   d. When they have bone metastases
   e. When they exhibit signs of pre-cachexia

Q.3 At what stages in their cancer pathway should patients be offered rehabilitation?
   a. Preventative and restorative phases
   b. Restorative and supportive phases
   c. Preventative, restorative and supportive phases
   d. Preventative, restorative, supportive and palliative phases

REFERENCES

Arends, J., Baracos, V., Bertz, H., Bozzetti, F., Calder, P., Deutz, N., …, & Weimann, A. (2017). ESPEN expert group recommendations for action against cancer-related malnutrition. *Clinical Nutrition, 36*(5), 1187–1196.

Aziz, N. M., & Bellizzi, K. (2008). Older survivors and cancer care. *Journal of the National Cancer Institute, 100*(1), 4–5.

British Geriatrics Society. (2018). *Frailty: what's it all about?* Retrieved from https://www.bgs.org.uk/resources/frailty-what%E2%80%99s-it-all-about (Accessed 2 September 2019).

Cancer Research UK. (2015a). *Most common cancers by age in females.* Retrieved from https://www.cancerresearchuk.org/health-professional/cancer-statistics/incidence/age#heading-Two (Accessed 2 September 2019).

Cancer Research UK (2015b). *Most common cancers by age in males.* Retrieved from https://www.cancerresearchuk.org/health-professional/cancer-statistics/incidence/age#heading-One (Accessed 2 September 2019).

Chamberlain, M. C. (2010). Neurotoxicity of cancer treatment. *Current Oncology Reports, 12*(1), 60–67.

Christensen, J. F., Jones, L. W., Anderson, J. L., Daugaard, G., Rorth, M., & Hojman, P. (2014). Muscle dysfunction in cancer patients. *Annals of Oncology, 25*(5), 947–958.

Cramp, F., & Byron-Daniel, J. (2012). Exercise for the management of cancer-related fatigue in adults. *Cochrane Database of Systematic Reviews, 11*, CD006145.

Department of Health. (2007). *Cancer reform strategy.* Retrieved from https://www.nhs.uk/NHSEngland/NSF/Documents/Cancer Reform Strategy.pdf (Accessed 2 September 2019).

Dietz, J. H., Jr. (1969). Rehabilitation of the cancer patients. *The Medical Clinics of North America, 53*, 607–624.

Fearon, K., Strasser, F., Anker, S. D., Bosaeus, I., Bruera, E., Fainsinger, R. L., …, & Baracos, V. (2011). Definition and classification of cancer cachexia: an international consensus. *The Lancet Oncology, 12*(5), 489–495.

Fialka-Moser, V., Crevenna, R., Korpam, M., & Quittan, M. (2003). Cancer rehabilitation. Particularly with aspects on physical impairments. *Journal of Rehabilitation Medicine, 35*(4), 153–162.

Gupta, Y., & Gupta, A. (2013). Glucocorticoid-induced myopathy: pathophysiology, diagnosis, and treatment. *Indian Journal of Endocrinology and Metabolism, 17*(5), 913.

Hershman, D. L., Lacchetti, C., Dworkin, R. H., Lavoie Smith, E. M., Bleeker, J., Cavaletti, G., …, & Loprinzi, C. L. (2014). Prevention and management of chemotherapy-induced peripheral neuropathy in survivors of adult cancers: American Society of Clinical Oncology clinical practice guideline. *Journal of Clinical Oncology, 32*, 1941–1967.

Kramer Mikkelsen, M., Nielsen, D. L., Vinther, A., Lund, C. M., & Jarden, M. (2019). Attitudes towards physical activity and exercise in older patients with advanced cancer during oncological treatment—a qualitative interview study. *European Journal of Oncology Nursing, 41*, 16–23.

Lipsett, A., Barrett, S., Haruna, F., Mustian, K., & O'Donovan, A. (2017). The impact of exercise during adjuvant radiotherapy for breast cancer on fatigue and quality of life: a systematic review and meta-analysis. *Breast, 32*, 144–155.

Loughney, L. A., Jack, S., Grocott, M. P. W., West, M. A., & Kemp, G. J. (2018). Exercise interventions for people undergoing multimodal cancer treatment that includes surgery. *Cochrane Database of Systematic Reviews, 12*(1), CD012280.

Macmillan (2013). *Throwing the light on the consequences of cancer and its treatment.* London. Retrieved from https://www.macmillan.org.uk/documents/aboutus/research/researchandevaluationreports/throwinglightontheconsequencesofcanceranditstreatment.pdf (Accessed 2 September 2019).

Macmillan. (2018a). *Physical activity for people with metastatic bone disease—guidance for professionals.* Retrieved from https://www.macmillan.org.uk/_images/physical-activity-for-people-with-metastatic-bone-disease-guidance_tcm9-326004.pdf (Accessed 2 September 2019).

Macmillan. (2018b). *Principles and guidance for prehabilitation within the management and support of people with cancer.* Retrieved from https://www.macmillan.org.uk/_images/prehabilitation-guidance-for-people-with-cancer_tcm9-353994.pdf (Accessed 2 September 2019).

Macmillan. (2019a). *Peripheral neuropathy.* Retrieved from https://www.macmillan.org.uk/information-and-support/coping/side-effects-and-symptoms/other-side-effects/peripheral-neuropathy.html (Accessed 2 September 2019).

Macmillan. (2019b). *Side effects and symptoms.* Retrieved from https://be.macmillan.org.uk/be/s-614-side-effects-and-symptoms.aspx (Accessed 2 September 2019).

Macmillan. (2019c). *Statistics fact sheet.* Retrieved from https://www.macmillan.org.uk/_images/cancer-statistics-factsheet_tcm9-260514.pdf (Accessed 2 September 2019).

McCrary, J. M., Goldstein, D., Sandler, C. X., Barry, B. K., Marthick, M., Timmins, H. C., …, & Park, S. B. (2019). Exercise-based rehabilitation for cancer survivors with chemotherapy-induced peripheral neuropathy. *Supportive Care in Cancer, 27,* 3849–3857.

McIsaac, D. I., Saunders, C., Hladkowicz, E., Bryson, G. L., Forster, A. J., Gagne, S., …, & McCartney, C. J. L. (2018). PREHAB study: a protocol for a prospective randomised clinical trial of exercise therapy for people living with frailty having cancer surgery. *BMJ Open, 8*(6), 1–8.

Milgrom, D. P., Lad, N. L., Koniaris, L. G., & Zimmers, T. A. (2017). Bone pain and muscle weakness in cancer patients. *Current Osteoporosis Reports, 15*(2), 76–87.

Moore, S. C., Lee, I. M., Weiderpass, E., Campbell, P. T., Sampson, J. N., Kitahara, C. M., …, & Patel, A. V. (2016). Association of leisure-time physical activity with risk of 26 types of cancer in 1.44 million adults. *JAMA Internal Medicine, 176*(6), 816–825.

National Institute for Health and Clinical Excellence (Great Britain). (2004). *Improving supportive and palliative care for adults with cancer, CSG4.* Retrieved from https://www.nice.org.uk/guidance/csg4, page 134 (Accessed 2 February 2019).

National Institute for Health and Clinical Excellence (Great Britain). (2016). *Multimorbidity: clinical assessment and management, NG56.* Retrieved from https://www.nice.org.uk/guidance/NG56 (Accessed 2 September 2019).

Owczarek, J., Jasińska, M., & Orszulak-Michalak, D. (2005). Drug-induced myopathies. An overview of the possible mechanisms. *Pharmacological Reports, 57*(1), 23–34.

Quaresma, M., Coleman, M. P., & Rachet, B. (2015). 40-year trends in an index of survival for all cancers combined and survival adjusted for age and sex for each cancer in England and Wales, 1971-2011: a population-based study. *The Lancet, 385*(9974), 1206–1218.

Roth, P., Happold, C., & Weller, M. (2015). Corticosteroid use in neuro-oncology: an update. *Neuro-Oncology Practice, 2*(1), 6–12.

Singh, V. A., Haseeb, A., & Alkubaisi, A. A. H. A. (2014). Incidence and outcome of bone metastatic disease at University Malaya Medical Centre. *Singapore Medical Journal, 55*(10), 539–546.

Segal, R., Zwaal, C., Green, E., Tomasone, J., Loblaw, A., & Petrella, T. (2017). Exercise for people with cancer: a systematic review. *Current Oncology, 24*(4), 290–315.

Silver, J. K., & Baima, J. (2013). Cancer prehabilitation. *American Journal of Physical Medicine & Rehabilitation, 92*(8), 715–727.

United Nations, Department of Economic and Social Affairs, Population Division. (2015). *Global cancer - facts and figures, 4th edn.* Retrieved from https://www.cancer.org/content/dam/cancer-org/research/cancer-facts-and-statistics/global-cancer-facts-and-figures/global-cancer-facts-and-figures-4th-edition.pdf (Accessed 18 April 2019).

Velthuis, M. J., Agasi-Idenburg, S. C., Aufdemkampe, G., & Wittink, H. M. (2010). The effect of physical exercise on cancer-related fatigue during cancer treatment: a meta-analysis of randomised controlled trials. *Clinical Oncology, 22*(3), 208–221.

West, H., & Jin, J. (2015). Performance status in patients with cancer. *JAMA Oncology, 1*(7), 998.

Winzer, B. M., Whiteman, D. C., Reeves, M. M., & Paratz, J. D. (2011). Physical activity and cancer prevention: a systematic review of clinical trials. *Cancer Causes and Control, 22*(6), 811–826.

World Health Organisation. (2017). *Mental health of older patients.* Retrieved from https://www.who.int/news-room/fact-sheets/detail/mental-health-of-older-adults (Accessed 29 April 2019).

51

Rehabilitation in Movement Disorders

Robert Iansek & Mary Danoudis

LEARNING OBJECTIVES

- Describe how malfunction occurs in common movement disorders
- Explain how to apply this information to movement strategy training
- Describe how to integrate the various rehabilitation approaches to individual patients
- Discuss the importance of a team approach to deliver comprehensive care for patients with movement disorders

CASE

Kimiko is an 83-year-old woman who has had Parkinson's disease (PD) for approximately 7 years. She takes L-dopa/benserazide 200/50 mg four times a day on a four-hourly interval. She lives alone in an independent living unit in a retirement village. She was referred by a neurologist to the day hospital for a programme of rehabilitation to improve her mobility. She had found that recently she was less physically active and that she had a fear of falling.

She had asked a friend to accompany her in the car which she drove to the hospital. Unfortunately, she got lost and had to go to the nearby police station to ask for directions. She had previously driven along the same route without any difficulties. She has had to get her medication prepacked by the chemist in order for her to remember to take the dose on time. She is still able to manage her finances but keeps all her bills in one location and has to check and recheck to make sure she does not forget to pay them when due.

This case study illustrates a common finding of PD-related cognitive issues. They represent difficulty of maintaining a task in readiness (cognitive set) as well as sequentially regulating the performance of the task (cognitive cues). Driving with a friend means that her attention is withdrawn from her intention and the destination (cognitive set is lost) and turning cues are reliant on basal ganglia (BG) function (cues are absent), which clearly is not working. Attention can only compensate while in use and withdrawal of attention for conversation means she gets lost. Similarly, the visual cues of a prepared medication pack with times acts as a reminder, as does checking the dates on her accounts. These issues are discussed in detail below.

INTRODUCTION

This chapter will discuss rehabilitative approaches for conditions affecting older people with movement disorders. The most common conditions include PD, Parkinson-related disorders (PRD) and frontal gait disorder (FGD). All these conditions involve the BG (part of the brain involved in voluntary movement and other functions; see Box 51.1 for a detailed description) and its connections in one or multiple ways. We will focus predominantly on PD, but the discussion would equally apply to the less common PRD and FGD. Rehabilitative approaches have been developed and used as an add-on to medications to improve movement, restore function and facilitate participation in work, family and society with the overall goal to optimise quality of life.

In general terms the basis of the rehabilitative approaches has been threefold:

- those that address the motor disturbance in PD
- those that optimise strength and endurance
- those that maintain an appropriate level of physical activity to enable easier everyday functions.

In addition, it has been suggested that rehabilitative approaches may have the capacity to alter the disturbed BG internal circuitry and, in that manner, modify the capacity to perform movement in a more normal manner. Lastly, rehabilitative mechanisms may alter dopamine (a chemical involved in transmitting signals in the brain) effects, perhaps through dopamine modifier functions. We will focus mainly on the first three mechanisms, but we will mention the others more in passing to ensure the reader is aware of all options.

All these conditions are complex, unfortunately not curable, progressive over time and associated with age-related conditions. Consequently, rehabilitation needs to be delivered in the context of a multidisciplinary team (MDT), or multiple teams, depending on the contact points. Examples include clinic, community and outreach. In addition, rehabilitation will be one of multiple interventions provided by each of the team members depending on the patient's needs.

PARKINSON'S DISEASE

PD is caused by a reduction of dopamine in the brain, due to degeneration of the neurons in the substantia nigra. This interferes with output to the motor cortical regions (that control movement) in two ways: disturbed selection and maintenance of a plan and disturbance in the sequential management of the plan (Iansek, Huxham, & McGinley, 2006; Morris et al., 2005).

BOX 51.1 Basal Ganglia Function

The basal ganglia (BG) are a group of nuclear structures located at the base of the brain which are connected with each other and with the cerebral cortex, as shown in Fig. 51.1 (Lanciego, 2012). Together they perform automatic functions based on the basal ganglia's connectivity with the specific area, or areas, of cerebral cortex. The BG are organised into two feedback loops. The input loop is composed of the corpus striatum (CS) and the substantia nigra (SN), and the output loop is composed of the two divisions of the globus pallidus (GP) and the subthalamic nucleus.

The BG automate movement (Marsden, 1982) or motor skills, enabling motor performance without the use of attention. To perform this function, the BG interrelate with the motor cortical regions: the supplementary motor area (SMA) and the pre-supplementary motor area (PSMA) (Wu, Chan, & Hallett, 2010).

The PSMA is involved with selection of movement plans and the SMA is involved in the maintenance of the plan and its sequential management. The BG enable these actions by maintaining both the selection and the plan in readiness as well as regulating its sequential management with the SMA in an online process. A change of intention terminates one plan and initiates another. In reality, multiple plans coexist and are thus automated simultaneously as the BG have a large functional reserve.

Attention control of movement utilises the premotor area, the cingulate gyrus and the cuneate gyrus, regulating movement by sensory feedback, predominantly visual in nature. It may work independently or in parallel to the automatic control, and there is a constant transition from one control mechanism to the other depending on the circumstances prevailing at the time of the performance of the task.

The usual motor features seen are tremor at rest, rigidity and bradykinesia (slow movement). Other signs can include reduced arm swing, small handwriting, a mask-like facial expression and reduced voice volume.

PD clinically is asymmetric, generally involving one side of the body at presentation and dominantly affecting this side throughout the disease course. The affected body part

will demonstrate a mismatch between the desired and actual amplitude, or speed, that was required to be maintained. This disparity is directly related to the degree of dopamine loss; the greater the dopamine loss the greater the disparity and the greater the reduction in overall amplitude of the plan. Movements thus become smaller and slower. Box 51.2 provides detailed information about neurological changes in PD.

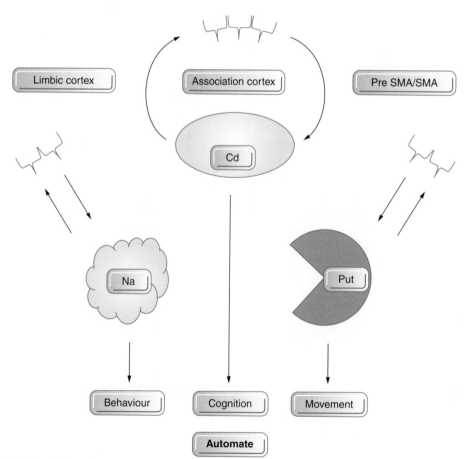

FIG. 51.1 Schematic representation of basal ganglia organisation into functional clinical entities based on reciprocal cortical connections. *Cd*, Caudate nucleus; *NA*, nucleus accumbens; *Put*, putamen; *SMA*, supplementary motor area.

BOX 51.2 Neurological Changes in PD

There may be disturbance in the sequential management of a task (Cunnington, Bradshaw, & Iansek, 1996). This manifests as an ever-reducing amplitude (sequence effect) inevitably resulting in a motor block for the movement (Iansek et al., 2006). The inability to adequately maintain plan selection can result in failure of plan initiation.

There is also an inability in patients with PD to appreciate the degree of their motor deficits (Ho, Iansek, & Bradshaw, 1999). It means that people with PD are unable to improve their motor mismatch voluntarily as they are unaware of the problem and its severity.

In this context, it is important to understand how attention control of movement interrelates with the impaired automatic control in PD. Attention control appears to have the capacity to augment automatic control by changing the intention and consequently re-planning the task, rather than influencing the task directly. The new programming is still using the BG supplementary motor area (SMA) control mechanisms, and it results in an inadequate improvement in amplitude. This is readily seen by asking patients to walk faster, write bigger or speak louder. This is easily done by the patient with improvement in amplitude, but the change never normalises the amplitude (Morris et al., 2005). If attention is withdrawn, the amplitude reduces back to the smaller uncompensated level.

At the same time, it is possible to utilise attention control to normalise movement in subjects with PD by providing sensory feedback (cueing) regarding normal movement amplitude. The most effective sensory feedback is usually visual but can be proprioceptive or auditory (Morris et al., 1996). This immediate improvement and normalisation of amplitude is easily elicited by demonstrating the correct amplitude and asking subjects to concentrate on performing the movement with that size. Once the correct amplitude is seen, the patient can continue to perform it without the visual guide as long as the subject is able to concentrate. If attention is diverted, then the movement reverts (Morris et al., 1996). This interaction between attention and automation occurs constantly and generally most patients perform better, but not normally, when they concentrate.

Executive dysfunction has been identified as the most prominent cognitive deficit in PD and involves impairment of working memory, sequencing, planning, initiation, impulse inhibition and reasoning (Caccappolo & Marder, 2010). With attention, patients are able to manage these tasks but possibly impaired by motor disturbances (Stolwyk et al., 2005).

BOX 51.3

Five guidelines to be used by therapists to assist in the design of strategies for each individual client based on the specific client needs and difficulties in activities of daily living.

1. Normal movement is possible in Parkinsonism
2. Break movements into component parts
3. Use attention to perform each component
4. Use cues to maximise the use of attention
5. Avoid simultaneous tasks

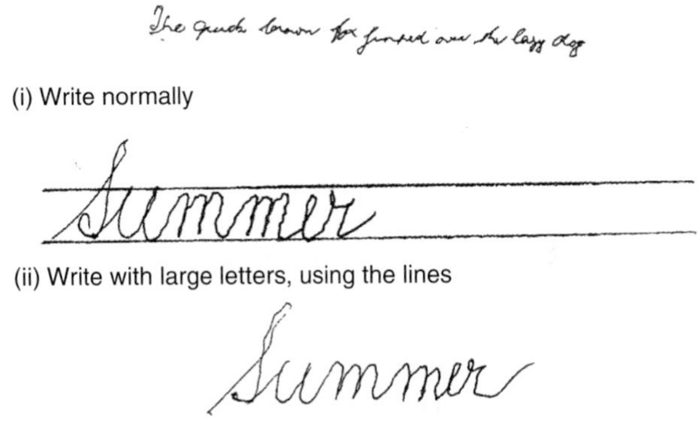

The quick brown fox jumped over the lazy dog

(i) Write normally

Summer

(ii) Write with large letters, using the lines

Summer

(iii) Write with large letters, after removing the lined paper

FIG. 51.2 Illustration of the use of attention with visual cues to determine amplitude of movement and the power of sustained attention when the cues are withdrawn.

REHABILITATION INTERVENTIONS TO HELP PARKINSON'S DISEASE

Movement Strategy Training

Movement strategy training is the prime rehabilitative approach delivered through the MDT as each discipline can apply the use of attention with external cues to indicate normal function (Morris, Martin, & Schenkman, 2010). The role of each therapist is to use this approach to teach patients and carers to perform tasks they find difficult. It needs to be emphasised that it is not a substitute for adequacy of medication adjustment. The two are delivered side by side by different team members but emphasised by all team members. Box 51.3 illustrates the guidelines all therapists should use to develop these strategies. These guidelines are based on the previously explained theory. Fig. 51.2 illustrates these principles as applied to normalisation of handwriting.

Exercise

An exercise programme is an essential part of any treatment plan for a person with PD (Mak et al., 2017). People with PD who undertake regular exercise have been shown to have better quality of life and function over the long term, compared to those who don't exercise or do so infrequently (Oguh et al., 2014). Animal models of PD and a growing body of research involving humans with PD suggest that regular exercise can induce neuroplasticity (remodelling of the brain) (Mak et al., 2017). Studies involving animal models of PD demonstrated a range of changes in the brain in response to exercise (Mak et al., 2017). The disease process itself was able to be slowed, suggesting a disease-modifying effect.

It is recommended that people with PD exercise regularly and undertake a minimum of 150 minutes of moderate intensity physical activity weekly (van der Kolk & King, 2013). Differing forms of exercise have been found to be effective at preventing or reversing the secondary consequences associated with PD (Shulman et al., 2013; Tomlinson et al., 2013). The core modes of exercise include training for aerobic/endurance, strength, balance and flexibility (Keus et al., 2007). The form of exercise depends on the individual's problems, their preferences and restrictions due to comorbidities. Exercise programmes may also include motor skill training through the practice of functional tasks that the individual finds problematic, such as bed mobility and transfers. Task-specific training along with improvements from strength, aerobic, balance and flexibility training work best to improve the person's overall functional abilities and lessen or limit their disabilities. Non-traditional forms of exercise, such as Tai Chi and dancing, have also been widely investigated and reviewed and have been shown to improve strength, mobility, balance and endurance (Kalyani et al., 2019; Ni et al., 2014). A recent review showed aquatic therapy exercise improved balance and functional mobility compared to land-based or usual care (Pinto et al., 2019).

Aerobic Training

Regular moderate to intense aerobic exercise during mid-life is associated with a lowered risk of developing PD (Ahlskog et al., 2011). In addition to the beneficial effects of aerobic exercise on fitness and function (Schenkman et al., 2012), there is increasing evidence for the positive effects on the disease process itself (Hirsch, Iyer, & Sanjak, 2016). A recent randomised clinical trial indicated that high-intensity aerobic and strengthening exercise is more effective at modifying disease severity than moderate to low intensity exercise in people with PD (Schenkman et al., 2018). High-intensity programmes may not suit everyone with PD as this is a disorder that largely affects older people who generally are sedentary and present with varying comorbidities. Individualised programmes based on the person's preferences and their capabilities are more likely to promote adherence. The intensity level can still be set to challenge the person and progressed as tolerated. The recommended aerobic training is $\geq$ 5 days weekly, 30 minutes per day (or 3 blocks of 10 minutes) of moderate intensity (van der Kolk & King, 2013). This can be achieved with moderately brisk walking, treadmill walking, cycling, dance or aqua therapy.

Progressive Strength Training and Flexibility Training

Progressive strength training in PD increases muscle strength, improves walking and reduces falls rate (Brienesse and Emerson, 2013; Morris et al., 2015). It is recommended that strength training be progressive and be performed twice weekly (van der Kolk & King, 2013). The recommended intensity is 8–12 repetitions at 60%–80% maximum effort, performing one to three sets. Muscle groups to target include the extensors of the trunk, shoulder girdle, hips and legs.

Flexibility exercises to counter the typical flexed posture associated with PD are ideally performed 2–3 days per week, targeting the flexor group of muscles of the neck, shoulder, trunk, and hip and knee. Aim for a 30-second stretch of each muscle group, repeating three times. In the early stages of PD, a general gym programme may be suitable, but in the later stages programmes need to be led by experienced physiotherapists and or exercise physiologists.

Balance

Balance re-training has been shown to improve postural control and improve walking and functional mobility (Allen et al., 2011). Research suggests that balance training combined with strength training is more effective at improving balance than balance exercises on their own (Keus et al., 2007). Tai Chi when used to train balance in PD improved postural control and reduced falls rate (Li et al., 2012). Movement strategy training along with falls prevention education was found to reduce falls rate in people with PD (Morris et al., 2015).

Parkinson-Related Disorders

These conditions (multiple system atrophy, progressive supranuclear palsy spectrum and corticobasal degeneration) present with similar clinical manifestations to PD initially but fail to respond to adequate doses of medication. They have a more rapidly progressive decline so that within 5 years, supervised care may be needed. Each has specific characteristics which aid in diagnosis and once this is apparent it is important to convey that information to the patient and family. The majority of patients have profound symptoms of movement slowing in most domains and become very reliant on movement strategy training from all the members of the MDT. In addition, supportive services are necessary as well as education of external service providers to enable home focussed living for as long as possible. Ongoing support is required in supervised care and for advice on palliative care options when necessary.

Frontal Gait Disorder

This condition is characterised by gait (walking pattern) and balance problems in the older age group with associated falls. Clinically it manifests as a wide base of support with short steps but quite good arm swing. Postural reflexes are typically disturbed or absent. It is associated with quite extensive small vessel strokes within the frontal subcortical white matter.

Pathophysiologically, the BG are disconnected from the leg area of the frontal somatosensory and supplementary motor areas of the cerebral cortex. This results in an inability to automatically regulate the size of the step to suit the environmental requirements. People with FGD can only walk with a limited range of step size with a compensated increased cadence. In a way it is similar to small-stepped gait in PD but with a wide base of support. However, there is no other clinical evidence of bradykinesia, tremor or rigidity, and the disturbance does not respond to medication. The approach to normalise walking is similar to PD. The patient is shown the correct step size and asked to concentrate on walking with the correct step size. It is best that this is practised with the use of a four-wheeled frame to eliminate fear of falling. In addition, individualised physiotherapy is directed to balance and generation of correct step size. In our programme, this is performed on an inpatient basis for 2–3 weeks, with individualised daily sessions with a trained physiotherapist and then hourly walking with a 'big step' strategy. At the end of training, the patient, if actively involved, will be able to walk normally without an aid. Regular maintenance therapy is required after discharge for 6 weeks and each subject is given specific daily exercises to maintain step length and balance. It is interesting that patients can maintain benefit for protracted periods as compared to PD which immediately reverts once attention is withdrawn.

SUMMARY POINTS

- Rehabilitation in movement disorders needs a multidisciplinary team, each member of which shares common roles as well as individual specialist roles
- Rehabilitation interventions need to be based on understanding basal ganglia function and malfunction in movement disorders
- The basal ganglia automates movement, behaviour, mood and cognition. It performs these tasks by selecting, maintaining and sequencing task components, all of which become impaired in Parkinson's disease and Parkinson-related disorders
- Guidelines enable therapists to design strategies specific to patient need, and these are applicable to all disciplines and to all malfunction domains. These strategies need to be delivered in combination with optimal medical and surgical therapy
- Other rehabilitative approaches include progressive strength training, underwater walking, underwater and on land balance training, exercise and aerobic training

MCQs

Q.1 Which functions does the basal ganglia automate?
  a. Movement
  b. Cognition
  c. Behaviour
  d. Mood
  e. All of the above

Q.2 Which one of the following is true about rehabilitation of movement disorders?
  a. Exercise has not been shown to be of benefit in the long term
  b. People with PD should undertake a minimum of 150 minutes of moderate intensity physical activity weekly
  c. Tai Chi and dancing have not been shown to be of benefit

  d. Moderate to low intensity exercise is best in people with PD
  e. Balance training exercises should ideally be done without strength training

Q.3 Which of the following gait patterns describes frontal gait disorder?
  a. A wide base of support with short steps but quite good arm swing
  b. A narrow base of support with short steps but quite good arm swing
  c. A narrow base of support with long steps
  d. Leaning to the front constantly
  e. None of the above

REFERENCES

Ahlskog, J. E., Geda, Y. E., Graff-Radford, N. R., & Petersen, R. C. (2011). Physical exercise as a preventive or disease-modifying treatment of dementia and brain aging. *Mayo Clinic Proceedings*, 86(9), 876–884.

Allen, N. E., Sherrington, C., Paul, S. S., & Canning, C. G. (2011). Balance and falls in Parkinson's disease: a meta-analysis of the effect of exercise and motor training. *Movement Disorders*, 26(9), 1605–1615.

Brienesse, L. A., & Emerson, M. N. (2013). Effects of resistance training for people with Parkinson's disease: a systematic review. *Journal of the American Medical Directors Association*, 14(4), 236–241.

Caccappolo, E., & Marder, K. (2010). Cognitive impairment in non-demented patients with Parkinson's disease. In M. Emre (Ed.), *Cognitive impairment and dementia in Parkinson's disease* (pp. 179–198). Oxford: Oxford University Press.

Cunnington, R., Bradshaw, J. L., & Iansek, R. (1996). The role of the supplementary motor area in the control of voluntary movement. *Human Movement Science*, 15, 627–647.

Hirsch, M. A., Iyer, S. S., & Sanjak, M. (2016). Exercise-induced neuroplasticity in human Parkinson's disease: What is the evidence telling us? *Parkinsonism & Related Disorders*, 22(Suppl 1), S78–S81.

Ho, A. K., Iansek, R., & Bradshaw, J. (1999). Regulation of parkinsonian speech volume: the effect of interlocuter distance. *Journal of Neurology Neurosurgery & Psychiatry*, 67(2), 199–202.

Iansek, R., Huxham, F., & McGinley, J. (2006). The sequence effect and gait festination in Parkinson disease: contributors to freezing of gait? *Movement Disorders*, 21(9), 1419–1424.

Kalyani, H. H. N., Sullivan, K. A., Moyle, G., Brauer, S., Jeffrey, E. R., Roeder, L., Berndt, S., & Kerr, G. (2019). Effects of dance on gait, cognition, and dual-tasking in Parkinson's disease: a systematic review and meta-analysis. *Journal of Parkinson's Disease*, 9(2), 335–349.

Keus, S. H., Bloem, B. R., Hendriks, E. J., Bredero-Cohen, A. B., & Munneke, M. (2007). Evidence-based analysis of physical therapy in Parkinson's disease with recommendations for practice and research. *Movement Disorders*, 22(4), 451–460, quiz 600.

Lanciego, J. L. (2012). Basal ganglia circuits: what's now and next? *Frontiers in Neuroanatomy*, 6, 4.

Li, F., Harmer, P., Fitzgerald, K., Eckstrom, E., Stock, R., Galver, J., Maddalozzo, G., & Batya, S. S. (2012). Tai chi and postural stability in patients with Parkinson's disease. *New England Journal of Medicine*, 366(6), 511–519.

Mak, M. K., Wong-Yu, I. S., Shen, X., & Chung, C. L. (2017). Long-term effects of exercise and physical therapy in people with Parkinson disease. *Nature Reviews Neurology, 13*(11), 689–703.

Marsden, C. D. (1982). The mysterious motor function of the basal ganglia: the Robert Wartenberg Lecture. *Neurology, 32*(5), 514–539.

Morris, M., Iansek, R., McGinley, J., Matyas, T., & Huxham, F. (2005). Three-dimensional gait biomechanics in Parkinson's disease: evidence for a centrally mediated amplitude regulation disorder. *Movement Disorders, 20*(1), 40–50.

Morris, M. E., Iansek, R., Matyas, T. A., & Summers, J. J. (1996). Stride length regulation in Parkinson's disease. Normalization strategies and underlying mechanisms. *Brain, 119*(Pt 2), 551–568.

Morris, M. E., Martin, C. L., & Schenkman, M. L. (2010). Striding out with Parkinson disease: evidence-based physical therapy for gait disorders. *Physical Therapy, 90*(2), 280–288.

Morris, M. E., Menz, H. B., McGinley, J. L., Watts, J. J., Huxham, F. E., Murphy, A. T., Danoudis, M. E., & Iansek, R. (2015). A randomized controlled trial to reduce falls in people with Parkinson's disease. *Neurorehabilitation and Neural Repair, 29*(8), 777–785.

Ni, X., Liu, S., Lu, F., Shi, X., & Guo, X. (2014). Efficacy and safety of Tai Chi for Parkinson's disease: a systematic review and meta-analysis of randomized controlled trials. *PLoS One, 9*(6), e99377–e199377.

Oguh, O., Eisenstein, A., Kwasny, M., & Simuni, T. (2014). Back to the basics: regular exercise matters in Parkinson's disease: results from the National Parkinson Foundation QII registry study. *Parkinsonism & Related Disorders, 20*(11), 1221–1225.

Pinto, C., Salazar, A. P., Marchese, R. R., Stein, C., & Pagnussat, A. S. (2019). The effects of hydrotherapy on balance, functional mobility, motor status, and quality of life in patients with Parkinson disease: a systematic review and meta-analysis. *PM& R, 11*(3), 278–291.

Schenkman, M., Hall, D. A., Barón, A. E., Schwartz, R. S., Mettler, P., & Kohrt, W. M. (2012). Exercise for people in early- or mid-stage Parkinson disease: a 16-month randomized controlled trial. *Physical Therapy, 92*(11), 1395–1410.

Schenkman, M., Moore, C. G., Kohrt, W. M., Hall, D. A., Delitto, A., Comella, C. L., …, & Corcos, D. M. (2018). Effect of high-intensity treadmill exercise on motor symptoms in patients with de novo Parkinson disease: a phase 2 randomized clinical trial. *JAMA Neurology, 75*(2), 219–226.

Shulman, L. M., Katzel, L. I., Ivey, F. M., Sorkin, J. D., Favors, K., Anderson, K. E., …, & Macko, R. F. (2013). Randomized clinical trial of 3 types of physical exercise for patients with Parkinson disease. *JAMA Neurology, 70*(2), 183–190.

Stolwyk, R. J., Triggs, T. J., Charlton, J. L., Iansek, R., & Bradshaw, J. L. (2005). Impact of internal versus external cueing on driving performance in people with Parkinson's disease. *Movement Disorders, 20*(7), 846–857.

Tomlinson, C. L., Patel, S., Meek, C., Clarke, C. E., Stowe, R., Shah, L., …, & Ives, N. (2013). Physiotherapy versus placebo or no intervention in Parkinson's disease. *Cochrane Database Systematic Review*(9), CD002817.

van der Kolk, N. M., & King, L. A. (2013). Effects of exercise on mobility in people with Parkinson's disease. *Movement Disorders, 28*(11), 1587–1596.

Wu, T., Chan, P., & Hallett, M. (2010). Effective connectivity of neural networks in automatic movements in Parkinson's disease. *Neuroimage, 49*, 2581–2587.

FURTHER READING

For more detailed explanation of multidisciplinary care:

Morris, M., & Iansek, R. (1997). *Parkinson's disease: a team approach.* Cheltenham [Vic.]: Southern Health Care Network.

Video clips associated with the article:

Iansek, R., & Danoudis, M. (2017). Freezing of gait in Parkinson's disease: its pathophysiology and pragmatic approaches to management. *Movement Disorders Clinical Practice, 4*, 290–297. (see Supplementary Materials)

For more detailed explanation of rehabilitation:

Iansek, R., & Morris, M.E. (2013) Rehabilitation in Parkinson's disease. In *Rehabilitation in movement disorders* (pp. 139–151). Cambridge University Press.

Guidelines for physiotherapy for PD, as well as for speech and language and occupational therapy:

European guidelines from ParkinsonNet. Retrieved from http://www.parkinsonnet.info/guidelines/guidelines-in-english.

52

Vestibular Rehabilitation

Dara Meldrum & Deirdre Murray

LEARNING OBJECTIVES

- List the most common vestibular problems and their causes in the older person
- Explain how the vestibular system contributes to balance and gaze stability (clear vision during head movement)
- Describe the effects of ageing on the vestibular system
- Recognise the common signs and symptoms of vestibular problems
- Describe the components of a vestibular rehabilitation programme and expected outcomes in the older person

CASE

Ann is an 87-year-old lady who fell at home 3 weeks ago when she was turning around in her kitchen. She could not describe any other circumstances of her fall, but she did not lose consciousness and remembered falling. Since the fall, she described decreased confidence and dizziness (non-spinning) when bending over and when walking. She did not have any spinning sensation when rolling over in bed. She had attended for rehabilitation two years previously and had been treated for benign paroxysmal positional vertigo (BPPV) which had resolved successfully with the Epley manoeuvre. She had also undergone balance and gait re-education and had been living at home independently since.

On examination, she had limited range of movement of her cervical spine. Her oculomotor examination was within normal limits for her age; normal smooth pursuit, saccades and vestibulo-ocular reflex cancellation. With visual fixation removed (using infrared goggles), she had no spontaneous nystagmus. She had no head shaking nystagmus. Her clinical head impulse test was normal. Positional testing was difficult due to limited cervical spine range of movement, so the bed was adjusted to a 30-degree head-down position to facilitate. She had a positive Dix-Hallpike test on the right (with right torsional and upward nystagmus), but she did not report a spinning sensation during the test, rather a 'dizziness'. Other positional tests were normal. She had impaired balance and a slow cautious gait (walking pattern).

Treatment consisted of three modified Epley manoeuvres, for the right posterior semicircular canal, performed during one treatment session, which were tolerated well. A week later, her dizziness was much improved, but she still reported unsteadiness. A repeat Dix-Hallpike test was negative and her balance was better. She was provided with a home exercise programme that included static and dynamic balance and gait exercises, the former included exercises with eyes closed and with an unstable surface. She was also prescribed a progressive resistance exercise programme for the major muscle groups of the lower limbs.

This case demonstrates that BPPV can present differently in the older person. It is not always accompanied by the usual spinning sensation with head movement. It also demonstrates that BPPV recurs, and that balance and gait can improve in older persons with an appropriately prescribed programme.

INTRODUCTION TO VESTIBULAR PROBLEMS IN THE OLDER PERSON

The vestibular system (one of the major systems involved in balance) is complex and has both sensory and motor roles in the control of balance, gait and eye movements. Dysfunction of the vestibular system increases with age, with over 80% of people experiencing it by the eighth decade (Agrawal et al., 2009). Dizziness is one consequence of vestibular dysfunction and is also common in older people, occurring in 33% in those over 70 years and 50% in those over 80 years (Jonsson et al., 2004). Dizziness in the older person is a diagnostic challenge; it is usually multifactorial with 62% of older persons having more than one identifiable cause. These commonly include vestibular problems, adverse effects of medications, cardiovascular causes (e.g. presyncope), psychological disease or stroke; consequently multidisciplinary input is important. Estimated percentages of vestibular dysfunction in older persons presenting to physicians with dizziness vary between 14% and 38% (Chau et al., 2015; Maarsingh et al., 2010).

Vestibular problems significantly increase the odds of falling and result in slower gait speed (Agrawal et al., 2009; Scheltinga et al., 2016). Other consequences are fear of falling, decreased balance confidence and reduced quality of life (Agrawal, Pineault, & Semenov, 2018; Marchetti et al., 2011). Vestibular dysfunction is often missed in older populations (Oghalai et al., 2000), resulting in a longer duration of

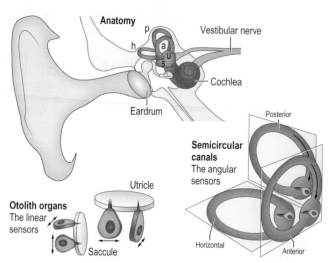

FIG. 52.1 The anatomy of the vestibular system and the orientation and pairing of the semicircular canals. (From Day BL, Fitzpatrick RC. The vestibular system. *Curr Biol.* 2015;15(15):R583–6, with permission.)

symptoms before receiving treatment (Liston et al., 2014). Furthermore, the older person with a vestibular problem is less likely to complain of vertigo than a younger individual, with feelings of 'unsteadiness' or 'about to lose balance' being common presenting symptoms (Liston et al., 2014). There is increasing evidence to suggest that recovery from acute vestibular disease in an older person is less complete, resulting in greater impairment in balance versus younger individuals.

Vestibular rehabilitation is a specialised form of physiotherapy that has a moderate to strong evidence base for reducing symptoms of dizziness and vertigo, improving balance and gait, and reducing the risk of falls. Older persons benefit from vestibular rehabilitation (Martins e Silva et al., 2016).

As vestibular dysfunction is highly prevalent in older people, incorporation of a vestibular rehabilitation programme should be considered in all patients presenting with dizziness, vertigo, falls or imbalance.

ANATOMY AND PHYSIOLOGY OF THE VESTIBULAR SYSTEM

The vestibular system is divided into peripheral and central components. The peripheral system is made up of three semicircular canals, two otoliths (the utricle and the saccule) and the vestibulocochlear nerve (Fig. 52.1) (Khan & Chang, 2013). The semicircular canals detect angular acceleration of the head (e.g. rotating the head from side to side or pitching the head forwards and backwards) and the otoliths use gravity to detect head tilt and linear acceleration (such as going up and down in a lift). The sensors of the vestibular system, hair cells, are in a structure called the cupula of the semicircular canals within an expanded area at one end of each canal, the ampulla (Fig. 52.1). In the otoliths, hair cells are covered with a layer of calcium carbonate crystals and during head acceleration or tilt, the shear of these crystals on the hair cells

activates them. Signals from the hair cells are conveyed via the eighth cranial nerve to the central vestibular system, located in the brainstem.

The three semicircular canals – horizontal, anterior and posterior – are named for their anatomical positions and are orientated at right angles to each other (Fig. 52.1). Each canal is paired functionally with a canal from the opposite side, forming three pairs: two horizontal canals, the right anterior and left posterior, and left anterior and right posterior. Each pair lies in the same plane. A head movement in the plane of a pair of canals will cause an excitation of one canal in a pair and an inhibition of the other. For example, if the head turns to the right, the right horizontal canal will be excited, and the left horizontal canal will be inhibited. The mismatch between excitation on one side and inhibition on the other side is interpreted as movement by the central nervous system. Diseases of the vestibular system can cause asymmetrical firing of the pairs and this in turn gives rise to the symptoms of vertigo/dizziness and to spontaneous nystagmus of the eyes.

Signals are decoded centrally to estimate head velocity and acceleration and to produce two main motor outputs: the vestibular ocular reflex (VOR) and the vestibulospinal reflex. The VOR is the fastest reflex in the human body which produces an eye movement that is equal in velocity and opposite in direction to a head movement. The VOR's function is to allow clear vision when the head is moving and when impaired, produces a visual blurring or jumping of the world during head movements, termed oscillopsia.

The vestibulospinal reflex plays a major role in facilitating balance reactions, particularly to recruit antigravity extensor muscles of the lower limbs. Other important connections of the vestibular system are to the cerebellum to coordinate movement and maintain balance, to the hippocampus for navigation and to the reticular activating system (for fear, flight and fright). There are also connections to the vomiting

TABLE 5.1　**Signs and symptoms of vestibular dysfunction.**	
Vertigo	Sensation of apparent movement of either the self or the environment, or distorted self-movement during an otherwise normal head movement. Commonly described as spinning in acute vestibular disease.
Dizziness	Feeling of abnormal spatial orientation without feeling of apparent movement, includes light-headedness.
Fall	Loss of postural stability from an upright, antigravity position or posture (e.g. standing or sitting), generally resulting in an uncontrolled, gravity-driven postural shift.
Unsteadiness	Feeling of being unstable without a directional preference (Bisdorff et al., 2009).
Nystagmus	Rhythmical oscillation of the eyes. In peripheral vestibular disease this usually consists of a slow eye movement in one direction followed by a fast corrective movement in the opposite direction. By convention the nystagmus is named by the direction of the fast movement, e.g. left beating horizontal nystagmus.
Anxiety	
Nausea/Vomiting	
Oscillopsia	Apparent jumping or bouncing of the visual environment during head movement, for example head movements during walking.

centre in the medulla. The consequences of vestibular disease are reflections of malfunctions of these pathways and are summarised in Table 52.1.

EFFECTS OF AGEING ON VESTIBULAR SYSTEM

After the age of 40 years, there is a 3% decline per decade in the number of vestibular neurons (Lopez, Honrubia, & Baloh, 1997). Hair cell loss occurs in the semicircular canals and in the otoliths, and VOR gains decline with age. Vestibular thresholds for detection of movement also increase with age, i.e. the system is less able to detect motion. Furthermore, as vestibular thresholds increase, failures on balance tests also increase which in turn are predictive of falling (Bermudez Rey et al., 2016).

COMMON VESTIBULAR DISORDERS IN THE OLDER PERSON

Vestibular disorders are also classified into being of peripheral or central origin.

Benign Paroxysmal Positional Vertigo

The commonest vestibular problem in the elderly is BPPV. This condition is easily treated by a skilled healthcare professional. In BPPV, the otoconia that are usually in the utricle become dislodged and move into one or more of the semicircular canals (Fig. 52.2A). The most common canal they enter is the posterior canal. The problem with the otoconia being in the canals is that the canals become sensitive to gravity. When the head goes into a position (for example, lying down), where gravity causes the otoconia to move in the canal, that canal is excited and signals movement even after the head has come to a stop. The individual will experience a short duration of spinning or dizziness until the otoconia drop to a resting position in the canal. BPPV can occur at any age and the incidence increases rapidly in the later decades of life (von Brevern et al., 2007). It is often missed in the older person. Two diagnostic tests – the Dix-Hallpike and the horizontal roll – identify BPPV and localise it to a specific semicircular canal.

Vestibular Neuritis

Vestibular neuritis is a viral infection, which is thought to be a re-activation of the herpes simplex virus, and most commonly affects the vestibular nerve and destroys hair cells (Strupp & Brandt, 2010). An acute onset of vertigo, disequilibrium and vomiting is followed by a 6–12 week period of gradual recovery through a process known as vestibular compensation (Curthoys, 2000). Although hair cells do not recover, adaptive central nervous system processes are able to compensate for unilateral vestibular loss, and there is an increased reliance on other sensory systems such as vision and proprioception. The non-affected side can also assist.

Meniere's Disease

Meniere's disease also affects the older person and is characterised by progressive hearing loss, tinnitus and attacks of vertigo, disequilibrium and often nausea and vomiting.

Presbystasis

Older persons have different levels of ability to cope with normal ageing of the vestibular system. A critical point where disequilibrium and dizziness may manifest themselves may be earlier in someone who has poor vision or other sensory or central nervous system problems. Presbystasis is the term given to age-related balance problems.

Central Vestibular Problems

These include stroke of the posterior circulation. As the incidence of stroke increases with age and up to 5% of those with acute vertigo presenting to an emergency department have a stroke, it should always be considered as part of the triage of acute vertigo. Concussion and migraine can also affect the vestibular system.

Bilateral Vestibular Disease

Bilateral loss of vestibular function occurs due to ageing, bilateral vestibular neuritis, autoimmune disorders and iatrogenic

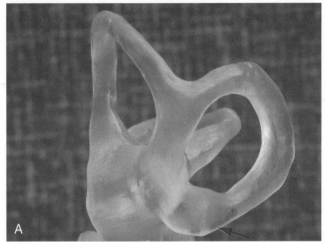

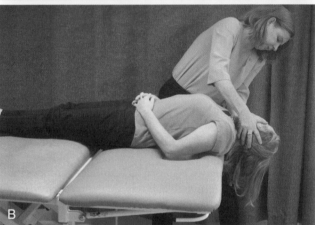

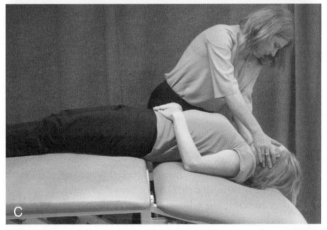

FIG. 52.2 (A) Benign paroxysmal positional vertigo (BPPV) showing otoconia that should be in the utricle migrated to the posterior semicircular canal, (B) the Dix-Hallpike test to diagnose BPPV, (C) Modified Dix-Hallpike used where cervical spine extension is limited.

causes such as aminoglycoside antibiotics and chemotherapy drugs (Leis, Rutka, & Gold, 2015; Prayuenyong et al., 2018).

APPROACH TO REHABILITATION

Rehabilitation of vestibular dysfunction in the older person should incorporate all of the essential components of vestibular rehabilitation in younger adults (Han, Song, & Kim, 2011).

These are summarised as gaze stability exercises, habituation exercises, gait and balance re-education and canal repositioning manoeuvres (See Resources section for more detail). Some modification in exercise intensity, modes or the level of challenge may be required depending on the person's ability. Additionally, a lower limb strengthening programme should be considered in older people due to the additional effects of sarcopenia (muscle loss) and the known benefits of combined strengthening and balance programmes in older people (Gillespie et al., 2012). Other practical falls prevention strategies should be considered in those who are at risk of falling.

BPPV, which is diagnosed using the Dix-Hallpike test (Fig. 52.2B) or horizontal roll test, should be treated with repositioning manoeuvres (Fig. 52.3), which may be modified if there is concern about extension of the neck. Once BPPV has resolved, the patient should undergo assessment of balance and gait and a vestibular rehabilitation programme commenced to address any problems with balance, residual dizziness or sensitivity to head positions.

A vestibular rehabilitation programme is prescribed based on a thorough assessment. Initially, a detailed subjective history is taken, including a description of the symptoms experienced, the nature of symptom onset (was it sudden/gradual/episodic) and the duration of the problem. Key questions about dizziness include whether the sensation of dizziness is constant or intermittent and whether it is provoked by activities or head positions. Orthostatic hypotension should be assessed (see Further reading below). BPPV is typically described as a brief, often intense, burst of vertigo which is aggravated by rolling over in bed or looking up to reach a high shelf, but this may not be described clearly. Other pertinent factors are changes in hearing, tinnitus, sensory changes in the face, headache and falls history.

The core elements of objective clinical assessment include the oculomotor examination, positional tests for BPPV, walking tests and objective balance testing. Infrared goggles are useful for observing nystagmus (Fig. 52.4). Referral for audiology laboratory assessments, such as videonystagmography (VNG) and the video head impulse test (vHIT), may be required to confirm vestibular loss.

Positional tests for BPPV are simple to perform and have high specificity for BPPV. The Dix-Hallpike test (Fig. 52.2B) involves placing the posterior semicircular canal into the position which promotes maximal movement of any otoconia present. The classic test does involve some extension and rotation of the cervical spine, but the same position of the canal can be achieved using lowering of a plinth or a pillow if there are any concerns regarding cervical spine extension (Fig. 52.2C).

The 10-m timed walk is a simple test requiring only a measured track and a stopwatch. The patient walks 10 m at their comfortable and maximal speeds, and both are recorded (Middleton, Fritz, & Lusardi, 2015). The modified Clinical Test for Sensory Organization of Balance (m-CTSIB) is a clinically accessible balance test which requires minimal time and basic equipment (a stopwatch and foam mat) (Shumway-Cook & Horak, 1986). It measures balance on a firm surface

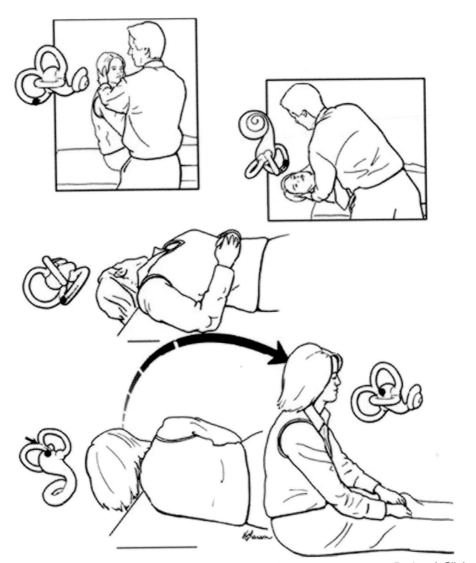

FIG. 52.3 Modified Epley manoeuvre. (From Noureldine M. *Neuroanatomy Basics: A Clinical Guide*, 1st edn, Elsevier; 2017, with permission.)

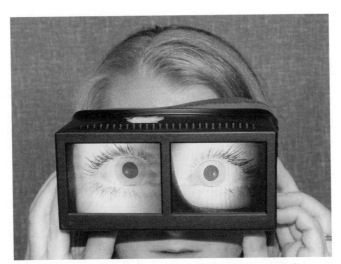

FIG. 52.4 Infrared goggles used in the vestibular assessment to observe nystagmus and other eye movements.

and on foam with eyes open and closed. More advanced balance testing such as computerised dynamic posturography should be used where possible.

An individualised treatment plan is developed based upon assessment findings.

BPPV is treated using canal repositioning manoeuvres (CRMs); the most commonly used is the modified Epley manoeuvre (Gold et al., 2014) (Fig. 52.3). This can result in an immediate resolution of the symptoms but often requires 2–3 treatment sessions and a patient should be followed up soon after the initial treatment (Bhattacharyya et al., 2017).

Rehabilitation of vestibular loss or hypofunction requires a programme of progressive exercise, and it is recommended that exercises are conducted frequently. For example, gaze stability exercises should be completed for short sessions 3–4 times per day (Hall et al., 2016). Balance exercises should be completed for 15 minutes, 5 days per week. Fifty hours of exercise are recommended for falls risk reduction (2 hours per week on an ongoing basis) (Sherrington et al., 2011).

In addition to the typical vestibular rehabilitation programme strengthening, falls prevention strategies and interventions to increase confidence are likely to be required in older people (Menant et al., 2018). Therefore, a multidisciplinary approach, including physiotherapy, nursing, occupational therapy, psychology, audiology as well as a geriatrician and ear/nose/throat specialist, is ideal.

SUMMARY POINTS

- The vestibular system has sensory and motor functions; therefore sensory symptoms such as dizziness and vertigo, as well as motor impairments in balance and gait, will occur with vestibular dysfunction
- When an older person complains of dizziness, vertigo or imbalance, the causes are likely multifactorial. An examination of the vestibular system should always be part of the evaluation
- Older people benefit from vestibular rehabilitation but ideally it should be provided by a therapist with specialist training
- Benign paroxysmal positional vertigo is common in the older person but is often undiagnosed and therefore not treated. When it is safe to do so, always perform the Dix-Hallpike test on the older person who has dizziness, vertigo or imbalance
- Vestibular system function declines with age and the decline across the senses requires a multifactorial approach that is different to younger persons. For example, leg strengthening exercises may be essential

MCQs

Q. 1 Which one of the following is a typical symptom of BPPV?
  a. A short spell of dizziness on rising quickly from a chair
  b. A short spell of vertigo when turning over in bed
  c. Feeling dizzy when watching an action movie
  d. Feeling dizzy when driving a car

Q.2 Which one of the following lists the core elements of vestibular rehabilitation?
  a. Standing, holding onto parallel bars while looking at a large letter, and practising sit to stand
  b. Habituation, gaze stability exercises and walking & balance exercises

  c. Stretching, strengthening and balance exercises
  d. Stationary bicycle, upper limb ergometry, range of motion exercises

Q.3 Assessment of the vestibular system should be considered in which one of the following situations?
  a. Only when a clear diagnosis of a vestibular disorder is made
  b. In any older person with imbalance or dizziness
  c. When syncope has been ruled out
  d. When an older person reports fatigue

REFERENCES

Agrawal, Y., Carey, J. P., Della Santina, C. C., Schubert, M. C., & Minor, L. B. (2009). Disorders of balance and vestibular function in us adults: Data from the national health and nutrition examination survey, 2001-2004. *Archives of Internal Medicine, 169*, 938–944.

Agrawal, Y., Pineault, K. G., & Semenov, Y. R. (2018). Health-related quality of life and economic burden of vestibular loss in older adults. *Laryngoscope Investigative Otolaryngology, 3*, 8–15.

Bermudez Rey, M. C., Clark, T. K., Wang, W., Leeder, T., Bian, Y., & Merfeld, D. M. (2016). Vestibular perceptual thresholds increase above the age of 40. *Frontiers in Neurology, 7*, 162.

Bhattacharyya, N., Gubbels, S. P., Schwartz, S. R., Edlow, J. A., El-Kashlan, H., Fife, T., …, & Corrigan, M. D. (2017). Clinical practice guideline: benign paroxysmal positional vertigo (update). *Otolaryngology Head and Neck Surgery, 156*, S1–S47.

Bisdorff, A., Von Brevern, M., Lempert, T., & Newman-Toker, D. E. (2009). Classification of vestibular symptoms: towards an international classification of vestibular disorders. *Journal of Vestibular Research, 19*, 1–13.

Chau, A. T., Menant, J. C., Hubner, P. P., Lord, S. R., & Migliaccio, A. A. (2015). Prevalence of vestibular disorder in older people who experience dizziness. *Frontiers in Neurology, 6*, 268.

Curthoys, I. S. (2000). Vestibular compensation and substitution. *Current Opinion in Neurology, 13*, 27–30.

Gillespie, L. D., Robertson, M. C., Gillespie, W. J., Sherrington, C., Gates, S., Clemson, L. M., & Lamb, S. E. (2012). Interventions for preventing falls in older people living in the community. *Cochrane Database of Systematic Reviews*, CD007146.

Gold, D. R., Morris, L., Kheradmand, A., & Schubert, M. C. (2014). Repositioning maneuvers for benign paroxysmal positional vertigo. *Current Treatment Options in Neurology, 16*, 307.

Hall, C. D., Herdman, S. J., Whitney, S. L., Cass, S. P., Clendaniel, R. A., Fife, T. D., …, & Woodhouse, S. N. (2016). Vestibular rehabilitation for peripheral vestibular hypofunction: an evidence-based clinical practice guideline: from the American Physical Therapy Association Neurology Section. *Journal of Neurologic Physical Therapy, 40*, 124–155.

Han, B. I., Song, H. S., & Kim, J. S. (2011). Vestibular rehabilitation therapy: review of indications, mechanisms, and key exercises. *Journal of Clinical Neurology, 7*, 184–196.

Jonsson, R., Sixt, E., Landahl, S., & Rosenhall, U. (2004). Prevalence of dizziness and vertigo in an urban elderly population. *Journal of Vestibular Research, 14*, 47–52.

Khan, S., & Chang, R. (2013). Anatomy of the vestibular system: a review. *NeuroRehabilitation, 32*, 437–443.

Leis, J. A., Rutka, J. A., & Gold, W. L. (2015). Aminoglycoside-induced ototoxicity. *CMAJ : Canadian Medical Association Journal, 187*, E52–E152.

Liston, M. B., Bamiou, D. -E., Martin, F., Hopper, A., Koohi, N., Luxon, L., & Pavlou, M. (2014). Peripheral vestibular dysfunction is prevalent in older adults experiencing multiple non-syncopal falls versus age-matched non-fallers: a pilot study. *Age and Ageing, 43*, 38–43.

Lopez, I., Honrubia, V., & Baloh, R. W. (1997). Aging and the human vestibular nucleus. *Journal of Vestibular Research, 7*, 77–85.

Maarsingh, O. R., Dros, J., Schellevis, F. G., Van Weert, H. C., van der Windt, D. A., ter Riet, G., & van der Horst, H. E. (2010). Causes of persistent dizziness in elderly patients in primary care. *Annals of Family Medicine, 8*, 196–205.

Marchetti, G. F., Whitney, S. L., Redfern, M. S., & Furman, J. M. (2011). Factors associated with balance confidence in older adults with health conditions affecting the balance and vestibular system. *Archives of Physical Medicine and Rehabilitation, 92*, 1884–1891.

Martins e Silva, D. C., Bastos, V. H., De Oliveira Sanchez, M., Nunes, M. K., Orsini, M., Ribeiro, P., Velasques, B., & Teixeira, S. S. (2016). Effects of vestibular rehabilitation in the elderly: a systematic review. *Aging - Clinical and Experimental Research, 28*, 599–606.

Menant, J. C., Migliaccio, A. A., Sturnieks, D. L., Hicks, C., Lo, J., Ratanapongleka, M., …, & Lord, S. R. (2018). Reducing the burden of dizziness in middle-aged and older people: a multifactorial, tailored, single-blind randomized controlled trial. *PLoS Medicine, 15*, e1002620.

Middleton, A., Fritz, S. L., & Lusardi, M. (2015). Walking speed: the functional vital sign. *Journal of Aging and Physical Activity, 23*, 314–322.

Oghalai, J. S., Manolidis, S., Barth, J. L., Stewart, M. G., & Jenkins, H. A. (2000). Unrecognized benign paroxysmal positional vertigo in elderly patients. *Otolaryngology-Head and Neck Surgery, 122*, 630–634.

Prayuenyong, P., Taylor, J. A., Pearson, S. E., Gomez, R., Patel, P. M., Hall, D. A., Kasbekar, A. V., & Baguley, D. M. (2018). Vestibulotoxicity associated with platinum-based chemotherapy in survivors of cancer: a scoping review. *Frontiers in Oncology, 8*, 363.

Scheltinga, A., Honegger, F., Timmermans, D. P., & Allum, J. H. (2016). The effect of age on improvements in vestibulo-ocular reflexes and balance control after acute unilateral peripheral vestibular loss. *Frontiers in Neurology, 7*, 18.

Sherrington, C., Tiedemann, A., Fairhall, N., Close, J. C., & Lord, S. R. (2011). Exercise to prevent falls in older adults: an updated meta-analysis and best practice recommendations. *New South Wales Public Health Bulletin, 22*, 78–83.

Shumway-Cook, A., & Horak, F. B. (1986). Assessing the influence of sensory interaction of balance. *Suggestion from the field. Physical Therapy, 66*, 1548–1550.

Strupp, M., & Brandt, T. (2010). Vestibular neuritis. In D. Z. E. Scott, & S. Z. David (Eds.), *Handbook of clinical neurophysiology.* Elsevier.

Von Brevern, M., Radtke, A., Lezius, F., Feldmann, M., Ziese, T., Lempert, T., & Neuhauser, H. (2007). Epidemiology of benign paroxysmal positional vertigo: a population based study. *Journal of Neurology, Neurosurgery, and Psychiatry, 78*, 710–715.

FURTHER READING

www.vestibular.org – useful resource for patients and professionals with patient educational leaflets

www.apta.org – The American Physical Therapy association has podcasts on the topic of vestibular rehabilitation and free patient education leaflets

www.brainandspine.org.uk – The Brain and Spine Foundation has a booklet on dizziness and balance problems for health care professionals and patients.

aVOR application – This is a mobile application about the vestibular system and eye movements. It is interactive and shows the anatomy, physiology and consequences of vestibular disease.

https://www.cdc.gov/steadi/pdf/Measuring_Orthostatic_Blood_Pressure-print.pdf – This is a useful document freely available from the Centre for Diseases Control to enable the assessment of orthostatic hypotension.

53

Rehabilitation in Dementia

Ellen McGough & Neva Kirk-Sanchez

LEARNING OBJECTIVES

- Describe the impact of dementia on cognition and function
- Describe the benefits of exercise and physical activity on brain health
- Identify person-centred approaches to rehabilitation for people with dementia
- Discuss rehabilitation strategies for behavioural, cognitive and motor training
- Describe strategies for increasing physical activity in people with dementia

CASE

Madeline is a 78-year-old lady who lives alone, and is having increasing difficulty with instrumental activities of daily living (IADLs). This includes managing her finances, planning meals and making appointments. She is often confused and has short-term memory problems. She has stopped many of her social outings. She has become isolated and anxious, and is worried that people are stealing her belongings, so she doesn't want carers coming into her apartment. She has fallen several times but not broken any bones, and she has bruises on arms and legs. Her walking has slowed and she has become more sedentary. She has a walking stick but forgets to use it when she leaves her apartment.

INTRODUCTION

Dementia is a syndrome characterised by progressive decline in cognitive function (e.g. memory, reasoning, communication) as well as behavioural and physical function. Alzheimer's disease is the most common cause of dementia, but there are other causes including Lewy body dementia, frontotemporal dementia and vascular dementia. Alzheimer's disease and related dementia (ADRD) can begin years or decades prior to clinical signs of dementia, often presenting as mild cognitive impairment (MCI). Individuals with MCI often have mild decline in memory, language and/or planning, and are at higher risk for developing dementia (Alzheimer's Association, 2019; Department of Health UK, 2009). Common assessments used to clinically screen patients for cognitive impairment include the Mini Mental Status Exam (MMSE), the Montreal Cognitive Assessment (MoCA) and the Addenbrooke's Cognitive Examination (Mathuranath et al., 2000).

Dementia has a profound impact on health, independence and maintenance of social relationships. As the disease progresses, people with dementia have limitations in ADLs, increased falls and fractures, and sedentary behaviour that further increases their risk for other health problems such as heart disease and diabetes. Individuals with dementia often need assistance from carers to complete daily activities. Barriers to independence include difficulty planning and scheduling appointments, keeping up with conversations and exercise groups, and learning or relearning skills and health information. The goal of rehabilitation is to increase participation in activities that are meaningful to the individual, promote a healthy lifestyle and improve quality of life. In addition, strategies to reduce burden on their carers are emphasised through education and access to resources for support (Afram et al., 2014).

COMMON IMPAIRMENTS IN PEOPLE WITH DEMENTIA

Cognition

Dementia is not a normal part of ageing, although the greatest risk factor for dementia is increasing age. Changes to brain cells begin years before the first sign of Alzheimer's disease in the brain region that affects short term and working memory, the hippocampus. Cognitive impairment in other types of dementia may present as problems with executive functions (processing and problem-solving), language and/ or working memory. Working memory is important for executive function, including awareness, planning, goal-setting, self-initiation and multitask (Alzheimer's Association, 2019). Thus, persons with dementia have difficulty learning skills, learning new routines and following recommendations from healthcare providers (e.g. medication regimes, dietary restrictions, exercise prescriptions). Daily function is also impacted, including difficulty with preparing meals, navigating transportation, managing finances, keeping up with conversations, and participating in physical and social activities.

Mood and Behaviour

Mood and behavioural changes are common in people with dementia. Common behavioural problems include agitation, aggressive behaviour, reduced inhibition, sleep disturbances, delusions and hallucinations. Changes in mood include anxiety, apathy (including loss of interest in food) and depression. Mood changes can strain family relationships and increase caregiver burden, making it difficult to care for individuals at home. Therefore, carer support, home services or nursing home care may be needed (Afram et al., 2014; Kratz, 2017). Psychologists and psychiatrists are crucial in providing guidance about management of behavioural disorders that impact quality of life in older adults and their caregivers.

Balance and Mobility

Compared to older adults without dementia, people with ADRD tend to have reduced balance and slower walking speed (Verghese et al., 2013). As they become less physically stable, physical fitness levels also decline, leading to progressive deconditioning and loss of function. Older adults with MCI are twice as likely to sustain an injurious fall as the general population of older adults (Muir, Gopaul, & Montero Odasso, 2012). Risk factors for falls in people with dementia include functional mobility limitations, slow walking speed, decreased ability to multitask and higher levels of depression (Ansai et al., 2017). Physiotherapists and occupational therapists play an important role in evaluating and treating functional mobility and fall risk. Evaluation during early stages can be useful in implementing programmes that prevent mobility decline, falls and injuries. Reliable assessments of functional mobility in older adults with dementia include the Six-Minute Walk Test, Timed Up and Go, and Berg Balance Scale (McGough et al., 2019).

REHABILITATION FOR PEOPLE WITH DEMENTIA

Rehabilitation is important for facilitating cognitive, physical and social activities, which contribute to the preservation of participation in meaningful activities (Kirk-Sanchez & McGough, 2014; McGough, Kirk-Sanchez, & Liu-Ambrose, 2017). Physiotherapy focuses on improving mobility via walking, balance and strength training, and on family/carer education for injury prevention. Improving physical fitness through physical activity programmes, completed with a partner or in a group, is also important for slowing disease progression (Kirk-Sanchez & McGough, 2014; McGough et al., 2017). Multicomponent programmes, motor skills training and cognitive training rehabilitation approaches, designed for people with dementia, are described in Table 53.1.

Multicomponent Programmes to Facilitate Participation

Rehabilitation includes treatments and strategies to promote a safe and healthy lifestyle for individuals with dementia and their caregivers. Adults with dementia are often unable to participate in the same physical and recreational activities as their peers due to cognitive impairment or behavioural and/or mobility problems. To implement and sustain effective

rehabilitation programmes for people with dementia (e.g. exercise, fall prevention), a cognitively intact partner may be needed (Teri, Logsdon, & McCurry, 2008). Participation of family or formal carers increases the chances that an activity or programme will be feasible and sustainable for people with dementia (Gitlin et al., 2018; Teri et al., 2012).

Teri and colleagues developed a comprehensive training programme designed to teach carers ways to improve affect and behaviour (Teri et al., 2012, 2018). An increase in positive mood and behaviours occurred in people with dementia after carers received the training (Teri et al., 2012, 2018). Promising evidence for improving behavioural issues and reducing functional decline has also been described by Gitlin and

---

TABLE 53.1   Rehabilitation interventions for people with dementia.

Multicomponent Programmes
Staff & Caregiver Training (STAR) (Teri et al., 2012)

- Realistic expectations
- Effective communication
- Activators, behaviours and consequences (A-B-C)
- Problem-solving for affective and behavioural problems
- Identifying, establishing and increasing pleasant events
- Understanding and altering environmental effectors
- Understanding and altering issues related to healthcare team and family/carer

Tailored Activity & Caregiver Training (Gitlin et al., 2018)

- Assessment by occupational therapist
- Customised activity programme
- Caregiver education

Preventing Loss of Independence through Exercise (PLIE) (Barnes et al., 2015)

- Repetition of the same basic sequences of events in each class
- Functional movements relevant to daily function and personal interests
- Slow pace and step-by-step instructions
- Participant-centred goal orientation
- Body awareness, mindfulness and breathing
- Positioning of group to facilitate social interaction
- Facilitation of positive emotions

Individualised Interventions
Motor Skills Training

- Task-based learning
- Practice and repetition
- Realistic environment
- Impairment-based exercise

Cognitive Skills Training

- Guided practice
- Errorless learning
- Techniques that use implicit memory
- Procedural learning

colleagues. The Tailored Activity Program involves assessment of the person with dementia by an occupational therapist to customise an activity programme and carer education. Study results reported a reduction in frequency and severity of behavioural symptoms and maintenance of ADLs after 4 months (Gitlin et al., 2018).

Mind-body therapies are becoming increasingly popular. Preventing Loss of Independence through Exercise (PLIE) is an integrative exercise programme for people with dementia that combines elements of conventional and complementary exercise modalities (e.g. Tai-Chi, yoga, Feldenkrais, dance therapy) and focuses on training procedural memory for basic functional movements while increasing mindful body awareness and facilitating social connection (Barnes et al., 2015). A functional mind-body programme includes focus on body awareness and movement memory, functional skill, social interactions with spontaneous sharing of personal stories or songs and techniques to reduce anxiety (Barnes et al., 2015). Seven guiding principles of PLIE are described in Table 53.1.

Motor Skills Training

Rehabilitation that incorporates implicit (procedural, task-based) teaching is more effective for people with dementia than explicit (declarative) teaching strategies that utilise memory techniques (Beaunieux et al., 2012). Explicit teaching strategies involve verbal instructions, demonstration of a step-by-step sequence, and written or auditory learning. Learning via traditional teaching techniques (e.g. listening, reading) is difficult even in early stages of dementia. Procedural learning, through active practice of tasks, is easier for people with dementia (van Halteren-van Tilborg, Scherder, & Hulstijn, 2007). Procedural learning encourages practice of automatic, well-practiced life skills (e.g. walking, rowing a boat, riding a bicycle). Although individuals in early stages of dementia can learn new motor tasks, their learning is slow and requires extensive practice and repetition. Research suggests that there is no single rehabilitation strategy that works best for all people with dementia (van Tilborg, Kessels, & Hulstijn, 2011). Instead, a combination of techniques that are tailored to the individual and their environment is likely to be most effective.

Individuals with dementia have preserved implicit memory related to well-learned tasks and life experiences, and these relatively intact memories can be used when teaching motor skills. However, they have difficulty in generalising their learning to performance of other skills. Therefore, a skill needs to be practised within an environment, and with the tool, that closely resembles the one that will be used by the individual in their daily life. For example, if a patient is trained in the use of a microwave, the device used during training should be the same as the one in the patient's household (van Halteren-van Tilborg et al., 2007). It has also been suggested that practice under dual-task conditions should be avoided in people with dementia, especially at advanced stages of disease.

Cognitive Training

Cognitive interventions for individuals with dementia focus on reality orientation (seasons of year, time of day, family members) and general cognitive stimulation that engage the individual with a range of activities and discussion in a group setting (Bahar-Fuchs, Clare, & Woods, 2013). Other techniques include the use of errorless learning strategies, in which corrections are made immediately to prevent inaccurate learning. Explicit teaching technique may be used during early stages to reinforce important cognitive skills, safety procedures, cooking procedures and navigating public transportation.

Cognitive training that is adjusted to the person's learning ability can support maintenance of general cognitive function in persons during early stages of dementia. Learning and cognitive stimulation may also positively impact well-being if the activities are appropriately challenging (Bahar-Fuchs et al., 2013). However, explicit teaching techniques that focus on improving a specific cognitive function (e.g. memory) can be frustrating for individuals with dementia, especially as their condition progresses. Neuropsychologists can clarify cognitive abilities through neuropsychological testing, followed by design and implementation of individualised cognitive training programmes of appropriate difficulty.

PHYSICAL ACTIVITY FOR PEOPLE WITH DEMENTIA

Higher physical activity is related to decreased risk of functional decline, decreased physical impairments and decreased risk of progression of chronic diseases such as ADRD. Physical activity positively affects brain health and cognitive function through a variety of pathways (Buchman et al., 2019). Improved brain health slows the decline of memory, learning, attention and executive function, and decreases depression and anxiety. Regular aerobic activity and resistance training are positively related to brain health and cognitive function. Regular exercise also improves physical fitness and mood, which further facilitates an active lifestyle (Kirk-Sanchez & McGough, 2014; McGough et al., 2017). Fig. 53.1 describes a model of the relationship between physical activity, motor function, non-motor functions (e.g. cognition, mood) and brain health.

Strategies for Increasing Physical Activity

Rehab programmes that combine cognitive and physical exercise have shown positive effects on global cognitive function, ADLs and mood in older adults with MCI or dementia. Multicomponent programmes also appear to be beneficial in reducing depressive symptoms and improving quality of life (Karssemeijer et al., 2017). Programmes that combine exercise and behavioural management techniques have been successfully administered as dyad activities with a cognitively intact partner (Teri et al., 2003, 2012). To facilitate and sustain increased physical activity levels, people with dementia will likely benefit from (1) instructions in easy-to-remember increments, (2) high repetition and practice, (3) a cognitively intact exercise partner, (4) written and visual memory cues, and (5) ensuring that the exercise is enjoyable (Teri et al., 2003). General strategies to increase physical activity in people with dementia are described in the Resources section.

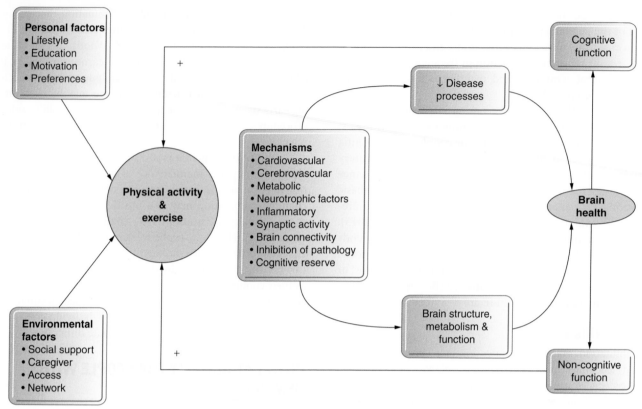

FIG. 53.1 Promotion of brain health: linking prediction, plasticity and participation. (McGough, E. L., Kirk-Sanchez, N., & Liu-Ambrose, T. (2017.) Integrating health promotion into physical therapy practice to improve brain health and prevent Alzheimer disease. *J Neurol Phys Ther, 41*(Suppl 3), S55–S62.).

CASE: INTERVENTION STRATEGIES FOR MADELINE

- Cognitive function: Use implicit teaching approach that draws from her life experience, but use written or auditory reminders to prevent errors (such as forgetting walking stick). Avoid didactic teaching strategies that may cause frustration.
- Behavioural function: Identify triggers of anxiety and social isolation. Identify ways to motivate Madeline to be more accepting of carers.
- Physical function: Use task-based motor training and an exercise routine including familiar and repetitive activities. Carer should support use of walking stick to increase physical activity. Educate Madeline and carer about use of supervised physical activity or group exercise programmes.

CONCLUSION

A comprehensive rehabilitation programme addresses cognitive, behavioural and physical domains of function in persons with dementia. A person-centred approach acknowledges the older person's life interests and can be utilised to facilitate activity and participation via individualised programmes. In persons with dementia, preserved memories and abilities can be leveraged to boost participation in exercise, social activities and ADLs. In particular, implicit or procedural learning strategies that reinforce existing capabilities and facilitate functional activity are recommended.

SUMMARY POINTS

- Rehabilitation strategies that work for the general population of older adults may be less effective for people with dementia
- Procedural learning activities (practising familiar and well-practiced tasks) are more effective and less frustrating for people with dementia than learning novel tasks and skills
- Motor skills training should involve repetition of specific functional tasks used by the individual in their daily life
- Functional training and education for carers is important in preventing fall-related injuries
- Inclusion of carers often improves participation in health promoting activities

MCQs

Q.1 In Alzheimer's disease and related dementia (ADRD), the most common form of dementia, the domain of cognition which is usually the first to be affected is:

a. Memory
b. Attention
c. Language
d. Visuospatial skills

Q.2 Which one of the following statements is true for people with ADRD?

a. Cognitive training programmes should use working memory strategies to learn new tasks
b. Using dual-task training is an effective strategy for enhancing motor learning
c. For people with ADRD, rehab programmes that combine cognitive and physical exercise have shown positive effects
d. People with ADRD are unable to learn new tasks

Q.3 Which of the following strategies is NOT effective for motor skills training for people with ADRD?

a. Memorisation of skill sequence
b. High repetition
c. Task-based learning
d. Carer involvement

REFERENCES

Afram, B., Stephan, A., Verbeek, H., Bleijlevens, M. H., Suhonen, R., Sutcliffe, C., …, & Hamers, J. P. (2014). Reasons for institutionalization of people with dementia: informal caregiver reports from 8 European countries. *Journal of the American Medical Directors Association, 15*, 108–116.

Ansai, J. H., De Andrade, L. P., Masse, F. A. A., Goncalves, J., De Medeiros Takahashi, A. C., Vale, F. A. C., & Rebelatto, J. R. (2017). Risk factors for falls in older adults with mild cognitive impairment and mild alzheimer disease. *Journal of Geriatric Physical Therapy, 42*, 1.

Alzheimer's Association. (2019). *Alzheimer's and dementia* [Online]. Retrieved from https://www.alz.org/alzheimers-dementia/what-is-alzheimers (Accessed 24 August 2019).

Bahar-Fuchs, A., Clare, L., & Woods, B. (2013). Cognitive training and cognitive rehabilitation for mild to moderate Alzheimer's disease and vascular dementia. *Cochrane Database of Systematic Reviews, 4*, CD003260.

Barnes, D. E., Mehling, W., Wu, E., Beristianos, M., Yaffe, K., Skultety, K., & Chesney, M. A. (2015). Preventing loss of independence through exercise (PLIE): a pilot clinical trial in older adults with dementia. *PLoS One, 10*, e0113367.

Beaunieux, H., Eustache, F., Busson, P., de la Sayette, V., Viader, F., & Desgranges, B. (2012). Cognitive procedural learning in early Alzheimer's disease: impaired processes and compensatory mechanisms. *Journal of Neuropsychology, 6*, 31–42.

Buchman, A. S., Yu, L., Wilson, R. S., Lim, A., Dawe, R. J., Gaiteri, C., Leurgans, S. E., Schneider, J. A., & Bennett, D. A. (2019). Physical activity, common brain pathologies, and cognition in community-dwelling older adults. *Neurology, 92*, e811–e822.

Gitlin, L. N., Arthur, P., Piersol, C., Hessels, V., Wu, S. S., Dai, Y., & Mann, W. C. (2018). Targeting behavioral symptoms and functional decline in dementia: a randomized clinical trial. *Journal of the American Geriatrics Society, 66*, 339–345.

Department of Health, UK. (2009). *Living well with dementia: a national dementia strategy* [online]. Retrieved from https://www.gov.uk/government/publications/living-well-with-dementia-a-national-dementia-strategy (Accessed 26 August 2019).

Karssemeijer, E. G. A., Aaronson, J. A., Bossers, W. J., Smits, T., Olde Rikkert, M. G. M., & Kessels, R. P. C. (2017). Positive effects of combined cognitive and physical exercise training on cognitive function in older adults with mild cognitive impairment or dementia: a meta-analysis. *Ageing Research Reviews, 40*, 75–83.

Kirk-Sanchez, N. J., & McGough, E. L. (2014). Physical exercise and cognitive performance in the elderly: current perspectives. *Clinical Interventions in Aging, 9*, 51–62.

Kratz, T. (2017). The diagnosis and treatment of behavioral disorders in dementia. *Deutsches Ärzteblatt International, 114*, 447–454.

Mathuranath, P. S., Nestor, P. J., Berrios, G. E., Rakowicz, W., & Hodges, J. R. (2000). A brief cognitive test battery to differentiate Alzheimer's disease and frontotemporal dementia. *Neurology, 55*, 1613–1620.

McGough, E., Kirk-Sanchez, N., & Liu-Ambrose, T. (2017). Integrating health promotion into physical therapy practice to improve brain health and prevent Alzheimer disease. *Journal of Neurologic Physical Therapy, 41*(Suppl 3), S55–S62.

McGough, E. L., Lin, S. Y., Belza, B., Becofsky, K. M., Jones, D. L., Liu, M., Wilcox, S., & Logsdon, R. G. (2019). A scoping review of physical performance outcome measures used in exercise interventions for older adults with Alzheimer disease and related dementias. *Journal of Geriatric Physical Therapy, 42*, 28–47.

Muir, S. W., Gopaul, K., & Montero Odasso, M. M. (2012). The role of cognitive impairment in fall risk among older adults: a systematic review and meta-analysis. *Age Ageing, 41*, 299–308.

Teri, L., Gibbons, L. E., McCurry, S. M., Logsdon, R. G., Buchner, D. M., Barlow, W. E., …, & Larson, E. B. (2003). Exercise plus behavioral management in patients with Alzheimer disease: a randomized controlled trial. *JAMA, 290*, 2015–2022.

Teri, L., Logsdon, R. G., & McCurry, S. M. (2008). Exercise interventions for dementia and cognitive impairment: the Seattle Protocols. *The Journal of Nutrition Health and Aging, 12*, 391–394.

Teri, L., Logsdon, R. G., McCurry, S. M., Pike, K. C., & McGough, E. L. (2018). Translating an evidence-based multicomponent intervention for older adults with dementia and caregivers. *Gerontologist, 60*, 548–557.

Teri, L., McKenzie, G., Logsdon, R. G., McCurry, S. M., Bollin, S., Mead, J., & Menne, H. (2012). Translation of two evidence-based programs for training families to improve care of persons with dementia. *Gerontologist, 52*, 452–459.

Van Halteren-Van Tilborg, I. A., Scherder, E. J., & Hulstijn, W. (2007). Motor-skill learning in Alzheimer's disease: a review with an eye to the clinical practice. *Neuropsychology Review, 17*, 203–212.

Van Tilborg, I. A., Kessels, R. P., & Hulstijn, W. (2011). How should we teach everyday skills in dementia? A controlled study comparing implicit and explicit training methods. *Clinical Rehabilitation, 25*, 638–648.

Verghese, J., Wang, C., Lipton, R. B., & Holtzer, R. (2013). Motoric cognitive risk syndrome and the risk of dementia. *The Journals of Gerontology Series A Biological Sciences and Medical Sciences, 68*, 412–418.

54

Rehabilitation in Peripheral Vascular Disease

Matthew Fuller, Rebecca Golder, Talia Lea & Fiona Murphy

LEARNING OBJECTIVES

- Describe important characteristics of the older population undergoing vascular surgery
- Explain in simple terms the common vascular operations
- Describe the approach to rehabilitation after vascular surgery

INTRODUCTION

Peripheral vascular disease (PVD) is a common problem involving narrowing or blockage of blood vessels, which causes symptoms from reduced circulation to the limbs (Fig. 54.1 shows the major arteries of the body). Vascular services are managing increasing numbers of older patients as the population ages and evidence accrues of the benefit from arterial vascular surgery in older people. This group of patients can have quite complex needs, due to often having multiple medical conditions. Partridge et al. (2015) found that among patients over 60 years old admitted for arterial vascular surgery, frailty and poor functional status were common. Frailty was associated with adverse postoperative outcomes (longer length of stay, postoperative infections, medical complications and adverse functional outcomes). Cognitive impairment or dementia was found in 68% of patients, the vast majority of which was previously unrecognised (Partridge et al., 2014).

This chapter describes common vascular surgical procedures and the individualised approach to management of rehabilitation afterwards. General guidance on rehabilitation for older people after surgery can be found in the Resources section.

CAROTID ENDARTERECTOMY

Carotid arteries are responsible for carrying blood to your head, brain and face. When plaque builds up in these arteries (atherosclerosis), it can lead to a stroke or a transient ischaemic attack (TIA). To reduce the risk of a stroke or TIA, a carotid endarterectomy can be performed to surgically remove this plaque. Patients normally present after experiencing a TIA or stroke, although some surgeons may treat asymptomatic stenosis that is found incidentally. For symptomatic patients, surgery should be performed within 14 days from the onset of symptoms; beyond this timeframe the benefits of the surgery compared with risk of further events are less certain.

An incision running vertically down the side of the neck is made, usually 7–10 cm in length. A cut is made along the artery and the plaque causing the narrowing is carefully removed (Fig. 54.2). A small plastic drain is placed in the neck for a short period to drain any blood and to reduce neck swelling after the operation.

For the first 12–24 hours, the patient will usually be nursed in a monitored bed for any signs or symptoms of a stroke or bleeding including numbness or weakness in the face, arm or leg; confusion or difficulty in talking or understanding speech; trouble seeing in one or both eyes; difficulty with walking, dizziness, or loss of balance and coordination. Early mobility is recommended, and postoperatively a team of therapists with an awareness of neurological symptoms can highlight any residual neurological issues.

Gentle range of movement (ROM) exercises should be provided for the neck and thorax, and the patient encouraged to pace their return to normal exercise tolerance. Due to a potential loss of sensation, men must be careful when shaving. Any patients with residual symptoms should be referred on to appropriate community teams. Expected length of stay is usually 24–48 hours.

ABDOMINAL AORTIC ANEURYSM

The aorta carries blood away from your heart to the rest of the body. Sometimes the walls can weaken and stretch outwards until they form a balloon shape. This is called an aneurysm; where it occurs informs the naming of the type of aneurysm, e.g. if it is in the abdominal section of the aorta it is referred to as an abdominal aortic aneurysm (AAA). The location and extent of the aneurysm combined with the frailty of the patient will make the surgery more or less complex, and hence the rehabilitation of these patients will be intervention-specific.

323

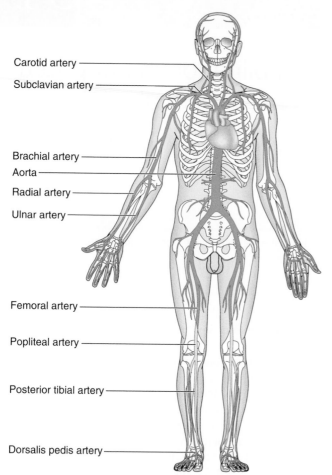

FIG. 54.1 Main arteries of the body. (From Innes, JA, Dover AR, Fairhurst K. *Macleod's Clinical Examination*, 14th edn. Elsevier; 2018, with permission.)

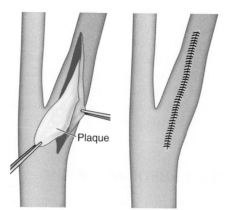

FIG. 54.2 Carotid endarterectomy. (From Sardar P, Chatterjee S, Aronow HD. Carotid artery stenting versus endarterectomy for stroke prevention: a meta-analysis of clinical trials. *J Am Coll Cardiol.* 2017;69(18):2266–75, with permission.)

Endovascular AAA Repair

Endovascular aneurysm repair (EVAR) is a minimally invasive 'keyhole' surgical procedure to repair an aneurysm. It is performed through a small incision in the groin. In EVAR,

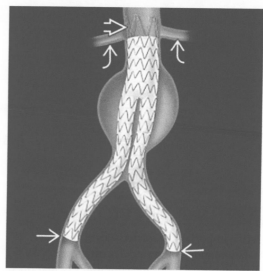

FIG. 54.3 EVAR (endovascular aneurysm repair) involves placing a stent (top of image) and graft (light area with broken lines) to bridge the ballooned section (dark area) of blood vessel. (From Moore WS, Ahn SS. *Endovascular Surgery*, 4th edn. Elsevier; 2011, with permission).

the aneurysm is repaired using a covered stent graft. The stent is used to 'bridge' the ballooned section of blood vessel, strengthening the artery and redirecting blood flow to prevent the aneurysm from bursting (Fig. 54.3).

Patients are allowed to sit out of bed and mobilise after approximately 6 hours. If possible an introduction to the therapy team prior to surgery is advised; patients should be encouraged to get up and walk around regularly, even on the day of surgery while they await their theatre slot to reduce the risk of postural hypotension (drop in blood pressure on rising) (Jevon, 2001). Explanation of the postoperative rehabilitation protocol should be provided to set expectations of early mobility and to put the patient at ease. Emphasis should be put on the need to have enough pain relief to be able to move comfortably and that not moving is counterproductive to their recovery.

Patients are often unprepared for the amount of groin pain they may experience from the cut-down or percutaneous puncture. Patients may also have burning sensations in the thighs if the nerves to the skin have suffered injury (neuropathic pain); these are often more pronounced in people who have had longer or more complex operations. It can be worth mentioning that although the patient has had keyhole surgery the size of keys can be very different! The use of 'when required' (PRN) pain relief and walking aids can help start the mobilisation process. The expected length of stay for this group of patients is 24–48 hours postoperation.

Complex Endovascular AAA Repair

Patients undergoing complex fenestrated (FEVAR) or branched (BEVAR) grafts will have much more of the aorta covered, requiring longer procedures. Although these procedures are still keyhole surgery, the operation is longer, and patients may require a spinal drain and more attachments than a standard EVAR. Spinal drains must be clamped before a patient can mobilise. Spinal ischaemia (reduced blood supply to the spinal cord) can happen acutely or several days postoperatively. Occasionally this may happen if the patient's blood pressure drops, which can happen when sitting the patient out of bed so should be observed for and reported to the surgical team immediately. The expected length of stay for this group of patients is 48–72 hours postoperation.

Open AAA Repair

An open AAA repair involves a longer operation and a longer recovery period, compared with the keyhole repair. It involves cutting open the abdomen to replace the aneurysmal segment with an artificial graft (Fig. 54.4). The main incision is vertical, from the top of the abdomen to the belly button.

The aorta is clamped and the diseased section opened; the artificial graft is then sown into place to exclude the aneurysm. The aorta is closed over the graft at the end of the operation to separate it from the overlying structures. This is a major operation and carries some risk.

As with any major open surgery, it is beneficial for patients to be seen by the physiotherapist from the first day of their operation to help them get moving, out of bed and to prevent chest complications. Pain is often an issue, and good control is essential to allow the patient to cough and clear their chest and to mobilise. The expected length of stay for this group of patients is 7–10 days postoperation.

Patients who are treated for emergency ruptured AAA with either open or endovascular repair may have greater rehabilitation needs. They will not have been optimised for surgery and the body will have suffered significant stress as a result of the sudden rupture and the associated blood loss. Following a repair of a ruptured aneurysm, it is common to still experience pain in the back and/or abdomen due to blood which sits in the abdominal cavity until the body reabsorbs it. This may hinder early mobilisation and require more pain medication. On rare occasions these haematomas may also compress femoral nerves with associated leg weakness.

AORTOILIAC OCCLUSION

The iliac artery supplies blood to the legs. Some people develop narrowing or blockages in the lower aorto-iliac arteries and will experience symptoms of reduced blood flow to the legs, either gradually or suddenly. To treat such occlusions, patients can have a procedure that involves making an incision in the abdomen to reach the aorta and also in the groins to reach the femoral arteries. A fabric tube graft in the shape of a pair of trousers is tunnelled under the skin and then sewn into the existing blood vessels, bypassing the blockages. Patients undergoing this operation present very much like an open AAA repair and the same therapy considerations should be contemplated.

Femoro-Femoral Bypass

When only one iliac vessel is blocked, it is possible to bypass the blockage using a graft from the healthy leg. The two femoral arteries at the top of the thighs are joined using a prosthetic graft which is tunnelled underneath the skin of the lower abdominal wall and then into the artery on the bad side (see Fig. 54.5). The arteries are accessed by cuts in the groin and tunnelled across the lower abdomen.

Lower Limb Bypass

There are different types of bypass in the lower limbs and these are all named by location. All bypass operations require a conduit to run from one location in the leg to another, and this can be made from the patient's own veins (preferred) or an artificial material. Where possible bypasses are tunnelled anatomically and joined together after measuring for length with the leg straightened, this is in order to allow freedom of movement. Operation notes should always be viewed prior to seeing the patient to take stock of any specific instructions; it is also important to have a dialogue with consultants to understand the patient's individual needs.

Almost all bypass operations will have the same ramifications for the patient: pain, swelling, loss of range and altered gait (walking pattern). Initially the patient may suffer with

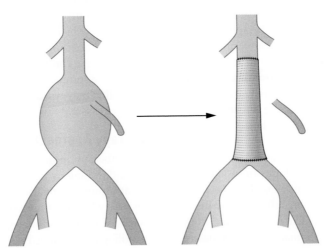

FIG. 54.4 The left shows an abdominal aortic aneurysm (AAA) and on the right the graft is in place in the middle section of the aorta. (From Cameron JL, Cameron AM. *Current Surgical Therapy*, 12th edn. 2017, with permission.)

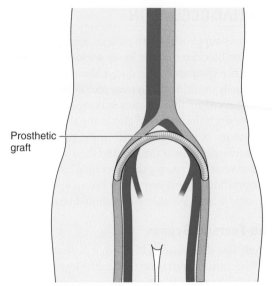

Prosthetic graft

FIG. 54.5 A femoro-femoral bypass involves bypassing the blockage using a graft from the healthy leg.

some 'reperfusion pain' when lowering the limbs from the edge of the bed; explaining that this is normal can be useful. This is pain related to tissues that were previously starved of blood supply suddenly receiving blood, causing a complex inflammatory response. If this happens, the patient may benefit from regularly lowering their legs off of the bed, and then elevating again. If the patient can tolerate standing for long enough to get to a chair, then doing this from a chair and foot stool is also worthwhile. Regular review of ROM, pain, temperature and ability to move the toes and foot should be undertaken in the first few days to assess for late onset compartment syndrome (an emergency caused by increased pressure from swelling, which can cut off the circulation), or graft occlusion. Any negative changes should be highlighted to the surgical team as a matter of urgency.

Swelling (oedema) is common in the legs after surgery because the tissues that are disturbed during the procedure produce fluid. This can take a few months to reduce, and in rare occasions never fully resolves. Patients will be told by their surgeon to keep the legs elevated, and by therapists to keep walking. These two instructions can seem counterintuitive to patients and cause confusion. It is important to acknowledge this, and explain that dependent sitting positions should be avoided. Walking regularly with a normal gait pattern utilises the muscle pumps of the calves to increase return of blood to the heart from leg veins; sitting with the legs elevated also helps and both are equally important.

Ankle ROM, especially in patients with fem-distal or ultra-distal bypasses, can be especially difficult due to swelling and pain on stretching the calf muscle which may have been disturbed during the operation, and/or suffered reperfusion injury. These patients are at particular risk of losing ROM and gait deviations longer term. Manual techniques, passive stretches, active assisted knee and ankle flexion and extension on the bed prior to mobilising can be useful to reduce oedema and pain, facilitate improved ROM and improve

gait. Patients tend to sit in the chair with the affected leg partially extended in front of them and the ankle pointed like a ballerina. In sitting, practising gentle knee flexion and extension and trying to bend the knee to bring the foot towards the chair, getting the foot flat on the floor and then putting pressure through the leg to push down into the floor can help further desensitise this painful movement and aid increases in available ROM.

Mobility will need to be encouraged. Walking aids and pain medication should be used as appropriate to promote a normal gait pattern with good heel-toe and step-through gait patterns. As the patient's pain and ROM improve, then walking aids should be weaned.

Referral for these patients to community teams is often sensible to monitor and progress ROM, mobility and wean walking aids. Patients' general fitness may have been adversely affected by their lower limb pain limiting their exercise tolerance and advice on exercise progression should also be provided.

FUNCTIONAL ASSESSMENTS

While early mobilisation is important, function should also be considered in the context of an individual's daily occupations. Encouraging getting out of bed for toileting or sitting out for personal care and eating a meal should also be used as part of therapeutic risk assessment and progression. Independence in these activities can be a motivating factor to improve engagement in therapy as patients will often see more purpose to these tasks. Goal setting is important to maintain active engagement in therapy. This can be completed collaboratively with the patient informally or by using validated tools.

Cognition

Cognitive impairment is common among older vascular patients (Partridge et al., 2014). Alongside other medical issues, there is a high risk of delirium for those patients undergoing surgery. Where appropriate or indicated it is useful to complete a cognitive screen prior to surgery to provide a baseline score from which to measure any potential changes. Patients at risk of delirium (e.g. pre-existing cognitive impairment, postoperative complications and critical care admission) require an appropriate management plan in place to prevent issues that may result from it such as falls, agitation, reduced engagement and functional deconditioning.

Therapy Approach

Early therapy input can be essential to prevent functional deconditioning as long as there is an adequate risk assessment around manual handling in place. Initially it may be necessary to use a more compensatory approach in the early stages of rehabilitation, e.g. use of more supportive manual handling aids such as hoists to focus on small goals such as being able to sit out of bed. This will contribute to optimising engagement with functional tasks such as eating, drinking and personal care.

Importantly it is essential to monitor and maintain patients once they have achieved a near baseline functionality as they have a tendency to have extended length of stay and a propensity for immobility and are therefore at risk of further physical decline.

Falls

There are many common factors which vascular patients share with other patients in relations to falls risk such as impaired physical function, cognitive impairment, decreased strength, balance and global weakness. There are further risk factors associated with vascular patients and falls to consider during admission. A large majority of these patients have peripheral neuropathy that can result in loss of sensory feedback or numbness, decreased balance or coordination and muscle weakness. Many patients also have diabetes and may have retinopathy which affects vision.

Depending on the surgery, the patient may have to wear specialist footwear to support wound healing by offloading a specific area of the foot. This footwear, which is often 'off the shelf' and not bespoke, can potentially be ill-fitting, cumbersome and negatively affect balance. The patient may require assistance with fitting/putting it on. A patient may also have attachments such as a urinary catheter, or a specialist dressing on their lower limb, that they are required to carry when mobilising, which can pose a further trip hazard. Due to dementia or postoperative delirium patients may forget to wear their specialist footwear, carry attachments or use their mobility aid whilst attempting to mobilise and complete functional activities.

To support with managing potential falls risks on the ward, it is recommended that therapists assess patients' function on admission and postoperatively and identify the most appropriate mobility or transfer aid and the level of assistance and technique required. This information should be clearly handed over to the ward staff. Completion of mobility charts placed above patients' beds can be very useful as a quick reference for all ward staff including type of footwear required if appropriate.

In summary, it is important to take a holistic approach when assessing patients and ensure there is a collaborative multidisciplinary assessment and decision making around patient care.

While it is essential to take a rehabilitative approach when dealing with functional decline and frailty, it should also be acknowledged that PVD is a long-term issue and requires life-long maintenance.

SUMMARY POINTS

- Older patients having surgery for peripheral vascular disease often have complex needs
- Rehabilitation should be tailored to the specific intervention as well as the individual's needs
- Frailty and cognitive impairment are common in this group and should be taken into account when making plans

MCQs

Q.1 After vascular surgery, which of the following is true?
　a. Patients should not walk for 2 days after a carotid endarterectomy
　b. Patients having an endovascular aneurysm repair (EVAR) are generally permitted to get out of bed 6 hours after surgery
　c. Rehabilitation needs after an emergency abdominal aortic aneurysm (AAA) are the same as those after planned (elective) surgery
　d. Patients should avoid elevating their legs after lower limb bypass surgery
　e. Walking aids should be avoided

Q.2 Regarding older people having vascular surgery, which of the following is true?
　a. There is a high risk of delirium, but it does not result in falls
　b. There is no role for therapy input prior to surgery
　c. Use of pain medication should be avoided due to side effects
　d. Not moving for a short period of time after surgery is an important part of recovery
　e. Goal setting is important to maintain active engagement

REFERENCES

Jevon, P. (2001). Postural hypotension: symptoms and management. *Nursing Times, 97*(3), 39–40.

Partridge, J. S. L., Dhesi, J. K., Cross, J. D., Lo, J. W., Taylor, P. R., Bell, R., Martin, F. C., & Harari, D. (2014). The prevalence and impact of undiagnosed cognitive impairment in older vascular surgical patients. *Journal of Vascular Surgery, 60*(4), 1002–1011e3.

Partridge, J. S. L., Fuller, M., Harari, D., Taylor, P. R., Martin, F. C., & Dhesi, J. K. (2015). Frailty and poor functional status are common in arterial vascular surgical patients and affect postoperative outcomes. *International Journal of Surgery, 18*, 57–63.

55

Amputee Rehabilitation

Jacqueline Stow

LEARNING OBJECTIVES

- List the causes of limb loss in the older person
- Explain the barriers to successful rehabilitation in older patients with amputation
- Describe the amputee rehabilitation pathway
- Explain how to assess rehabilitation potential and list predictors of successful prosthesis use

Amputee rehabilitation aims to enable the person with limb loss to return to previous functional activities. This may involve using a prosthetic limb to aid mobility and improve participation in home and community activities.

CAUSES OF AMPUTATION IN OLDER PEOPLE

Over 75% of lower limb amputations occur in patients over the age of 65 years (Clark, Blue, and Bearer 1983; Fletcher et al., 2001) and the numbers are increasing. The main cause of limb loss in this group is peripheral vascular disease (PVD) accounting for 90%, with trauma, tumours and infections contributing to lesser degree. Many of these patients with PVD have associated diabetes (30%) (Thiruvoipati, Kielhorn, & Armstrong, 2015).

For many people, successful rehabilitation means returning to walking. Research has demonstrated that only 36% of single-sided older vascular amputee patients are successfully fitted with a prosthesis (Cumming, Barr, & Howe, 2006; Fletcher et al., 2001). For older people amputation can be a poor prognostic indicator for survival and the duration of time spent using a prosthetic limb is often short. The median survival of people over 65 years with a major lower limb amputation is approximately 1.5 years. Those who are considered suitable for prosthetic rehabilitation have a better median survival of 3.5 years (Fletcher et al., 2001).

CHALLENGES TO SUCCESSFUL REHABILITATION

Many older patients do not achieve a high functional level of mobility using a prosthesis. Only 25% of patients over 50 years with a transfemoral amputation achieve functional community walking and this decreases with age (Fortington et al., 2012; Steinberg, Sunwoo, & Roettger, 1985). This percentage improves with more distal (further along the limb) amputation and 50% of transtibial amputees are successful with community mobility. Fig. 55.1 shows sites for lower limb amputation. Rehabilitation to return the older person to independent walking following limb loss has challenges that are particular to this population (Lee & Costello, 2018). These specific challenges include:

1) Higher burden of chronic disease

Older people have a higher incidence of coexisting health problems such as heart disease, cardiac failure, chronic kidney disease and chronic obstructive pulmonary disease (COPD) (Cumming et al., 2006). These contribute to reduced physical fitness, stamina and exercise tolerance and limit the patient's capacity to regain lost fitness.

PVD is a multisystem disease and affects cardiac and cerebrovascular circulation. Cognitive impairment is highly prevalent making it more difficult for an older person to learn the new skills required to use a prosthesis effectively and safely (Lee & Costello, 2018). Vascular disease is likely to be present in the remaining limb causing ischaemic ulcers and claudication and limiting both walking tolerance and weight-bearing.

Degenerative arthritis (more prevalent in older people) can lead to weakness, increased falls risk, limited tolerance of walking due to pain, reluctance to perform essential exercise programmes and hastening of joint contractures.

Neurodegenerative diseases (dementia, Parkinson's disease) and strokes are more prevalent in the older population and pose difficulties for successful rehabilitation. An older person may be mobile with these conditions prior to amputation but find it extremely difficult to use a prosthetic limb following amputation.

Visual impairment will increase risk of falls and impact on independent care of the residuum (portion of the limb remaining) and prosthesis. Hearing impairment may mimic cognitive impairment and may reduce effectiveness of therapeutic input.

Sarcopenia (age-related muscle loss) is more common in over 65s and poses difficulties for rehabilitation. It increases the likelihood of pressure sores and dependency on care.

Osteoporosis may make an older patient more vulnerable to fractures if they fall while undergoing rehabilitation.

2) Mobility restriction prior to amputation

Many older amputees are deconditioned prior to commencing rehabilitation (see Chapter 21 Avoiding Deconditioning).

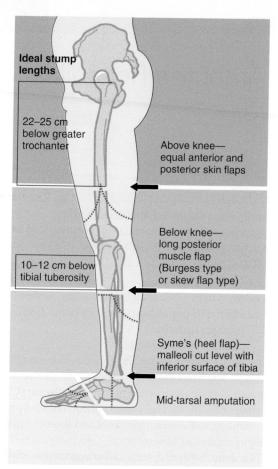

Ideal stump lengths

22–25 cm below greater trochanter

10–12 cm below tibial tuberosity

Above knee— equal anterior and posterior skin flaps

Below knee— long posterior muscle flap (Burgess type or skew flap type)

Syme's (heel flap)— malleoli cut level with inferior surface of tibia

Mid-tarsal amputation

FIG. 55.1 Sites for lower limb amputations. (From Quick CRG, Reed JB, Harper SJF, Saeb-Paersy K. *Essential Surgery: Problems, Diagnosis and Management*, 5th edn. Elsevier; 2014, with permission.)

The progressive decline in their mobility because of vascular disease is a significant contributor to this process. Patients often report progressive symptoms (claudication, painful ischaemic ulcers) increasingly restricting their ability to walk over a period of years. The reduced mobility contributes to the higher frequency of joint contractures seen in older patients. Delayed wound healing, failure to perform an appropriate exercise programme post-amputation, arthritis and the effects of ageing on musculoskeletal tissue also encourages the formation of joint contractures. Deconditioned patients frequently have weakness of the upper limbs which can make transfers and use of gait aids more challenging.

3) Higher risk of falls and reduced balance

Older patients are more likely to have an increased risk of falling which is compounded by limb loss. Conditions which increase this risk include arthritis, muscle weakness, impaired balance, orthostatic hypotension (postural drops in blood pressure), polypharmacy and medication side effects.

4) Increased skin fragility

Older patients have more vulnerable skin, increasing risks of pressure sores and skin breakdown with prosthesis use.

REHABILITATION PATHWAYS

All the above factors reduce the likelihood of successful rehabilitation, so amputee rehabilitation for the older person is best delivered as part of an integrated care multidisciplinary programme, with rehabilitation commencing prior to amputation and continuing throughout that person's life.

PREHABILITATION

Prior to amputation, prehabilitation focuses on minimising deconditioning to promote recovery and return to independence following amputation. Education should be provided concerning complications that would impact on return to walking and an exercise programme established to prevent contractures and deconditioning. Expectations need to be addressed to ensure patients have achievable goals. For most patients, returning to activities as before is unfortunately unlikely.

Information regarding home adaptations to ensure wheelchair accessibility can be provided and appropriate carers arranged to ensure timely discharge after surgery.

Serial amputation (transtibial followed by transfemoral) should be avoided in older patients as this increases length of time spent immobile and leads to deconditioning. Preservation of joints is important to maximise rehabilitation potential and so assessing the most distal level at which healing is likely to occur is vital to determine the best level of amputation.

POST-AMPUTATION REHABILITATION

Following amputation, the focus of rehabilitation is the restoration of independence with personal care and mobility. Older patients have a higher risk of postoperative complications and death after surgery. Early mobilisation will decrease their risk of immobility-related complications. Independence with transfers is key to reducing immobility and restoring independence with self-care. A supervised exercise programme to maintain strength, balance and joint range is required. Training to enable independent wheelchair use will restore mobility. Optimisation of health and fitness after surgery will enable patients to reach their maximum rehabilitation potential.

Post-amputation falls are frequent in older patients. They are likely to occur early in the course of recovery. The contributing factors include phantom sensations, drowsiness from pain medications, urinary frequency and delirium. The consequences of a fall can be very deleterious. Fractures or wound breakdown will delay prosthetic rehabilitation.

Patients require oedema management of their residuum to reduce wound breakdown, and infection as delayed wound healing will lead to slower prosthetic rehabilitation and increased deconditioning. Patients will need appropriate postural management to reduce likelihood of hip and knee contractures and require a suitably aligned stump board on their wheelchair. A patient will usually be provided with a shrinker stocking (see Fig. 55.2) to aid oedema management once sutures or staples are removed.

It is recommended that patients have a fully wheelchair accessible home even if they achieve a high level of mobility

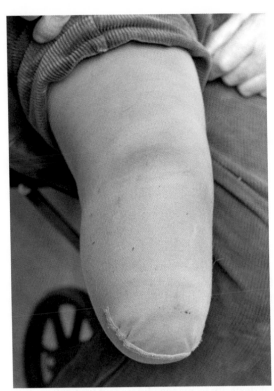

FIG. 55.2 A stump shrinker sock applied over a transtibial amputation stump. (From Loftus I, Hinchcliffe RJ. *Vascular and Endovascular Surgery: A Companion to Specialist Surgical Practice*, 6th edn. Elsevier; 2019, with permission.)

with their prosthesis. This is to ensure that despite changes in health they can continue to manage independently in their home.

ASSESSING REHABILITATION POTENTIAL

Rehabilitation potential is assessed through a multidisciplinary process and a prosthetic prescription established in keeping with the anticipated activity level. All patients should be considered for prosthetic rehabilitation, and the decision regarding appropriateness is determined by their health, level of motivation, home supports and personal goals (Davies & Datta, 2003). An older person may have the potential to walk with a prosthetic limb but not to achieve their desired goals. A lack of agreement between the goals considered realistic by the rehabilitation team and the patient's desired rehabilitation outcome can lead to a patient becoming dissatisfied and abandoning prosthetic use.

Barriers to prosthetic rehabilitation include cognitive impairment, reduced exercise tolerance due to comorbidities, joint disease, condition of remaining foot (ulceration and neuropathy) and hip and knee contractures (Spruit-van Eijk et al., 2012).

The level of amputation will impact on rehabilitation potential. Amputees with preserved knee joint (transtibial amputation) will achieve a higher level of mobility than a transfemoral amputee. Most older patients are unable to achieve functional walking with a prosthesis following transfemoral

amputation due to the high-energy expenditure in walking. The additional energy expenditure over and above normal gait is 40% to 60% for a unilateral transtibial amputee, 60% to 100% for a bilateral transtibial amputee and 90% to 120% for a transfemoral amputee.

The older person with a transfemoral amputation will need to be able to stand without assistance on their remaining leg in order to be able to use a prosthesis. The ability to balance without arm support correlates positively with greater functional independence. Most will need supervision to ensure safety when walking with a prosthesis. The situation is different for transtibial amputees where most people benefit from receiving a prosthesis and can return to limited walking. Even if walking is not a goal due to restricted exercise tolerance or the condition of their remaining foot, the below knee prosthesis may improve ease of transfers.

Cognitive impairment is a major barrier to independent prosthesis use and can be particularly challenging when the patient lacks insight into the impact on their success and safety in managing a prosthesis. Prosthetic rehabilitation requires the learning of new skills, and the ability to problem solve and adapt to changing situations. An older person may only be deemed safe to use the prosthesis under direct supervision (therapeutic walking) which may mean that those living alone without social supports would not be considered suitable.

Contractures of hip and knee will reduce gait efficiency, socket comfort and even prevent prosthesis fitting. The absence of flexion contractures has been shown to be an important predictor of successful prosthetic rehabilitation and likely reflects patient motivation, engagement in exercise programme and cognitive abilities. Knee flexion contracture of 30 degrees is the maximal limit for the fitting of a prosthesis, and hip flexion contractures of more than 15 degrees make prosthesis fitting difficult and increase dependency on a walking aid such as a frame. A PPAM (Pneumatic Post-Amputation Mobility) Aid (temporary leg) and Femurett (an adjustable training prosthesis device) are useful tools to assess rehabilitation potential and aid the patient to develop insight into achievable prosthetic goals and improve muscle strength and balance (see Fig. 55.3).

In those older patients where prosthetic rehabilitation is not appropriate, the focus of rehabilitation is to optimise their ability to function independently in their own home as a wheelchair user. Many older people can function safely from a wheelchair with limited supports where they would require continuous supervision and assistance as a prosthesis user. Powered wheelchairs may offer considerably improved mobility while preserving joints and reducing exertion.

PROSTHETIC REHABILITATION

Once appropriate, prosthetic rehabilitation should provide prosthesis fitting and intensive goal-directed therapy under the auspices of a multidisciplinary team. The prosthetic prescription will depend on several factors including the level of the amputation, anticipated activity level, condition of

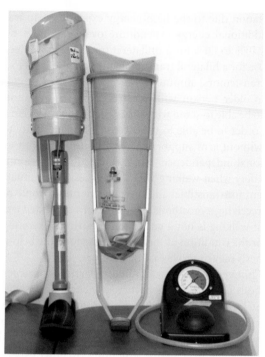

FIG. 55.3   A selection of early walking aids: Femurette (left) and pneumatic post-amputation mobility aid (PPAM Aid; centre). A foot pump to inflate the PPAM Aid is shown on the right. (From Loftus I, Hinchcliffe RJ. *Vascular and Endovascular Surgery: A Companion to Specialist Surgical Practice*, 6th edn. Elsevier; 2019, with permission.)

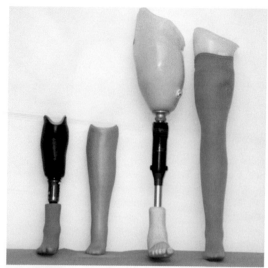

FIG. 55.4   Modular endoskeletal prostheses for transfemoral and transtibial amputation, with and without cosmetic covers. (From Loftus I, Hinchcliffe RJ. *Vascular and Endovascular Surgery: A Companion to Specialist Surgical Practice*, 6th edn. Elsevier; 2019, with permission.)

the residuum, condition of the other remaining limb, the patient's dexterity and goals (see Fig. 55.4 for examples of prostheses). Rehabilitation should include therapeutic interventions to improve core stability, gait pattern, control of the prosthesis and balance. Patients should receive training in all functional activities of daily living (ADLs) and management of falls. Education regarding skin care, hygiene and care of the prosthesis is also an important component of rehabilitation.

Prosthetic Prescription

In the older person, safety when walking is an important consideration when determining appropriate prosthetic prescription. The stability of the patient during stance phase is essential to ensure safety. Many older patients do better with a knee that can be used in a locked position. Prosthetic feet and ankles should have less movement and provide increased stability. The weight of the prosthesis affects walking speed and energy expenditure and so in older patients lighter components should be selected. Older patients with transfemoral amputations frequently have contractures at the hip and weak hip adductors. A prosthesis with hip joint with pelvic band and waist belt (RPB, rigid pelvic band) provides improved rotational stability and makes walking safer and more stable. Ease of donning must be considered as patients may lack the

manual dexterity to manage liners and find cotton socks and belt easier to use. The steps involved in donning should not be too complicated to facilitate success despite cognitive changes. Predicted activity level can help guide choice of prosthetic components in prosthetic prescription. The K Level classification of activity level is used by many prosthetic providers.

MONITORING OUTCOMES

Measuring outcomes is important to evaluate interventions and effectiveness of service provided. Outcome measures need to be easy to perform and show responsiveness. The SIGAM (Special Interest Group in Amputee Medicine) mobility scale is a simple and useful tool to demonstrate level of mobility achieved following rehabilitation and to evaluate if outcomes are maintained. Other tools that are in frequent use are the Timed Up and Go (TUG); L-test; 2-minute or 6-minute walk test. All measure balance, agility and gait speed, and reflect overall level of mobility with a prosthesis. The Barthel score, although not developed for the amputee, is a useful tool in assessing the level of assistance needed with ADLs and mobility and is particularly useful in those patients not using a prosthesis. There are numerous other outcome tools that are more complicated to administer but may be useful, including the Amputee Mobility Predictor, Locomotor Capability Index 5 and Houghton Scale.

Patients need access to ongoing multidisciplinary review to ensure mobility levels are maintained and to provide for future prosthetic needs. This also provides review of changing needs as some patients subsequently through increasing frailty or deteriorating health are no longer able to safely use a prosthesis.

SUMMARY POINTS

- Peripheral vascular disease is the leading cause of amputation in the older population with diabetes contributing to the development of this condition
- Age alone is not an absolute contraindication to prosthetic limb prescription; however, it does influence the chances of successful rehabilitation
- Older patients with an amputation require a multidisciplinary approach to rehabilitation as they have additional challenges due to medical conditions, deconditioning and the effects of ageing
- Both prehabilitation and post-amputation rehabilitation are important to ensure the best outcomes
- Successful use of a prosthesis is not possible in every older amputee; however, almost all will benefit from rehabilitation to increase independence in transfers and learn wheelchair skills

MCQs

Q.1 Useful outcome measures in evaluating rehabilitation outcome in older amputees are
  a. SIGAM
  b. Timed Up and Go (T.U.G.)
  c. Two-minute walk test
  d. Locomotor Capability Index 5
  e. All of the above

Q.2 The predominant reason for amputation in the older person is
  a. Bone tumours
  b. Septicaemia
  c. Trauma
  d. Peripheral vascular disease
  e. Osteomyelitis

Q.3 Which of the following factors increases the complexity of rehabilitation of older amputees?
  a. Cognitive impairment
  b. Joint contractures
  c. Multiple comorbidities
  d. Skin fragility
  e. All of the above

REFERENCES

Clark, S. C., Blue, B., & Bearer, J. B. (1983). Rehabilitation of the elderly amputee. *Journal of the American Geriatrics Society, 31*, 439–448.

Cumming, J., Barr, S., & Howe, T. E. (2006). Prosthetic rehabilitation for older dysvascular people following a unilateral transfemoral amputation. *Cochrane Database of Systematic Reviews, 1*, CD005260.

Davies, B., & Datta, D. (2003). Mobility outcomes following unilateral lower limb amputation. *Prosthetics and Orthotics International, 27*, 186–190.

Fletcher, D. D., Andrews, K. L., Butters, M. A., Jacobsen, S. J., Rowland, C. M., & Hallett, J. W. (2001). Rehabilitation of the geriatric vascular amputee patient: a population-based study. *Archives of Physical Medicine and Rehabilitation, 82*, 776–779.

Fortington, L. V., Rommers, G. M., Geertzen, J. H., Postema, K., & Dijkstra, P. U. (2012). Mobility in elderly people with a lower limb amputation. *Journal of the American Medical Directors Association, 13*, 319–325.

Lee, D. J., & Costello, M. C. (2018). The effect of cognitive impairment on prosthesis use in older adults who underwent amputation due to vascular-related etiology: a systematic review of literature. *Prosthetics and Orthotics International, 42*, 144–152.

Spruit-van Eijk, M., van der Linde, H., Buijck, B., Geurts, A., Zuidema, S., & Koopmans, R. (2012). Predicting prosthetic use in elderly patients after major lower limb amputation. *Prosthetics and Orthotics International, 36*, 45–52.

Steinberg, F. U., Sunwoo, I., & Roettger, R. F. (1985). Prosthetic rehabilitation of geriatric amputee patients: a follow-up study. *Archives of Physical Medicine and Rehabilitation, 66*, 742–745.

Thiruvoipati, T., Kielhorn, C. E., & Armstrong, E. J. (2015). Peripheral artery disease in patients with diabetes: epidemiology, mechanisms, and outcomes. *World Journal of Diabetes, 6*(7), 961–969.

FURTHER READING

Fleury, A. M., Salih, S. A., & Peel, N. M. (2013). Rehabilitation of the older vascular amputee: a review of the literature. *Geriatrics & Gerontology International, 13*(2), 264–273.

56

Lymphoedema Rehabilitation

Helen Mackie & Vaughan Keeley

LEARNING OBJECTIVES

- Describe how to recognise lymphoedema, why it occurs and associated conditions
- Explain why persistent limb swelling in the older person should not be ignored
- Explain how wounds/ulcers, skin breakdown or leakage do not heal without the control of tissue oedema

- Plan proactive management of skin care, mobilisation, physiotherapy and specific lymphoedema therapy including compression
- Describe how management of lymphoedema and chronic oedema results in improved function, reduced frequency of cellulitis episodes and improved quality of life

CASE

Bob was 72 years old when he was diagnosed with prostate cancer. He underwent radical prostatectomy (removal of prostate and surrounding lymph nodes), followed by radiation therapy. Now over 10 years later, he remains cancer free. In the years after surgery, he noticed his right thigh was bigger. His family doctor advised him to watch it. During the next 5 years, he gained weight and the right calf and foot slowly swelled and then began to leak. He used sanitary pads taped to his leg to 'mop up' the leakage. He became socially isolated and less mobile. Over the following 3 years, he suffered 4 episodes of cellulitis (infection of the leg tissue under the skin) requiring intravenous antibiotics. He gained a further 32 kg and found it difficult to get in and out of bed, so he slept in a chair. During his fourth hospital admission for cellulitis, aged 80 years, secondary lymphoedema was diagnosed.

Bob was referred to a dermatologist and a lymphoedema therapist, who worked together to reduce the leg size with a combination of skin hygiene, lymphoedema decongestive massage, multilayer bandaging and mobility exercises. Bob was placed on daily low-dose preventive antibiotic for 1 year. The leakage stopped and the size of Bob's leg reduced, and he was fitted with compression hosiery. Bob is now regularly reviewed for effective compression garments and skin care monitoring by the community nurse. He lost weight with better nutrition and exercise. He sleeps in his bed at night. He has stopped the antibiotics and has had no cellulitis-related hospital admissions for the last 3 years.

WHAT IS LYMPHOEDEMA?

Lymphoedema is where excess fluid collects in tissues (often the legs) causing swelling, due to a problem with the lymphatic system (see Fig. 56.1). The lymphatic system is made up of a vast network of open-ended lymphatic capillaries, collector lymph vessels and multiple lymph nodes (commonly called 'glands') carrying lymph fluid back into the venous blood circulation system. This body system is involved in several functions including tissue fluid balance (homeostasis) and immunity (innate and adaptive).

Generally, lymphoedema is divided into primary and secondary types. Primary lymphoedema is due to a genetic abnormality of the lymphatic system that may present as swelling at birth, in childhood, adolescence or later in life. Secondary lymphoedema occurs as a result of damage to a previously normal lymphatic system, for example, following cancer treatment, infection, injury and venous disease.

In addition, the intrinsic pumping of the lymph collector vessels which allows lymph to flow against gravity shows an age-related decrease. This is most marked in women after menopause and it progresses with advancing age (see Fig. 56.2). Reduced lymph flow speed causes lymph pooling (Unno et al., 2011).

HOW DOES LYMPHOEDEMA USUALLY OCCUR?

Clinically there are two main circumstances where lymphoedema occurs and affects the older person:

1. The older person with lymphoedema that developed at a younger age.

   Older people may present with lymphoedema associated with the treatment of cancers such as breast, pelvic or melanoma, which are now increasingly survivable into old age. This unfortunate complication of a survived cancer treatment has increasingly become a life-long disability, and its management can become more and more onerous for the older person or their carers. Primary lymphoedema that developed earlier in life will continue into older age. Lymphoedema has traditionally been considered to be a chronic oedema due to specific lymphatic failure. Lymphatic structures age and lymphatic function declines with age so a previously stable lymphoedema may deteriorate late in life.

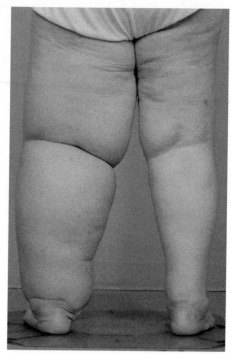

FIG. 56.1 This patient has lymphoedema of their left leg, many years after cancer treatment. (From Gurtner GC, Neligan PC. *Plastic Surgery. Volume 1: Principles*, 4th edn. Elsevier; 2018, with permission.)

2. The older person who develops lymphoedema/chronic oedema.

In the older person who develops chronic swelling, there are commonly a number of co-existing causative factors which have not traditionally been associated with the diagnosis of lymphoedema; the term chronic oedema has been coined to describe this clinical picture. This reconceptualising of the term lymphoedema to chronic oedema can tip the balance toward a more proactive rehabilitative management for older people with persisting swelling mostly of the feet, ankle and legs.

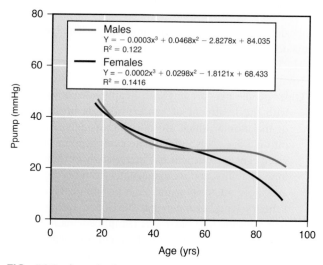

FIG. 56.2 Lymphatic pump pressure and ageing. (From Unno et al. 2011.)

Complex age-related anatomical, biochemical and functional change in the lymphatic system can result in decreased ability to transport bacteria to the draining lymph node and increased permeability of the lymphatic vessel can allow escape of bacteria into surrounding tissue (Zolla et al., 2015). This along with decreasing ability of the ageing immune system to control infections increases the risk of cellulitis.

COLD Concept: Chronic Oedema - Lymphatic Deficient

The term **chronic oedema** is an umbrella description of abnormal swelling of tissues persisting for more than 3 months (Moffatt et al., 2003). It has been used to standardise the definition of chronic swelling in research studies. Increasingly the terms lymphoedema and chronic oedema are being used synonymously and are intrinsically linked, as a revised understanding of the physiology of oedema formation recognises that all chronic oedema is caused by failure of the lymphatic system (Mortimer & Rockson, 2014). In this new model, all fluid which has been filtered into the tissue space from the capillary is drained by the lymphatic system with no reabsorption of fluid into the venous end of the capillary. Oedema occurs if the function of the lymphatic system is impaired or if a normal lymphatic system is draining at its maximum capacity but this is inadequate to cope with high capillary filtration (e.g. in venous hypertension). Therefore, in all chronic oedema there must be either inadequate or deficient lymphatic function in that area of swelling.

Several causes of chronic oedema particularly apply to the older person including:
- cancer treatment-related oedema
- dependency oedema: oedema associated with inactivity and immobility, e.g. due to neurological conditions or arthritis
- venous oedema: oedema mainly caused by the venous insufficiency
- obesity-induced lymphoedema
- oedema associated with chronic heart failure
- oedema due to advanced disease, e.g. cancer, respiratory and liver diseases.

Several of these causes may occur concurrently in the individual older person who presents with chronic leg oedema.

HOW LYMPHOEDEMA AFFECTS MOBILITY AND FUNCTION

Chronic oedema can affect people of all ages. However, Moffatt et al. (2016) found that it is 7 times more prevalent in older people. In this study, the estimated frequency of chronic oedema is roughly 4 people per 1000 in the general population, and 29 people per 1000 among people aged 85 years and over.

Lymphoedema is frequently unrecognised or erroneously considered to be an inevitable consequence of ageing, resulting in diagnostic delay and inappropriate or inadequate treatment. If untreated, this swelling has impacts on mobility and skin health, and increases falls risk (Mortimer & Levine, 2017).

Chronic oedema can have a profound effect on people's quality of life and their ability to engage in normal daily activities. It also has a significant impact on health service resources as patients can have multiple hospital admissions for cellulitis.

Effective treatment includes promoting self-management of chronic oedema/lymphoedema and the correct use of bandages and stockings. Exercise is one of the most important factors of the 'Four cornerstones of care', i.e. skin care, movement, simple lymphatic drainage and compression.

HOW TO UNDERTAKE LYMPHOEDEMA REHABILITATION

All management begins with recognition of the condition followed by a holistic assessment, seeking to identify the underlying cause(s) and contributing factors.

a) History:

Features of the oedema: e.g. site(s), duration, precipitating factors.

General health history: past conditions including cancer treatment, thyroid problems, trauma, deep vein thrombosis (DVT).

Medications which may cause/contribute to oedema, e.g., calcium channel blockers which slow intrinsic lymph pumping, steroids/NSAIDs (non-steroidal anti-inflammatories)/pregabalin which cause fluid retention.

Home and care circumstances: mobility and activity level; always check sleeping position and sitting times.

b) Physical examination:

General examination: cardiac, respiratory, abdominal looking for general causes of oedema.

Specific examination of the oedematous area: site and extent of oedema. Take off the socks! – pitting test, Stemmer sign (see Fig. 56.3).

Regular weighing: a sudden increase likely to be caused by right heart failure.

c) Investigations:

Consider:

Blood screen including full blood count, thyroid function tests, B natriuretic peptide (to assess for possible heart failure), kidney function, liver function and protein/albumin, if history/examination suggests a general cause of swelling.

Chest x-ray, echocardiography, venous Doppler and CT (computed tomography scan) of abdomen/pelvis, if history/examination suggests underlying cause, e.g., heart failure, venous disease, intra-abdominal malignancy.

Lymphoscintogram: if underlying primary lymphoedema is a possibility (rarely needed in older people).

ICG (indocyanine green) lymphography: to examine superficial lymphatic anatomy and function which may help to influence treatment.

THERAPEUTIC AND COMMUNITY OPTIONS FOR LYMPHOEDEMA REHABILITATION

Self-management support through a partnership between the person and their care provider prepares, supports and ultimately empowers the person to manage their health and ongoing care. Giving people knowledge and confidence to manage their condition is more likely to alter behaviour, and there is good evidence that improved self-efficacy is associated with better clinical outcomes.

Older persons who have stable lymphoedema should have a coordinated treatment plan that allows for review and modification for age changes. The management of lymphoedema may vary according to the severity of the condition – treatment should be responsive to patient needs over time. The role of compression garments extends to the long-term management of lymphoedema. The effectiveness of compression garments to maintain the gains made by other components of lymphoedema therapy depends on the appropriate choice

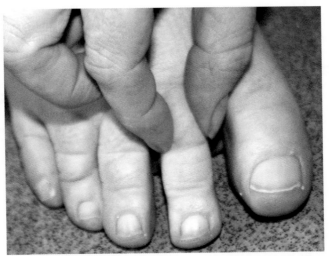

FIG. 56.3 Stemmer sign for lymphoedema is the inability to pick up a fold of skin over the proximal digit of the second toe. A negative sign is normal. A positive sign is found in many cases of lymphoedema.

of garment and the adherence of the person in wearing them. Putting on compression garments is difficult, and loss of joint flexibility, arthritis and skin fragility make this more problematic for the older person. Use of alternate options such as pumps or Velcro compression wraps and gaining carer support is important.

In the older person some simple physical issues can be addressed to avoid lymph stasis such as avoidance of prolonged sitting, a short rest in the lying position with legs in elevation, encouragement and access to activity and simple exercise. Exercises such as Tai Chi where there is an emphasis on slow rhythmic movement coordinated with breathing are suggested. Any and all exercise, from walking, seated exercise in a group or at-home exercise regimen, can be beneficial. Skin cleaning is important including between toes, and the use of antifungals if needed. The daily use of moisturisers and protection of fragile skin from injury and pressure is essential.

People with lymphoedema experience a significantly heightened risk of cellulitis in the affected body area. Cellulitis is caused by spreading bacterial infection of the skin, resulting in redness, pain and lymphangitis. Treatment requires antibiotics. Cellulitis is the most common cause for hospitalisation in people with lymphoedema. The treatment of cellulitis in lymphoedema may differ from conventional cellulitis. Cellulitis most commonly occurs in one leg; it must be distinguished from stasis dermatitis, common in the older person and associated with longstanding redness of both legs, itching and skin pigmentation without being unwell (see Chapter 40 Skin Care and Podiatry). Treatment of stasis dermatitis may require the use of cortisone (steroid) cream; however, elevation, exercise and light garment compression are also part of the management of the chronic oedema associated with this condition.

Cellulitis is a risk factor both for lymphoedema development and for lymphoedema deterioration. Cellulitis can lead to obstruction and damage of the lymphatic system that predisposes people to recurrent cellulitis. Effective conservative management of lymphoedema has been shown to significantly reduce the frequency of cellulitis.

SUMMARY POINTS

- Recognition of lymphoedema, its effects and cause are important aspects of caring for older people
- Lymphoedema/chronic oedema has consequences such as skin breakdown, reduced mobility and reduced quality of life
- Lymphoedema/chronic oedema can be treated by a combination of exercise and elevation, appropriate compression and ongoing community support for the patient and carers

MCQs

Q.1 Cellulitis and stasis dermatitis in the legs can be distinguished by
  a. The redness of the legs
  b. The heat of the skin of the legs
  c. The presence of fever
  d. The irritability of the skin

Q.2 Which of the following may cause chronic oedema in older people?
  a. Primary lymphoedema
  b. Breast cancer treatment
  c. Obesity
  d. Multiple sclerosis
  e. All of the above

REFERENCES

Moffatt, C. J., Franks, P. J., Doherty, D. C., Williams, A. F., Badger, C., Jeffs, E., Bosanquet, N., & Mortimer, P. S. (2003). Lymphoedema: an underestimated health problem. *Quarterly Journal of Medicine*, 96(10), 731–738.

Moffatt, C. J., Keeley, V., Franks, P. J., Rich, A., & Pinnington, L. (2016). Chronic oedema: a prevalent health care problem for UK health services. *International Wound Journal*, 14, 772–781.

Mortimer, P., & Rockson, S. (2014). New developments in clinical aspects of lymphatic disease. *The Journal of Clinical Investigation, 124*(3), 915–921.

Mortimer, P., & Levine, G. (2017). *Let's talk lymphoedema*. London: Elliott and Thompson Ltd.

Unno, N., Tanaka, H., Suzuki, M., Yamamoto, N., Mano, Y., Sano, M., Saito, T., & Konno, H. (2011). Influence of age and gender on human lymphatic pumping pressure in the leg. *Lymphology*, 44, 113–120.

Zolla, V., Nizamutdinova, I. T., Scharf, B., Clement, C. C., Maejima, D., Akl, T., …, & Santambrogio, L. (2015). Aging-related anatomical and biochemical changes in lymphatic collectors impair lymph transport, fluid homeostasis, and pathological clearance. *Aging Cell*, 14, 582–594.

57

Cardiac Rehabilitation

Eoin Fahy

LEARNING OBJECTIVES

- Describe the role of cardiac rehabilitation as a treatment for older people with heart disease
- Explain the structure and components of cardiac rehabilitation
- List the indications and contraindications for cardiac rehabilitation

INTRODUCTION

Heart disease comes in many forms with cardiovascular disease (CVD), heart failure (HF) and valvular heart disease (VHD) being the most common types of cardiac problems affecting people across the globe. CVD refers to hardening and narrowing of blood vessels that can lead to limitation of blood flow to the major organs. HF occurs when the hearts ability to pump or circulate blood is reduced. VHD occurs when the valves of the heart become either stenosed (narrowed) or incompetent (leaky). CVD remains the biggest cause of death worldwide with nearly 18 million people dying from CVD in 2016 (WHO, 2017). Our understanding of heart disease has dramatically improved over the past century with major advancements mostly occurring in the past 40 years. This has allowed us to develop therapies and interventions that are particularly guided towards the prevention and treatment of heart disease.

With an ageing population there has been and will continue to be an increased number of people who are affected by cardiac disease. Our improving ability to treat these diseases successfully with medications and sometimes surgeries means that people who may have died from cardiac causes in the past are now living longer. Our goals as healthcare professionals should be not only to help people to live longer but also to live better quality lives, free from disability that might be associated with any disease. Improving symptoms associated with heart disease is a key goal of all cardiac treatments.

CASE

Jacob is an 83-year-old man living alone in a suburban area. He owns a dog and used to walk him near his home on a daily basis. His medical history includes diabetes, high blood pressure and prostate problems. He used to smoke but gave up 10 years ago.

Jacob has taken the dog out for a walk one day when he is forced to stop before he can get to the shop. He feels a heavy chest pressure and becomes very breathless. He also starts to sweat profusely. A neighbour can see that Jacob is unwell and calls an ambulance.

The nurse and then the doctor in the local emergency department tell Jacob that he has 'had a heart attack' and needs to be admitted to the hospital for treatment. They give him some tablets and injections and Jacob's chest pressure stops after about 1 hour. He meets one of the cardiology doctors who tells him he will need a coronary angiogram. After the procedure, she tells Jacob that she 'put in two stents' which should help him. The doctor mentions a few times how important it will be to take his medications and that his diabetes needs to be better controlled.

Later that day, Jacob meets a nurse who works with cardiac rehabilitation (CR) in the hospital. She asks Jacob about his medical history and explains what happened to Jacob in more detail. Jacob realises that he had been experiencing similar symptoms to a milder degree in the 6 months before his heart attack. He had thought it was indigestion and 'getting old'. He had stopped walking his dog because he felt he 'wouldn't make it'. The nurse tells Jacob that he was experiencing angina.

The nurse mentions that he is overweight. Jacob agrees and says the weight gain is mostly recent, since he stopped walking. She tells him about the hospital CR programme that they would recommend starting in about 6 weeks' time. The following day he is discharged from the hospital. It is 4 days since his heart attack.

HEART DISEASE

The concept of risk factors for heart disease is extremely important. It is useful to think of risk factors as being modifiable or non-modifiable. Age, sex and family history (or genetics) are non-modifiable risks and play a large part in increasing the risk of developing heart disease. Modifiable or behavioural risks include tobacco use, unhealthy diet, physical inactivity and excessive use of alcohol. The behavioural risks have a large part to play in the development of high blood pressure and high cholesterol. These behavioural risks are the obvious and likely best targets for intervention to reduce a person's risk of developing heart disease.

Medical advances directed towards the treatment of heart disease have been impressive. This includes medicines or drugs for treatment of blood pressure and high cholesterol. While these drugs are very effective in treating these cardiac risks, changing the behavioural risks is often as effective at reducing the risk of heart disease (Yusuf et al., 2004).

CARDIAC REHABILITATION

One of the mainstays of therapy used to be the prescription of bed rest, often for up to 6 weeks after an initial heart attack or heart surgery. This unfortunately led to a number of immobility-related complications, which could range from thrombosis (clotting) and infections to depression and anxiety. In the 1960s evidence began to emerge that supported the early use of mobilisation and exercise after acute cardiac problems (Saltin et al., 1968). Gradually the medical and cardiology community began to embrace CR as a very important tool in prolonging and improving quality of life in patients with cardiac disease (Mampuya, 2012). The use of CR is most common in people who have undergone cardiac surgery (coronary artery bypass grafting or valve surgery); however, its role is expanding. It plays a key role in treatment of people after myocardial infarction (heart attack), people with HF and people who have undergone percutaneous coronary interventions (PCI, otherwise known as stenting). There has been a significant increase in older people undergoing minimally invasive cardiac procedures such as valve replacements performed via keyhole procedures (transcatheter aortic valve implantation or TAVI) in the past decade. These people will also certainly benefit from CR programmes.

CR has evolved from mostly exercise-based interventions to a comprehensive and more holistic approach to treating cardiac disease. It has been shown conclusively that CR can prolong life and certainly improve quality of life after heart attacks or cardiac surgery (Wannamethee, Shaper, & Walker, 2000). Regular sustained physical activity can improve cholesterol levels, blood pressure, diabetes control and weight. CR programmes usually include smoking cessation advice and support for patients, offering a further benefit to people's health. Various informal and formal interventions are used to improve the psychological health. Mood disorders such as depression and anxiety are extremely common after cardiac events and cardiac surgery. CR offers a unique chance to identify and treat mood disorders in the early period after a cardiac illness (Milani & Lavie, 2007). Often the structure and regular follow-up with CR will allow the identification of problems specific to an individual such as issues with medication side effects or other non-cardiac health problems.

STRUCTURE

Most CR programmes include three to four phases.

Phase 1: The in-hospital part of the programme. This occurs soon after the initial cardiac event or cardiac surgery. The main goals are:
- Explanation of the cardiac problem
- Identifying risk factors
- Smoking cessation
- Symptom management
- Advice on diet, medications and exercise
- Psychological support, stress management and relaxation techniques
- Advice on return to regular activity and exercise.

Phase 2: This is the immediate post discharge phase. Often telephone contact is maintained with the CR team. Any issues with medications or questions about cardiac disease or procedures can be addressed. It is a useful time for reinforcement of the advice given in hospital during phase 1. Some programmes include an information session in the hospital for people and their families.

Phase 3: This is the outpatient phase. Usually 10–30 sessions are organised over a 6- to 12-week period. People meet with nurses, physiotherapists, dieticians and doctors if needed. Family are often encouraged to attend. The goals are:
- Improving exercise tolerance
- Improving confidence
- Reducing symptoms
- Reducing blood pressure and cholesterol
- Reducing tobacco use
- Improving quality of life
- Help to return to normal activities of daily living, including work.

The exercise aspect of CR is often guided by a physiotherapist. The initial exercises tend to take the form of light 'aerobic type' including stretching and stepping type activity. Depending on the person's physical ability, it progresses gradually to 'jogging on the spot' or 'jumping-jacks'. Treadmills can be used for longer walking circuits. In some cases swimming can be used. Each person will have an exercise programme tailored to their abilities. People are advised to continue the physical activity in their own time, in between classes. Over the course of the entire CR programme most people would expect to see a significant increase in the amount of physical activity that they can perform.

Phase 4: This is the maintenance phase. After the outpatient programme is completed, people are often encouraged to attend local exercise classes or to undertake exercise programmes at home. The goal is to maintain the lifestyle changes addressed in the earlier phases.

INDICATIONS FOR CR

The indications for CR are summarised in Table 57.1. Usually people are selected or referred after a heart attack or surgery that has required a stay in hospital. However, it is important to consider referral of people who may have more long-term cardiac problems that are usually addressed in an outpatient setting.

CONTRAINDICATIONS FOR CR

There are fewer absolute contraindications for CR than people may think. The risk of a serious cardiac event (such as death or heart attack) during CR is estimated at one event per 60,000–80,000 hours of exercise (Thompson

TABLE 57.1	Summary of indications for referral to cardiac rehabilitation.
SETTING	**INDICATION**
Inpatient	Cardiac surgery (coronary bypass grafting, valve replacement, cardiac transplantation)
	Cardiac arrest (after treatment of underlying cause)
	Acute myocardial infarction ('heart attack' with or without PCI/ 'stenting')
	Acute heart failure (after optimising medical therapy)
	TAVI and mitral valve interventions
Outpatient	Angina
	Heart failure with New York Heart Association class II and III symptoms

et al., 2007). Age is not a contraindication to CR. Reduced mobility is also not a barrier to CR, and it is important to inform older people that the exercise aspects of CR will be suited to the individual's needs. A person who mobilises with a walking stick will not be given the same exercises as a long distance runner! A history of falls should also not stop an older person from attending CR and in fact the programme may help to reduce the risk of falling by improving general strength and mobility. Mild or moderate cognitive

impairment is also not a reason to avoid CR, and again some evidence exists that it may help to improve cognition (Smith et al., 2010). The advanced stages of some diseases will make CR impractical for some older people. This would include severe dementia (where people have significant functional limitations in communication, memory or attention) and people who are completely immobile for other medical reasons. An issue that may seem like a contraindication at first may only need encouragement and creative therapies to make it less of a barrier. For example, people with joint or obesity problems may do well with swimming pool-based exercises. Educating older people and their families should help dispel myths that can exist surrounding CR.

CARDIAC REHABILITATION IN OLDER PEOPLE

CR has been shown to be as beneficial in an older population as in a younger population. In some studies the benefits of rehabilitation were more pronounced in older people. Improvements in exercise tolerance, symptom burden, psychological health and reduction in the risk of death from cardiac disease are seen despite a person's age. The older person is more prone to deconditioning related to acute illness and the related hospital stay. CR plays an enhanced role in avoiding these complications in this group of people. Frailty is not necessarily a contraindication to CR and in fact many of the aspects of frailty can be improved with a rehab programme (Fig. 57.1).

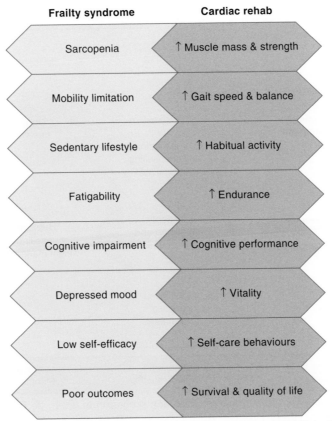

FIG. 57.1 Evaluating and treating frailty in cardiac rehabilitation. (From Afilalo J. Evaluating and treating frailty in cardiac rehabilitation. *Clin Geriatr Med.* 2019;35(4):445–57, with permission.)

Despite these clear benefits, participation in CR programmes is often very poor. This is even more pronounced in older people. Referral rates from healthcare professionals can unfortunately be quite low, particularly for the older population. Advice and encouragement to participate is often not strong enough. Explanations as to the role and benefits of CR are often short and insufficient. If older people and their families are not educated about the structure and importance of CR, then incorrect ideas about life after cardiac disease may persist. Fig. 57.2 offers a summary of structure and benefits of CR. The idea that one should rest after a heart attack or heart surgery may persist amongst an older person's family despite medical evidence to the contrary. People may feel they are 'too old' to participate or that the benefit may not be clear, particularly as concrete goals such as returning to work may be less likely to be a driving force for an older person.

Even when older people are referred to CR, they are less likely to attend than younger people. This is often due to a combination of other medical problems (arthritis, lung disease or mobility issues) that people feel might affect their ability to participate. Social and family support or lack of the same can also affect an older person's likelihood of attending CR. Many older people do not drive, and other transport arrangements can be complicated.

Careful consideration of issues unique to the older population should allow us to develop strategies to combat the traditionally poor attendance at CR. Encouraging participation from families is a useful strategy to address some of the barriers to CR that older people may face.

CASE Conclusion

Six weeks after Jacob's heart attack, he attends the first session of his CR programme in the local hospital. Before commencing the programme, a gentle exercise stress test is performed on a treadmill. The proposed plan is two sessions per week for 8 weeks. Travel to the hospital is difficult as Jacob does not drive anymore and so his family has arranged to help him with transport. At the sessions he meets nine other people who have had similar cardiac problems. Their ages range from 45 years old up to 87 years old. The people attending the programme are given talks by nurses, physiotherapists and dieticians once a week. Exercise sessions are tailored to each person's physical ability. Advice is given on smoking cessation, diet and exercise. Mood and sexuality are also discussed. Following the 16 sessions, the exercise treadmill test is repeated. Most of the people involved note a significant improvement in exercise tolerance, mood and confidence. They often describe an improved understanding of their various cardiac conditions and feel they can apply what they have learned in the rehabilitation programme their lives.

The final input from the CR team is organisation of maintenance of the lifestyle changes that each person has made. Jacob is offered an exercise programme in the local gym. Advice is also given on a home exercise programme. The class in the gym is mostly made up of older people with cardiac disease, many of whom have attended the same CR as Jacob.

Six months after the heart attack, Jacob is back walking his dog on a daily basis. He is no longer limited by his angina symptoms when he walks. While he does get very rare minor 'reminders' of his angina symptoms if he exerts himself very significantly, he is not bothered by the symptoms in his daily life. His family note that he is more active and more 'like his old self'.

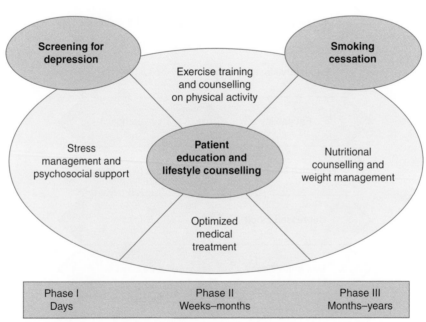

FIG. 57.2   Components of a cardiac rehabilitation programme. (From de Lemos J, Ormland T. *Chronic Coronary Artery Disease: A Companion to Braunwald's Heart Disease,* 1st edn. Elsevier; 2018, with permission.)

SUMMARY POINTS

- Cardiac rehabilitation (CR) improves quality of life and helps people live longer after developing cardiac disease
- Improvements in exercise tolerance, confidence, quality of life and adherence to medical therapy have been consistently reported
- Attendance at CR is often poor, and this is more pronounced in older people
- Older people may have complex reasons for not attending CR but absolute contraindications to CR are few
- Education and awareness can improve attendance at CR in all age groups

MCQs

Q.1 Which of the following is a modifiable risk factor for heart disease?
  - **a.** Age
  - **b.** Family history
  - **c.** Gender
  - **d.** Physical exercise
  - **e.** All of the above

Q.2 Which of the following is true about bed rest after heart attack or heart surgery?
  - **a.** It is the best approach to improve recovery
  - **b.** It is not recommended as it can slow recovery and lead to complications
  - **c.** It improves mood
  - **d.** It improves quality of life
  - **e.** All of the above

Q.3 Which of the follow is true about cardiac rehabilitation in older people?
  - **a.** It is safe and effective
  - **b.** It is often poorly attended because of low referral rates and limited education about the benefits
  - **c.** It is suitable for people with mild or moderate dementia
  - **d.** It improves exercise tolerance and quality of life
  - **e.** All of the above

REFERENCES

Mampuya, W. M. (2012). Cardiac rehabilitation past, present and future: an overview. *Cardiovascular Diagnosis and Therapy, 2*(1), 38–49.

Milani, R. V., & Lavie, C. J. (2007). Impact of cardiac rehabilitation on depression and its associated mortality. *American Journal of Medicine, 120*, 799–806.

Saltin, B., Blomqvist, G., Mitchell, J. H., Johnson, R. L., Jr., Wildenthal, K., & Chapman, C. B. (1968). Response to exercise after bed rest and after training. *Circulation, 38.* VII1–78.

Smith, P. J., Blumenthal, J. A., Hoffman, B. M., Cooper, H., Strauman, T. A., Welsh-Bohmer, K., Browndyke, J. N., & Sherwood, A. (2010). Aerobic exercise and neurocognitive performance: a meta-analytic review of randomized controlled trials. *Psychosomatic Medicine, 72*, 239–252.

Thompson, P. D., Franklin, B. A., Balady, G. J., Blair, S. N., Corrado, D., Mark Estes, N. A., ..., American Heart Association Council on Nutrition, Physical Activity, and Metabolism; American Heart Association Council on Clinical Cardiology; American College of Sports Medicine. (2007). Exercise and acute cardiovascular events placing the risks into perspective: a scientific statement from the American Heart Association Council on Nutrition, Physical Activity, and Metabolism and the Council on Clinical Cardiology. *Circulation, 115*, 2358–2368.

Wannamethee, S. G., Shaper, A. G., & Walker, M. (2000). Physical activity and mortality in older men with diagnosed coronary heart disease. *Circulation, 102*, 1358–1363.

World Health Organisation. (2017). *Cardiovascular diseases fact sheets* [Online]. Retrieved from https://www.who.int/en/news-room/fact-sheets/detail/cardiovascular-diseases-(cvds) (Accessed 29 April 2019).

Yusuf, S., Hawken, S., Ounpuu, S., Dans, T., Avezum, A., Lanas, F., ..., & Lisheng, L. (2004). Effect of potentially modifiable risk factors associated with myocardial infarction in 52 countries (the INTERHEART study): case-control study. *Lancet, 364*, 937–952.

58

Pulmonary Rehabilitation

Lisa Jane Brighton & Matthew Maddocks

LEARNING OBJECTIVES

- Describe the typical structure and content of pulmonary rehabilitation
- Explain the benefits of pulmonary rehabilitation for people with chronic lung disease
- Describe the challenges to consider when delivering pulmonary rehabilitation for older people with chronic lung disease

CASE

Gareth is an 85-year-old man living with chronic obstructive lung disease (COPD) and frailty, and a history of diabetes. He lives on his own in a first-floor apartment since his wife Silvia died a few years ago. He has no family that live close by but keeps in touch with a few friends by phone. Given these circumstances, his mobility and independence are of great importance to him, as he relies on himself to get by day to day.

Over the past year, Gareth's health had deteriorated: he has lost weight, felt increasingly breathless and fatigued, and found it difficult to motivate himself to get out and about. Having seen his respiratory doctor, he was referred for an outpatient pulmonary rehabilitation programme at the local community centre. Gareth hadn't been to pulmonary rehabilitation before and didn't know what to expect, but he was willing to try anything if it might help improve how he was feeling.

INTRODUCTION

As people with chronic respiratory disease age, they are at increased risk of falls, exacerbations (a period of significant worsening of symptoms; sometimes known as 'flare-ups') and hospitalisations (Hunter et al., 2016; Montserrat-Capdevila et al., 2015; Roig et al., 2011). They report higher levels of disability and breathlessness, and when admitted to hospital they present with higher disease severity, lower performance status (degree of activity) and more medical conditions than their younger counterparts (Stone et al., 2012). Together these factors contribute to reduced physical activity and general deconditioning of bodily systems. This can be associated with reduced muscle mass and function (known as sarcopenia) and increased vulnerability to stresses on their health (frailty). As a result, older people with chronic respiratory disease commonly experience reduced capacity for exercise and poorer levels of physical function.

On a background of optimal medical management, pulmonary rehabilitation provides an opportunity to address some of the contributing factors to poor health (e.g. breathlessness, deconditioning) through improvements in muscle function and efficiency (Spruit et al., 2013). Combined with integrated support for continued self-management, this can improve long-term outcomes and people's ability to manage and live well alongside their chronic lung disease.

PULMONARY REHABILITATION

Pulmonary rehabilitation is defined as a comprehensive programme of exercise and education for people with chronic lung disease. Based on a thorough assessment of the individual, it takes a tailored approach to improving their short- and long-term physical and psychological health.

Target Population

Pulmonary rehabilitation is designed for anyone with a chronic lung condition who reports being limited by their breathlessness. Typically, this includes those with scores of 3 to 5 on the Medical Research Council (MRC) Dyspnoea Scale (Table 58.1), and/or those reporting functional limitation.

The most common group of people referred for pulmonary rehabilitation are those living with COPD (Yohannes & Connolly, 2004). Most of the early evidence was built in this group. However, there is rapidly increasing evidence that the principles and benefits of pulmonary rehabilitation apply across a range of chronic lung conditions, including but not limited to interstitial lung disease, bronchiectasis, cystic fibrosis, asthma, pulmonary hypertension, lung cancer, lung volume reduction surgery and lung transplantation (Spruit et al., 2013). Pulmonary rehabilitation is relevant across all stages of disease (Takigawa et al., 2007) and regardless of comorbidities (Naz et al., 2018). This includes people recently hospitalised for an acute exacerbation of their illness, where it is recommended that people be referred at the point of

TABLE 58.1   MRC dyspnoea scale.

Score	Description
1	Breathless only with strenuous exercise
2	Short of breath when hurrying on the level or up a slight hill
3	Slower than most people of the same age on a level surface or have tostop when walking at my own pace on the level.
4	Stop for breath walking 100 meters or after a few minutes walking at my own pace on the level.
5	Too breathless to leave the house

discharge and start within the following 4 weeks (Bolton et al., 2013).

Service Structure and Setting

People are most often referred for pulmonary rehabilitation by healthcare professionals such as respiratory (lung) doctors or general practitioners (Spruit et al., 2014). Programmes are often delivered in groups in hospital outpatient settings. However, with variations in local set-ups and resources, some teams deliver pulmonary rehabilitation within inpatient, community and home environments (Spruit & Wouters, 2019).

Guidance describes pulmonary rehabilitation as comprising at least twice-weekly supervised exercise sessions over at least 6 weeks (British Thoracic Society, 2014), and in practice programme duration often extends to 8 to 12 weeks (Spruit et al., 2014). Combined with delivery of educational and behaviour change components, people typically spend between 1 and 2 hours at each session.

Pulmonary rehabilitation should be delivered by an interdisciplinary team, in order to meet the multidimensional needs of people with chronic lung conditions. This includes primarily lung doctors, dieticians, nurses and physiotherapists, but can also involve social workers, occupational therapists, psychologists and pharmacists (Spruit et al., 2014).

Content
Initial Assessment

Comprehensive assessment is an essential starting point for any pulmonary rehabilitation programme. This allows the team to ensure safety of the intervention (e.g. checking for important cardiovascular comorbidities, considering previous injury), assess whether supplemental oxygen may be helpful and individualise the prescription of exercise. This should include using established tools to measure exercise capacity (e.g. six-minute walk test), breathlessness (e.g. MRC Dyspnoea Scale, Borg Dyspnoea Scale) and health status (e.g. Chronic Respiratory Questionnaire), to monitor subsequent progress.

Exercise Training

Exercise training is a cornerstone of pulmonary rehabilitation. The most common types of exercise used are strength training (e.g. using handheld weights) and aerobic training (e.g. using stationary cycling, treadmill walking). A combination of both is preferable as this can lead to better results than either strategy can achieve alone (Benton & Swan, 2006).

Exercise prescription can be individualised to each person's ability and goals and adjusted over time. This will include progressively increasing the intensity and/or duration as their performance improves, but also tailoring back if it becomes too burdensome. Where people find it difficult to achieve their target exercise duration, evidence supports using interval training: where the individual switches between short, high-intensity training and periods of rest or low-intensity training (Spruit et al., 2013).

Education, Behaviour Change and Self-Management

Alongside tailored exercise, pulmonary rehabilitation includes structured education. This element of pulmonary rehabilitation includes information sharing, supporting long-term self-management and behaviour change. This means working collaboratively between professionals, people living with chronic lung disease and their caregivers to ensure a shared understanding of important elements of living with and managing their illness (Box 58.1).

While some of these components may be taught by the core pulmonary rehabilitation team, this can also be an opportunity for teams to bring in additional relevant expertise – for example, linking with speech and language therapists or palliative care specialists. Those delivering the educational components must consider how well the content will suit people with lower education levels, health literacy or cognitive ability (Blackstock & Evans, 2019), as these are common and important factors in chronic respiratory conditions (Roberts, Ghiassi, & Partridge, 2008; Yohannes et al., 2017). Providing written materials on these topics is recommended.

Final Assessment and Ongoing Support

Towards the end of pulmonary rehabilitation, those participating should have the opportunity to have their exercise

BOX 58.1   Suggested Educational Topics for Pulmonary Rehabilitation (Blackstock & Evans, 2019)

- Normal lung anatomy and physiology
- Pathophysiology of chronic respiratory disease
- Communicating with healthcare providers
- Interpreting medical tests
- Breathing strategies
- Secretion clearance techniques
- Role of medications including oxygen therapy
- Effective use of respiratory devices
- Benefits of exercise and physical activity
- Energy conservation during daily living
- Healthy food intake
- Irritant avoidance
- Early recognition and treatment of exacerbations
- Leisure activities
- Coping with chronic lung disease

capacity, breathlessness and health status reassessed. This allows people to see the progress they have made and can inform a personalised plan for their ongoing exercise maintenance. This plan should specify and encourage continuation of strength and aerobic exercises and provide information on local services that may support them (e.g. gyms, walking clubs).

WHAT ARE THE BENEFITS OF PULMONARY REHABILITATION?

The clinical effectiveness of pulmonary rehabilitation is well established for people living with COPD, both when their disease is stable and when they have recently experienced an exacerbation.

Stable Disease

For people with stable COPD, the pooled findings of 65 randomised controlled trials demonstrate significant improvements across multiple domains following pulmonary rehabilitation (McCarthy et al., 2015). In questionnaires following pulmonary rehabilitation, people report feeling less symptomatic, less limited by their illness and having greater quality of life. People also demonstrate improvements in exercise capacity, and on average can walk an additional 44 m in a six-minute walk test at the end of pulmonary rehabilitation. In all cases, these differences exceed established minimum clinically important differences, signifying a change that is noticeable and valuable to the participant.

When asked to describe their experiences of pulmonary rehabilitation in interviews, participants talk about increased physical abilities, having more energy and feeling less restricted by their breathlessness. As a result, people become more confident to undertake activities they previously depended on others for, feel more able to engage in more social activities and describe a more positive self-image (Jones et al., 2018).

Post-hospitalisation for an Exacerbation

For people undertaking pulmonary rehabilitation after being in hospital for an exacerbation of COPD, a review of 20 randomised controlled trials also showed substantial clinical benefits (Puhan et al., 2016). Again, people reported feeling less symptomatic and less limited by their symptoms. They could also walk on average an extra 62 m in a six-minute walk test by the end of pulmonary rehabilitation.

Considering concerns around the safety of pulmonary rehabilitation soon after a hospitalisation, this review also examined hospital readmissions and mortality. Data from up to 810 individuals showed a significant impact of pulmonary rehabilitation on reducing hospital readmissions, with no significant difference in mortality. Of note, the findings were variable, potentially due to variations in programme delivery and individual study quality. Adverse events were rare (a single event across five studies with 278 participants in total), suggesting it is safe as well as beneficial to participate in pulmonary rehabilitation following an acute exacerbation.

Impact on Clinical Practice

The benefits seen in research studies have also been seen in real-life practice, captured in the National Pulmonary Rehabilitation Audit for England and Wales. This audit included over 7000 people with COPD attending 210 different programmes (representing over 90% of eligible services). Here, 83% of individuals completing pulmonary rehabilitation had improved functional exercise capacity (63% achieving more than the minimum clinically important difference), and 74% had improved health status (31% achieving more than the minimum clinically important difference; Fig. 58.1) (Steiner & Roberts, 2016). Combined with evidence of cost-effectiveness (Griffiths et al., 2001), pulmonary rehabilitation is now understood as one of the most high value and beneficial approaches to managing COPD, following flu vaccinations and smoking cessation (Zoumot, Jordan, & Hopkinson, 2014).

CONSIDERATIONS FOR THE OLDER PERSON WITH CHRONIC LUNG DISEASE

Influence of Age and Frailty

While there is no evidence that participants' age predicts outcomes of pulmonary rehabilitation, syndromes such as sarcopenia and frailty are common in older people with chronic lung disease. Living with sarcopenia does not seem to impact on completion of, or outcomes following, pulmonary rehabilitation. Importantly, the improvements in skeletal muscle mass, handgrip strength and gait speed following pulmonary rehabilitation can result in some people no longer meeting the definition for sarcopenia (Jones et al., 2015).

For people living with frailty, the picture is more complex. Within this group, pulmonary rehabilitation still results in significant improvements in breathlessness, strength, exercise capacity, health status and mood (Blindenbach et al., 2017; Maddocks et al., 2016). In fact, they tend to experience greater benefit than others, likely as a result of lower baseline health and greater scope for improvements. Similar to sarcopenia, improvements in handgrip strength, gait speed, physical activity and reduced feelings of exhaustion contribute to some participants no longer meeting the criteria for frailty following pulmonary rehabilitation (Maddocks et al., 2016; Mittal et al., 2015) (Fig. 58.2). Individuals living with frailty alongside the lung condition therefore have the potential to gain a lot from pulmonary rehabilitation. However, while factors associated with ageing do not seem to affect outcomes of pulmonary rehabilitation, there is evidence that they may affect the extent to which people attend and complete the programmes.

Approximately 40% of those referred for pulmonary rehabilitation do not complete it (Steiner et al., 2017), and those living with frailty have twice the odds of not completing pulmonary rehabilitation (Maddocks et al., 2016). Evidence from people living with COPD and older people living with frailty suggest common barriers that may be more prevalent or exaggerated in this group. For example, people with COPD report challenges around lack of perceived benefit

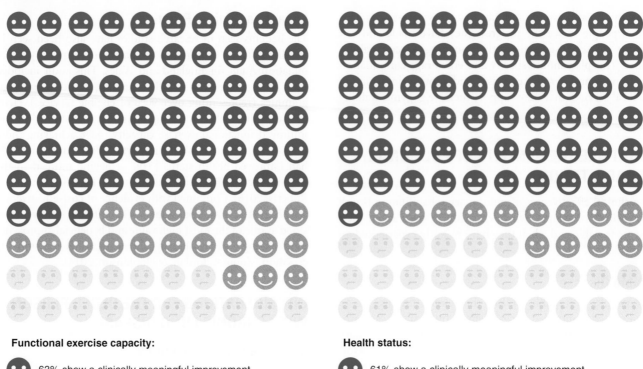

Functional exercise capacity:

63% show a clinically meaningful improvement

20% show a small improvement

17% show no improvement or get worse

Health status:

61% show a clinically meaningful improvement

13% show a small improvement

26% show no improvement or get worse

FIG. 58.1 Clinical response for patients completing pulmonary rehabilitation in the National Pulmonary Rehabilitation Audit for England and Wales (Adapted from Steiner & Roberts, 2016).

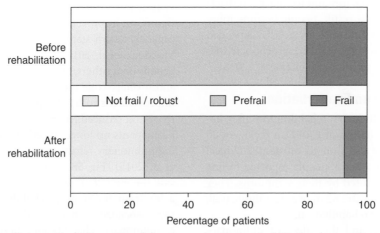

FIG. 58.2 Changes in frailty status following pulmonary rehabilitation in people with COPD (Adapted from Maddocks et al., 2016).

and fear of worsening symptoms (Sohanpal et al., 2015), and older people living with frailty report disengagement with exercise due to a perceived inevitability of frailty in older age (D'Avanzo et al., 2017). Travel is also a commonly reported barrier by people with COPD (Keating, Lee, & Holland, 2011), and many over the age of 80 years report difficulties travelling to where programmes are based

(Holley-Moore & Creighton, 2015). Moreover, people describe difficulty attending or completing rehabilitation due to the burden of symptoms and medical conditions (Sohanpal et al., 2015), which often increase in older age. Considering their potential to benefit, maximising support for older people with chronic lung disease to participate in pulmonary rehabilitation is a high priority.

CASE CONCLUSION

Gareth attended pulmonary rehabilitation twice a week for 8 weeks. He described it as 'killer' at first – he felt tired and achy after the first sessions and felt like he'd only just recovered before the next one. However, as time went on and he kept attending, this tiredness happened less and less. He felt stronger, more energetic, and like his breathing was a bit better than before. The educational component had given him more confidence managing his inhalers, and a clearer idea of what to do if he found himself in a crisis with his breathing.

Although at first Gareth had been worried about whether he should be doing this at his age, he was reassured and encouraged by the physiotherapist that it didn't matter how old he was, so long as he could take part. Having finished the programme, he is keen to continue exercising at home, and looks forward to attending again in the future.

SUMMARY POINTS

- Living with chronic lung disease in older age is associated with low levels of exercise capacity and function
- Pulmonary rehabilitation is multicomponent intervention, centred around exercise and education, relevant to people with a variety of chronic lung conditions
- Pulmonary rehabilitation can improve exercise capacity, function and health-related quality of life in stable and post-exacerbation periods of respiratory disease
- Delivery of pulmonary rehabilitation must consider the challenges prevalent in older age such as frailty, increasing illness burden and comorbidities, and difficulties travelling, especially as this group can benefit greatly from completing this intervention

MCQs

Q.1 What is the typical structure and delivery of pulmonary rehabilitation?
- a. Exercise delivered twice weekly over at least 6 weeks by a multidisciplinary team
- b. A multicomponent programme comprising exercise, education, behaviour change and self-management strategies, delivered twice weekly over at least 6 weeks by a multidisciplinary team
- c. An exercise programme delivered twice weekly over at least 6 weeks by physiotherapists
- d. A multicomponent programme comprising exercise, education, behaviour change and self-management strategies, delivered twice weekly over at least 6 weeks by physiotherapists

Q.2 What are the benefits of pulmonary rehabilitation for people with chronic lung disease?
- a. It improves how people feel about their health and symptoms
- b. It improves people's functional exercise capacity
- c. It's cost-effective
- d. All of the above

Q.3 What are some challenges to consider when delivering pulmonary rehabilitation for older people with chronic lung disease?
- a. People who are older have worse outcomes from pulmonary rehabilitation
- b. People with other medical conditions cannot participate in pulmonary rehabilitation
- c. Supporting people to participate alongside symptom burden, comorbidities, frailty, and travel difficulties
- d. Those living with sarcopenia and/or frailty cannot benefit from pulmonary rehabilitation

REFERENCES

Benton, M. J., & Swan, P. D. (2006). Addition of resistance training to pulmonary rehabilitation programs: an evidence-based rationale and guidelines for use of resistance training with elderly patients with COPD. *Cardiopulmonary Physical Therapy Journal, 17*, 127–133.

Blackstock, F. C., & Evans, R. A. (2019). Rehabilitation in lung diseases: 'education' component of pulmonary rehabilitation. *Respirology, 24*, 863–870.

Blindenbach, S., Vrancken, J. W. F. A., Van Der Zeijden, H., Reesink, H. J., Brijker, F., Smalbrugge, M., & Wattel, E. M. (2017). Effects of geriatric COPD rehabilitation on hospital admissions and exercise tolerance: a retrospective observational study. *Tijdschrift voor Gerontologie en Geriatrie, 48*, 112–120.

Bolton, C. E., Bevan-Smith, E. F., Blakey, J. D., Crowe, P., Elkin, S. L., Garrod, R., Walmsley, S., & British Thoracic Society Pulmonary Rehabilitation Guideline Development Group, on behalf of the British Thoracic Society Standards of Care Committee (2013). British Thoracic Society guideline on pulmonary rehabilitation in adults. *Thorax, 68*, ii1–ii30.

British Thoracic Society. (2014). Quality standards for pulmonary rehabilitation in adults. Retrieved from https://www.brit-thoracic.org.uk/quality-improvement/quality-standards/pulmonary-rehabilitation/ (Accessed May 2019).

D'avanzo, B., Shaw, R., Riva, S., Apostolo, J., Bobrowicz-Campos, E., Kurpas, D., Bujnowska-Fedak, M., & Holland, C. (2017). Stakeholders' views and experiences of care and interventions for addressing frailty and pre-frailty: a meta-synthesis of qualitative evidence. *PLoS One, 12*, e0180127.

Griffiths, T. L., Phillips, C. J., Davies, S., Burr, M. L., & Campbell, I. A. (2001). Cost effectiveness of an outpatient multidisciplinary pulmonary rehabilitation programme. *Thorax, 56*, 779–784.

Holley-Moore, G., & Creighton, H. (2015). *The future of transport in an ageing society.* London, UK: International Longevity Centre-UK. Retrieved from https://www.ageuk.org.uk/global-assets/age-uk/documents/reports-and-publications/reports-and-briefings/active-communities/rb_june15_the_future_of_transport_in_an_ageing_society.pdf (Accessed May 2019).

Hunter, L. C., Lee, R. J., Butcher, I., Weir, C. J., Fischbacher, C. M., Mcallister, D., Wild, S. H., Hewitt, N., & Hardie, R. M. (2016). Patient characteristics associated with risk of first hospital admission and readmission for acute exacerbation of chronic obstructive pulmonary disease (COPD) following primary care COPD diagnosis: a cohort study using linked electronic patient records. *BMJ Open, 6*, e009121.

Jones, R., Muyinda, H., Nyakoojo, G., Kirenga, B., Katagira, W., & Pooler, J. (2018). Does pulmonary rehabilitation alter patients' experiences of living with chronic respiratory disease? A qualitative study. *International Journal of Chronic Obstructive Pulmonary Disease, 13*, 2375–2385.

Jones, S. E., Maddocks, M., Kon, S. S. C., Canavan, J. L., Nolan, C. M., Clark, A. L., Polkey, M. I., & Man, W. D. C. (2015). Sarcopenia in COPD: prevalence, clinical correlates and response to pulmonary rehabilitation. *Thorax, 70*, 213.

Keating, A., Lee, A., & Holland, A. E. (2011). What prevents people with chronic obstructive pulmonary disease from attending pulmonary rehabilitation? A systematic review. *Chronic Respiratory Disease, 8*, 89–99.

Maddocks, M., Kon, S. S., Canavan, J. L., Jones, S. E., Nolan, C. M., Labey, A., Polkey, M. I., & Man, W. D. (2016). Physical frailty and pulmonary rehabilitation in COPD: a prospective cohort study. *Thorax, 71*, 988–995.

McCarthy, B., Casey, D., Devane, D., Murphy, K., Murphy, E., & Lacasse, Y. (2015). Pulmonary rehabilitation for chronic obstructive pulmonary disease. *Cochrane Database of Systematic Reviews, 2*, CD003793.

Mittal, N., Raj, R., Islam, E., & Nugent, K. (2015). Pulmonary rehabilitation improves frailty and gait speed in some ambulatory patients with chronic lung diseases. *The Southwest Respiratory and Critical Care Chronicals, 3*, 2–10.

Montserrat-Capdevila, J., Godoy, P., Marsal, J. R., Barbé, F., & Galván, L. (2015). Risk of exacerbation in chronic obstructive pulmonary disease: a primary care retrospective cohort study. *BMC Family Practice, 16*, 173.

Naz, I., Sahin, H., Varol, Y., & Kömürcüoğlu, B. (2018). The effect of comorbidity severity on pulmonary rehabilitation outcomes in chronic obstructive pulmonary disease patients. *Chronic Respiratory Disease, 16*, 1479972318809472.

Puhan, M. A., Gimeno-Santos, E., Cates, C. J., & Troosters, T. (2016). Pulmonary rehabilitation following exacerbations of chronic obstructive pulmonary disease. *Cochrane Database of Systematic Reviews, 12*, CD005305.

Roberts, N. J., Ghiassi, R., & Partridge, M. R. (2008). Health literacy in COPD. *International Journal of Chronic Obstructive Pulmonary Disease, 3*, 499–507.

Roig, M., Eng, J. J., MacIntyre, D. L., Road, J. D., Fitzgerald, J. M., Burns, J., & Reid, W. D. (2011). Falls in people with chronic obstructive pulmonary disease: an observational cohort study. *Respiratory Medicine, 105*, 461–469.

Sohanpal, R., Steed, L., Mars, T., & Taylor, S. J. (2015). Understanding patient participation behaviour in studies of COPD support programmes such as pulmonary rehabilitation and self-management: a qualitative synthesis with application of theory. *NPJ Primary Care Respiratory Medicine, 25*, 15054.

Spruit, M. A., Pitta, F., Garvey, C., Zuwallack, R. L., Roberts, C. M., Collins, E. G., & Wouters, E. F. M. (2014). Differences in content and organisational aspects of pulmonary rehabilitation programmes. *European Respiratory Journal, 43*, 1326.

Spruit, M. A., Singh, S. J., Garvey, C., Zuwallack, R., Nici, L., Rochester, C., & Wouters, E. F. (2013). An official American Thoracic Society/European Respiratory Society statement: key concepts and advances in pulmonary rehabilitation. *American Journal of Respiratory and Critical Care Medicine, 188*, e13–e64.

Spruit, M. A., & Wouters, E. F. M. (2019). Organizational aspects of pulmonary rehabilitation in chronic respiratory diseases. *Respirology, 24*, 838–843.

Steiner, M., Mcmillan, V., Lowe, D., Holzhauer-Barrie, J., Mortier, K., Riordan, J., & Roberts, C. (2017). *Pulmonary rehabilitation: an exercise in improvement. National Chronic Obstructive Pulmonary Disease (COPD) Audit Programme: clinical and organisational audits of pulmonary rehabilitation services in England and Wales.* London: Royal College of Physicians.

Steiner, M. C., & Roberts, C. M. (2016). Pulmonary rehabilitation: the next steps. *The Lancet Respiratory Medicine, 4*, 172–173.

Stone, R. A., Lowe, D., Potter, J. M., Buckingham, R. J., Roberts, C. M., & Pursey, N. J. (2012). Managing patients with COPD exacerbation: does age matter? *Age and Ageing, 41*, 461–468.

Takigawa, N., Tada, A., Soda, R., Takahashi, S., Kawata, N., Shibayama, T., & Takahashi, K. (2007). Comprehensive pulmonary rehabilitation according to severity of COPD. *Respiratory Medicine, 101*, 326–332.

Yohannes, A. M., Chen, W., Moga, A. M., Leroi, I., & Connolly, M. J. (2017). Cognitive impairment in chronic obstructive pulmonary disease and chronic heart failure: a systematic review and meta-analysis of observational studies. *Journal of the American Medical Directors Association, 18*, 451e1–451e11.

Yohannes, A. M., & Connolly, M. J. (2004). Pulmonary rehabilitation programmes in the UK: a national representative survey. *Clinical Rehabilitation, 18*, 444–449.

Zoumot, Z., Jordan, S., & Hopkinson, N. S. (2014). Emphysema: time to say farewell to therapeutic nihilism. *Thorax, 69*, 973.

59

Trauma in Older People

George Peck & Meenakshi Nayar

LEARNING OBJECTIVES

- Describe the changing patterns of trauma in older people
- List factors that contribute towards increased mortality in older trauma patients
- Describe the most common body injuries in older people
- Describe elements of rehabilitating the older person with polytrauma that are challenging

---

CASE

Zuzanna is an 83-year-old lady who presents to the emergency department (ED) as a 'major trauma call' having fallen down 10 stairs at home. She is on anticoagulation (blood thinner medication) for atrial fibrillation (irregular heartbeat) and has chronic obstructive pulmonary disease (COPD). The following injuries are identified on admission:
- Right-sided rib fractures from 3rd to 7th
- Large right-sided pneumothorax
- Grade II liver laceration
- Right non-displaced superior pubic ramus fracture
- Left fractured clavicle
- Small left-sided subdural haemorrhage

She is usually independently mobile and is keen to get home as soon as possible.

INTRODUCTION

In the last two decades, the rising average age of populations in developed societies has led to significant shifts in the patterns of trauma admissions. The incidence of traumatic injury in older people has risen in absolute numbers and as a percentage of national trauma admissions.

Seriously injured adults are described as having suffered from 'major trauma'. This is measured on a scale known as the Injury Severity Score (ISS) which scores injuries from 1 to 75, the latter being the most serious. Patients who have an ISS > 15 are defined as having suffered from major trauma. Centralisation of trauma management has been shown to improve outcomes internationally. In England, patients with major trauma are now 20% more likely to survive their injuries since the implementation of regional trauma networks in 2012. Ambulance services now transfer patients with suspected major trauma directly to regional major trauma centres where multispeciality services can cater for the immediate management of severe injuries across multiple body sites. Trauma units provide support for large numbers of less severely injured patients and can transfer patients to major trauma centres if necessary.

In 2017, more than 50% of all Trauma Audit and Research Network (TARN) eligible patients (those with major traumatic injuries) were 60 years of age or older (TARN, 2017). Major trauma was once dominated by young or middle-aged patients involved in traffic collisions, but now low-level falls (<2 m) are the most common mechanisms of injury, with most injuries occurring in a person's own home (Kehoe et al., 2015).

TRAUMA OUTCOMES IN OLDER PEOPLE

Older people are more likely to die from trauma than younger people who sustain similar mechanisms and severity of injury. Many factors are thought to contribute towards this (see Fig. 59.1):
- Frailty is an independent risk factor for death or complications in older trauma (Khan et al., 2019). Mortality is five times higher in older trauma patients who are moderately frail or above compared to non-frail patients (Cheung et al., 2017) (see Chapter 4 Frailty).
- Seemingly trivial mechanisms can cause significant injury in older patients but may not trigger on pre-hospital or ED trauma triage protocols resulting in delayed imaging, missed injuries and admission under inappropriate care pathways which can have effects on outcome.
- Pre-existing high blood pressure and the use of certain medications, such as beta-blockers, can mask the normal physiological responses to bleeding or shock making the diagnosis of serious injury more challenging. This also contributes towards under-triage.
- Many older patients are prescribed anticoagulants which predispose to greater bleeding tendency after trauma. Polypharmacy is also known to be associated with increased mortality.
- Comorbidities (medical conditions) can be exacerbated during admission, and in-hospital complications such as cardiovascular events or pneumonia are much more common in older patients affecting more than a third of trauma admissions (Sammy et al., 2016).

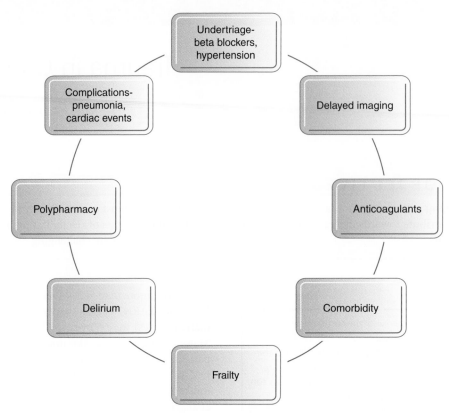

FIG. 59.1 Multiple factors contributing towards increased mortality in older patients with trauma.

- Delirium is common in older trauma patients and is associated with increased in-hospital morbidity, complications and length of stay. This can also impact on engagement with early therapy input with resultant effects on deconditioning.

Older people are less likely to make a good functional recovery after major trauma than younger people. Pre-existing frailty contributes towards this and is associated with increased length of hospital stay, discharge to a rehabilitation or nursing facility and lower health status at one year after injury (de Munter et al., 2019; Joseph et al., 2016; Maxwell et al., 2016). Delirium can persist for days to weeks after injury, and it is important that older patients are afforded enough time to reveal their rehabilitation potential. Many older patients benefit greatly from specialist rehabilitation services and make significant recoveries. For those that survive major trauma the majority express positive opinions about surviving their injuries and their quality of life even in the presence of functional impairment (Koizia et al., 2019).

There is growing recognition internationally that trauma systems must adapt their practices to provide the best care for older trauma patients. In the UK, new financial measures (tariffs) were instituted by the National Trauma Network aiming to incentivise increased geriatrician input to major trauma centres in England. Similarly, trauma triage protocols and bespoke guidelines for older patients, such as the 2018 London Major Trauma System Elderly Major

Trauma Guidelines (Centre for Trauma Sciences, 2018), are available to help optimise care.

MANAGEMENT OF POLYTRAUMA

The head is the most common body site injured in older adult trauma, occurring in approximately 85% of patients. Blunt chest injury occurs in up to 25% of patients; rib fractures, pneumothorax, haemothorax and pulmonary contusion being the most common injuries. Spinal, pelvic, limb and abdominal injuries each occur in <10% of patients (see Fig. 59.2).

Brain injuries, limb injuries and spinal injuries are discussed in other chapters so here we focus on blunt chest trauma and abdominal injuries.

Blunt Chest Trauma
Rib Fractures

Rib fractures are the commonest blunt chest injury in older patients. They can occur after seemingly trivial falls and up to 50% are missed on plain x-rays. They can be extremely painful causing impaired coughing, impaired deep breathing and voluntary splinting. Consequently, pneumonia is a common complication.

Often several ribs in the same region are broken at the same time. If three or more contiguous ribs are broken at

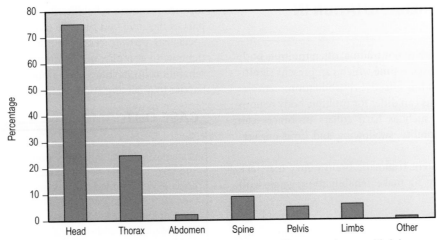

FIG. 59.2 Prevalence of body area injured in patients ≥60 years of age with injury severity score >15. (From TARN, 2017, with permission.)

two different places, this can result in what is known as a flail segment. This can cause paradoxical chest wall movement with inspiration which impedes effective respiration. Patients with significant chest wall deformities can be considered for surgical fixation to restore effective chest wall movement (Swart et al., 2017). Significantly displaced sternal fractures may also benefit from surgical fixation.

The most crucial element in the early rehabilitation of rib fractures is to provide adequate pain relief to facilitate deep breathing and coughing and thus to prevent complications such as pneumonia and respiratory failure. This also allows patients to move more freely around the bed and engage in physiotherapy as well as minimising deconditioning. Most trauma units have dedicated rib fracture pathways to guide management. Effective analgesia (pain control) can be achieved through a variety of methods:

- Non-invasive analgesia:
  o Oral morphine or oxycodone
  o Intravenous patient-controlled analgesia (PCA)
- Invasive analgesia:
  o Paraspinal blocks
  o Serratus anterior blocks
  o Erector spinae blocks
  o Epidural analgesia

In patients with severe pain, prompt escalation to invasive analgesia is crucial. Epidurals can provide excellent analgesia, but vigilance is required for side effects such as hypotension. Lying and standing blood pressures should be monitored when patients begin to mobilise.

Regular deep breathing exercises have been shown to prevent atelectasis (lung tissue collapse) and pneumonia in some older surgical populations although evidence for benefit in trauma is lacking. Some patients can be taught how to use incentive spirometer devices, and vital capacity or peak expiratory flow measurement can also be useful to monitor for deterioration or response to treatment (Brown & Walters, 2012). Some centres use devices that provide positive airway pressure to help keep the lungs open, assist in airway recruitment and

prevent atelectasis, although further studies are required to confirm meaningful benefit (Udekwu et al., 2017).

Pneumothorax and Haemothorax

Pneumothorax (air within the pleural cavity) and haemothorax (blood within the pleural cavity) commonly accompany rib fractures. Some small pneumothoraces can be managed conservatively, but often pneumothorax or haemothorax will require chest drain insertion to allow the lung to re-expand and blood or fluid to drain effectively. Early mobilisation is usually still possible, but chest drain tubing and bottles must be kept below the level of the chest to allow effective drainage and lung re-expansion. These are typically removed after the lung has re-expanded or any effusion/haemothorax has been drained.

Pulmonary Contusion

Approximately 19% of older patients with blunt chest trauma have pulmonary contusion. This is characterised by injury to the lung tissue itself, similar to bruising. Haemorrhage and swelling of the lung tissue can cause collapse and consolidation of the lung segment. Pulmonary contusions can worsen after admission and are associated with higher rates of complications and mortality (Bader et al., 2018).

Abdominal Trauma

Abdominal trauma accounts for <5% of older major traumatic injuries. Blunt abdominal trauma most commonly affects the liver and spleen, with diaphragmatic rupture, mesenteric and renal injuries less common.

Liver and spleen injuries are graded I–V according to severity, and patients with active bleeding or haemodynamic instability may require urgent surgical or radiological intervention (Stassen et al., 2012). Most injuries are however managed conservatively with observation. Repeat imaging may be required after 24–48 hours. During this time modest mobilisation with careful monitoring should still be encouraged to prevent deconditioning and atelectasis.

KEY ASPECTS OF REHABILITATION IN POLYTRAUMA

As one would expect with major trauma, often multiple body sites are affected at the same time which can present significant challenges in providing effective rehabilitation:

- Weight-bearing status can differ for multiple body regions
- Spinal precautions such as hard collars or braces can impede balance, mobility, swallowing and limit engagement with therapy
- Patients with coexistent traumatic brain injury may lack the cognitive ability to make rehabilitation gains with other injuries
- Delirium is common

In the early stages of admission, the prevention of in-hospital medical problems (e.g. pneumonia) and deconditioning are crucial whilst the immediate management of different injuries is clarified and actioned. Individualised rehabilitation should be initiated as soon as possible and, once patients no longer require specialist care at a major trauma centre, prompt repatriation back to their local trauma unit allows recovery closer to home with easier access to local rehabilitation facilities and social services.

The British Society for Rehabilitation Medicine guidelines (2013) recommend that all patients with major traumatic injuries receive a rehabilitation prescription and this forms part of national best practice tariffs in the UK. Rehabilitation specialists provide crucial input to trauma centres, and patients with complex needs often require referral to specialist rehabilitation facilities. Age alone should never be seen as a barrier to accessing appropriate rehabilitation.

CASE OUTCOME

Zuzanna had a chest drain inserted on admission for her pneumothorax, and her anticoagulation was reversed immediately. The pain from her rib fractures was severe, and a thoracic epidural was inserted to allow pain-free deep respiration. Her liver contusion, pelvic fracture and clavicle fracture were managed non-operatively. The orthopaedic team allowed her to fully weight-bear on her pelvis, and she was given a collar and cuff for her clavicle fracture. She was able to transfer to a chair with assistance on day 2 of her admission. She had mild delirium which was proactively managed. On day 3 her pneumothorax had resolved and her chest drain was removed. By day 4 she was able to take a few steps with assistance. On day 6 her epidural was removed, and she was converted to oral painkillers. She progressed well with physiotherapy and was discharged home on day 10 with a re-ablement care package and community physiotherapy. The cause of her fall was fully investigated while she was an inpatient and anti-coagulation was recommenced on discharge.

SUMMARY POINTS

- Polytrauma in older people is increasing
- Mortality is higher in older compared to younger people despite similar mechanisms and severity of injury
- Effective pain relief in the early stages of injury is crucial to encourage prompt mobilisation and prevent in-hospital medical problems
- Rehabilitation in polytrauma can be complex but should be initiated as soon as possible
- Older people with polytrauma and delirium may require a longer time for recovery before a decision about rehabilitation potential is made

MCQs

Q.1 The most common site of injury in older adult major trauma is:
- a. Spine
- b. Chest
- c. Head
- d. Abdomen

Q.2 The most common mechanism of injury in older adult major trauma is:
- a. Road traffic collision
- b. Fall >2 m
- c. Self-inflicted injury
- d. Fall <2 m

REFERENCES

Bader, A., Rahman, U., Morris, M., McCormack, J. E., Huang, E. C., Zawin, M., Vosswinkel, J. A., & Jawa, R. S. (2018). Pulmonary contusions in the elderly after blunt trauma: incidence and outcomes. *Journal of Surgical Research, 230,* 110–116.

British Society for Rehabilitation Medicine. (2013). Specialist rehabilitation in the trauma pathway: BSRM core standards Version 1.4 – October 2013. Retrieved from https://www.bsrm.org.uk/publications/publications (Accessed 25 April 2019).

Brown, S. D., & Walters, M. R. (2012). Patients with rib fractures: use of incentive spirometry volumes to guide care. *Journal of Trauma Nursing, 19*(2), 89–91. quiz 92-3.

Centre for Trauma Sciences; London Major Trauma System – Management of elderly major trauma patients – second edition (2018). Retrieved from http://www.c4ts.qmul.ac.uk/downloads/london-major-trauma-system-elderly-trauma-guidancesecond-editiondecember-2018.pdf (Accessed 25 April 2019).

Cheung, A., Haas, B., Ringer, T. J., McFarlan, A., & Wong, C. L. (2017). Canadian Study of Health and Aging Clinical Frailty Scale: does it predict adverse outcomes among geriatric trauma patients? *Journal of the American College of Surgeons, 225*(5), 658–665.

de Munter, L., Polinder, S., van de Ree, C. L. P., Kruithof, N., Lansink, K. W. W., Steyerberg, E. W., & de Jongh, M. A. C. (2019). Predicting health status in the first year after trauma. *British Journal of Surgery, 106*(6), 701–710.

Joseph, B., Phelan, H., Hassan, A., Orouji Jokar, T., O'Keeffe, T., Azim, A., …, & Rhee, P. (2016). The impact of frailty on failure-to-rescue in geriatric trauma patients. *Journal of Trauma and Acute Care Surgery, 81*, 1150–1155.

Kehoe, A., Smith, J. E., Edwards, A., Yates, D., & Lecky, F. (2015). The changing face of major trauma in the UK. *Emergency Medicine Journal, 32*(12), 911–915.

Khan, M., Jehan, F., Zeeshan, M., Kulvatunyou, N., Fain, M. J., Saljuqi, A. T., O'Keeffe, T., & Joseph, B. (2019). Failure to rescue after emergency general surgery in geriatric patients: does frailty matter? *The Journal of Surgical Research, 233*, 397–402.

Koizia, L., Kings, R., Koizia, A., Peck, G., Wilson, M., Hettiaratchy, S., & Fertleman, M. B. (2019). Major trauma in the elderly: frailty decline and patient experience after injury. *Trauma, 21*(1), 21–26.

Maxwell, C. A., Mion, L. C., Mukherjee, K., Dietrich, M. S., Minnick, A., May, A., & Miller, R. S. (2016). Preinjury physical frailty and cognitive impairment among geriatric trauma patients determine postinjury functional recovery and survival. *Journal of Trauma and Acute Care Surgery, 80*(2), 195–203.

Sammy, I., Lecky, F., Sutton, A., Leaviss, J., & O'Cathain, A. (2016). Factors affecting mortality in older trauma patients-a systematic review and meta-analysis. *Injury, 47*(6), 1170–1183.

Stassen, N. A., Bhullar, I., Cheng, J. D., Crandall, M., Friese, R., Guillamondegui, O., …, & Kerwin, A. (2012). Nonoperative management of blunt hepatic injury: an Eastern Association for the Surgery of Trauma practice management guideline. *Journal of Trauma and Acute Care Surgery, 73*(5 suppl 4), S288–S293.

Swart, E., Laratta, J., Slobogean, G., & Mehta, S. (2017). Operative treatment of rib fractures in flail chest injuries: a meta-analysis and cost-effectiveness analysis. *Journal of Orthopaedic Trauma, 31*(2), 64–70.

TARN (Trauma Audit and Research Network). (2017). Major trauma in older people. Retrieved from www.tarn.ac.uk/content/downloads/3793/Major%20Trauma%20in%20Older%20People%202017.pdf (Accessed 25 April 2019).

Udekwu, P., Patel, S., Farrell, M., & Vincent, R. (2017). Favorable outcomes in blunt chest injury with noninvasive bi-level positive airway pressure ventilation. *The American Surgeon, 83*(7), 687–695.

60

Traumatic Brain Injury

Aine Carroll

LEARNING OBJECTIVES

- Describe the commonest causes of traumatic brain injury (TBI) in older people
- Explain the difference between primary and secondary brain injury
- Describe predictors of poor outcomes in patients with TBI
- Describe the different models of post-TBI rehabilitation

CASE

Patrick, an 83-year-old man, tripped on his dog while bringing his wife breakfast in bed upstairs which was his usual routine after taking his anticoagulant (blood thinner medication) for atrial fibrillation (irregular heartbeat). He banged his head and although initially alert, gradually became drowsy and lost consciousness. He was taken by ambulance to the local emergency department (ED) where his Glasgow Coma Scale (GCS) was 7 (indicating a low level of consciousness). A CT scan of his brain revealed an acute subdural haematoma (bleed into the lining of his brain), and he was transferred to the neurosurgical unit for surgery to remove the blood (evacuation). He was transferred back to the initial hospital and referred to local rehabilitation services.

INTRODUCTION

According to the World Health Organization, traumatic brain injury (TBI) will be the commonest cause of death and disability by the year 2020. It is estimated that 10 million people are affected annually by TBI (Hyder et al., 2007). TBI is defined as 'An alteration in brain function, or other evidence of brain pathology, caused by an external force' (Menon et al., 2010). Sometimes referred to as a silent epidemic (Centers for Disease Control and Prevention, 1999), there is an often neglected subgroup: older adults with TBI. Problems resulting from TBI are often not immediately visible, and patients with TBI and their families tend not to be very vocal. The term 'silent' further reflects the common underestimation of the actual incidence and that society is often unaware of the impact of TBI (Koskinen & Alaranta, 2008; Prince et al., 2015).

CAUSES

Falls are the leading cause of TBI for older adults (51%), and motor vehicle crashes (MVCs) (pedestrian or driver/passenger) are second (9%). Assaults account for 1%, and all other known causes account for 17%, although more than 21% of TBIs in older adults are from unknown causes (Thompson, McCormick, & Kagan, 2006).

The differences in mechanisms of injury compared to younger people are thought to be due to age-related brain atrophy (shrinkage), the presence of other medical conditions, greater use of anticoagulants for other medical problems and reduced free radical clearance (Borkar et al., 2011; Harvey & Close, 2012; Susman et al., 2002; Thompson et al., 2006).

This is likely to have significant impacts on present and future acute hospital and rehabilitation resources (Court-Brown & Clement, 2009). It has been shown that the majority of older people with TBI can be rehabilitated successfully and discharged home, where they may even resume employment and driving (Dijkers et al., 2013).

MECHANISM OF INJURY

Primary injury consists of the initial damage directly resulting from the mechanical forces affecting the cerebral tissues. Secondary injury refers to the cascade of cellular and molecular processes initiated by the primary injury. In addition, secondary injury can also be the result of damage to the brain due to low blood sugar, low blood pressure or low oxygen levels and raised intracranial pressure resulting in cerebral ischaemia (lack of blood supply). Depending on the mechanism of injury, brain damage can be localised (for example, a collection of blood within the brain) or more generalised (for example, swelling of the whole brain).

The commonest type of problem in older patients is an acute subdural hematoma (ASDH), where a clot of blood develops between the surface of the brain and the dura mater, the brain's tough outer covering. These are reported to be 4 times larger in older people and produce twice the mass effect (the blood causes surrounding areas of brain tissue to be compressed and injured), compared with younger patients (Howard et al., 1989).

MANAGEMENT OF TRAUMATIC BRAIN INJURY

The management of TBI has become much more standardised and evidence based since the publication of international and national guidelines covering many aspects of care. There is good evidence to show the survival benefits of patients with severe head injury being treated in a neurosurgical centre, and there is a strong case to be made for transferring and treating all patients with severe head injury in a 24-hour neurosurgical centre setting. Trauma systems describing a whole organisation of trauma care as a continuum from prevention to rehabilitation and community reintegration have been shown to improve access to care and reduce length of stay and have demonstrated significant improvements in quality and processes of care. However, many countries struggle to implement such systems due to human and technical resource issues.

OUTCOME FOLLOWING TRAUMATIC BRAIN INJURY

The relationship between acute structural damage demonstrated on brain imaging and severity of impairment/disability is weak. Glasgow Coma Scale (GCS) scores on admission (Teasdale & Jennett, 1974), length of coma or post-traumatic amnesia (PTA) are commonly used measures of survival and/or severity but are only weakly related to long-term patient outcome. Some patients initially classified as 'severe' will make a complete and rapid recovery, while others initially classified as 'mild' may have enduring neuropsychiatric sequelae that

may have a catastrophic effect on family relationships and societal participation. The Full Outline of UnResponsiveness (FOUR) score is a relatively new score which has yet to be used widely but showed early promise as it can be rated in intubated patients (Sadaka, Patel, & Lakshmanan, 2012).

CONSEQUENCES OF TRAUMATIC BRAIN INJURY

The consequences of TBI are many and varied but mainly depend on the nature and location of the injury. As can be seen from Table 60.1, the wide-ranging deficits following TBI can have a devastating impact on an individual's biopsychosocial functioning. These problems not only affect the individual themselves but also the immediate family, the extended family, friends, colleagues, etc.

HOW DOES RECOVERY HAPPEN AFTER TRAUMATIC BRAIN INJURY?

It is generally accepted that acquired brain injuries initiate a cascade of regenerative events that last for at least several weeks, if not months. Initial recovery (first 3–6 months) happens as the brain swelling decreases and blood flow and brain chemistry improve. In later recovery, a second mechanism is neural plasticity or relearning (Chen, Epstein, & Stern, 2010; Nudo, 2011; Overman & Carmichael, 2014). Experimental evidence indicates that relearning can be helped through several external conditions, including medication, electrical stimulation and environmental stimulation (Turolla et al., 2018).

TABLE 60.1   Consequences of traumatic brain injury.

PHYSICAL	COMMUNICATION	COGNITIVE	BEHAVIOURAL/EMOTIONAL	LIFESTYLE
Motor deficits	**Language deficits**	**Impairment of:**	**Emotional lability**	**Unemployment/ financial hardship**
Paralysis	Expression	Memory	Poor initiation	Loss of pre-injury roles; loss of independence and purpose
Alterations in muscle tone	Reception	Attention	Mood change	Lack of transportation alternatives and social isolation
Ataxia/incoordination	Dysarthria	Perception	Adjustment problems	Inadequate recreational opportunities
Sensory deficits	Dyslexia	Problem-solving	Aggressive outbursts	Difficulties in maintaining interpersonal relationships and marital breakdown
Visual/auditory impairment	Dysgraphia	Insight	Disinhibition	
Dysphagia		Safety awareness	Inappropriate sexual behaviour	
Epilepsy		Self-monitoring	Poor motivation	
Others: headache, fatigue, pain, etc.		Social judgement	Psychosis	
			Other neuropsychiatric issues	

Adapted from Turner-Stokes, L. (Ed.). (2003). *Rehabilitation following acquired brain injury: national clinical guidelines*. Royal College of Physicians.

Patients recover after TBI in two different, but related, ways:

a) A reduction in the extent of neurological impairment which results from spontaneous neurological recovery.

b) Improved ability to perform daily functions within the limitations of their physical impairments. The ability to perform these tasks can improve through adaptation and training in the presence or absence of natural neurological recovery. This is thought to be the element of recovery on which rehabilitation exerts the greatest effect.

More research is required to encourage more clinicians, rehabilitation engineers and neuroscientists to work together to further dissect the neural mechanisms underscoring functional recovery after acquired brain injuries and translate these findings into novel therapies (Turolla et al., 2018).

REHABILITATION

There is now strong evidence to show that rehabilitation in specialist settings for people with traumatic brain or spinal cord injury and stroke is effective and provides value for money in terms of reducing length of stay in hospital and reducing the costs of long-term care (Turner-Stokes, 2005, 2008; Turner-Stokes et al., 2005). Early transfer to specialist centres and more intense rehabilitation programmes are cost effective, the latter particularly in the small group of people who have high care costs due to very severe brain injury. Clinical and cost-benefits are similar for people with severe behavioural problems following brain injury (Duarte et al., 2018; Oddy & da Silva Ramos, 2013; Worthington et al., 2006). Continued coordinated multidisciplinary rehabilitation in the community improves long-term outcomes and can help to reduce hospital re-admissions.

There is also consensus on how effective rehabilitation should be delivered (Turner-Stokes, 2003). However, most of this evidence is in relation to younger adults and not older people. As neurological recovery following TBI occurs over an extended period, it is fundamental that different patients need different input at the various stages of the rehabilitation process.

An essential feature of this model is the need for smooth transition between services. This necessitates excellent communication and sharing of information between services so that patients experience a seamless continuum of care.

The important challenge is to make sure that each patient can access the right service by the right team at the right time.

MAIN STAGES OF REHABILITATION

The following are adapted from the British Society of Rehabilitation Medicine (BSRM) Core Standards for Specialist Rehabilitation, October 2014.

Hyperacute/Acute Rehabilitation

Rehabilitation should start as soon as possible, including during the acute stages of intensive care in hospital. Interventions at this stage focus on reducing impairment and preventing secondary complications, such as contractures, malnutrition, pressure sores, pneumonia, etc., and managing any acute behavioural complications.

Such rehabilitation needs multidisciplinary input from a comprehensive medically led rehabilitation team on the neurosciences/trauma system site.

Subacute Rehabilitation

As the patient starts to recover, a period of intensive inpatient rehabilitation may be required to enable a successful transition from hospital to home or community. Subacute or post-acute rehabilitation primarily addresses regaining mobility and independence in self-care to allow the individual to manage safely at home. Interventions at this stage focus on improving activity and independence, i.e. reducing activity limitation.

Post-acute rehabilitation requires direct transfer from the neurosciences centre to an appropriate post-acute neurorehabilitation service that meets the criteria for such a service. Specialist rehabilitation is the total active care of patients with a complex, disabling condition by a multiprofessional team who have undergone recognised specialist training in rehabilitation, led or supported by a consultant trained and accredited in rehabilitation medicine.

Ambulatory Outpatient Specialist Rehabilitation

Ambulatory care services allow continuation of structured rehabilitation programmes following in-patient treatment in acute or sub-acute health facilities. An outpatient specialist rehabilitation programme can facilitate earlier transition of care or discharge from inpatient settings. These services can also avoid hospitalisation. Early Supported Discharge stroke rehabilitation programmes are an example of ambulatory care.

Community Rehabilitation

Community-based specialist rehabilitation teams provide interdisciplinary rehabilitation, ideally with a case management approach, and therapy support to patients with stable complex needs usually after single incident neurological conditions, usually in an outpatient or home setting. The interdisciplinary team case manages, and coordinates multiagency referral and ongoing care, often on a life-long basis. This phase of rehabilitation concentrates on extended activities of daily living, social integration and return to work or education. Interventions focus on enhanced participation, improved quality of life, psychological adjustment and carer stress (Turner-Stokes, 2003).

ONGOING CARE FOR HIGHLY DEPENDENT PATIENTS

A growing number of patients are surviving severe TBIs with complex disabilities and high care requirements. Some may have ventilatory support requirements or disorders of consciousness. These individuals will require 24-hour care and ideally should be engaged in 'slow-stream' multi- or interdisciplinary rehabilitation over a period of many years to facilitate their optimal recovery.

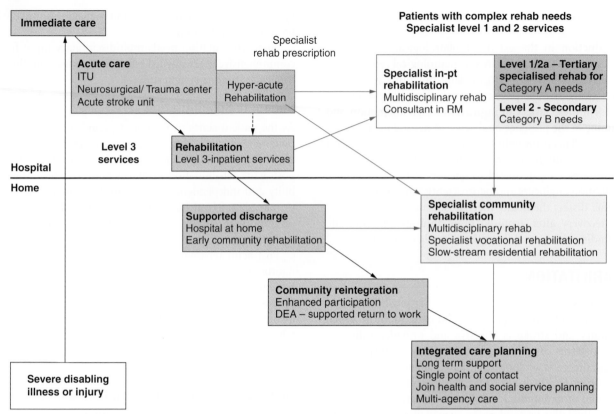

FIG. 60.1 Pathway for patients with severe disabling illness or injury. (Adapted from British Society of Rehabilitation Medicine (2013). *Specialist Rehabilitation in the Trauma Pathway: BSRM Core Standards.*)

Whilst the pathway described in Fig. 60.1 provides a useful illustration of the need for different services at different stages, with seamless continuity of care, the real-world picture is often much more complex. Patients progress through the different stages at different rates. Patients with a mild TBI who do not require acute hospital admission may transition straight to services in the community. A small minority with very severe injury, complex disability and perhaps disorder of consciousness may spend many months in hospital and require long-term care. Individuals with brain injury may also need to re-access services at different points in time as their needs change over time. Within each stage a range of different service providers are involved, who must coordinate their interventions, and these services may change their input depending on the stage of rehabilitation (Turner-Stokes, 2003).

Ideally, there will be a range of community rehabilitation options available, including home-based rehabilitation, outpatient rehabilitation programmes, community re-entry programmes, comprehensive day treatment programmes, residential community reintegration programmes and neurobehavioural programmes. They may also include supported living programmes, independent living centres and vocational rehabilitation (Turner-Stokes, 2003).

CURRENT SITUATION

There are often no clear pathways of care for TBI for all age groups. This results in patients with TBI who do not require neurosurgical intervention often being admitted under the care of surgeons with little or no training or experience of managing the medical complications of TBI or the complex disabilities associated with them.

Recent research by Dijkers et al. suggests the selection process for rehabilitation may be biased towards not admitting frail older patients with severe TBI (Dijkers et al., 2013).

Traditional medical rehabilitation environments often do not foster partnerships with persons with TBI or their families and carers. The importance of appreciating long-term family needs and other quality of life issues should not be underestimated.

MANAGED CLINICAL REHABILITATION NETWORKS

Clinical networks are more commonly being viewed as an important strategy for increasing evidence-based practice and improving models of care. Managed clinical networks (MCNs) facilitate re-design, quality improvement, strategy and planning across pathways. Teams work across department boundaries, teams, units and divisions and achieve their results through consensus and collaboration by enabling clinicians with differing levels of expertise, patients and service managers to work together to deliver safe, effective and person-centred care.

The essential components of MCNs are:

- Excellent clinical governance and quality assurance structures
- Excellent relationships and communication between all key stakeholders

- Distributed leadership
- Multidisciplinary approach and participation of all players
- Education and training for staff and service users
- Continuing Professional Development for staff
- Research & development
- Demonstration of value for money.

Although well established in some countries such as Scotland, this approach is emerging in a number of different countries as a preferred approach to the planning, design and provision of services that can work in parallel with a trauma system to improved processes and efficiency and improve quality, experience and outcomes.

CONCLUSION

TBI is a frequent but diverse condition that can impact on all aspects of life. With the ageing population and the increase in the rate of TBI in acute care as people age, prevention strategies targeted at the older adult population are vital.

Decreasing the burden of injuries is among the main challenges for public health in this century, and health and care services need to prepare for an increasing number of older adults with the sequelae of TBI. All clinicians providing services to patients with TBI should have competencies in screening, diagnosing and managing these potentially life-long conditions. Like younger people, older people with TBI can be rehabilitated successfully, and discharged back to the community. Clear pathways of care within a trauma system are required to optimise resource utilisation and outcome and any trauma system should have pathways based on the needs and not the age of patients.

CASE CONCLUSION

Patrick had emergency evacuation of his ASDH followed by specialist rehabilitation. He made an excellent recovery and after 6 months was able to resume his breakfast in bed rituals.

SUMMARY POINTS

- TBI is common and impacts on many aspects of a person's life
- Relearning (neural plasticity) accounts for some of the recovery after TBI and this can be facilitated by timely and appropriate rehabilitation
- Rehabilitation reduces activity limitation and improves participation
- The majority of rehabilitation services for older persons with TBI fall short of international recommendations
- There is a need for investment to provide adequate resources for the design and implementation of appropriate care pathways for all patients with TBI

MCQs

Q.1 The commonest cause of traumatic brain injury (TBI) in older people is:
   a. Road traffic collision
   b. Sports
   c. Assault
   d. Falls
   e. Industrial accidents

Q.2 The most common type of injury in TBI in older people is:
   a. Epidural haematomas
   b. Parenchymal contusions
   c. Traumatic axonal injury

   d. Acute subdural haematoma
   e. Diffuse cerebral oedema

Q.3 Essential components of a managed clinical network include
   a. Excellent clinical governance and quality assurance structures
   b. Excellent relationships and communication between all key stakeholders
   c. Multidisciplinary approach and participation of all players
   d. Education and training for staff and service users
   e. All of the above

REFERENCES

Borkar, S. A., Sinha, S., Agrawal, D., Satyarthee, G. D., Gupta, D., & Mahapatra, A. K. (2011). Severe head injury in the elderly: risk factor assessment and outcome analysis in a series of 100 consecutive patients at a Level 1 trauma centre. *The Indian Journal of Neurotrauma, 8*, 77–82.

British Society of Rehabilitation Medicine (2013). *Specialist rehabilitation in the trauma pathway: BSRM core standards.*

Chen, H., Epstein, J., & Stern, E. (2010). Neural plasticity after acquired brain injury: evidence from functional neuroimaging. *PM&R, 2*, S306–S312.

Centers for Disease Control and Prevention. (1999). *Traumatic brain injury in the United States: a report to Congress.* Atlanta, GA: US Department of Health and Human Services.

Court-Brown, C. M., & Clement, N. (2009). Four score years and ten. An analysis of the epidemiology of fractures in the very elderly. *Injury, 40,* 1111–1114.

Dijkers, M., Brandstater, M., Horn, S., Ryser, D., & Barrett, R. (2013). Inpatient rehabilitation for traumatic brain injury: the influence of age on treatments and outcomes. *NeuroRehabilitation, 32,* 233–252.

Duarte, A., Bojke, C., Cayton, W., Salawu, A., Case, B., Bojke, L., & Richardson, G. (2018). Impact of specialist rehabilitation services on hospital length of stay and associated costs. *The European Journal of Health Economics, 19,* 1027–1034.

Harvey, L. A., & Close, J. C. T. (2012). Traumatic brain injury in older adults: characteristics, causes and consequences. *Injury, 43,* 1821–1826.

Howard, M. A., Gross, A. S., Dacey, R. G., & Winn, H. R. (1989). Acute subdural hematomas: an age-dependent clinical entity. *Journal of Neurosurgery, 71,* 858–863.

Hyder, A. A., Wunderlich, C. A., Puvanachandra, P., Gururaj, G., & Kobusingye, O. C. (2007). The impact of traumatic brain injuries: a global perspective. *NeuroRehabilitation, 22,* 341–353.

Koskinen, S., & Alaranta, H. (2008). Traumatic brain injury in Finland 1991-2005: a nationwide register study of hospitalized and fatal TBI. *Brain Injury, 22,* 205–214.

Menon, D.K., Schwab, K.P., Wright, D.W., Maas, A.I., Demographics and Clinical Assessment Working Group of the International and Interagency Initiative toward Common Data Elements for Research on Traumatic Brain Injury and Psychological Health (2010). Position statement: definition of traumatic brain injury. *Archives of Physical Medicine and Rehabilitation,* 91, 1637–1640.

Nudo, R. J. (2011). Neural bases of recovery after brain injury. *Journal of Communication Disorders, 44,* 515–520.

Oddy, M., & Da Silva Ramos, S. (2013). The clinical and cost-benefits of investing in neurobehavioural rehabilitation: a multi-centre study. *Brain Injury, 27,* 1500–1507.

Overman, J. J., & Carmichael, S. T. (2014). Plasticity in the injured brain: more than molecules matter. *The Neuroscientist, 20,* 15–28.

Prince, M. J., Wu, F., Guo, Y., Robledo, L. M. G., O'Donnell, M., Sullivan, R., & Yusuf, S. (2015). The burden of disease in older people and implications for health policy and practice. *The Lancet, 385,* 549–562.

Sadaka, F., Patel, D., & Lakshmanan, R. (2012). The FOUR score predicts outcome in patients after traumatic brain injury. *Neurocritical Care, 16,* 95–101.

Susman, M., DiRusso, S. M., Sullivan, T., Risucci, D., Nealon, P., Cuff, S., Haider, A., & Benzil, D. (2002). Traumatic brain injury in the elderly: increased mortality and worse functional outcome at discharge despite lower injury severity. *Journal of Trauma and Acute Care Surgery, 53,* 219–224.

Teasdale, G., & Jennett, B. (1974). Assessment of coma and impaired consciousness: a practical scale. *The Lancet, 2,* 81–84.

Thompson, H. J., McCormick, W. C., & Kagan, S. H. (2006). Traumatic brain injury in older adults: epidemiology, outcomes, and future implications. *Journal of the American Geriatrics Society, 54,* 1590–1595.

Turner-Stokes, L. (2003). *Rehabilitation following acquired brain injury: national clinical guidelines.* London: Royal College of Physicians.

Turner-Stokes, L. (2005). The national service framework for long term conditions: a novel approach for a "new style" NSF. *Journal of Neurology Neurosurgery and Psychiatry, 76,* 901–902.

Turner-Stokes, L. (2008). Evidence for the effectiveness of multi-disciplinary rehabilitation following acquired brain injury: a synthesis of two systematic approaches. *Journal of Rehabilitation Medicine, 40,* 691–701.

Turner-Stokes, L., Nair, A., Sedki, I., Disler, P. B., & Wade, D. T. (2005). Multi-disciplinary rehabilitation for acquired brain injury in adults of working age. *Cochrane Database of Systematic Reviews, 12,* CD004170.

Turolla, A., Venneri, A., Farina, D., Cagnin, A., & Cheung, V. C. K. (2018). Rehabilitation induced neural plasticity after acquired brain injury. *Neural Plasticity, 2018,* 6565418.

Worthington, A. D., Matthews, S., Melia, Y., & Oddy, M. (2006). Cost-benefits associated with social outcome from neurobehavioural rehabilitation. *Brain Injury, 20,* 947–957.

FURTHER READING

Coronado, V. G., Thomas, K. E., Sattin, R. W., & Johnson, R. L. (2005). The CDC traumatic brain injury surveillance system: characteristics of persons aged 65 years and older hospitalized with a TBI. *The Journal of Head Trauma Rehabilitation, 20,* 215–228.

Duffau, H. (2006). Brain plasticity: from pathophysiological mechanisms to therapeutic applications. *Journal of Clinical Neuroscience, 13,* 885–897.

Kolakowsky-Hayner, S. A., Miner, K. D., & Kreutzer, J. S. (2001). Long-term life quality and family needs after traumatic brain injury. *The Journal of Head Trauma Rehabilitation, 16,* 374–385.

Roozenbeek, B., Maas, A. I., & Menon, D. K. (2013). Changing patterns in the epidemiology of traumatic brain injury. *Nature Reviews Neurology, 9,* 231.

World Health Organization. (2017). *Rehabilitation in health systems.*

61

Spinal Injury

Thomas Nathaniel Bryce & Matthias Linke

LEARNING OBJECTIVES

- Describe common causes and mechanisms of spinal cord injury for an older individual
- Describe basic expected functional outcomes by neurological level of injury

- Explain how secondary conditions related to spinal cord injury can affect the rehabilitation of an older individual with spinal cord injury
- Describe tenodesis action, how to promote it, and how it can improve function

CASE

Ralph is an 84-year-old man who slipped in his bathroom, lost his balance, struck his forehead on the sink and fell to the floor from where he could not get up. His wife called emergency services, and he was taken to the local trauma centre where he was found to have greater weakness in the hands and arms than in his legs. Imaging revealed multilevel cervical spondylosis and abnormal signal within the cervical spinal cord indicating a spinal cord injury (SCI). He underwent emergent cervical decompression and after a few days was transferred to an acute SCI rehabilitation centre where he underwent physiotherapy, occupational therapy, speech therapy and psychological counselling by therapists and nurses who had experience in caring for persons with SCI to ensure his best possible outcome.

Upon rehabilitation admission he was found to be voiding (passing urine), but only smaller amounts and more frequently than before the fall. He was also incontinent of stool. An ultrasound bladder scan revealed urinary retention, and he was begun on intermittent catheterisation. Over a few weeks he regained the ability to void with control and had low post-void residual volumes so he did not need catheterisation anymore. In order to control the bowel incontinence, he was started on a daily mini-enema which triggered a regular bowel movement at a time that was convenient for him and the staff alleviating his need for incontinence wear. When standing in therapy he was initially lightheaded and his blood pressure was found to be dropping on standing. This orthostatic blood pressure was treated with compression stockings, an abdominal binder and a medication to raise his blood pressure called midodrine that he took 1 hour before his therapy sessions. As he became stronger the medications were no longer needed.

In therapy although the strength in his legs was graded as good (4/5 on manual muscle testing), he could not walk initially due to impaired trunk balance. However, with balance training and walking training initially with body weight support using a harness or with a platform walker with his hands attached with straps to the walker, he improved and was ultimately able to walk unassisted. His hands improved slowly as did the strength in his shoulders, but by the time of discharge to home he still needed some assistance for dressing his upper body and bathing. With adaptive equipment including a sock donner, dressing stick, long-handled shoehorn and a long-handled sponge provided by the occupational therapist, he was able to dress his lower extremities and put on his shoes himself. He returned home needing only minimal assistance for bathing and dressing.

SPINAL CORD INJURY IN OLDER INDIVIDUALS

In the United States, the incidence of traumatic SCI in older individuals (> 65 years) approaches 90 cases per million as compared to 54 cases per million for all ages. There is an increasing incidence of traumatic SCI in older adults that is not seen in any other age group throughout the world (Noonan et al., 2012). SCI in older individuals is most commonly the result of a 'low fall' or a fall from less than 1 m above the ground. In addition to a relatively minor trauma such as a fall at home or in the street, it may also occur after a low-velocity collision. The mechanism is commonly due to hyperextension of the neck in a person with a narrowed cervical canal due to spondylosis or degenerative arthritis of the spine whereupon the spinal cord is pinched between a hypertrophied ligamentum flavum and anterior vertebral body osteophytes. The typical presentation is weakness of the hands more than the legs and variable bowel and bladder dysfunction. The presentation is known as central cord syndrome due to the injury to the centre of the spinal cord (see Fig. 61.1). Older individuals may also develop SCI due to compression of the spinal cord by metastatic cancer originating most commonly from the prostate, breast, lung or kidney (Heary & Filart, 2002). SCI from cancer is more likely to occur at the thoracic level leaving the arms unimpaired.

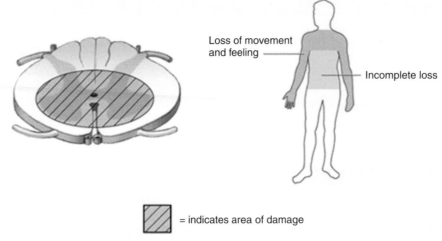

Loss of movement
and feeling

Incomplete loss

= indicates area of damage

FIG. 61.1   Central cord syndrome. (Adapted from Armstrong, Eickstaedt, & Reeves, 2014.)

PROGNOSIS FOR RECOVERY AFTER SCI IN OLDER INDIVIDUALS

Individuals who are older have a worse prognosis for recovery than their younger counterparts. In one study, when groups of individuals younger than 50 years of age were compared to groups of older individuals with the same severity of SCI, almost twice the number of individuals in the younger group were walking at 1 year who started with non-functional strength (less than grade 3/5 on motor testing for most muscles); however, for those with functional strength (more than grade 3/5 on motor testing for most muscles) nearly all in both groups were walking at 1 year (Burns et al., 1997). Nearly all individuals who have incomplete injuries of all severities are generally expected to improve over time. The typical pattern of neurological improvement with regards to gains in motor score is characterised by the greatest changes within the first 3 months, lesser changes over the next 3 months with even lesser changes thereafter with a plateauing at 1 year. Therefore it is essential that active rehabilitation efforts (and not just maintenance therapies) need to be continued throughout this timeframe.

NEUROLOGICAL ASSESSMENT OF INDIVIDUALS WITH SCI

All individuals who sustain a SCI should undergo an assessment of neurological function using the International Standards for Neurological Classification of Spinal Cord Injury (ISNCSCI) (InSTeP International Standards Training Program, n.d.). Comprehensive online e-learning modules (InSTeP) are available through the American Spinal Injury Association (ASIA) website (InSTeP International Standards Training Program, n.d.). The procedure includes a systematic evaluation of all the dermatomes and extremity myotomes. Because SCI usually affects the spinal cord at a discrete site, determining the last intact sensory and motor level can reliably and accurately determine a neurological level of injury.

Derived neurological characteristics of any SCI which are near universally accepted include the Neurological Level of Injury (NLI) and the ASIA Impairment Scale (AIS) (Box 61.1). Use of the NLI and AIS, which provide in combination a gross description of an individual's muscle function, sensation and completeness or incompleteness of injury, is a way to effectively communicate a person's neurological status in a concise manner facilitating communication between team members.

BOX 61.1   ASIA Impairment Scale (AIS) Is Determined According to the Letters A Through E

A = Complete. No sensory or motor function is preserved in the sacral segments S4-S5.

B = Sensory Incomplete. Sensory but not motor function is preserved below the neurological level and includes the sacral segments S4-S5 (light touch [LT] or pin prick [PP] at S4-S5 or deep anal pressure [DAP]) AND no motor function is preserved more than three levels below the motor level on either side of the body.

C = Motor Incomplete. Motor function is preserved at the most caudal sacral segments for voluntary anal contraction (VAC) OR the patient meets the criteria for sensory incomplete status (sensory function preserved at the most caudal sacral segments S4-S5 by LT, PP or DAP), and has some sparing of motor function more than three levels below the ipsilateral motor level on either side of the body. (This includes key or non-key muscle functions to determine motor incomplete status.) For AIS C, less than half of key muscle functions below the single NLI have a muscle grade ≥3.

D = Motor Incomplete. Motor incomplete status as defined above, with at least half (half or more) of key muscle functions below the single NLI having a muscle grade ≥3.

E = Normal. If sensation and motor function as tested with the ISNCSCI are graded as normal in all segments, and the patient had prior deficits, then the AIS grade is E. Someone without an initial SCI does not receive an AIS grade.

Using ND: To document the sensory, motor and NLI levels, the ASIA Impairment Scale grade, and/or the zone of partial preservation (ZPP) when they are unable to be determined based on the examination results.

TABLE 61.1 Expected functional outcomes by NLI.

ACTIVITY	C4	C5	C6	C7	C8-T12
Self-feeding	D	IA	IA	IA	I
Upper body dressing	D	A	I	I	I
Lower body dressing	D	D	A	I or A	I
Level transfers	D	A	I	I	I
Bed mobility	D	A	A	I	I
Wheelchair mobility	IP	IP	IM (indoors)	IM	IM

A, Assistance needed; *D*, dependent; *I*, independent; *IA*, independent with adaptive equipment; *IM*, independent manual wheelchair; *IP*, independent power wheelchair.

Determining the NLI will help determine appropriate functional goals for an individual with SCI. Published functional outcomes stratified by NLI such as can be found in the Consortium for Spinal Cord Medicine Clinical Practice Guideline entitled 'Outcomes Following Traumatic Spinal Cord Injury' can help guide realistic goal setting (Consortium for Spinal Cord Medicine Clinical Practice Guidelines. Paralyzed Veterans of America, n.d.). This prognostic information of expected outcomes tempered by an individual's personal characteristics (body habitus, level of conditioning, etc.), mental state and medical conditions should be communicated to patient and family in order that everyone has realistic expectations for rehabilitation. Table 61.1 shows the expected level of assistance needed as well as medical equipment to assist mobility and ADLs.

SECONDARY CONDITIONS RELATED TO SCI IN OLDER INDIVIDUALS

Older individuals (>65 years) have higher rates of complications, including pneumonia, respiratory insufficiency, pulmonary embolism, renal stones and gastrointestinal bleeding than persons who are younger (Scivoletto et al., 2003). However, treatment of individuals in specialised SCI centres has been shown to reduce these complications (Scivoletto et al., 2003).

Bowel and Bladder Issues

Bowel motility, reflexes and external anal sphincter volition are often impaired in persons with SCI, a condition called neurogenic bowel; this can lead to constipation and incontinence. Similarly, bladder muscle contractions, reflexes and external urinary sphincter volition may be affected in persons with SCI, a condition called neurogenic lower urinary tract dysfunction; this can lead to urinary retention or incontinence. Occupational therapists should work closely with rehabilitation nurses to address bowel and bladder management issues especially as they relate to urinary self-catheterisation technique, reaching to perform digital stimulation to trigger bowel evacuation, clothing management after toileting and use of adaptive or other durable medical equipment such as suppository inserters, catheter insertion clamps, clothing aids and commodes.

Low Blood Pressure

A drop in blood pressure with upright activity, or orthostatic hypotension, resulting from autonomic nervous system changes due to SCI is especially common in older individuals with cervical SCI. Symptoms can include dizziness, lightheadedness, confusion, impaired vision and even syncope. Use of an abdominal binder (or girdle) and lower extremity compression garments can assist in mitigating the drop in blood pressure. Medications can be added by the physician to help raise blood pressure if needed (e.g. midodrine, an alpha agonist). Hypotension often resolves during the recovery process and the need for ongoing use of compression garments and medications should be periodically re-examined. Many older individuals have been prescribed antihypertensive medications prior to their injury, and therefore will need close blood pressure monitoring during the rehabilitation process to ensure that medication dosage is titrated appropriately should orthostatic hypotension become apparent.

Autonomic Nerve Problems

Autonomic dysreflexia is another manifestation of dysregulation of the autonomic system in persons with SCI. It is usually triggered by a noxious stimulus below the neurologic level of the injury, most commonly a distended bladder or bowel. The individual presents typically with a severe headache, elevated blood pressure, flushing of the skin, piloerection and sweating above the level of injury. The elevated blood pressure can lead to heart attack or stroke especially in older individuals who are more likely to have underlying heart disease so the cause needs to be quickly identified and addressed as the symptoms will disappear if the noxious stimulus is removed reducing the risk of further comorbidity.

Effects of Traumatic Brain Injury

Concomitant traumatic brain injury occurs frequently with SCI due to falls. As this can affect the cognition of the individual and the ability of the individual to learn new tasks, it will affect the approach of the treatment team (see Chapter 60 Traumatic Brain Injury) (Sachdeva et al., 2018). Older individuals, especially those with more severe functional impairments, may also be affected by perceived burden on family and other loved ones who may themselves be unable to provide physical assistance.

Pressure Area Damage

The risk of pressure injuries increases both with increasing time since injury and chronological age, especially for those over 50 years of age (Chen, Devivo, & Jackson, 2005). Pressure injuries typically occur in an individual who is not able to perform an adequate pressure relief of the skin and tissues overlying bony prominences such as the heels, sacrum, greater trochanters and ischium. Care should be taken to ensure a pressure relieving wheelchair cushion or bed support surface is provided to those who are unable to perform adequate pressure relief themselves as is recommended in most clinical practice guidelines including the Consortium for Spinal Cord Medicine Clinical Practice Guideline entitled 'Pressure Ulcer Prevention and Treatment Following Spinal Cord Injury' (Garber, 2014). Individuals with impaired sensation and/or mobility should be educated how to inspect areas of the body that are at risk for pressure injury every day.

GOALS AND TREATMENT APPROACHES IN SCI REHABILITATION

Rehabilitation of all individuals with significant SCI that affects mobility and other secondary conditions of SCI such as neurogenic bowel and neurologic lower urinary tract dysfunction optimally should be conducted by a team that includes at a minimum a physician with expertise in SCI, physiotherapists and occupational therapists with experience in SCI, a rehabilitation nurse who is familiar with bowel and bladder management, and a psychologist. Individuals treated in a specialised SCI centre have increased overall survival rates, decreased complication rates, fewer pressure injuries, decreased length of hospital stays, greater functional gains during rehabilitation, a greater likelihood of home discharge and lower rehospitalisation rates (Bergman, Yarkony, & Stiens, 1997; DeVivo et al., 1990). The goal of rehabilitation is to enable the individual to become as independent as possible with the best quality of life as the impairments that limit the function of the patient allow. Educating the individual with SCI on how to advocate for themselves and direct their care helps them regain control of their surroundings even if there are significant functional limitations. The rehabilitation process is ultimately a life-long endeavour to improve and maintain function.

When assessing functional goals of someone with SCI, underlying degenerative joint disease or osteoarthritis become relevant as they can impact the achievement of optimal functional outcomes. They usually manifest as joint pain with movement or limited range of motion and are common in older individuals. When the treatment team is considering ordering a wheelchair for mobility, it is important to keep in mind that an older individual with secondary conditions such as arthritis of the shoulders, which can affect wheelchair propulsion, or coronary or respiratory disease, which can affect exercise tolerance, may be much more independent using power mobility than a manual one.

Hand function usually limited by weakness and sensory loss in someone with a SCI may be further limited by arthritis in the older individual. Training in the use of tenodesis action may be necessary to provide a person with at least anti-gravity (>3/5) wrist extension strength but poor finger flexor strength and functional hand grasp and lateral pinch to allow performance of activities of daily living independently. Tenodesis action occurs as the fingers and thumb naturally flex with wrist extension; a tenodesis grasp capitalises on this to allow an individual without active finger and thumb flexion to grasp and pinch objects during active wrist extension. Unlike someone with a stroke who may need to have their hand splinted with their fingers extended for anti-spasm treatment, the individual in whom a tenodesis grasp is needed is encouraged to develop thumb and finger flexor tendon shortening to assist with a tenodesis grasp. Additionally, adaptive equipment will be unique to the patient's functional level with built up handles or a universal cuff utilised to facilitate independence when needed.

Prevention of the adverse effects of secondary conditions such as contractures, pressure injuries and syncope related to orthostatic hypotension is essential to the rehabilitation process. Education of the individual and family with a daily stretching programme for all joints to maintain range of motion and prevent contracture, how to perform pressure reliefs, how to properly position to avoid pain and pressure on bony prominences, as well as techniques to avoid sudden drops in blood pressure is essential.

Adjustment to impairments and disability after SCI needs to be addressed by the rehabilitation team. Psychological support to adjust to life-altering injury can be provided by all members of the team including if available psychologists, peer counsellors and SCI support groups. The prevalence of major depression in persons with SCI at any one time is approximately 20%, of whom 15% have suicidal ideation (Hoffman et al., 2011). Older individuals may also be affected by perceived burden on family and medical comorbidities. Providing educational resources can foster continued learning.

▌ SUMMARY POINTS

- All individuals who sustain SCI should undergo an assessment of neurological function using the International Standards for Neurological Classification of Spinal Cord Injury (ISNCSCI)
- Compared to younger counterparts, older individuals and their caregivers need to be more vigilant for the development of pneumonia, respiratory insufficiency, pulmonary embolism, renal stones, gastrointestinal bleeding, cognitive impairment and pressure injuries
- Older individuals with SCI are more likely to consider power mobility devices compared to younger individuals with the same NLI and severity of injury
- Individuals treated in specialised SCI centres have increased overall survival rates, decreased complication

rates, fewer pressure injuries, decreased length of hospital stays, greater functional gains during rehabilitation, a greater likelihood of home discharge and lower rehospitalisation rates

MCQs

Q.1 What is the most common type of spinal cord injury in the elderly?
  a. Complete tetraplegia
  b. Incomplete tetraplegia
  c. Complete paraplegia
  d. Incomplete paraplegia

Q.2 Which of the following allows one to determine a neurological level of injury?
  a. Modified Ashworth Scale
  b. Manual Muscle Testing
  c. International Standards for Neurological Classification of Spinal Cord Injury
  d. Barthel Index

Q.3 What is tenodesis action in an individual with SCI?
  a. An inflammation of a tendon
  b. Adhesions of two tendons
  c. Infection of a tendon
  d. Flexion of the fingers with wrist extension

REFERENCES

Armstrong, K., Eickstaedt, J., & Reeves, R. (2014). Care for the rehospitalized patient with chronic spinal cord injury. *Hospital Medicine Clinics, 3,* e270–e292.

Bergman, S. B., Yarkony, G. M., & Stiens, S. A. (1997). Spinal cord injury rehabilitation. 2. Medical complications. *Archives of Physical Medicine and Rehabilitation, 78,* S53–S58.

Burns, S. P., Golding, D. G., Rolle, W. A., Jr., Graziani, V., & Ditunno, J. F., Jr. (1997). Recovery of ambulation in motor-incomplete tetraplegia. *Archives of Physical Medicine and Rehabilitation, 78,* 1169–1172.

Chen, Y., Devivo, M. J., & Jackson, A. B. (2005). Pressure ulcer prevalence in people with spinal cord injury: age-period-duration effects. *Archives of Physical Medicine and Rehabilitation, 86,* 1208–1213.

Consortium for Spinal Cord Medicine. (n.d.). Clinical Practice Guidelines. Paralyzed Veterans of America. Retrieved from https://www.pva.org/publications/clinical-practice-guidelines (Accessed January 6, 2019).

DeVivo, M. J., Kartus, P. L., Stover, S. L., & Fine, P. R. (1990). Benefits of early admission to an organised spinal cord injury care system. *Paraplegia, 28,* 545–555.

Garber, S.L. (2014). Pressure ulcer prevention and treatment following spinal cord injury: a clinical practice guideline for health-care professionals, 2nd edn. Retrieved from: https://www.aci.health.nsw.gov.au/__data/assets/pdf_file/0004/387535/03.-CPG_Pressure-Ulcer.pdf.

Heary, R. F., & Filart, R. (2002). Tumors of the spine and spinal cord. In S. Kirshblum, D. I. Campagnolo, & J. A. DeLisa (Eds.), *Spinal cord medicine* (pp. 480–497). Philadelphia, PA: Lippincott, Williams and Wilkins.

Hoffman, J. M., Bombardier, C. H., Graves, D. E., Kalpakjian, C. Z., & Krause, J. S. (2011). A longitudinal study of depression from 1 to 5 years after spinal cord injury. *Archives of Physical Medicine and Rehabilitation, 92,* 411–418.

InSTeP International Standards Training Program. (n.d.). American Spinal Injury Association. Retrieved from: https://asia-spinalinjury.org/learning/ (Accessed 6 January 2019).

Noonan, V. K., Fingas, M., Farry, A., Baxter, D., Singh, A., Fehlings, M. G., & Dvorak, M. F. (2012). Incidence and prevalence of spinal cord injury in Canada: a national perspective. *Neuroepidemiology, 38,* 219–226.

Sachdeva, R., Gao, F., Chan, C. C. H., & Krassioukov, A. V. (2018). Cognitive function after spinal cord injury: a systematic review. *Neurology, 91,* 611–621.

Scivoletto, G., Morganti, B., Ditunno, P., Ditunno, J. F., & Molinari, M. (2003). Effects on age on spinal cord lesion patients' rehabilitation. *Spinal Cord, 41,* 457–464.

FURTHER READING

Burns, S. P., & Hammond, M. C. (2009). In *Yes you can! a guide to self-care for persons with spinal cord injury,* (4th edn.). Washington, DC: Paralyzed Veterans of America.

Washington PV of AESN, DC20006-35171-800-424-8200USA. Publications: Consumer Guides. https://www.pva.org/publications/consumer-guides. (Accessed 12 November 2018).

Reeve Foundation. *Paralysis resource guide - living with paralysis.* Retrieved from: https://www.christopherreeve.org/living-with-paralysis/free-resources-and-downloads/paralysis-resource-guide (Accessed 12 November 2018).

62

Rehabilitation for People with Progressive Neurological Conditions

Paul Carroll

LEARNING OBJECTIVES

- Explain how health services and professionals can support patients with progressive neurological conditions
- Describe the approach to goal setting and rehabilitation in patients with progressive neurological conditions

- Describe how family and friends can support the rehabilitation process

In deep gratitude to the generosity of spirit of the people with progressive neurological conditions with whom I have had the privilege to work.'

INTRODUCTION

This chapter presents and explores some ideas and challenges in the practice of rehabilitation for and with people with progressive neurological conditions (PNCs).

The primary aim is not to give complex detail of specific conditions, but to encourage the reader to consciously consider and cultivate the quality of presence and thinking that you bring to the moments you share with a person who has been affected by a difficult disease.

There is a wide range of topics that are important to know about when working with people with PNCs, many of which are covered in other chapters including palliative care and advance care planning, rehabilitation goals and loneliness.

SOME IDEAS AND REFLECTIONS ON REHABILITATION SERVICES FOR PEOPLE WITH PNCs

Seeing the Service from the Service User Perspective and the Service Provider

There is a wide breadth of PNCs such as multiple sclerosis, Parkinson's disease, motor neurone disease and Alzheimer's disease. Some of these conditions will have challenges in common and some will present their own unique challenges.

There is a very large number of people living with a PNC. There is likewise a large number of people who live alongside the person and who witness the challenges, try their best to offer support and often suffer with them.

When people want help, they look for it in a way that is accessible, available in good time, respectful and genuinely interested. People in need of help will not separate out parts of the help they need – diagnosis, medication, imaging, rehabilitation, palliative care, etc. – these are inventions of health system organisation and their histories. Services need to take the perspective of the person needing help and consider what barriers have to be overcome to allow someone to access the help they need. The dispersed location and lack of communication between services can make life much harder for people looking for help.

Society – Achievement and Failure

Our societies are improving but have a long way to go in offering equality of opportunity to people with disabilities. There is widespread non-intentional exclusion. The values and lack of values present in societal culture may be taken into the rehabilitation service environment by those who use the services and those who work there. When someone has been given a PNC diagnosis, there can be a tendency of the 'well' to look at them differently and for the individual to be lost sight of through the distraction of medical fact, pity and the changes arising from the condition. There is opportunity in services for people with PNCs to convey alternative messages such as a sense of possibility, hope and value.

Rehabilitation Definition

Rehabilitation tends to be described as a biopsychosocial practice. In palliative care a biopsychosociospiritual model is put forward. This is a wider framework and one that seems appropriate for rehabilitation in progressive conditions.

For the purposes of this chapter, rehabilitation can be defined as the helping of another with respect, collaboration and creativity, in their efforts to gain and keep independence, to develop understanding of their condition, to achieve goals, meaning and expression of their individuality, to experience the breadth of human experiences including happiness, hope and peace of mind, and to stay as healthy as possible. This latter factor includes helping people with symptoms and experiences that can be deeply intrusive and distressing such as pain, fatigue, incontinence and anxiety.

Rehabilitation Is Not a Standalone Activity

Rehabilitation can tend to be conceived of and configured as a process to take place following diagnosis and disease treatment. Services that someone with a PNC may need to draw on tend to be located in different sites, adding to the challenge for people needing help. This is not the way help should be configured – rehabilitation should be integrated within the fabric of service throughout and not be something that follows in series.

Professionals and teams should seek to develop working relationships and resources for people with PNCs. These conditions can give rise to a wide range of problems including incontinence, mental ill health, pain, sleep disorder, osteoporosis, respiratory weakness, cardiac disease, and global or specific physical weakness or deconditioning, and it is deeply helpful to have integration of professionals with these skill sets.

Rehabilitation Model and Trajectory of Change

The most common experience that professionals working in rehabilitation services acquire is working with people where their illness event is a one-off, for example as in a stroke. In PNCs there is a profound difference in the journey – the condition will at some stage most likely worsen and the person with the condition and their family must live their lives with this prospect. Uncertainty, for example around extent and rate of progression, will tend to be very hard to deal with.

This fundamental difference brings several important consequences. In progressive conditions, the work of appraisal, goal formulation and rehabilitation plans may need to be made repeatedly as the condition evolves. Rehabilitation practice for PNCs usually tends to be more complex than that for one-off conditions.

Rehabilitation working and the inherent natural hoping held by patients, families and professionals fits with one-off conditions, whereas in PNCs the working and hoping required is often against the grain of the trajectory of the condition.

Self-knowledge can be important for self-care. Insight tends to be important in this. Insight and adjustment can often be immensely difficult for people to achieve – for very good reason as they can tend to be very hard tasks cognitively and emotionally to begin to do. This challenge will tend to be present both in one-off neurological conditions and with PNCs. The process of rehabilitation itself – learning how one's body has changed through feedback from physiotherapy and other staff, learning to use new aids, getting changes made at home and talking through experiences can mediate a gradual growth of insight. Sometimes healthcare professionals are impatient for insight building or can even get frustrated by the lack of development of it. In both categories of condition cognitive and communication impairment may occur that can hinder someone developing insight. In both, distress within the person and their family can influence insight and self-protection can arise as someone, in order to get through that day or time phase, may need to avoid the envisaging of future problems. In addition someone with a PNC may have only just begun to understand their condition when it changes again. When considering someone's insight it is important to turn the insight microscope back on ourselves – thus to consider how much do we have insight into what it is like to live with the challenges with which that person is living such as chronic pain, living by one's bladder and the omnipresent vista of deterioration.

Disease-Specific Services and Services with Wider Breadth

In some PNCs service has developed around the diagnosis. Motor neurone disease is a good example. There are benefits to this model, e.g. service users are well known to that service and an excellence in practice is built up. However, the development of diagnosis-specific services is not feasible for every PNC. There is a need for resource and expertise sharing. Within neurological rehabilitation systems currently, there are relatively developed services for people who have had a stroke but often very little rehabilitation for those with multiple sclerosis, dementia or Parkinson's disease. Some difficulties are shared across conditions and require specialist expertise including neuro-urology, behavioural medicine and mental health, assistive technology, specialist seating, social work and family therapy. An economy of scale approach to service configuration is vital as it allows the development of such services at one location and this can be of immense benefit to people with PNCs and their families in terms of convenience and timely collaboration between specialists.

Local and Regional – the Need for Both to Work and Develop Together

Local services can get to know a service user in their home context, and being able to visit someone in their home can give much rich information and connection. Well-resourced regional or national services are in the majority of cases hospital-based, and thus have access to specialist expertise and equipment such as imaging and neurophysiology. It is good practice for services already established to take interest in and form connections with colleague services and then consider how they may form more organised networks in order to bring about cohesive joint working between the local and regional service in order to help those needing assistance more effectively. Such a network may allow greater opportunity for education, research and resource sharing.

Age and Maintaining Health

One person aged 70 years may be working and doing marathons, and another may be frail and have a sedentary lifestyle. This variation may arise from a wide range of factors including poverty, lifestyle factors such as smoking and exercise, genetic factors and richness of social support. These same factors may also be present for people with PNCs and have impact on their health. Someone with a PNC is more likely to be caught in poverty because of not being able to work and will often lack opportunity to exercise. Someone with a PNC may more likely be alone as they may not have had the chance to develop relationships and have families, or the relationships they did have may have become altered or severed due to factors arising from the condition. Loneliness can be a factor and health professionals can be a major point of social/human contact.

Many PNCs will shorten life span or have the potential to shorten life span. This can be hard to predict at an individual level even through there may be research evidence of life-shortening risk factors in a given population. It is important to hold in mind both the chronological age of a person but also think in terms of years potentially remaining and not get stuck on an age number as a major determinant of rehabilitation goals. Some PNCs present the risk of an earlier death, and it is important to stand back and consider how best to assist someone taking into account the hopes and goals they may be holding in the present, but also the possible disease trajectory.

WORKING WITH PEOPLE WITH PNCS AND THEIR FAMILIES AND FRIENDS

Both Goals and No Goals

Contemporary rehabilitation tends to be heavily goal based in practice and in its theoretical framework. This is needed in situations where the challenges are many, complex and at times overwhelming as is often the case when a condition is progressing. Rehabilitation as a process needs to be more than this; however, it should be both goal based and goal free, where there is time and space to live in the moment. We do not live our lives directed only by goals but take it for granted that we go for a meal, spend time at a game or watch the sea. Goal-free time does not mean the leftover time between or after therapy sessions where people are in their wheelchair or bed on a ward, spectators of a service around them, but having a culture that recognises that joy, entertainment and recreation are essential human experiences and that these are still essential and possible when someone has a progressive condition.

Rehabilitation Beyond the Usual Formula

As mentioned above, it is important to have professionals who work creatively such as art and music therapists and those who work with the aim of recreation and enjoyment. People with PNCs may also benefit from assistive technology. This may be simple or more sophisticated such as eye-gaze technology and environmental controls.

The milieu or atmosphere in a service can make a major difference. Sometimes people with a PNC may avoid using a service because they do not want to see someone who may be further down the path of disease progression. The presence and impact of other staff such as catering, cleaning and administration can be large and the simple kindness of staff can transform low moments. The role of chaplaincy can also be valuable.

Animals, plants and access to outdoor spaces in a rehabilitation environment can touch people in ways that no psychotherapy can (see Fig. 62.1).

All these things are especially important in progressive conditions where someone may need to come back again and again over many years. Some places elicit anxiety when people approach them.

Working with Hope

Hope is an essential human experience and is a deep motivator of behaviour. Hope and hoping will often be deeply challenged by a PNC, and it is a really important factor to be aware of in this field.

Maintaining hope can be very hard when there is loss after loss. It is normal that hope may falter and disappear at times. If hopelessness is sustained, there can be loss of interest in life, reduced motivation to care for self and the development of profound depression and grief.

When listening to someone expressing their hopes, it may seem that some of these are unrealistic. Sometimes people are well aware that their hopes are unrealistic, but the hopes

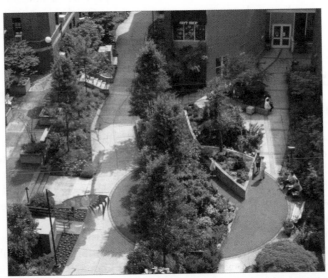

FIG. 62.1 An example of an outdoor 'Healing Garden' area in a rehabilitation centre. (From Burton A. Gardens that take care of us. *Lancet Neurol.* 2014;13(5):447–8, with permission.)

they hold play the role of a lifebuoy in keeping them going. Consider carefully before you challenge someone's unrealistic hopes if they are not having any negative consequences on them or the people around them.

If there is a specific loss, for example of a job, there can be a generalisation of hopelessness from this lost singular hope. It can be helpful to assist someone with reflecting on this specific lost hope in order to restore a more generalised or trait-like hopefulness. This may also be relevant when working with family members and friends.

It can often be helpful to ask someone explicitly about their hopes, goals and beliefs. Often these will be merged into one and asking may help someone with a PNC to begin to appreciate they are holding a composite of hope, goal and belief. This can be helpful where a hope is being held as a goal and this goal is markedly unrealistic. Someone may through distinguishing the difference between a hope and a goal begin to find a place in their mind for their hope yet engage pragmatically with appropriate guidance that may be offered.

Sometimes someone with a PNC or their family member is right in their hope in achieving something, and it is the professional or team that has got it wrong. Sometimes a team can exude a sense of hopelessness without knowing this and this can tend to occur if a professional or team is tired.

Advance Care Planning

Exploring ceilings of treatment, for example whether to resuscitate, should be considered in rehabilitation settings. It is usually overlooked. If there is uncertainty and lack of expertise in how to do this, then forming a collaboration with palliative care will likely be helpful. Discussing such topics is not at odds with rehabilitation. Both rehabilitation and palliative care can fit well together and some people may find it easier to discuss such topics in a rehabilitation context than being referred to a distinct palliative care service. In a rehabilitation context, the support of a speech and language therapist and knowledge of someone's cognitive strengths and weaknesses can make a big difference to the person understanding more fully the implications of what is being discussed.

Working with Families

Working with families and close friends is a large part of the work of rehabilitation in the context of PNCs. They can be an immense source of support; however, in some instances they can also be sources of distress for the person with the PNC. For example, a family that is resolutely positive may not allow space for the person to express grief or frustration. The impact of distress in a family on a person with a PNC needs to be appraised with wisdom. Having a PNC does not mean someone cannot fulfil a role of support for others. An essential part of the realisation of loving relationships is the offering comfort to another and the love, companionship and reassurance that someone with a PNC can offer to a partner or family member should not be underestimated. However, professionals can play an important role in making sure someone with a PNC and their partner or close family members do not become lost under the pressures and stresses associated with the condition.

Much fear and anxiety can arise in family members about a PNC. It is important to ask what people know or believe about a condition. Fear and anxiety can come across as anger, and can be a cause of someone not taking on information correctly. Negative information may be remembered more easily. On occasion people will take only the positive, however, and not seem to hear information that does not fit with their hopes and beliefs.

Emotion will tend to spread naturally across people. Thus states such as hope, anxiety and anger will tend to travel between family members. It is important a team keep the person with the progressive condition as their primary focus and to maintain their working form in the face of pressure. Processes such as goal setting, team meetings and family meetings can help.

Your Presence

Do not underestimate your presence. Even if you feel you have little to say, your interest in someone as a person and your presence may lift up another person and give them solace. The presence we bring to each encounter is important. People with PNCs may have vulnerability, and the poorly hidden impatience or boredom on a professional's part can be crushing. Gentleness, humility and patience can have a power to help someone keep going in a way that may make no rational sense, yet they do and they are priceless for this reason.

▌ SUMMARY POINTS

- There are many people who have a PNC or live with someone with such a condition. The number of such conditions is wide
- PNCs cause serial losses of ability, can denude people of their dignity and self-belief and value in their eyes and in the eyes of others, and cause people to be in positions where they are dependent on others and not able to achieve things most take for granted
- Services need to be configured around people who need the service – this means different professionals working together as a broader team

- Rehabilitation needs to be holistic
- Rehabilitation in the context of PNCs has differences with that for one-off conditions arising from the progressive nature of the condition and the changing picture associated with it as well as the uncertainty and anticipation of progression
- It is possible to help someone in profound ways even if it is not possible to cure or fully treat a condition. Rehabilitation should be a key part in helping people with PNCs live more fully and more comfortably

MCQs

Q.1 Which of the following symptoms can occur due to a progressive neurological condition?
- a. Mental ill health
- b. Pain
- c. Sleep disorder
- d. Osteoporosis
- e. All of the above

Q.2 Which one of the following actions is appropriate to consider during the rehabilitation of patients with progressive neurological conditions?
- a. Keeping the family at a distance
- b. Avoiding discussions about death
- c. Advance care planning
- d. Sticking rigidly to goals
- e. Discouraging hope

63

Rehabilitation in the Community

Sujo Anathhanam & Eileen Burns

LEARNING OBJECTIVES

- Describe various models of rehabilitation in community settings
- Identify the key benefits of delivering rehabilitation in the community
- Discuss the challenges associated with providing care for older people in these environments

CASE

Mary Jo, an 80-year-old retired teacher, suddenly developed severe chest pain one afternoon whilst shopping. She was rushed to hospital. A myocardial infarction (heart attack) was diagnosed, and she underwent emergency stenting. After the procedure, Mary Jo developed pneumonia, delirium and atrial fibrillation (an irregularity in the heartbeat). She spent some time on the coronary care unit and then moved to Ward 12, a general cardiology ward. She had now been in bed for nearly 3 weeks, was catheterised and had developed a pressure ulcer on her left heel. She felt exhausted and was only able to transfer out of bed with a standing aid and moderate assistance from two ward physiotherapists. However, she was motivated to get better and the ward's multidisciplinary team felt that she would benefit from continued rehabilitation.

Two days later, Mary Jo was informed that a bed had become available at Silver Tree Intermediate Care Centre; she moved there that evening and spent the following 5 weeks there. Silver Tree Intermediate Care Centre was a 35-bedded unit in a suburban area, five miles away from her home. Mary Jo was seen by the physiotherapist there the day after arrival who discussed her goals with her. Mary Jo wanted to be able to live alone again, take responsibility for her personal care and get back to her hobbies including shopping and gardening. She had previously mobilised independently at home but used a three-wheeled walker outside. She found Silver Tree to be a quieter environment than the acute hospital. She ate her meals with other residents in the communal dining room, had her own room and was able to sleep better. When her family members visited, they were able to take her out into the unit's gardens and found parking easier than at the acute hospital. Mary Jo

received daily nursing care and was regularly reviewed by the unit's physiotherapist and occupational therapist. She was also reviewed three times by a geriatrician who visited the unit weekly. She undertook a detailed review of Mary Jo's medication, stopping her quinine and antihistamines, weaning down amiodarone and increasing her diuretics (water tablets). Her kidney function started to deteriorate and this was kept under review with weekly blood tests. The geriatrician discussed the possibility of re-admission to hospital and cardiopulmonary resuscitation with her. Mary Jo was happy to be transferred to hospital if needed but wanted time to talk about resuscitation with her family. The team discussed her goals and progress in the weekly multidisciplinary team meetings.

After 3 weeks, Mary Jo was managing to transfer and mobilise with a Zimmer frame. Her pressure ulcer was being dressed by the nurses and was felt to be improving. Her catheter was removed but she was left with a sensation of urgency when needing the toilet. The occupational therapist undertook a home visit with Mary Jo. Although this went well, Mary Jo struggled with the stairs so subsequently decided to have a stairlift installed. On discharge, her care was handed over to the local 'neighbourhood team'. Her therapy outcome measures (TOM) scores are shown in Table 63.1 (see also Chapter 22 Measuring Progress With Rehabilitation). A district nurse visited Mary Jo at home to dress her heel and the community physiotherapists are continuing to work with Mary Jo. Her daughter lives opposite her and is currently undertaking her shopping and heavier chores around the house. Mary Jo hopes to continue rehabilitation at home and reach a point where she no longer requires the Zimmer frame and can transfer into and out of a car so she can go shopping.

WHY PROVIDE REHABILITATION IN COMMUNITY SETTINGS?

Hospitalised older people with frailty do not rapidly 'bounce back' from illness and are especially susceptible to complications including falls, pressure ulcers, adverse drug events and healthcare-associated infections which can lengthen their recovery (Rothschild, Bates, & Leape 2000). Against the backdrop of an ageing population and reductions in hospital beds, it is unsurprising that acute hospitals are under pressure. Whilst healthcare systems and their funding vary across the globe, international policy objectives are similar. Most

TABLE 63.1 Mary Jo's therapy outcome measure (TOM) scores at admission and discharge from Silver Tree Intermediate Care Centre.		
	AT ADMISSION	AT DISCHARGE
Impairment	2.5	4
Activity	2.5	4
Participation	3	5
Well-being	5	5

TOM scores can be used by a range of professionals and each dimension is scored from 0 to 5, with 0 representing the worst possible scenario and 5 the best score (Enderby & John, 2015).

developed countries are exploring ways of 'working differently' with an emphasis on providing more care in the community and reducing dependence on hospital care.

Offering 'step-down' rehabilitation within community settings may mean that older people recovering from illness and injury are not competing with the needs of more unwell inpatients and are more likely to receive holistic care catered to their needs. In Mary Jo's case, we can see that the calmer environment of Silver Tree Intermediate Care Centre provided a suitable setting for her to achieve her goals and progress her independence. A hairdresser visited this unit, pets were allowed and Mary Jo was able to eat in the dining room, enabling social interactions with other residents, all contributing to a more 'homely' environment than Ward 12. Simultaneously, this transfer of care contributed to ensuring flow through the acute hospital and enabled another patient to access the cardiology ward in their time of need. 'Step-up' services aim to avoid hospital admission altogether for a selected group of older people but must amalgamate rapid clinical assessment and diagnosis with a rehabilitation component.

WHAT DOES REHABILITATION IN THE COMMUNITY LOOK LIKE?

Intermediate Care

The concept of intermediate care originated in the UK and was first described within the NHS plan (Department of Health, 2000) and later in the National Service Framework for Older People (Department of Health, 2001). Intermediate care bridges the gap between hospital and home, pulling together a range of staff from the community and social services as well as geriatricians and general practitioners. Its aims are to help people avoid being admitted to hospital unnecessarily, to be as independent as possible after a stay in hospital and to avoid admission to long-term care unless absolutely needed (NHS Benchmarking Network, 2017). Most community rehabilitation is provided under the umbrella of intermediate care services within the UK. The National Institute of Health and Care Excellence (NICE) recognises four broad types of intermediate care as outlined in Fig. 63.1 (NICE, 2017). Around the world, a mixture of publicly and privately funded 'hospital at home', 'community rehabilitation' and 'post-acute

care' services are available with similar underlying aims and principles to intermediate care.

Mary Jo was transferred from the acute hospital trust to bed-based intermediate care and then discharged to the home-based intermediate care service within her locality. Bed-based intermediate care is typically provided within care homes, community hospitals or standalone intermediate care facilities (Age UK, 2019). Most service users in bed-based intermediate care settings have been stepped down from hospital as they are no longer acutely unwell but have not yet recovered to the point of being able to look after themselves at home. The composition of the multidisciplinary team can vary but usually includes nursing staff, physiotherapists, occupational therapists, pharmacists and social workers. Clinical leadership is typically provided by a visiting geriatrician or general practitioner. A minority of units have speech and language therapists, dieticians or mental health workers based onsite (NHS Benchmarking, 2017).

A key disadvantage of providing rehabilitation in a bed-based setting is that it involves a move from hospital to yet another unfamiliar environment. This is particularly relevant for the 44% of people in bed-based rehabilitation with cognitive impairment as such a move may precipitate delirium (Holditch, 2018). Home-based rehabilitation is superior in this regard and can lead to greater involvement of family members, but space for equipment and therapy may be limited and can in some cases place extra demands on families (Forster & Young, 2011). Clinical leadership in home-based rehabilitation teams is usually provided by therapists. Reablement services do not have medical or therapy input but instead employ social care staff who can help support older people with personal care, activities of daily living and practical tasks for a time-limited period with the aim of enabling them to develop the practical skills and confidence to carry out these tasks themselves. The reablement approach has its roots in UK home care and has been associated with a decrease in subsequent social care use (Glendinning et al., 2010).

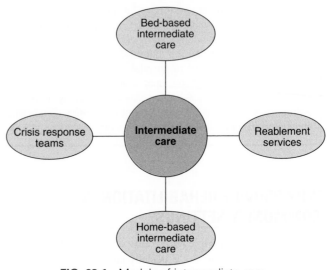

FIG. 63.1 Models of intermediate care.

But is the 'step-down' transfer of older people to community rehabilitation settings safe? A review of the evidence from 32 studies across 12 countries found that people discharged home with services similar to the above had a shorter length of stay in hospital than those having usual care (Gonçalves-Bradley et al., 2017). Reassuringly, death rates were no different, readmission rates were similar, service users were less likely to be admitted to institutional care and tended to be more satisfied with their care. There was insufficient evidence to draw firm conclusions on cost savings. The evidence-base for 'step-up' services is limited by the small size of individual trials. However, a review of the evidence from 16 studies across seven countries suggested that home-based treatment and admission avoidance did not affect readmission rates or death rates and may reduce the chances of living in residential care in 6 months (Shepperd et al., 2016). Excluding the cost of informal care, admission avoidance strategies may be less expensive than admission to hospital but the impact on caregivers has not been adequately studied.

In 2017, the majority of intermediate care service users in the UK were discharged home (69% from bed-based, 80% from home-based and 83% from reablement services) and showed a 35% improvement in dependency score (NHS Benchmarking, 2017). The proportion of patients returning to acute hospitals from bed-based intermediate care was 12%, and a smaller proportion was discharged to long-term care facilities. At one point during Mary Jo's stay, her kidney function worsened; hence the possibility of readmission to the acute hospital for more intensive medical management was discussed. As hospitalisation is not an uncommon event, it is crucially important that treatment escalation plans and decisions about the appropriateness of transfers are in place.

Geriatric Day Hospitals

The concept of the geriatric day hospital originated in the UK and spread to the United States, Canada, Australia and New Zealand. However, many geriatric day hospitals in the UK have now closed. By housing a team of multidisciplinary professionals 'under one roof', the geriatric day hospital was well placed to deliver comprehensive geriatric assessment and rehabilitation for visiting service users. The major disadvantages of this model were the costs and perceived inefficiency involved in transportation of older people to and from these units. A review of the evidence showed that these units were no more effective than other types of well-coordinated geriatric care and at least as or more expensive (Brown et al., 2015). More recently, there has been renewed interest in using geriatric day hospitals as a setting for ambulatory assessment of older people but this is primarily for the purposes of admission avoidance rather than ongoing rehabilitation.

Rehabilitation of Care Home Residents

Older people living in residential and nursing homes are often assumed to have little 'rehabilitation potential', but this does not necessarily hold true. A review of 67 trials suggested that physical rehabilitation for long-term residents may be effective, leading to small improvements in disability, but concluded that larger trials were required to draw firmer conclusions (Crocker et al., 2013). A common clinical scenario is the older person from a care home who falls and presents to hospital with a fracture requiring surgery or a cast. Such patients are usually discharged back to their care home often without any formal rehabilitation support. A small Canadian study showed that a 10-week outreach rehabilitation programme helped users achieve better mobility than the group who received usual post-fracture care (Beaupre et al., 2019). This is an area where further research would be of value.

TRANSITIONS TO AND FROM COMMUNITY SETTINGS

It is recommended that people are transferred to intermediate care within 2 days of referral (NICE, 2017). This is to ensure that they are able to make maximal gains from rehabilitation and are not 'stranded' in hospital. Safe transition between hospital and community settings can be a challenge, with multiple opportunities for communication to go awry. During Mary Jo's hospital admission, new medications had been started, plans had been made for an outpatient cardiology review and the subject of cardiopulmonary resuscitation had been broached. Most, but not all, of this information was available to the team caring for Mary Jo at Silver Tree. The development of shared electronic health and social care records or interoperable systems can present significant logistical challenges and information governance issues but can go some way towards reducing information loss (Holder et al., 2018).

Mary Jo was given written information about Silver Tree on arrival to the unit but may have felt less apprehensive about the move she been given more information pre-transfer. Sample patient information leaflets can be found online (for example, Leeds City Council, 2019).

Upon discharge from bed-based intermediate care, it is again of fundamental importance that information is shared between the bed-based and home-based teams and with Margaret's GP and social worker. Older people with complex conditions are at high risk of readmission. Treatment escalation plans, decisions about the appropriateness of hospitalisation and any self-care or 'rescue' plans should be clearly documented and shared.

SUMMARY POINTS

- Older people are at heightened risk of adverse events in hospital and sometimes prefer to remain in their own homes and receive care in their local communities

- As demand on acute hospitals increases, there has been an international policy focus on reducing length of stay and delivering rehabilitation services in the community

- Older people can benefit from rehabilitation in community hospitals, standalone intermediate care facilities, day hospitals or can be visited by teams in their own homes and care homes
- There is more evidence for the benefit of 'step-down' services than 'step-up' services. In the former, older people have usually been assessed and treated in an acute hospital and are then transferred to a community setting for recovery and rehabilitation. In the latter, older people may avoid admission to hospital altogether

MCQs

Q.1 Transferring older people from acute hospitals to community rehabilitation settings is thought to:
   a. Reduce length of stay in the acute hospital and result in healthcare cost savings
   b. Reduce length of stay in the acute hospital with no effect on mortality or readmission rate and decrease the likelihood of admission to long-term care
   c. Reduce length of stay in the acute hospital but increase the likelihood of death or admission to long term care
   d. Reduce length of stay in the acute hospital but increase the readmission rate

Q.2 Avoidance of acute hospital admission and treating older people in their own homes or in bed-based community rehabilitation settings is thought to:
   a. Result in increased mortality rates and carer strain
   b. Be the preferred option of all older people
   c. Be suitable for a cohort of older people if clinical assessment and diagnostic facilities are offered as well as rehabilitation
   d. Be less cost-effective than admission to an acute hospital

REFERENCES

Age UK. (2019). *Factsheet 76, Intermediate care and reablement* [online]. London: Age UK. Retrieved from https://www.ageuk.org.uk/globalassets/age-uk/documents/factsheets/fs76_intermediate_care_and_reablement_fcs.pdf (Accessed 10 July 2019).

Beaupre, L. A., Magaziner, J. S., Jones, C. A., Jhangri, G. S., Johnston, D. W. C., Wilson, D. M., & Majumdar, S. R. (2019). Rehabilitation after hip fracture for nursing home residents: a controlled feasibility trial. *The Journals of Gerontology Series A, Biological Sciences and Medical Sciences, 74*(9), 1518–1525.

Brown, L., Forster, A., Young, J., Crocker, T., Benham, A., & Langhorne, P. (2015). Medical day hospital care for older people versus alternative forms of care. *Cochrane Database of Systematic Reviews, 6*, CD001730.

Crocker, T., Forster, A., Young, J., Brown, L., Ozer, S., Smith, J., …, & Greenwood, D. C. (2013). Physical rehabilitation for older people in long-term care. *Cochrane Database of Systematic Reviews, 2*, CD004294.

Department of Health. (2000). *The NHS plan. A plan for investment. A plan for reform* [online]. London: Stationery Office. Retrieved from: https://webarchive.nationalarchives.gov.uk/20130124064356/ http://www.dh.gov.uk/prod_consum_dh/groups/dh_digitalassets/@dh/@en/@ps/documents/digitalasset/dh_118522.pdf (Accessed 11 August 2019).

Department of Health. (2001). *National service framework for older people* [online]. London: Department of Health. Retrieved from https://assets.publishing.service.gov.uk/government/uploads/system/uploads/attachment_data/file/198033/National_Service_Framework_for_Older_People.pdf (Accessed 11 August 2019).

Enderby, P., & John, A. (2015). *Therapy outcome measures for rehabilitation professionals* (3rd edn.). Guildford: J&R Publications.

Forster, A., & Young, J. (2011). Community rehabilitation for older people: day hospital or home-based services. *Age and Ageing, 40*(1), 2–4.

Glendinning, C., Jones, K., Baxter, K., Rabiee, P., Curtis, L., Wilde, A., Arksey, H., & Forder, J. (2010). *Home care re-ablement services: investigating the longer-term impacts (prospective longitudinal study)* [online]. University of York Social Policy Research Unit. Retrieved from https://www.york.ac.uk/inst/spru/research/pdf/Reablement.pdf (Accessed 11 August 2019).

Gonçalves-Bradley, D. C., Iliffe, S., Doll, H. A., Broad, J., Gladman, J., Langhorne, P., Richards, S. H., & Shepperd, S. (2017). Early discharge hospital at home. *Cochrane Database of Systematic Reviews, 6*, CD000356.

Holder, H., Kumpunen, S., Castle-Clarke, S., & Lombardo, S. (2018). *Managing the hospital and social care interface: Interventions targeting older adults* [online]. London: Nuffield Trust. Retrieved from https://www.nuffieldtrust.org.uk/files/2018-03/hospital-and-social-care-interface-final-web.pdf (Accessed 11 August 2019).

Holditch, C. (2018). *National Audit of Intermediate Care 2018: Key Findings* [online]. NHS Benchmarking Network. Retrieved from http://www.careengland.org.uk/sites/careengland/files/NAIC%202018findings%20FINAL.pdf (Accessed 10 July 2019).

Leeds City Council. (2019). *Recovery hubs for older people* [online]. Leeds: Leeds City Council. Retrieved from https://www.leeds.gov.uk/residents/health-and-social-care/adult-social-care/care-homes-and-housing-options/recovery-hubs-for-older-people (Accessed 14 July 2019).

National Institute for Health and Care Excellence. (2017). *Intermediate care including reablement* [online]. London: National Institute for Health and Care Excellence. Retrieved from https://www.nice.org.uk/guidance/ng74/resources (Accessed 10 July 2019).

NHS Benchmarking Network. (2017). *National Audit of Intermediate Care* [online]. London: NHS Benchmarking Network. Retrieved from https://www.nhsbenchmarking.nhs.uk/naic-resources-key-documents (Accessed 10 July 2019).

Rothschild, J. M., Bates, D. W., & Leape, L. L. (2000). Preventable medical injuries in older patients. *Archives of Internal Medicine, 160*(18), 2717–2728.

Shepperd, S., Iliffe, S., Doll, H. A., Clarke, M. J., Kalra, L., Wilson, A. D., & Gonçalves-Bradley, D. C. (2016). Admission avoidance hospital at home. *Cochrane Database of Systematic Reviews, 9*, CD007491.

64

Palliative Rehabilitation

Emily Stowe

LEARNING OBJECTIVES

- Describe the key principles of rehabilitation in palliative care
- Explain who delivers palliative care in different settings
- Describe goal setting and treatment planning in palliative care
- Explain the psychological impact of living with a palliative diagnosis and the impact on rehabilitation

CASE

Dorothy is a 76-year-old lady with breast cancer which has metastasised to her lung and bones. It is not curable and she is being treated palliatively. She has bone metastases in her spine, pelvis and right femur, for which she has had radiotherapy. Her main symptoms are pain in her right hip which is restricting her mobility, significant fatigue and breathlessness on exertion. She is currently able to walk about 50 yards with a wheeled frame before she needs to sit down. She is fairly bright in mood most of the time but is struggling emotionally with the restrictions her functional impairments are placing on her. She lives in her own home and has carers twice a day to help with personal care. Her son lives nearby and visits most days to see her. Until recently she was still driving and was very involved in local village life, including an active social life and collecting her grandchildren from school each day.

WHAT IS PALLIATIVE CARE?

The World Health Organization defines palliative care as 'an approach that improves the quality of life of patients and their families facing the problems associated with life-threatening illness, through the prevention and relief of suffering by means of early identification and impeccable assessment and treatment of pain and other problems, physical, psychosocial and spiritual' (World Health Organization, 2019).

Palliative care is available to anyone with life-limiting illness, not just those with cancer, for example motor neurone disease, chronic obstructive pulmonary disease, heart failure or kidney failure. There is also increasing interest in developing models of care for those who may be termed older adults with frailty and multiple comorbidities (Help the Hospices Commission into the Future of Hospice Care, 2013). Historically palliative care was associated with the care of people in the last days or weeks of life; however, an individual can receive palliative care at any point from the diagnosis of a life-limiting condition to death.

WHO PROVIDES PALLIATIVE CARE?

Palliative care is provided by two distinct groups of health and social care professionals:

- Those who provide day to day care of people in their homes, care homes or hospitals (for example, community allied health professionals, GPs and district nurses)
- Specialist palliative care professionals who are usually based within a hospice or specialist team in a hospital or community setting.

An individual patient's requirements for specialist palliative care will depend upon how complex their health and care needs are and whether the generalist health and social care professionals are able to meet these needs. Professionals working with the older patient in any environment need to be aware of the specific needs of patients with a palliative diagnosis.

Specialist palliative care teams are usually multidisciplinary, often consisting of doctors, nurses, physiotherapists, occupational therapists, psychologists, chaplains and social workers. Most hospices provide services in both inpatient and outpatient settings, as well as community-based services. It is useful for rehabilitation professionals to know what services are available in their local area and how to refer on when appropriate.

In Dorothy's case, she is likely to have some input from her local hospice to help support her with complex pain management and emotional support, possibly accessing outpatient or day services. However, she is also likely to have contact with her general practitioner, district nursing team, community physiotherapists and occupational therapists to help her manage her functional limitations at home. All of these professionals can have a positive impact on her palliative rehabilitation and therefore her quality of life.

WHAT IS PALLIATIVE REHABILITATION?

The terms 'palliative care' and 'rehabilitation' may appear to be two opposite ends of a spectrum. However, it must be remembered that a palliative diagnosis does not mean that

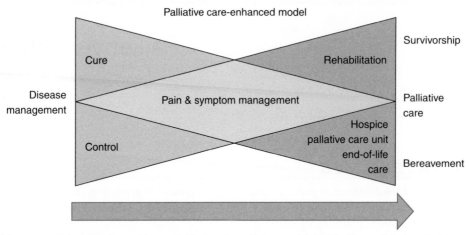

FIG. 64.1 Rehabilitation within a Palliative Care-Enhanced Model. (From Cristian A. *Central Nervous System Cancer Rehabilitation*, 1st edn. Elsevier Inc; 2019, with permission.)

an individual has lost all ability to improve or maintain their function. Fig. 64.1 shows where rehabilitation fits within the Palliative Care-Enhanced Model. Palliative rehabilitation is usually delivered by allied health professionals with a speciality in palliative care.

'Rehabilitative palliative' care is a slightly different term, describing an approach, taken by a whole multidisciplinary team to the provision of care to an individual and has been described as follows:

'Rehabilitative Palliative Care aims to optimise people's function and wellbeing and to enable them to live as independently and fully as possible, with choice and autonomy, within the limitations of advancing illness. It is an approach that empowers people to adapt to their new state of being with dignity and provides an active support system to help them anticipate and cope constructively with losses resulting from deteriorating health' (Tiberini & Richardson, 2015).

GOAL SETTING AND TREATMENT PLANNING IN PALLIATIVE REHABILITATION

For healthcare professionals who are new to palliative care or for whom palliative care is just one part of the care they provide in their day to day work, goal setting and planning treatment can be the biggest challenge. As rehabilitation professionals we are usually focused on restoring function to as near to pre-morbid state as possible and this can be difficult to adapt in the face of progressive deterioration. Goal setting within palliative care should be focused on what is meaningful and important to an individual, rather than being focused on a professional's agenda. It may be helpful to ask questions such as:

- What would you like to be able to do?
- What do you usually enjoy doing?
- What are you happy to have help with?
- Who or what is important to you? (Eva, 2013)

These types of questions enable people to really focus on what is significant to them and basing rehabilitation care

planning around the answers will help to facilitate adherence to treatment.

It is important to recognise the difference between hopes and goals. Goals can be SMART (specific, measurable, achievable, realistic and time-bound) and can provide focus, both for patients and their healthcare team. However, when asked what their goals are, people will often state activities that healthcare professionals feel are unrealistic within their current limitations. These may be better described as hopes.

Hopes are things that someone would like, but may not have complete control over (Eva, 2013). For example, I may make a goal to save 5% of my income each month towards paying for a holiday at the end of the year, but hope that I win the lottery in the meantime! Both hopes and goals can be useful for people living with a palliative diagnosis as they can provide a sense of optimism for the future, alongside acknowledgment of the challenges they face at the present time. It can be useful within a rehabilitation context to recognise both hopes and goals. Research has suggested that supporting older adults to adjust to transitions and losses as well as maintaining relationships and spiritual connections may help them maintain hope and deal with their experiences (Duggleby et al., 2012).

Different types of goals may be appropriate at different stages of someone's disease and the focus of treatment may shift along with these goals (Tiberini & Richardson, 2015). Descriptions of the different stages and goals that may be set for Dorothy are provided in Table 64.1.

Treatment planning in palliative care can be difficult, particularly for those with less experience in working with people who are dying. With the older adult this can be further complicated by having multiple medical conditions. Professionals often find it difficult to plan for an uncertain future – do we push for improvement in a patient who may never improve? Are we creating false hope by providing a rehabilitation programme? However, the very nature of having an uncertain future means that prognosis could be longer than we expect, therefore avoiding rehabilitation can mean that

TABLE 64.1 Potential rehabilitation goals.

STAGE OF DISEASE	GOAL
Restorative Goals – aim to restore patients to previous level of function	To be able to walk to local school (approximately 300 yards) to collect my grandchildren within 2 weeks
Preventative Goals – attempt to prevent avoidable deterioration in function related to disease or treatment processes	To continue to walk 50 yards twice a day (to the end of the garden and back) – ongoing
Supportive Goals – focus on maximising function, independence and participation in meaningful activities alongside disability	To ask a friend to give me a lift to meet up with a group of friends twice a week for coffee and cake – ongoing
Palliative Goals – involve supporting people to adapt to and come to terms with irreversible changes in function	To purchase mobility scooter and gain confidence in using it, to a point at which I feel confident to pick up my grandchildren from school on it – within 3 weeks

those with potential to improve or maintain function miss out on this vital opportunity. A balanced view of 'hoping for the best, whilst planning for the worst' can be useful in these scenarios. For example, giving someone a functional exercise programme to strengthen their legs if they have become weaker in their transfers, whilst also providing appropriate equipment, aids and support so that if transfers continue to worsen, they can remain safe and secure in their daily activities. Where appropriate, patients' families should be involved in this process to ensure they understand what rehabilitation is aiming to achieve and why.

PSYCHOSOCIAL AND SPIRITUAL NEEDS OF OLDER ADULTS IN PALLIATIVE CARE

Living with a palliative diagnosis can cause significant psychological, social and spiritual distress, not only for the person living with the condition, but for their family, friends and loved ones. Impending death can cause people to experience a range of emotions and they may swing very rapidly between two seemingly opposite emotions, such as denial and acknowledgement. Whilst you may expect that knowing one's time is short would create great pain and sadness, for some it can bring peace and an opportunity to reflect on the positive aspects of their life.

When designing rehabilitation programmes, it is important to try to explore how the individual is feeling, to acknowledge that a range of emotions may be 'normal' and to

provide space for the person to express this. Asking someone to self-manage and take on a home exercise programme when they are in a state of despair and collapse is likely to fail. If there is significant distress, other health professionals such as psychologists, psychotherapists or chaplaincy services may need to support the patient through this, either alongside or before a physical rehabilitation programme for it to have maximum benefit. However, for many people, a kind, trustworthy and empathic listening ear may be sufficient to help them to cope with their emotions. It is therefore important for rehabilitation professionals to develop some basic listening and counselling skills to enable them to provide a level of psychological support whilst also having an awareness of local services they can refer on to for more support if required.

MAKING ADAPTATIONS FOR PALLIATIVE PATIENTS

Many patients with a palliative diagnosis will have difficulties with symptoms such as breathlessness or fatigue. These may be caused by their primary diagnosis or by other medical conditions. These need to be accounted for within a rehabilitation programme, e.g. by adjusting repetitions of exercises or providing additional opportunities for rest breaks in daily activities. Some non-pharmacological interventions that may be helpful for these symptoms are described in Table 64.2.

TABLE 64.2 Non-pharmacological management of breathlessness and fatigue.

BREATHLESSNESS	FATIGUE
Breathing techniques such as rectangular breathing or pursed lip breathing	Activity pacing advice
Handheld fan	Prioritising activity
Fatigue and activity management	Exercise (adapted to the individual)
Positioning to ease breathlessness	Relaxation techniques
Relaxation techniques or mindfulness	Information on sleep hygiene
Equipment provision	Equipment provision

REHABILITATION AT THE END OF LIFE

For some patients it may be appropriate for rehabilitation professionals to be involved in their care in their last few days or weeks of life. This may be, for example, to facilitate discharge to their preferred place of death or to provide management of symptoms such as pain, breathlessness or troublesome secretions. It may also be that a professional who has been involved in someone's care can provide ongoing psychological support to the patient and their family, even if they are not providing any rehabilitation. It is vitally important that access to rehabilitation professionals at this point in life is rapid and uncomplicated to ensure that needs are met in a timely fashion. It is also helpful for professionals to be aware of local bereavement support services to be able to direct patients' friends or family to if required.

SUMMARY POINTS

- Palliative care is for anybody with a life-limiting illness, not just cancer and can be applicable at an early stage of the disease
- It is important to adjust rehabilitation goal setting and treatment planning to ensure that patient preferences are prioritised, allowing space for hopes alongside more realistic goals
- The psychological impact of living with a life-limiting diagnosis must be acknowledged, and professionals should ensure they provide an appropriate level of support
- Non-pharmacological interventions for specific symptoms such as breathlessness and fatigue can be helpful in palliative patients

MCQs

Q.1 Palliative care improves the quality of life of patients and their families by means of assessment and treatment of which of the following problems?
  a. Physical problems
  b. Psychosocial problems
  c. Spiritual problems
  d. All of the above
Q.2 Who provides palliative care?
  a. Specialist hospices
  b. District nurses
  c. All healthcare professionals who may be involved in care
  d. Specialist teams
Q.3 Rehabilitation goals in palliative care can be broken down into the following stages:
  a. Restorative, preventative, supportive, palliative
  b. Rehabilitative, preventative, supportive, deteriorating
  c. Restorative, prehabilitative, sensitive, palliative
  d. Prehabilitative, specific, palliative, terminal

REFERENCES

Duggleby, W., Hicks, D., Nekolaichuk, C., Holtslander, L., Williams, A., Chambers, T., & Eby, J. (2012). Hope, older adults and chronic illness: a metasynthesis of qualitative research. *Journal of Advanced Nursing, 68*(6), 1211–1223.

Eva, G. (2013). Goal setting. In J. Taylor, R. Simader, & P. Nieland (Eds.), *Potential and possibility: rehabilitation at end of life* (pp. 39–41). Munich, Germany: Urban and Fischer.

Help the Hospices Commission into the future of hospice care. (2013). *Future needs and preferences for hospice care: challenges and opportunities for hospices* [online]. London: Hospice UK. Retrieved from https://www.hospiceuk.org/docs/default-source/ default-document-library/future-needs-and-preferences-for-hospice-care-challenges-and-opportunities-for-hospices.pdf (Accessed 28 January 2019).

Tiberini, R., & Richardson, H. (2015). *Rehabilitative palliative care. Enabling people to live fully until they die: a challenge for the 21st century.* London: Hospice UK. Retrieved from https://www. hospiceuk.org/what-we-offer/clinical-and-care-support/rehabilitative-palliative-care/resources-for-rehabilitative-palliative-care (Accessed 28 January 2019).

World Health Organization. (2019). *WHO definition of palliative care* [online]. World Health Organization. Retrieved from https://www.who.int/cancer/palliative/definition/en/ (Accessed 28 January 2019).

65

The Ageing Athlete

Howard J. Luks

LEARNING OBJECTIVES

- Explain how older athletes can maintain their level of fitness

- Describe the particular needs of older athletes in rehabilitation

CASE

Cathy is a 76-year-old woman who has been running for decades. She loved to run for many different reasons, but she was finding it increasingly challenging to finish a course in the allotted time. She had no intention of stopping and was very interested in addressing strategies to help her maintain her running habits deep into her elder years. She said "Trail running has long been my happy place. Actually, any form of running enables me to start my day invigorated and ready to go. Regular exercise has so many upsides".

INTRODUCTION

With population ageing comes a certain increase in the amount of ill health. However, it also brings a growing number of older people who maintain fitness for longer than ever before. This brief chapter focuses on those older people who have been particularly athletic and still possess such prowess in older age. They may have particularly high rehabilitation goals. They may have injuries that occur more usually in people many years younger due to their high levels of physical activity. This demonstrates the need for individualising their rehabilitation approach.

Exercising so that we can live longer is a draw for a few. Most master athletes exercise because they have to. They thrive on the hormone rush that follows, they thrive on the brain clearing effects of a walk/run through the trees. Older athletes are just as driven as younger superstars. They thrive on the thrill of a race, regardless of pace. They thrive on the way it makes them feel, and they will go to any length to protect their time on the road or the trail.

Plainly stated, you have to make it to a certain age to become a master athlete; it sounds cruel, but it is true. A Western lifestyle and diet are not likely to help you achieve that milestone. You cannot outrun, outexercise or medicate away a bad diet. Fad diets are the rage, but typically do not lead to sustained lifestyle changes. Eating real food, less of it, and getting enough fibre in your diet to support your gut is clearly advantageous. The earlier in life that you focus on your diet and lifestyle, the more likely you are to have the ability to become a master athlete.

THE EFFECT OF AGEING ON THE MUSCULOSKELETAL SYSTEM: SARCOPENIA

During our more formative years, we laced up and ran outside. We did not worry about balance, strength, muscle tone and energy. As the athlete ages, these become very important issues to address proactively. Sarcopenia is the process of age-related muscle loss. Starting in our 30s, we begin to lose a percentage of our muscle mass each and every year. Muscle mass is not only critical to performance, but also predicts longevity and a longer healthspan. Simply put, your healthspan is the number of years that you live relatively disease free, free of neurocognitive decline and free of a chronic disease burden which threatens your quality of life. A longer lifespan does not necessarily equal a longer healthspan (see Fig. 65.1).

Resistance exercise is a must for the ageing athlete. A short well-balanced programme consisting of calf exercises, squats, bridges, biceps curls and shoulder exercises is critical to both reverse the changes of sarcopenia and maintain our current muscle mass. As we age our body has a harder time making enough protein to suit our needs. Our nutritional requirement for protein increases as we age. Unless you suffer from kidney disease, the average master athlete should be getting a minimum of 1.4–2 g of protein per kilogram of body weight. A contemporary body of research shows that the timing of that protein intake is not critical. So, you do not need to bring that protein shake with you to the gym or track.

THE EFFECTS OF AGEING ON THE MUSCULOSKELETAL SYSTEM: BALANCE

As we age, our ability to balance and stabilise ourselves diminishes. This is a far more serious problem than most people realise. While chronic disease sets us up for a diminished healthspan, injuries sustained as the result of a fall and the downtime to recover from those injuries significantly affect

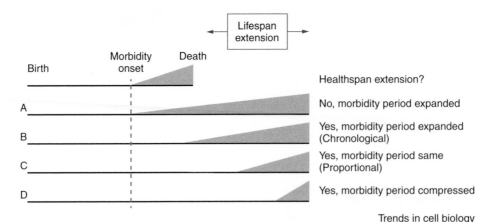

FIG. 65.1 Longer lifespan does not always equal longer healthspan. In some cases, morbidity (illness from medical conditions) is expanded. The preferred option is to have compression of morbidity into the last phase of life. (From Hansen M, Kennedy BK. Does longer lifespan mean longer healthspan? *Trends Cell Biol.* 2016;26(8):565–8, with permission).

our health and longevity. Diminishing our fall risk starts with an active balance training programme. These do not need to be elaborate gym-based programmes. There are plenty of balance exercises we can perform in the comfort of our home. Standing on one leg for 30 seconds can be challenging enough. When that becomes easy, perturb the system; start to move your arms around while one leg is raised. You will notice an improvement in your balance and control within a few weeks. Switch legs every minute. Carry small cans or weights in your hands when body weight alone becomes too easy. You will feel more surefooted and confident after these exercises. Your fall risk will diminish with this programme, and you will have diminished the risk of injury after a fall with your resistance exercise programme.

REHABILITATION AFTER INJURY OR ILLNESS

Which Exercise is Best?

Simply put, the best exercise is the one that you will enjoy and continue pursuing because you enjoy it. Different exercises offer different benefits. Research shows that we only need to walk for 15–20 minutes a day to start to see the benefits of exercise (Piercy et al., 2018). For many of us that might be enough. For others, it will not be. Many love to swim. Swimming provides an excellent combined aerobic and resistance-based exercise. You will maintain muscle mass, improve your heart function, lower your blood pressure, lower your cholesterol and improve your glucose management with any aerobic exercise programme. Cycling and running are also great exercise programmes. They offer the same benefits of other aerobic exercises, but you will still need to work on balance and resistance exercises.

Rest Is a Relative Term

"You should rest." How many times have you heard that? From an orthopaedic perspective, the term rest is a relative term. If you are used to running 30 miles/week and something bothers you, then "rest" might mean running on 10–15

miles per week. If you are used to running 10-minute miles, then you may need to run 12-minute miles. The same goes for resistance training. Absolute rest and ceasing all activities is almost never necessary. You will lose the aerobic or strength benefits of your training very rapidly. A few weeks of no activity and you are set back months in terms of the level you were training at.

Understanding Recovery Is Critical

The concept of recovery is poorly understood. Have you noticed that the day after a particularly long walk, ride or jog your heart rate is a little higher, or perhaps you are a little short of breath? Your body is telling you that it needs to have a lighter day. Recovery, just like rest, is a relative issue. If you rode your bike 40 miles the day before, then a recovery ride might only be 4 miles. If you jogged 5 miles, then a recovery day might be a 1-mile walk. At least 1 or 2 days a week you should let your body completely rest from resistance or pushing your aerobic thresholds. That does not mean you cannot hike or take a walk. It simply means that you need to let your heart and muscles recover and repair themselves from your activity over the past week.

Does Exercise Cause Arthritis?

No, exercise does not cause arthritis. Quite the opposite; runners have a lower incidence of arthritis when compared to a matched group of less active peers. It turns out that your cartilage or the cushioning in your knees thrives on the cyclical loading of running. If you already have osteoarthritis or some degeneration in your knee, then let pain be your guide. It may be best to cross train with swimming or cycling if your arthritis is advanced enough that running simply hurts too much to pursue.

Is It OK to Exercise with Pain?

This is a very important issue for the older athlete. Many will have discomfort with certain activities. More often than not you should not stop exercising. There are no overuse tendon issues that are treated with rest. Our tendons can start to bother us for many reasons, but stopping an exercise programme is rarely in your best interest. Stopping your exercises will result in loss of heart health, loss of muscle mass, loss of endurance and often make it harder to get back into your exercise programme. Aches and pains are often just a mild annoyance or nuisance. Exercise or physiotherapy is often the best way to address them. Again, rest is rarely the right answer. Now that comes with a caveat. If you think of a pain scale from 0 to 10, with 0 being no pain; if you have pain during activity and you would rate it under 4 then it is generally okay to continue exercising. If you have pain that concerns you, then you should see your practitioner. If you do choose to see a doctor, you must remember to ask if rest is necessary. If they say yes, then ask how long, and what are the potential downsides of not resting. For example, groin pain with certain exercises could potentially indicate a stress fracture of the hip. You should not exercise with a stress fracture of your hip. But groin pain can also be due to a muscle strain. The best treatment for a muscle strain is to stretch and strengthen it. So do not be afraid to ask your doctor pointed questions about what they believe the source of your pain is, how are they going to prove it and whether or not continuing to exercise puts you at risk of developing a more serious injury.

In the end, the vast majority of senior athletes do not need to stop their exercises for mild aches and pains. You want to avoid potentially problematic issues like a stress fracture, but you never want the risk of the treatment to be higher than the risk of the injury. So take it upon yourself to ask what your doctor believes might be the cause of your pain. Have them clarify if any further tests are needed. Ask them if rest is absolutely needed. You will need a solid plan and goal if you aim to continue your happy exercise pursuits for years to come.

SUMMARY POINTS

- Exercise is critical to achieving our best possible health; the best exercise is the one you enjoy doing
- Speak with your doctor to be sure you can start an exercise programme
- Age-related muscle loss can be corrected, but it requires resistance exercises
- Balance training is critical to minimise the risk of falling
- Physiotherapy is often effective at treating the pain associated with degenerative tears

MCQs

Q.1 Which of the following is important for older athletes?
   a. Resistance exercises
   b. Balance training
   c. Appropriate protein intake
   d. Maintaining a healthy diet
   e. All of the above

Q.2 Which of the following is true about exercise for older athletes?
   a. Pain is not a deterrent
   b. Absolute rest is healthy

   c. Physiotherapy can help with pain from degenerative disease
   d. Exercise should be avoided in the presence of arthritis
   e. A few weeks of no activity helps with recovery after minor injury

REFERENCES

Piercy, K. L., Troiano, R. P., Ballard, R. M., Carlson, S. A., Fulton, J. E., Galuska, D. A., George, S. M., & Olson, R. D. (2018). The physical activity guidelines for Americans. *JAMA, 320*(19), 2020–2028.

Planning for Discharge

66

Discharge Planning: When, How and Who?

Adam Gordon & Elinor Burn

LEARNING OBJECTIVES

- Describe the process of discharge planning for a patient undergoing rehabilitation
- Explain the role of different team members in the discharge planning process
- Identify the variety of factors that can delay discharge and explain how to proactively address these
- List the different discharge destinations and how each can affect planning
- Outline features of the discharge documentation and communication of the plan to relevant parties

CASE

June, an 80-year-old lady, was admitted to hospital after falling at home. She sustained a pubic ramus fracture (in her pelvic bone). She had always been independent and managed to look after herself, with her son visiting twice a week to deliver food and check on her.

Once admitted, June struggled to get out of bed or to the toilet due to pain. She made slow progress with the therapy staff in hospital. She moved to an intermediate care facility in a community hospital.

Upon arrival, the multidisciplinary team (MDT) conducted a full assessment with June. She was determined to return home, valued her independence and felt an important part of her community through her role as a neighbourhood watch coordinator. She was assessed to have capacity to make decisions about her discharge destination. The MDT set a predicted date of discharge (PDD) for 14 days after admission and told Jean and her family about this.

Jean's son had concerns about her falls risk and some forgetfulness. He reported occasional 'near misses' when she had tripped over hazards at home, infrequent episodes of missed medication doses and forgotten meals in recent weeks.

Potential solutions to the safety concern were discussed with June and her son. A home visit was performed by an occupational therapist (OT). They made suggestions about carer support and some home adaptations. Her son still had concerns but accepted that this was the best compromise taking account of June's ambitions to return to her previous life.

In preparation for discharge, a dosette box adherence aid for her medications was organised. A discharge letter from her rehabilitation facility was written to her GP highlighting the need to review her cognition in the future, and to consider a memory service referral if appropriate.

June was able to be discharged back to her own home.

WHY DO IT?

Discharge planning is crucial when coordinating services for patients' return to home. Successful planning allows health and social care needs to be met on discharge, and can enable continuation of medical and rehabilitation care in the community to minimise disruption as patients move between hospital and home. Effective planning can reduce the length of hospital stays and the likelihood of readmission (Shepherd et al., 2004).

Hospital stays are often associated with a reduction in functional ability, such as the ability to wash and dress independently. This can be due to a sudden change in the abilities of an individual following an acute medical illness, or a consequence of deconditioning related to the demands of a hospital stay. Patients often require modifications to community support arrangements even if they had comprehensive care before. This can be temporary, whilst a patient rehabilitates and recovers, or more permanent. Successful discharge planning improves patient and carer satisfaction (Nazareth et al., 2001; Weinberger, Oddone, & Henderson, 1996) when patients are central to the process.

WHEN TO DO IT?

Discharge planning should begin at the point of admission and efforts should escalate closer to the end of the inpatient stay (Bowker, Price, & Smith, 2012).

Defining and sharing a PDD early in the stay is important to manage expectations and coordinate efforts. It sets a timescale so the MDT can coordinate rehabilitation efforts and discharge planning. It can also help set and manage patient and family expectations and enable them to prepare emotionally and practically for discharge.

The PDD should be revised, and the revised date shared, if medical status or progress with rehabilitation changes. When the PDD is changed all team members, the patient and their carers must be informed and the rationale for change explained. For families and patients preparing for discharge, uncertainty generated by bringing discharge forward can be tempered by explanation of how this reflects, for example, more rapid recovery. If discharge is delayed, it is important to realise that this can cause disappointment and to explain the need for a longer stay and how the patient will benefit.

In many healthcare sectors, there is emphasis on planning with patients for discharge earlier in their recovery trajectory than would have traditionally been possible. The Discharge to Assess (or Transfer to Assess) model takes account of extensive rehabilitation resources available in the community. Traditionally initial assessment, with delineation of rehabilitation and recovery goals, would happen in an inpatient setting. Discharge to Assess asserts that once a patient is medically stable, they can move either to their own home or a community rehabilitation setting, where a better understanding of their rehabilitation needs can be established. This approach is new to many patients and their families, and careful explanation is required.

HOW TO DO IT?

Communicate

Begin by discussing the wishes for discharge **with the patient** and their family or carers. Because patients receiving rehabilitation are often dependent upon support from families on discharge from hospital, principles of relationship-centred care (Table 66.1) can be a useful to guide discussions, recognising that addressing the needs of family carers can be important to supporting and maintaining a patient on discharge. This avoids the tendency of medical discharge planning to be reductive and focussed on pathology and deficits.

At a more practical level, patients and families are important sources of collateral history about functioning and lifestyle prior to the current illness. Understanding the extent and nature of change in function can shape discharge plans.

Take a Holistic Approach

The International Classification of Functioning, Disability and Health (Gladman, 2008) is useful when developing a discharge plan, as it is throughout rehabilitation (Table 66.2).

Discharge decisions can be complicated and involve a complex understanding of clinical risk. Assessment of a patient's mental capacity (see Chapter 20 Brain Health and Mental Capacity) is often important and should be guided by relevant laws. It is important to review the home environment and any new care needs (see Chapter 68 The Home Environment Assessment, and Chapter 69 Home Supports) to judge environmental adaptations and support that may be needed.

Traditionally discharge planning meetings (see Chapter 67 Care Planning Meetings) were central to discharge discussions. In fast-paced modern healthcare settings, these can be cumbersome to organise and are possibly best reserved for particularly difficult discussion around complicated or expensive changes to care. The principles that guide good

TABLE 66.1	The Senses Framework - A model of relationship-centred care (Nolan, 2006).
SENSE	**QUESTIONS TO ASK** **WHAT DOES THE PATIENT AND CARER NEED....**
Safety	...to feel safe physically, psychologically and existentially?
Belonging	...to feel part of a valued group, to maintain or form important relationships?
Continuity	...to be able to make links between their past, present and future?
Purpose	...to enjoy meaningful activity and to feel their goals are valued?
Achievement	...to achieve the goals that they value?
Significance	...to feel that they 'matter' and are accorded value and status?

TABLE 66.2	The ICF framework in discharge planning.
ICF DOMAIN	**IMPORTANCE IN DISCHARGE PLANNING**
Body structure and function	What specific accommodations are required to take account of abnormality of body structure or function? Examples might include catheter or stoma care, or specific dressings.
Activity	What support or adaptations does the patient require to engage in both basic (e.g. personal hygiene, eating, mobility) and extended (e.g. cooking, cleaning, driving) activities of daily living?
Participation	What support or adaptations does the patient require to participate in important activities and social interactions (e.g. sports, hobbies, social events, going to church)?
Environment	What sort of environment does the patient have to live in upon discharge? This includes the built environment and the availability of family and peer support, both of which can be a barrier or facilitator to discharge planning.
Personal	How do the patient's personality and beliefs affect discharge planning? Are they determinedly independent and likely to push help away, or do they prefer lots of help and assistance?

discharge planning meetings – multidisciplinary representation, open and transparent communication, honesty about prognosis and anticipated outcomes, and empowering patients and families to take part in shared decisions – should also guide the more flexible, iterative conversations that define modern discharge planning. Discharge discussions should cover risk of readmission to hospital, the contexts in which this might be appropriate, and circumstances which can be managed effectively in the community (Chu & Pei, 1999).

Discussion about rehabilitation after discharge (see Chapter 72 Continuing Rehabilitation at Home) is important to manage expectations. Patients should be told that recovery takes time. Discharge to a community setting often represents continuation of a rehabilitation process, rather than "discharge from rehabilitation".

A frequently neglected step in discharge planning is advance care planning (see Chapter 74 Advance Care Planning), which can be used to understand wishes about future treatment. Discharge from hospital can be an emotionally and cognitively challenging time and professionals should resist the temptation to "force" advance care planning discussions. In most health services, there are community-based colleagues who can take conversations forward later, particularly if prompted by discharge paperwork.

WHO IS INVOLVED?

MDT members need to understand how they each contribute to the broader endeavour of discharge planning, and the need to consult with each other before making promises to patients or their relatives. Table 66.3 outlines the roles.

POTENTIAL DELAYS

Discharge planning can be disrupted by sudden changes in circumstance. It is important that professionals, patients and carers do not see these as defeat but, rather, as part of

---

TABLE 66.3 Multidisciplinary team members and roles in discharge planning.

Patient	Central to the decision making and the focus of care
Family or caregiver	Support the wishes and decision making, and may become their advocate
Doctor	Manage medical issues, optimise treatments, encourage shared decision making and authorise the discharge. In most healthcare settings, have final responsibility for the patient.
Nurse	Often have the most comprehensive overview of patient care. Act as an important coordinator of care and discharge planning. Role in therapy, e.g. through skill rehearsal. Act as a point of contact for patient and relatives on behalf of the MDT. Educate about medication and current nursing needs. Liaise with community nursing services, or nurses at step-down rehabilitation facilities.
Social worker	Assess social care needs and organise an appropriate care package. This can extend to advice on care homes if needed. Can advise on financial implications of care. Often attend to safeguarding issues. Role in crisis management and can plan ahead for periods of respite care if a need is anticipated.
Physiotherapist	Improve physical functioning, address adaptation and prevention methods (e.g. for falls), provide motivation and rehearse skills. Evaluate patient's progress and identify when they have reached a plateau or when further therapy can be performed in the community.
Occupational therapist	Assess functional status and environment (e.g. with a home visit) and identify ways that an individual can adapt to maintain their function. Assess memory and impact of any cognitive impairment.
Pharmacist	Advise on all aspects of prescribing. Particularly useful in polypharmacy. Can organise adherence aids and ensure these are supported by community pharmacists on discharge.
SLT (speech and language therapist)	Assessment of swallowing and communication disorders. Advise patients and families of alternatives (diet formulations, communication boards, non-verbal methods). May liaise with community-based SLT services regarding ongoing rehabilitation needs.
Dietician	Assess nutritional problems and create tailor-made plans for the individual to encourage intake. May send patient home with specific dietetic interventions and a plan for community follow-up.
Clinical psychologist	Assess behaviour, design cognitive interventions, aid in adjusting to health challenges. Provide psychological therapy interventions.
Discharge coordinator	Act as a liaison between ward staff, wider MDT and community care givers, and are important in complex discharges. Not present in all systems.
GP or community care coordinator	Lead caregivers after discharge. It is important that they are involved with discharge decisions and are aware of the planned follow-up.

ill health, rehabilitation and recovery. Timely recognition, management and mitigation are core competencies for a rehabilitation team.

Some common delays include:

- Health

A change in mobility status, e.g. non-weight-bearing after a fracture, or a change in cognitive status, e.g. new brain injury can define new care needs to be considered during discharge planning.

Inpatient stays are associated with a risk of hospital-acquired infection, e.g. pneumonia, and the development of delirium. These complications can create a sudden delay to planned discharge.

- Failure to recognise care needs

Acute admissions to hospital can be the result of a crisis situation. Simple solutions, e.g. a single piece of equipment or slight change to existing care package, can sometimes solve these problems, mitigating the need for prolonged rehabilitation. Nursing needs may require care adjustment or education rather than rehabilitation.

Medically unwell patients or those in need of end-of-life care should be identified for care to continue in the correct setting. Dementia alone is not a reason to decline rehabilitation, but different approaches and techniques are required (see Chapter 53 Rehabilitation in Dementia).

- Finance

Government policies on welfare, disability, housing and care shape care delivery. In socialised health and social care settings, rationing of community services can reduce immediate availability and create delay. In fee-for-service settings, patients and families may require time to adjust to required expenditure. Even where patients and families do not have to pay, a change in caregiving responsibilities can have financial implications which can take time to work around.

- Change in needs and abilities

Care needs can change over the course of rehabilitation. This can lead to reconfiguration of a previously established discharge plan with subsequent delay.

- Resources

Waiting for space in rehabilitation or reablement services, for household modifications or for new accommodation can all result in delay in resource-constrained health and social care systems.

- Communication or lack of shared understanding

Discharge planning can be filled with difficult decisions, and deliberation over complex choices can create delay. Understanding patient and family perspectives, frequent and open communication, and management of expectations from the point of admission onwards are key to good, supportive care and can avoid delays caused when patients or families become overwhelmed.

DISCHARGE DESTINATIONS

A change in functional ability may require a change in care support, home adaptation, community nursing care or longer-term care placement (Department of Health, 2007).

Potential options include:

- Returning home with no additional care
- Returning home with help from family
- Returning home with help from a home care service
- Intermediate care at home (rehabilitation in a home setting)
- Residential intermediate care (rehabilitation either in a care home or community hospital)
- Long-term care home (nursing home) (see Fig. 66.1).

Most developed health and social care economies have discharge options similar to those described above, although the precise terminologies may differ between countries. The decision about which discharge destination best suits patient needs will be based upon specific rehabilitation goals, the configuration of medical and allied health professionals required to deliver them, and the preferences and personal circumstances of patients and families.

Rehabilitation in settings other than hospital is comparable in terms of outcomes and likely to be both cheaper and associated with equivalent or higher levels of patient

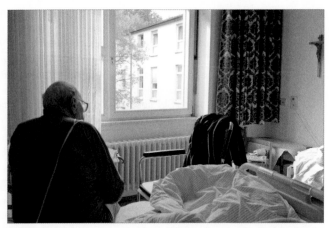

FIG. 66.1 Nursing homes provide care for those whose needs cannot be met at home. (From Stewart,R. Reducing depression in nursing homes: so little, so late. *Lancet.* 2013 29;381(9885):2227–8, with permission.)

satisfaction (Oliver, 2014). It is important that these are recognised as venues for the specialised care, rather than a mechanism to move patients out of hospital.

PRACTICALITIES FOR HEALTH STAFF

Prior to Discharge

Prepare all discharge communications. Inpatient assessments and rehabilitation plans should be communicated in a comprehensive way to all relevant community stakeholders. Remember to include care home staff in discharge communications as they will be pivotal in supporting day-to-day care delivery after discharge. If local policies demand explicit consent to include these team members, then establish this with the patient. If patients lack capacity to consent to sharing of their information, it is almost always in their best interests to share relevant information with community-based colleagues who will be providing support.

Where possible, written information should be supported by verbal handover.

Getting Ready to Go Home

Equipment and supplies such as mobility aids, home adaptations and assistance devices need to be in place or arranged for delivery. Time to prepare the home space ready for discharge is essential and should not be underestimated. This includes creating space for new equipment, moving items that can cause falls and ensuring that there is a place for family to sit near their relative. It may be necessary to a place to store medication, particularly regulated drugs such as morphine, if the medication regimen has changed.

Other changes, such as new diet consistencies and appropriate foods, and mobility and transfer advice, should be verified with patients, families and carers prior to discharge.

At the point of discharge, follow-up appointments should be identified. These should be included in a complete discharge letter, which should be ready at the time the patient leaves hospital. There can be human error and inaccuracies in these discharge letters (Dawson, Iyengar, & Ferguson, 1998). The MDT can contribute to discharge letters to minimise this. Where possible, one comprehensive summary is preferable to multiple communications.

TOP TIPS

- Start planning from the beginning of the admission
  - Establish and communicate PDD to the full MDT, the patient and their families.
  - Communicate and explain any changes to PDD.
- Communication
  - Team members need to make decisions about discharge collaboratively, recognising each others' competencies and expertise. No team member should make promises to a patient or their family without understanding others' perspectives.
  - The Senses Framework is a useful way to ensure patient and family perspectives are taken on board and that discharge planning does not become reductive and medical.
- The International Classification of Functioning, Disability and Health is a useful framework to establish and discuss discharge planning needs.

SUMMARY POINTS

- Discharge planning helps to improve the coordination of care and services after an inpatient stay, and the transition back to community living
- Successful planning requires anticipation of potential hurdles through proactive problem solving, thorough information gathering and involvement of the correct members of staff
- Close collaboration between the patient, family/caregivers and the whole MDT is crucial

MCQs

Q.1 Discharge planning decisions should be informed by:
   a. The patient's wishes
   b. The ability of the family to support the patient
   c. The environment in which the patient is required to live
   d. Physical deficits and the ability of community-based teams to support these
   e. All of the above

Q.2 Which of the following is true about discharge planning?
   a. It can reduce readmission rates
   b. It leads to longer times before discharge
   c. Families should be involved at the end of the process
   d. Community or primary care teams are not usually involved
   e. A change in health status should not affect it

REFERENCES

Bowker, L., Price, J., & Smith, S. (2012). Rehabilitation. In: *Oxford handbook of geriatric medicine* (pp 71–99). Oxford: Oxford University Press.

Chu, L. W., & Pei, C. K. W. (1999). Risk factors for early emergency hospital readmission in elderly medical patients. *Gerontology*, 45, 220–226.

Dawson, R., Iyengar, N., & Ferguson, C. J. (1998). How good are interim discharge summaries? A prospective audit. *Annual Royal College Surgery England*, 80, 229–231.

Department of Health. (2003). *Discharge from hospital: pathway, process and practice.* Retrieved from http://www.wales.nhs.uk/sitesplus/documents/829/DoH%20-%20Discharge%20Pathway%202003.PDF.

Department of Health. (2007). *National framework for NHS continuing healthcare and NHS-funded nursing care.* Retrieved from https://www.events.england.nhs.uk/upload/entity/30215/national-framework-for-chc-and-fnc-october-2018-revised.pdf.

Gladman, J. R. F. (2008). The International Classification of Functioning, Disability and Health and its value to rehabilitation and geriatric medicine. *Journal of the Chinese Medical Association, 71*(6), 275–278.

Nazareth, I., Burton, A., Shulman, S., Smith, P., Haines, A., & Timberal, H. (2001). A pharmacy discharge plan for hospitalized elderly patients—a randomised controlled trial. *Age Ageing, 30*, 33–40.

Nolan, M., Brown, J., Davies, S., Nolan, J., & Keady, J. (2006). The SENSES framework: improving care for older people through a relationship-centred approach. University of Sheffield.

Oliver, D., Foot, C., & Humphries, R. (2014). *Making health and care systems fit for an ageing population.* London: King's Fund.

Shepherd, S., Parkes, J., McClaren, J., & Phillips, C. (2004). Discharge planning from hospital to home. *Cochrane Database System Review, 1*, CD000313.

Weinberger, M., Oddone, E. Z., & Henderson, W. G. (1996). Does increased access to primary care reduce hospital readmissions? Veterans Affairs Cooperative Study Group on Primary Care and Hospital Readmission. *New England Journal Medicine, 334*, 1441–1447.

FURTHER READING

Age UK 'going into hospital' resource: www.ageuk.org.uk/health-wellbeing/doctors-hospitals/hospital-discharge-arrangements/.

Age UK factsheet about Hospital Discharge: https://www.ageuk.org.uk/globalassets/age-uk/documents/factsheets/fs37_hospital_discharge_fcs.pdf.

Carers UK 'planning the discharge process' resource: www.carersuk.org/help-and-advice/practical-help/coming-out-of-hospital/discharge-planning.

'Hospital to Home' resource pack for all professional sectors that have a role in hospital discharge for older people: housinglin.org.uk/hospital2home_pack/.

Independent Neurorehabilitation Providers Association (INPA). (2019). *Neurorehabilitation in the UK.* Retrieved from https://www.in-pa.org.uk/neurorehabilitation-in-the-uk/.

Katikireddi, S. V., & Cloud, G. C. (2008). Planning a patient's discharge from hospital. *BMJ, 337*, a2694.

New, P. W., Jolley, D. J., Cameron, P. A., Olver, J. H., & Stoelwinder, J. U. (2013). A prospective multicentre study of barriers to discharge from inpatient rehabilitation. *The Medical Journal of Australia, 198*(2), 104–108.

NHS Information for patients leaving hospital: www.nhs.uk/NHSEngland/AboutNHSservices/NHShospitals/Pages/leaving-hospital.aspx.

NHS practical support for carers: www.nhs.uk/CarersDirect/guide/practicalsupport/Pages/hospital-discharge.aspx.

The British Red Cross 'Independent living' services for people when they face a crisis in their daily lives: www.redcross.org.uk/What-we-do/Health-and-social-care/Independent-living.

67

Care Planning Meetings

Richard Wong

LEARNING OBJECTIVES

- Describe core roles of different health professionals in the care planning setting
- Explain the interprofessional approach as a way of integrating the roles of the multiprofessional members
- Outline an effective structure for meeting content and scheduling and the skills and culture for effective collaboration
- Explain the reasons for potential conflict in care planning between the various parties (professionals and stakeholders) and approaches to managing it

The process of devising a tailored discharge plan for rehabilitation patients, most with underlying frailty and multimorbidity, has already been described in Chapter 66. It can bring about modest reductions in length of hospital stay and subsequent emergency readmission as well as improving patient satisfaction (Gonçalves-Bradley et al., 2016). With patients often receiving input from a variety of disciplines and professionals, there are risks to communication and the smooth coordination of care. Indeed, in the United Kingdom, an independent report into the care of older people in the NHS (National Health Service) highlighted failures in discharge planning, particularly around communication, as a key problem (Abraham, 2011). Developing an effective alliance between the various health and social care professionals can reduce such problems, with the evidence suggesting that there are synergistic gains to be made from good interdependent as opposed to independent working (Gage, 1998).

MULTIPROFESSIONAL COLLABORATION – INTERDISCIPLINARY APPROACH

The hallmark of good care planning is the manner in which professionals from various disciplines work together to effect better patient outcomes. Traditionally, true collaborative working was reserved for patients with the most challenging or complex needs with the majority of patients otherwise receiving central administration of care from a physician who might direct nursing and therapy assessments for a patient without much cross-discipline dialogue. Evolving models have since recognised the value of a more collaborative approach for all patients through multiprofessional team meetings; this allows for checks on safety and quality from the wider team and gives rise to natural learning and development across established disciplines with consequent blurring of boundaries that each professional might bring to their assessment process (e.g. physiotherapists and occupational

therapists both being able to assess someone for falls risks, nurses and therapists being able to proposition the ideas of adverse prognosis and counselling patients/family members accordingly) – this is the *Interdisciplinary* approach.

MEETING FREQUENCY AND REQUIRED INFRASTRUCTURE

Most care planning discussions begin within the multiprofessional team setting, whilst additional minicase conferences involving patients/families may occur where there are complexities. Trends are towards a more dynamic multiprofessional dialogue to maintain momentum in care and discharge planning. Thus daily 'Board Rounds' have been promulgated in the UK by the NHS (Emergency Care Intensive Support Team, 2011) and professional bodies (Royal College of Physicians & Royal College of Nursing, 2012), with rounds taking place away from the main clinical area, around a "patient-at-a-glance" whiteboard or screen, facilitating focused, collaborative decision-making.

In acute environments, such rounds are usually short; individuals stand if that facilitates the pace of discussions. In rehabilitation settings, daily board rounds are equally valuable for efficiency and effectiveness of care and discharge planning, but the pace will need to accommodate discussing patient goals and progress in greater detail. Teams might undertake a full daily board round or have one to two in-depth board rounds each week and shorter "business-like" discussions on remaining days. The aim is consistency, including the timing of rounds.

Technology enablers include videoconferencing and systems that record outputs from meetings, logging functional and discharge goals, relevant tasks required to achieve these and decisions on care escalation with key data accessible for "at-a-glance" viewing during meetings. The alternative is a large well-maintained "patient at-a-glance" whiteboard with relevant headings, situated away from public sight.

ROLES WITHIN THE MULTIPROFESSIONAL, INTERDISCIPLINARY TEAM

A list of personnel from the multiprofessional team and a summary of actions they may undertake in preparation for and during care planning meetings are included in the Resources section of this book. Core disciplines would typically include a physician with competencies in managing frail older people (this could be a geriatrician or an internist/general practitioner with appropriate competencies), nurse, physiotherapist, occupational therapist and social worker. Personnel with specific remits on discharge may also be present and have either backgrounds in social or health care (e.g. specialist discharge nurses). Significant structural and cultural re-organisation needs to take place for such teams to have maximum effectiveness, and this will often involve establishing colocation of offices and information/process sharing.

There may also be a role for a range of other healthcare professionals (e.g. pharmacists) or charitable organisations to be involved on a periodic basis in order to assist with selected patients and to maintain awareness amongst the multiprofessional team of relevant support services.

CONDUCTING EFFECTIVE MEETINGS

It is important to be mindful at the outset that the patient is the focus of the care planning meeting; very often the complexities of the health and social care system and also of patient and carer needs mean that it can be easier to look at the most expedient processes that suit the system rather than the patient.

Important foundational principles will support greater effectiveness of the multiprofessional team meetings. Among these are clear leadership and direction of the team, open communication, appropriate infrastructure and resources to support the team, supportive climate (trust, valuing contributions) and systems to monitor performance and outcomes (Nancarrow et al., 2013). There is also a recognition that building effective non-technical skills (NTS) within a healthcare team can improve effectiveness, developing the domains of social (communication, leadership, teamwork), cognitive (situational awareness – see Fig. 67.1, decision-making, mental readiness) and personal resource skills (stress, time and fatigue management) (Ellis & Sevdalis, 2019).

Leadership of the team commonly comes from the physician, but this does not necessarily have to be the case. The skills that are required to be effective include an ability to keep a clear focus and on track through complex discussions, to maintain an appropriate pace of the meeting, be methodical in gaining contributions from the various disciplines, ensuring they feel respected and their opinions have been heard. They will need to be able to deal with conflicting opinions and foster a healthy discussion over the differences that will eventually lead to a broad consensus of opinion. The leader might allocate other tasks during the meetings (e.g. recording of information and plans) or this could be something that is rotated around the rest of the team.

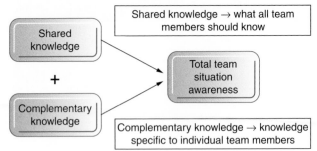

FIG. 67.1 Components of team situation awareness. Members come with shared knowledge and/or complementary knowledge; by the end of the meeting or board round there should be total team situation awareness. (From Crozier MS, Ting HY, Boone DC, et al. Use of human patient simulation and validation of the Team Situation Awareness Global Assessment Technique (TSAGAT): a multidisciplinary team assessment tool in trauma education. *J Surg Educ.* 2015;72(1):156–63, with permission).

A standard and rigorous approach to the meeting helps consistency and typically involves:
- Introducing new or unfamiliar members, explaining their roles and making them feel welcome.
- Critically evaluating the progress for each patient on a daily basis (based on NHS Improvement recommendations) (NHS Improvement, 2017):
  - What information do we need to progress their physical status and function?
  - Is there an activity or discussion that will helpfully progress rehabilitation, eventual discharge or mutual understanding of the patient's further requirements?
  - Review whether progress has been so limited or outlook so poor/uncertain, that arrangements need to be made to discuss limited prognosis and escalation care plans with the patient/family?
- For each patient the physician summarises the medical problems at stake. This should be limited to a list of background comorbidities that might influence long-term function, long-term care delivery and prognosis. A resume may follow about acute medical/surgical problems that have been a factor in recent decompensation of function and where the individual is in the recovery process, anticipated timescales for completion of key treatments and even if not fully recovered, at what stage they may be stable for input from the multiprofessional team. If it is felt that the acute medical problem is unlikely to fully resolve and will significantly impact on prognosis, this needs to be communicated to the wider team so that any necessary functional and adaptive assessments can occur to progress the patient for transition from hospital for supportive/palliative care in the community.
- Nursing feedback is gained on any problems experienced with care delivery (toileting, continence, skin integrity, mood and anxiety, oral intake, swallowing, cognition, behavioural symptoms) and discussions raised on what might be required to address them.
- Therapists outline any information gained around baseline physical function if not already established and comment

on progress with rehabilitation goals and barriers to improvement that might warrant wider input (e.g. fatigue, anxiety, pain).

- The social worker/specialist discharge nurse may highlight known concerns raised from previous contact with community care agencies, provide updates on progress with arranging social care packages or care home placement or where appropriate, provide constructive challenge around existing discharge goals that have been set by the rest of the team.

- Once feedback has been collated and documented, the team works together to agree or clarify the overall aims for the patient (attainment of a treatment or functional goal, place of discharge and required support). A pre-existing aim may need revision if the latest evidence suggests it is no longer as appropriate. Setting an aim might involve balancing varied views. A therapist may feel they are making serial gains with a patient and desire continuation of inpatient therapy. However, a physician who is mindful of a significant life-limiting condition in the same patient, combined with information from a nurse who ascertained that the patient was desperate to be at home, might suggest a compromise of earlier discharge home (for patient satisfaction and quality of life) and if necessary continuing aspects of therapy at home. Such outcomes exemplify team members not only providing objective input from their professional stance but also acting as patient advocates.

- The next steps required to achieve these aims are outlined, and if there are codependencies of actions, then these should be documented in a logical sequential order along with allocation of responsibility for each of these tasks. This provides a comprehensive handover brief that can be picked up by any incoming professionals to the team and allows the relevant information to be sourced from the right person if required. Expected timeframes for completion of steps should be documented (e.g. delivery dates for equipment, dates for case conference meetings with patient/family and members of the multidisciplinary team). Where barriers to the completion of any of these steps is identified in advance, it is helpful to identify lines of escalation. It is also helpful to allocate responsibility for feeding plans back to the patient/family whenever there is an initial indication of the direction of care or where the care direction changes so that a 'sense check' can be undertaken with them, allowing any issues to be identified at an early stage.

- For each patient, ensure some thought has been given to the right levels of medical care escalation, including resuscitation status; this is usually directed by the physician but may be prompted by experienced nursing or therapy staff too.

DEALING WITH CONFLICTS

It is inevitable that disagreements will arise when teams are planning complex discharges for their patients. Sometimes there will be differences between team members and other times between the team and the patient or family. Rehabilitation often involves trying to help patients and families remain hopeful whilst preparing them for scenarios that may be disappointing. Moreover, there may be justifiable differences of professional opinion over best treatment strategies or potential for improvement when dealing with patients with a significant degree of health and functional complexity. Each professional will be uniquely shaped by their training and past clinical experiences which will bring a lot to bear on their approach; well-trained professionals who are thinking critically will sometimes come to differing opinions.

Good leadership includes helping the whole team to keep the patient as the focus of discussions and looking towards *all* aspects of life that may contribute to their 'best interests' (safety may be one aspect but so too may a degree of autonomy). This may better define the course of action but given the often significant degrees of uncertainty, agreement to trial a certain course of action and review at a certain stage might help to allay any concerns within the group.

Conflict with patient/carer decisions can have heterogeneous roots. Sometimes it reflects a lack of understanding or understandable denial responses. At times, financial issues are at stake whilst at other times it is a genuine outcome of an imperfect health and social care system with inadequate resources to deal with very complex health and social care needs and carer burnout/strain. There is no definitive solution to this, but generally professionals need to take great care to listen to the concerns of their patient/family. This requires one-to-one time and selecting the appropriate professional to answer those queries. Where this is not satisfactorily addressed, a review and discussion by a second person from the team may help ensure that no concerns have been missed.

DISAGREEMENTS BETWEEN PATIENTS AND FAMILY

Increasingly encountered is variance between patient and family wishes. A typical scenario is a patient wanting to be discharged back to their own home whilst their family harbour safety concerns and prefer discharge to a nursing home; this is often on a background of the patient having cognitive impairment. The concept of assessing the patient's mental capacity for this decision is addressed in Chapter 20 (Brain Health and Mental Capacity). Although the principles of mental capacity are relatively straightforward, the practice of it in reality is often complex and in contentious situations a second opinion may be required. If a patient is deemed to have capacity for this decision and the family have qualms with it, then it will become incumbent on them to discuss all options together and agree on a plan between them; this may require more compromise from one party. Ultimately discussions need to respect the patient's right to self-determination, putting in place steps to monitor and support on discharge where concerns persist. If however the patient is found to lack capacity for this decision, then local laws need to be followed, e.g. to make decisions based on best interests or by a power of attorney.

Where differences between patient and family over decisions on discharge are encountered, it is helpful to allocate a member of the multiprofessional team to manage discussions. Convening with the family away from the main meeting enables detailing of the concerns, evaluation of the likelihood of them surfacing on discharge and exploration of actions that might mitigate such concerns (e.g. isolating the gas stove to reduce fire risks if returning home). Second opinions from other physicians and/or escalation to senior personnel in social services or discharge teams remain other options where an impasse has been reached. To see top tips for effective care planning meetings, refer to the Resources section at the end of the book.

SUMMARY POINTS

- Effective care planning meetings will often demonstrate interprofessional working with blurring of traditional professional roles in the decision-making process. This allows for cross-professional checks on decisions as well as professional development
- Meeting daily in an agreed format allows for dynamic, critical evaluation of patient progress
- Resources are required to support effective teams, including IT infrastructure and support for team development (non-technical skills)

- Disagreements over care planning decisions do not signify failure; amongst a wide range of factors there are complexities of patient background, balancing autonomy versus safety and accommodating different professional backgrounds and training
- Approaches to managing disagreements include keeping the patient central to the decisions, gathering further information if required and maintaining clear lines of communication with relevant stakeholders

MCQs

Q.1 Which of the following is true about care planning meetings?
a. Blurring the lines across professions is part of effective meetings
b. Daily board round should consist of an in-depth discussion of patient management
c. Doctors should always lead these meetings
d. Therapists should not consider any issues related to pain
e. Overall aims should not be discussed with patients

Q.2 Which of the following approaches is best when dealing with conflict?
a. Clear concise criticism of the party that is believed to be wrong
b. Avoid compromise as this shows weakness
c. Professionals need to take great care to listen to concerns
d. Mental capacity should be checked immediately
e. Allocate a different person to liaise for each meeting

REFERENCES

Abraham, A. (2011). *Care and compassion? Report of the Health Service Ombudsman on ten investigations into NHS care of older people.* [online]. London: The Parliamentary and Health Service Ombudsman (HMSO). Retrieved from https://www.ombudsman.org.uk/sites/default/files/2016-10/Care%20and%20Compassion.pdf (Accessed 12 February 2016).

Ellis, G., & Sevdalis, N. (2019). Understanding and improving multidisciplinary team working in geriatric medicine. *Age and Ageing, 48*(4), 498–505.

Emergency Care Intensive Support Team. (2011). Effective approaches in urgent and emergency care. Paper 1: Priorities within acute hospitals. [online]. Retrieved from https://www.england.nhs.uk/wp-content/uploads/2013/08/prior-acute-hosp.pdf (Accessed 3 June 2012).

Gage, M. (1998). From independence to interdependence. Creating synergistic healthcare teams. *Journal of Nursing Administration, 28*, 17–26.

Gonçalves-Bradley, D., Lannin, N., Clemson, L., Cameron, I., & Shepperd, S. (2016). Discharge planning from hospital. *Cochrane Database of Systematic Reviews, 1*, CD000313.

Nancarrow, S., Booth, A., Ariss, S., Smith, T., Enderby, P., & Roots, A. (2013). Ten principles of good interdisciplinary team work. *Human Resources for Health, 11*, 19.

NHS Improvement. (2017). *The SAFER patient flow bundle.* [online]. Retrieved from https://improvement.nhs.uk/documents/633/the-safer-patient-flow-bundle.pdf (Accessed 25 January 2018).

Royal College of Physicians & Royal College of Nursing. (2012). *Ward rounds in medicine: principles for best practice.* London, UK: Royal College of Physicians. [online]. Retrieved from https://www.rcplondon.ac.uk/projects/outputs/ward-rounds-medicine-principles-best-practice (Accessed 10 February 2016).

68

The Home Environment Assessment

Kate McGoldrick

LEARNING OBJECTIVES

- Describe the purpose of assessing a patient's home environment
- Explain the difference between the Environmental Assessment Visit and the Home Assessment Visit
- List the physical and cognitive components assessed when undertaking an Environmental or Home Assessment Visit
- Explain the role of the recommendations and how these may impact upon the individual and others living in the property

It is the role of the occupational therapist (OT) to promote independence and function with everyday tasks or activities which are important to the individual, and to ensure they are able to carry out these tasks at home or return home to live as safely as possible.

Whilst OTs assess and treat individuals within the hospital setting, there can be numerous benefits to assessing the patient's home environment either with the patient present or without the patient being present.

Both of these visits hold their own value which will be explained in more depth.

ENVIRONMENTAL ASSESSMENT

Environmental assessments are usually carried out in the presence of a relative, or written consent would be gained from the patient for the therapist and a colleague to access the property unaccompanied.

An environmental assessment would usually occur if the patient was unable to attend along with the therapist. For example, if it was likely that the patient would require the provision of moving and handling equipment for transfers or mobility such as a hoist, or an electric profiling bed or a wheelchair, where it was not already available.

The purpose of an environmental assessment is to assess the home environment for a clearer picture of the layout, gauge the size of the rooms and the distances the patient would be expected to mobilise or to establish the equipment already available and potential aids or adaptations that may be required to facilitate a safe discharge.

It can also be useful in enabling the therapist to assess the style of staircase or type of banisters or rails fitted or required for discharge.

HOME ASSESSMENT VISIT

A Home Assessment Visit (HAV) is led by an OT. The patient is taken out to their home for approximately 1 hour to assess physical and/or cognitive function within their home environment.

Reasons for Conducting HAVs

HAVs are usually considered if a patient's functional capabilities are significantly different to their reported pre-admission level and there are concerns raised by the patient themselves, their family or by the multidisciplinary team regarding how they will manage at home.

Where an individual has sight loss, their own familiar home environment would be a more appropriate setting to assess their functional ability and identify any equipment or support needs.

For other patients, a HAV can be organised to help them form a decision if there have been concerns regarding their ability to function at home and they are contemplating a move into a care home. A visit can help to stimulate discussion based on their current ability mobilising and transferring within the familiar home setting rather than assumptions being made by the multidisciplinary team based upon their functional ability within the safe clinical environment.

Internal/External Access Considerations

Consideration needs to be given to the patient's ability to access the home prior to the visit being agreed to ensure they would manage external or internal stairs upon arrival.

Access to the property would also be assessed if there was a requirement for the patient to use a wheelchair both within and outside of the property. This would allow for provisions to be put in place to have doorways widened or for ramps to be installed.

Transfers, Mobility and Falls Risks

Whilst on the HAV the patient would be assessed transferring on and off their bed, chair and toilet and the bathing or showering facilities would be assessed with a view to recommending equipment to optimise function or safety, if required. The patient would be assessed mobilising on the carpet, taking into consideration the pile of the carpet or the type of floor covering (a thick luxury carpet may be difficult to push a wheeled Zimmer frame across or add increased resistance for a self-propelled wheelchair). In addition, the therapist would consider the patient's use of a mobility aid on that particular flooring with a view to optimising safety (see Fig. 68.1). Things to consider would include the condition of the carpet, the thread, frayed areas which may pose a trip hazard or could potentially get caught in a mobility aid and recommending this be replaced or temporarily taped down.

If there were rugs or mats on the floor, an assessment would be made on an individual basis to establish if these posed a risk for the patient, e.g. trip hazard or a potential risk of sliding.

Door thresholds would be assessed. If raised, the therapist would consider how these may interfere with a mobility aid or a kitchen trolley and whether or not they may present as a trip hazard to the individual.

The space available to the individual to manoeuvre would be assessed, and recommendations could be made to reconfigure furniture in a bid to optimise function if necessary. The type of walking aid may need to be reconsidered, e.g, a standard wheeled Zimmer frame may need to be replaced with a narrow wheeled Zimmer frame. Rails may need to be installed if there is insufficient space to mobilise or turn with an aid within the confined space. Likewise, recommendations

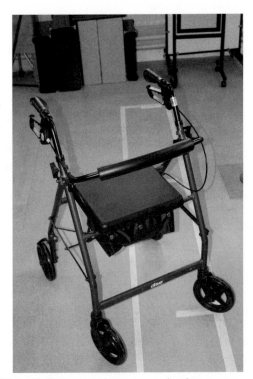

FIG. 68.1 Patients may be assessed using a new mobility aid on various surfaces to ensure suitability. This four-wheeled walker may be easier to use on hard surfaces, but can sometimes roll forward unexpectedly and increase falls risk. (From Bradley SM, Hernandez CR. Geriatric assistive devices. *Am Fam Physician*. 2011;84(4):405–11, with permission.)

may be made for a door to be rehung to open in or out if it would optimise access to a room.

Stairs

Assessing patients within their own environment and on their own stairs can be of significant value compared with a routine set of 'safe' stairs within the hospital setting that physiotherapists would traditionally take patients on during inpatient rehabilitation. Some aspects which would be considered include step height and depth, carpet thread, floor covering, banisters, turns and angles, foot placement and the potential need for a stairlift if the patient experienced difficulty mobilising on the stairs, or was unable to use them (see Fig. 68.2).

If there was an existing stairlift installed within the property, the therapist would assess the physical and cognitive element for the patient transferring on and off safely in addition to the cognitive aspect of operating the stairlift controls safely.

As it would not be considered safe to use moving and handling equipment at the top of a flight of stairs, consideration would need to be given to single-level living either up or downstairs if the patient required handling aids to transfer.

The therapist would assess the patient's ability to attend to day-to-day activities within the home safely including the physical aspects of lifting, reaching, carrying and turning.

The HAV offers the therapist and the patient the opportunity to walk-through daily tasks such as getting up from bed to access the toilet or commode, positioning of equipment to optimise function and ensuring there is sufficient space to manoeuvre a walking aid. It is important to be mindful that some older people may downplay the difficulties or the challenges they experience at home if they are private in nature. At other times people could simply lack insight into the difficulties experienced. A HAV can be a useful tool for facilitating an independent assessment of the patient's function in the home environment whilst also considering both the patient and their family's concerns.

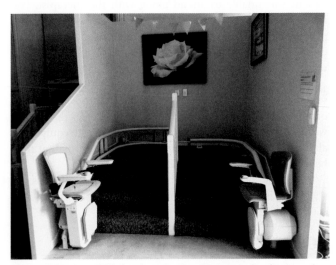

FIG. 68.2 A stairlift in place in the therapy suite for practice purposes.

Due Consideration Towards a Spouse/Relative Sharing the Home

Although the HAV is primarily undertaken to assess the patient under your care, it is also important to consider how any recommendations may impact on a spouse or others living within the home. For example, would raising the height of the bed or the chair hinder access by a patient's wife who was of short stature? Or would the patient's husband agree to a referral being made to the community occupational therapy team to consider bathroom renovations to optimise access for bathing or showering?

Whilst it is difficult if you feel there have been obvious signs that a patient or family have not been coping before admission from those observations made during the HAV, it is usually the aim of the multidisciplinary team to support a safe discharge as best we can by ensuring the patient has access to the necessary equipment and support services within the community.

RECOMMENDATIONS FOLLOWING AN ENVIRONMENTAL OR HOME ASSESSMENT VISIT

It is considered good practice to recap at the end of the visit with those present, whether it's the patient on their own or with family/carers, any key issues raised from having assessed the patient in their home or from undertaking an assessment of the environment alone.

There should be time built into the visit to allow for questions or concerns to be addressed. Either during the visit if appropriate or once the report is compiled, a list of identified issues along with the corresponding recommendation should be documented alongside the named person responsible for actioning them. For example, it may have been agreed that the patient's daughter will remove a rug in front of the fireplace or reconfigure the bedroom furniture to enable her mother to access her side of the bed with the newly provided walking aid. Or it could be the responsibility of the OT to arrange for a grabrail to be installed next to the toilet or make a referral to the community occupational therapy team to investigate options for making the property wheelchair accessible. Timescales for each action should be agreed, and it would be customary to acknowledge whether each of the identified recommendations was essential or not to facilitate a safe discharge.

COGNITION AND HAVs

A HAV can be very useful in assessing a patient's cognitive ability which can be used to enhance standardised assessments or alternative cognitive testing. Usually the therapist would consider the patient's level of orientation within their home environment by ensuring they were able to locate rooms, identify belongings and even identify family members within photos.

Considering the safety of the patient and optimising their function would usually be the key goals when assessing an individual within their home. Often the patient would be asked to prepare a hot drink and a light snack. This allows the therapist to assess the individual using electrical appliances and ensure they are able to operate power sockets, gas hobs, ovens or fires safely. This also allows the therapist to assess the patient's ability to plan and sequence the task, manoeuvre safely within the home, reach high and low units, and assess their ability to transport items either between work surfaces or between rooms.

There is an abundance of aids, adaptations and devices available to promote and enhance safety within the home environment. Telecare devices such as flood detectors, linked smoke detectors and heat detectors to name a few can help to maintain the safety of an individual who may be at risk of leaving a tap on or forgetting to switch off the cooker. Gas isolation units, locked medication safes, kettle cradles and kitchen trolleys are some other adaptations and aids which can be used to promote safety.

A patient can be assessed operating their door entry system to ensure they could allow entry for visitors or consideration could be given to the need to have a key safe to be fitted. In addition, patients can be assessed operating their telephone which can contribute to assessing memory and problem-solving skills, and the therapist can if required ensure the patient can hear the doorbell or telephone ring if there were concerns relating to hearing. Requests can be made to Sensory Impairment Teams for consideration of flashing lights or loop systems to compensate for the identified difficulties.

At times, a HAV can reveal signs of poor medication adherence if there is a build-up of unused boxes of medication or if there were inconsistencies within old blister packs within the property. In this circumstance it is important to raise this with the patient's family who can return unused medications to the pharmacy for safe disposal at the same time as highlighting this with the multidisciplinary team who arrange for community follow-up reviews to check adherence.

From experience, it tends to be individuals with no family contacts or those with relatives who are not living within close proximity where more concerns are uncovered from carrying out assessments within their home. In some cases, assessing the home environment can give an indication of how the patient was coping at home prior to admission in terms of cleanliness, a tidy environment or standard of living, and sometimes it can even disclose signs of hoarding (see Fig. 68.3).

MENTAL CAPACITY AND HAVs

Ultimately, recommendations can be made following a HAV to promote the safety and independence of the patient, and it should be used as a collaborative assessment tool with the individual. However, patients are under no obligation to action or adhere to any of the suggestions if they have mental capacity to make this decision.

If a patient has been assessed as lacking mental capacity for this decision and they are not in agreement to action or adhere to any recommendations, then it would usually be a multidisciplinary decision alongside involvement of family to establish and agree the risks involved with not adhering

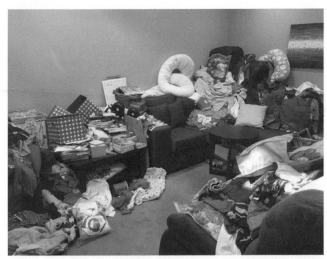

FIG. 68.3 An example of a room full of clutter, which may suggest hoarding behaviour. (From Crone C, Norberg MM. Scared and surrounded by clutter: the influence of emotional reactivity. *J Affect Disord*. 2018;235:285–92, with permission.)

to recommendations and whether this would impact on the patient's ability to return home. The safety of the individual would likely be the first consideration.

HAV CASE EXAMPLES

- A patient required a pulpit frame to mobilise during her inpatient stay. From speaking with her son, a HAV was agreed to measure access after he informed the therapist that his mother's flat was not large enough to accommodate that particular frame. A visit was carried out, and measurements were taken which were satisfactory. The lady was discharged home with the pulpit frame to mobilise independently.
- A patient whose daughter lived in another country and who had no other family nearby reported that her mother was coping well at home with no difficulties or concerns about physical/functional capabilities. During the admission the

patient was found to be cognitively impaired and required supervision to mobilise. A HAV was carried out, and there was an infestation around the foot of her lounge chair, in the bedroom carpet and in her bed. A professional decision was made to refer the patient to social work for an assessment of her care needs even though her family felt the house was not too bad and would be agreeable to replacing carpets and furniture if required to facilitate a return home. The visit highlighted signs of the patient not managing well before admission.

- A family raised concern over their father's ability to remain safe at home due to excessive alcohol intake, reduced mobility, poor lighting and an abundance of furniture within his home. Although the family had acknowledged and raised these concerns with their father, he was dismissive of their concern. The family requested a HAV as they felt their father may adhere to a healthcare professional making similar recommendations more than his family. Following the visit, the patient agreed to the family arranging an electrician to install more ceiling lights and remove and reposition furniture to optimise safer mobility around his home.
- A patient reported managing well at home yet their family raised lots of concerns with their mobility, transfers and demands placed upon relatives and neighbours while also turning homecare staff away. Within the ward the patient's mobility was poor and they were highly anxious with a fear of falling. The family reported that this was not new. A HAV was carried out, and the patient took 50 minutes to mobilise a short distance, was panicking, fearful and anxious. There were discrepancies between how the patient stated they were managing before admission and what they anticipated they would manage upon discharge compared with their presentation on the visit. It was felt that the patient lacked insight into the existing difficulties, and this raised further questions over the individual's cognitive functioning. Further cognitive tests were completed which supported a diagnosis of dementia. A referral was made to social work to commence an assessment of their care needs.

SUMMARY POINTS

- It is the role of the occupational therapist to promote function, independence and safety, enabling older people to remain within their own home for as long as possible
- Environmental and Home Assessment Visits allow for a richer understanding of how the individual functions, compared to the safe clinical environment within the hospital setting

- The Home Assessment Visit can be a useful tool for assessing patients with a visual, cognitive or physical impairment
- There are a variety of aids and adaptations available to support individuals to live independently and safely within their home environment
- Recommendations should be made, where possible in collaboration with the patient and their family/carer

MCQs

Q.1 What are the reasons for conducting a HAV?
- a. To enable the occupational therapist to decide if the patient should return home or not
- b. To contribute towards decision-making relating to the patient's future care needs

- c. It allows the occupational therapist to organise equipment or adaptations without the need to involve the patient, their family or the multidisciplinary team
- d. To assess the patient's spouse or family members at home

Q.2 What considerations should be given to patients with mobility difficulties?
  a. Distances they would be expected to mobilise between rooms
  b. Floor coverings in place, e.g. type, quality and condition of carpet
  c. Space for moving and handling aids
  d. All of the above

Q.3 Why are HAVs beneficial for patients with cognitive impairment?
  a. They can be used to enhance standardised assessments or alternative cognitive testing
  b. It allows the occupational therapist to assess orientation
  c. They can be used to assess the individual operating their own familiar appliances and ensure they are able to operate power sockets, gas hobs, ovens or fires safely
  d. All of the above

FURTHER READING

Atwal, A., & McIntyre, A. (2013). *Occupational therapy and older people*, 2nd edition. Retrieved from: https://onlinelibrary.wiley.com/doi/book/10.1002/9781118782835.

Preston, J., & Edmans, J. (2016). *Occupational therapy and neurological conditions*. Retrieved from: https://onlinelibrary.wiley.com/doi/book/10.1002/9781119223719.

Royal College of Occupational Therapists. (2019). *Adaptations without delay: a guide to planning and delivering home adaptations differently*. Retrieved from: https://www.rcot.co.uk/adaptations-without-delay.

Royal College of Occupational Therapists. (2020). Occupational therapy in the prevention and management of falls in adults: practice guideline, 2nd edition. Retrieved from: https://www.rcot.co.uk/practice-resources/rcot-practice-guidelines/falls.

69

Home Supports

Kate McGoldrick

LEARNING OBJECTIVES

- Explain why home support services might be required
- Identify types of support services are available
- Describe the benefit to the individual and family

There is a strong drive towards supporting individuals to remain in their own home safely for as long as possible. There are many reasons why returning home remains the preferred choice for many people: primarily due to familiarity and comfort, sentimental value, home being a place of safety and home offering a degree of autonomy. For many individuals, choosing to remain at home can be viewed as empowering, and offers them a level of control which they may not have within a formal care setting. Utilising and drawing on as much community support available enables an individual's (at times complex) care needs to be met and this can prevent people from feeling isolated, lonely, vulnerable or unsafe. The financial implications to both the individual and/or the health service of supporting someone to remain in their own home can also be significantly less than funding for a formal care setting.

HOMECARE

Homecare services can offer support for simple as well as complex care needs. The level of support offered tends to be assessed on a case-by-case basis and would usually be bespoke to address the care needs of the individual. Carers can attend individually, or in a pair, usually where there are moving and handling needs identified. Homecare services can be accessed for support throughout the day and sometimes overnight, depending on the health service. In some circumstances, overnight carers could be organised where the individual has toileting or skin care needs which would place them at a higher risk of skin breakdown or harm if they were to be left unattended at night.

Homecare services can help individuals by providing care that meets their needs within their own home and usually consists of the following:

Personal care
- Showering, bathing or washing
- Dressing
- Grooming
- Catheter care or stoma care
- Skin care

- Specialist feeding – either 1:1 physical assistance to feed or continued verbal prompts or encouragement to ensure food is consumed.

Transfers and mobility
- Assistance getting in or out of bed
- Mobilising between rooms
- Accessing the toilet
- Emptying the commode

Domestic tasks
- Food and drink preparation
- Medication prompt
- Shopping
- Laundry

Homecare can offer a period of enhanced support to a patient initially upon discharge from hospital. The support can be temporary in conjunction with recovery or it can be a long-term support service.

Homecare services can be organised to work around a patient's pre-arranged weekly schedule such as requesting no lunch visit on a Wednesday if they attend a day centre, or no morning visit on a Saturday if they would prefer a lie-in or if their family visit to offer assistance.

Depending on the service provision within the area of residence, for some individuals the maximum level of homecare support can be insufficient in meeting their ever-increasing needs. Examples would be if there were concerns over skin integrity and the individual required two-hourly positional turns, or if they were unable to tolerate sitting up in a chair for several hours between homecare visits. Likewise, if there were issues around continence and the individual was likely to require a higher level of support, then this needs to be considered before establishing if the individual can be supported sufficiently at home to meet their individual needs.

Overnight care needs tend to pose most concern for individuals wishing to remain in their own home rather than consider a move into a care home. With the last homecare visit of the day being as early as 7:00 pm and the first visit of the day potentially being as late as 10:00 am in some cases, there is a possibility of the patient being alone at home overnight for up to 15 hours. For those reliant on support for mobility, transfers, continence care, skin care or feeding, this could put the individual at risk of injury or harm.

Managing the expectations of the individual or their family around the services available is of significant importance in ensuring a sustainable and safe discharge is organised. For some patients the lack of control they have over the times of their homecare visits or the lack of control over the tasks they would like assistance with may not meet their needs fully or may cause them unnecessary distress.

There are sometimes options available for private homecare services which could be utilised separately to government-funded homecare or as an add-on to supplement it. However, these can be costly, and assumptions should not be made that individuals would be able to sustain such cost on a short or long-term basis. For some individuals, employing private carers may be a viable option to supplement homecare if they wish to remain living safely at home for as long as possible. For others, private homecare services may be able to meet their expectations better than a government-funded homecare service with regards to times of visits, tasks undertaken and the duration of the visit.

Access for carers also needs to be considered; where the patient is immobile or unable to access the door to let carers in, then a key box could be considered. A key box (or key safe) is a strong metal box which can be drilled to concrete or wood usually outside the property. A set of house keys are stored within the key box and can be accessed by homecare services by pressing a combination code. A remote door entry system could be another option for consideration if the individual experienced mobility difficulties and would struggle or not manage to mobilise to open the door to carers independently.

TELECARE

Telecare is the use of technologies such as remote monitoring and emergency alarms to enable an individual to remain at home as safely and for as long as possible.

There are a variety of devices such as pendant or wrist alerts and falls detectors which can either be touch-activated or self-activating if a fall is detected (see Fig. 69.1). The benefits include increased confidence and peace of mind for the individual and their relatives knowing there is a system or plan in place to raise an alarm and seek urgent assistance if they required help.

Raising an urgent alarm reduces the risks involved with a potential long lie or urgent help not being sought, which can have significant consequences on the individual's medical and functional status and recovery.

There are devices designed for those who live with a carer that can ring or vibrate through a pager carried by the carer. These can be linked to bed and chair alarms or door exit sensors.

For patients who experience problems with memory, there are smoke detectors, heat detectors and flood detectors which can raise an alarm to the central call centre in the event of an electrical appliance or taps being left on.

Individuals who are at risk of wandering or who have difficulties with orientation may benefit from a Global Positioning

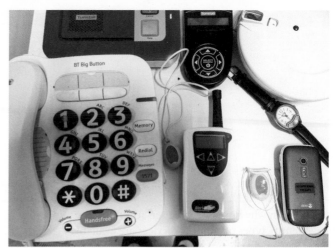

FIG. 69.1 A range of telecare equipment including large button phones, pendant alarm and pager monitoring system.

System (GPS) tracking device. Such devices can offer a degree of independence for someone who may be at risk of not finding their way back if they go out alone or for those who are at risk of leaving home unaccompanied, or who could get up overnight disorientated and attempt to go out alone.

Notifications can be raised with a central alarm centre or with a family member who will respond accordingly or the emergency services could be contacted if there were no local responders available.

In addition to telecare devices specifically designed to support individuals to remain in their own home, as safely and for as long as possible – there are also advances in technological devices widely available on the commercial market such as smart speakers which can be used to make phone calls, control lights/door locks/appliances, change the temperature, answer questions, set timers and control the television.

All of these devices can give the individual and their family the independence to remain at home, with added piece of mind to help optimise their function and maintain their safety.

SHOPPING SERVICES

For individuals who are unable to attend to their own shopping or for those who do not have family support for such tasks, there are services available which can be organised, usually for a fee. Whilst online shopping services may suit some tech-savvy older people, there are many who would prefer to pick up the telephone and speak to someone to place an order or write down a list of items that they need which could be collected in person.

HOT FOOD DELIVERY SERVICES

There are also Meals on Wheels services available to deliver hot meals to individuals within their own home once a day at an additional fee to the service user. This type of service can be organised for a short period of time, for example to support someone over a period of ill health or when other support services are down, such as family going on holiday.

An interesting initiative by one service was developed to incorporate social interaction within the community setting where an individual is connected with someone in their local community who prepares an extra portion of a hot meal to be shared together. This type of service works towards reducing feelings of loneliness and isolation for individuals with limited social connections or for those who are housebound.

HOME SAFETY FIRE CHECK

A referral to the fire service for a home safety fire check can be valuable for some older people who have undergone a home assessment visit, and concerns have been highlighted. If there are signs of hoarding, clutter, older heating systems, electric heaters, immobility or a general concern about vulnerability, contacting the fire service can be worthwhile.

With a home safety fire check, the fire officer from a local fire station would attend the individual's home to carry out an assessment of the property, help the individual formalise an escape plan, supply and install smoke, heat and carbon monoxide alarms.

This service also registers that individual or family on the fire service's register enabling them to identify the property as having a vulnerable adult should an alarm be raised.

BEFRIENDING/VOLUNTEER SERVICES

There are telephone services offering daily or weekly calls for older people living alone at home. As people age it can become more difficult to maintain social connections. Life events such as bereavement, retirement or family moving away can leave people feeling lonely and isolated.

Having strong social connections can help people deal with stressful situations, promotes good mental health, enhances self-esteem and can support longevity and good brain health.

For some individuals this is an important service to reduce feelings of loneliness, to increase social interaction and to build relationships which can be missing if someone is unable to leave their home due to e.g. reduced mobility. These services can offer emotional support at difficult times and can also raise an alert to a nominated family member if a call goes unanswered.

For some individuals a telephone service works well however, for others who prefer face-to-face contact a befriending service may be more appropriate in meeting their needs in enhancing social contact. A volunteer is usually matched with the individual where possible with similar likes and interests and regular visits are agreed either weekly, fortnightly or monthly.

The befriender could visit someone at home, or for individuals who are more mobile, the befriender or volunteer could accompany them on outings to a local café or shops.

This service is also valuable in enabling carers a period of respite for a few hours or time away to attend to essential tasks such as shopping or banking.

COMMUNITY TRANSPORT

Getting to appointments or accessing the community can be a concern for some older people who experience difficulties with their mobility. Tasks such as attending the shops or visiting someone in hospital can prove difficult for individuals who do not have the confidence or the ability to access public transport to help them live independently. This can lead to feelings of isolation, loneliness and reduced independence.

Voluntary services are available in some areas to collect individuals from their home and take them out in either their own vehicles or in some cases adapted vehicles to attend appointments or to attend community activities.

HOME LIBRARY SERVICE

Reading and listening to books for many older people can be an enjoyable and relaxing pastime and can also help reduce feelings of loneliness and isolation. However, for individuals who experience difficulty mobilising or who are unable to get to their local library there are services available where the books, talking books or in some case films can be brought to the older person at home.

Preferences can be highlighted by requesting specific books or books can be selected based upon the individual's taste. Books are then delivered and uplifted on an agreed date.

In the UK, the Royal National Institute of Blind People (RNIB) also offer a free talking book service for those with sight loss to enable them to gain access through various devices such as USB sticks or digital downloads.

HANDY PERSON SERVICE

Practical support is available in some areas to help with small repairs and DIY (Do it Yourself) jobs around the home.

This assistance can be vital to help an individual maintain their home and improve safety measures within their home environment. The handy person or DIY service can assist with tasks which may be unsafe for an individual to perform themselves or which may put them at risk of injury or harm such as changing lightbulbs, turning mattresses and fitting curtain rails. Minor repairs can also be undertaken such as fixing door locks, repairing taps or installing key safes.

In many areas an individual would be expected to pay for the materials required for the work undertaken, but the labour and time may be free for people over 65 years.

▮ SUMMARY POINTS

- Home support services can be utilised to enable an older person to remain in their own home safely for as long as possible

- Home supports offer a wide variety of practical support to older people living in their own home

- Home support services can reduce feelings of loneliness and isolation in older people

- Home support services can optimise older people's independence, enabling them to access community services that they may not have been able to access alone

MCQs

Q.1 For what reason would an individual likely wish to remain in their own home rather than consider a move to a care setting?
  a. To maintain an element of autonomy
  b. For familiarity and sentimental value
  c. Home can be a place of safety and comfort
  d. For financial reasons
  e. All of the above

Q.2 What is the purpose of telecare?
  a. To eliminate all risk
  b. Offers practical support to an individual living in their own home
  c. To alert all neighbours if there is a risk of fire

  d. Surveillance of older relatives without telling them
  e. All of the above

Q.3 Why are befriending and volunteer services of value to older people?
  a. Social interaction can be reduced if individuals are unable to leave their home due to reduced mobility
  b. Life events such as bereavement, retirement or family moving away can reduce social circles
  c. Strong social connections can enhance self-esteem
  d. Social interaction stimulates brain function and can support longevity
  e. All of the above

FURTHER READING

Atwal, A., & McIntyre, A. (2013). *Occupational therapy and older people*, 2nd edition. Retrieved from: https://onlinelibrary.wiley.com/doi/book/10.1002/9781118782835.

Preston, J., & Edmans, J. (2016). *Occupational therapy and neurological conditions.* Retrieved from: https://onlinelibrary.wiley.com/doi/book/10.1002/9781119223719.

Royal College of Occupational Therapists. (2019). *Adaptations without delay: a guide to planning and delivering home adaptations differently.* Retrieved from: https://www.rcot.co.uk/adaptations-without-delay.

Royal College of Occupational Therapists. (2020). *Occupational therapy in the prevention and management of falls in adults: practice guideline, 2nd edition.* Retrieved from: https://www.rcot.co.uk/practice-resources/rcot-practice-guidelines/falls.

Informal Care

Hannah Gallagher

INTRODUCTION

Informal caregivers are family, neighbours and friends taking an active role in looking after a person's care needs, such as helping to prepare meals or washing and dressing. There are around seven million carers in the UK, 1 in 10 people (Carers UK, 2015), and for many rehabilitation is a part of what they do every day. This chapter considers some elements of care that aid recovery. It is written with both the carer and the healthcare professional in mind. Those who work in caring for older people know that health is often about getting the basics of care right, but how much time do health professionals spend working with the carer? Central to this is an understanding that the informal carer often becomes an expert in the person being cared for. They should not be seen as a substitute physiotherapist, dietician or nurse, but their expertise in knowing the person and their changing needs and abilities is vital for successful rehabilitation. I am writing from the perspective of a doctor with some experience and clinical knowledge but also as a carer who initially had little understanding of how much physical and mental work was involved. I have included elements of my grandmother's story (with her consent) to demonstrate some of the complexity and challenges involved.

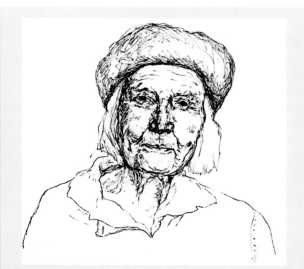

FIG. 70.1 Drawing of Margaret by her granddaughter Ellen Gallagher.

She called out repeatedly to express a distress she could not articulate and was unable to derive any benefit from inpatient therapy.

We took her home without much of a plan but an expectation that these might be her final weeks. Unexpected progress happened when what we knew about Gran's history and personality balanced with treatment and care given.

Gran is now 94. She has not been admitted to hospital since. Important progress has been made, but caring remains difficult and full of uncertainty. Rehabilitation in someone with globally ailing health is not a linear process, and recovery from some illnesses is only partial.

Now when I hear the phrases 'no-rehab potential' or 'new baseline' in acute medical settings (sometimes conveyed in a well-meaning but clunky family update) I wince. Families and carers need realistic expectations of the future, but also encouragement that, with the right support, progress can be made (see Chapter 9 Rehabilitation Potential and Selection for Rehabilitation).

CASE: LOOKING AFTER GRAN

At 92, Margaret (Fig. 70.1) had been living on her own, walking to the shops every day, managing her own housework and finances. One day a neighbour found her unwell in the street. She spent a night in hospital but insisted on returning home. From that point her cognitive and physical health started to decline. As a family we were optimistic we could care for her in her own home.

Six months later she broke her hip, and the consequences were catastrophic. The operation, sleepless nights, pain, repeated catheterisations, skin breakdown, medication burden and infection left her delirious and unable to walk unaided.

REHABILITATION AND CAREGIVING AT HOME

"People . . . are underprepared for their recovery or for life after their illness or injury" (British Red Cross, 2019).

The day of discharge can be daunting. Patients may have had weeks of having their food brought to them, been prompted to dress, go to the toilet, move and sleep. The first days at home require a reconditioning for all involved to manage day-to-day tasks out of the clinical environment. "Home to the Unknown" (British Red Cross, 2019) highlights how difficult discharge can be with patients feeling abandoned and unprepared and recounts instances in which carers were offered little support or guidance in how to meet care needs whilst encouraging recovery.

The following sections look briefly at what a caregiver can practically do, encouraging them to tap into what they already know about the person being cared for, and also highlights professional involvement that may help. See the Resources section at the end of the book for more detail.

Ears, Eyes and Mouth

Dentures, hearing aids and glasses are often overlooked or misplaced in the hospital. Their impact on rehabilitation can be far-reaching.

Dentures, for example, may affect not only what a person can eat but also their speech and self-confidence. Without dentures, Gran is quiet, withdrawn and her accent changes. With dentures in she is far more likely to talk to the doctor and join conversation.

An up-to-date glasses prescription might be what is needed to keep a person orientated and participating in the activities around them.

Prompt regularly but be aware of how the person responds. We tried hearing aids but at 94, Gran was used to a quieter world. They lasted a few minutes before demands of "cut me off!" were made.

Food and Drink

Food can be a meaningful part of recovery. Aim to sit at a table where possible, ideally within smelling distance of the food being cooked to help with appetite. Engaging in tasks, even small acts like holding the recipe page open at an old favourite, choosing from a menu or watching the process might bring back some autonomy and interest. Set the table simply and allow plenty of time to eat.

Seek professional input if there are concerns about eating in a person with dementia. The book "Practical Nutrition and Hydration for Dementia-Friendly Mealtimes" gives advice both carers and professionals may find useful (Martin, 2019).

Continence

New incontinence is common in hospital but should not be considered normal (see Chapter 35 Bladder and Bowel Problems). If there is no lasting medical reason, ongoing work at home to regain continence should be encouraged with advice from the healthcare team before discharge and in the community.

The process of getting used to using a toilet again can be confusing for the person and stressful for the caregiver. Expect progress to take time and aim for a routine of regular prompting to use the toilet through the day. Change incontinence pads in the toilet area and always explain what is happening, maximising privacy as able. If there is no bowel output for more than a day or two, think about using a laxative.

Skin

Skin breakdown must be taken seriously (see Chapter 40 Skin Care and Podiatry). This is a signal that there are bigger problems with the rest of the body. Food, drink and continence are keys to maintaining good skin integrity. Incontinence and poor mobility are major risks, causing damage within a few hours. This should be planned for, with community team involvement before the first sign of redness if someone's mobility or continence has deteriorated.

Washing and Dressing

The temptation when someone is unwell is to do everything for them, but even small actions can lead to deconditioning (losing skills through lack of use, see Chapter 21 Avoiding Deconditioning) and increasing dependence.

Be led by the person as to how much help they need and offer them a choice of their own clothes. Offer each article and see how far they can manage rather than automatically putting it on for them. Even when very confused they should have the chance to express their wishes about how often they wash. A daily shower might be normal to younger generations but not necessarily to someone born in 1925.

Sleep

Poor sleep can be a significant problem when caring for an older person (see Chapter 32 Sleep and Fatigue).

Sleeping tablets may only offer false hope or create problems for the following day such as drowsiness, unsteadiness, falls and confusion, as their effect can last for longer than 8 hours.

Check that the sleepless person is not in pain, needing to go to the toilet or worried about something that can be addressed. Depression or anxiety can disrupt sleep at any age; if as a carer you suspect mood is part of the problem, raise with their doctor as treating it may be the key.

For further practical tips on sleep hygiene in people with dementia, guides such as those produced by the Alzheimer's society may help (Alzheimer's Society, 2019).

Movement

Physiotherapy and occupational therapy teams are best placed to advise on specific activities. Carers can use their knowledge of what the person enjoys to complement this.

If there is an unexpected deterioration in mobility, be suspicious of new medications as many commonly used drugs can impair walking in older people.

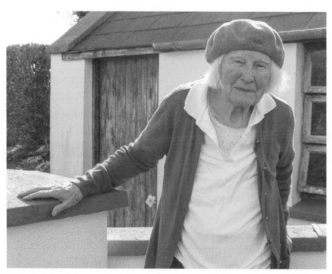

FIG. 70.2 Margaret on a visit to her childhood home, enjoying sharing memories of the farm.

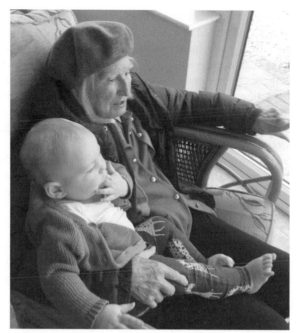

FIG. 70.3 Margaret in conversation with her great-grandson Owen.

Some leave hospital without ongoing active physiotherapy, as physical or cognitive limitations suggest formal input will not lead to measurable improvements.

Ongoing movement, however, remains essential for physical and mental health. This can start small and be increased. A person nursed in bed and confused may be able to follow instruction to brush their hair, stretch out to reach possessions that interest them or more actively dress themselves. For those that can walk, moving the chair a bit further from the bed or walking around the house each day can over time lead to improvements that might not have been predicted in hospital assessments (Fig 70.2).

Cognition

Confusion is common during episodes of ill health (usually delirium – see Chapter 30 Cognitive Problems) and impacts on all areas of care. Approaches to care may help to mitigate the impact on relationships.

There have been times that Gran has told me she felt lost, speaking of the past as 'when I was alive'. Revisiting things she enjoyed in the past helps her feel more grounded. Looking at an old cookbook, Gran is the expert in the conversation and when visited by great grandchildren she engages confidently with them (Fig. 70.3).

It is not always this easy. The "therapeutic lie" (to lie in an attempt to reassure) has never been a useful tool with Gran. Feil's work on validation explores ways in which carers of those with dementia can listen with empathy in these moments to "validate" the feelings of the concerned person (Feil & deKlerk-Rubin, 2012). Feil suggests mirroring a person's tone and movements to build trust.

One agitated night, Gran was trying to get out into the street to call for her son (who was in another country). When something like this happens, the impulse is to cheerily tell her he is coming and that everything is okay. In that moment she might settle but on some level she knows this is not true,

she loses trust and her behaviour eventually escalates. The alternative, of showing her that I understand the situation is serious, that we are in it together and that nights can be frightening, is more likely to help her relax and talk about what is worrying her.

CARER HEALTH

The caring role often has a negative impact on the carer's own health. In taking on responsibility for another's health needs, they may sacrifice their own.

The UK State of Caring Report (2018) surveyed 7397 carers. Approximately 72% of respondents reported mental ill health and 61% reported physical ill health as a result of their role. The De-Stress study surveyed 200 spousal carers of people with dementia in Ireland, and about 37% reported clinically significant depressive symptoms (Brennan et al., 2017).

Burnout is a term often used to describe occupational stress. Its use here acknowledges the work aspect of the caring role and places chronic stress in this context. Burnout is a three-factor syndrome in which people experience exhaustion, cynicism (sometimes referred to as depersonalisation) and feelings of ineffectiveness (Maslach & Leiter, 2016).

There are services to support carers but the professional's awareness and ability to facilitate or signpost to appropriate local voluntary and state services is important as carers, particularly early on in a care role, may be unaware of what they are entitled to.

General practitioners in the UK have a carer's register; carers may be offered flexible appointments and their needs may be included in case discussions with social services. This may be a route for referral and involvement from the charity sector. They are entitled to a needs assessment provided by the local council. Assessments may lead to financial or practical support such as help with taxi fares or suggesting therapeutic activities for the carer. The assessment must be requested, which relies either on an informed healthcare professional telling the caregiver about it or the individual seeking out the assessment for themselves by contacting their local social services.

Services for caregivers are available online from charities such as Carers UK. Collaborative projects which use carer experience, such as that developed by Newcastle University's "Dementia Care: Staying Connected and Living Well", are a useful educational resource for carers.

CONCLUSION

Professionals only get glimpses of the home life of the cared for and the caregiver. This chapter has revealed some of the ways in which caregivers enable rehabilitation. Understanding the breadth of work and the impact this can have on the caregiver's life should prompt the professional to reflect on their own practice and how they can support and signpost services for caregiver health.

SUMMARY POINTS

- Caregivers in engaging in the ordinary acts of day-to-day care should acknowledge the power of their actions in enhancing a person's capacity for recovery
- The great satisfaction that comes with progress will at times be countered by real moments of difficulty and despair; preparing for how you will cope through those hard times and seeking support is vital
- Health professionals should reflect on how they can best support caregivers

ACKNOWLEDGEMENTS

We would like to thank Ellen Gallagher for the illustration of Margaret Gallagher, and Katherine, Mary, Gerard and Sheelagh Gallagher and Carmel Staunton for reflections on the caregiver's experience.

REFERENCES

Alzheimer's Society. (2019). *Sleep disturbance and waking up at night*. Retrieved from https://www.alzheimers.org.uk/about-dementia/symptoms-and-diagnosis/sleep-and-night-time-disturbance (Accessed 8 March 2019).

Brennan, S., Lawlor, B., Pertl, M., O'Sullivan, M., Begley, E., & O'Connell, C. (2017). *De-Stress: A Study to Assess the Health & Wellbeing of Spousal Carers of People with Dementia in Ireland*. Dublin: The Alzheimer Society of Ireland.

British Red Cross. (2019). *Home to the unknown: getting hospital discharge right*. Retrieved from https://www.redcross.org.uk/about-us/what-we-do/we-speak-up-for-change/more-support-when-leaving-hospital/getting-hospital-discharge-right (Accessed 8 March 2019).

Carers UK. (2015). *Facts about carers*. Retrieved from https://www.carersuk.org/news-and-campaigns/press-releases/facts-and-figures (Accessed 8 March 2019).

Carers UK. (2018). *State of caring 2018*. Retrieved from https://www.carersuk.org/for-professionals/policy/policy-library/state-of-caring-2018-2 (Accessed 8 March 2019).

Feil, N., & deKlerk-Rubin, V. (2012). *The validation breakthrough* (3rd edn.). Baltimore: Health Professions Press.

Martin, L. (2019). *Practical nutrition and hydration for dementia-friendly mealtimes* (1st edn.). London: Jessica Kingsley.

Maslach, C., & Leiter, M. P. (2016). Understanding the burnout experience: recent research and its implications for psychiatry. *World Psychiatry, 15*, 103–111.

Newcastle University. *Dementia care: staying connected and living well*. Retrieved from https://www.futurelearn.com/courses/dementia-care (Accessed 1 April 2019).

71

Loneliness

Anna Lewis & Tahir Masud

LEARNING OBJECTIVES

- Describe the concept of loneliness
- List the negative impacts of loneliness on physical and psychological well-being and on health and social care services
- Identify potential interventions available to address loneliness and explain how we can make them more accessible to patients

CASE

Franz has had a prolonged stay in an acute hospital followed by residential rehabilitation. He is not yet back at baseline mobility, and although community input is planned, he is unlikely to return to his pre-admission level of function. His wife recently died and he has no local family. He no longer drives and misses the close personal contacts he used to enjoy. The community team feel that his lack of motivation and isolation is affecting his progress now that he is back at home.

WHAT IS LONELINESS?

Mother Teresa is said to have quoted: "the greatest disease in the West today is not TB or leprosy; it is being unwanted, unloved, and uncared for. We can cure physical diseases with medicine, but the only cure for loneliness, despair, and hopelessness is love..." (Tiwari, 2013).

Although there seems to have been a recent interest in loneliness, it is not a new concept and was first defined in 1981 (Perlman & Peplau, 1981). Surprisingly, the incidence of loneliness has actually changed very little over the past few decades (Patel, Wardle, & Parikh, 2019).

Although the terms loneliness and social isolation are often used interchangeably, they mean slightly different things. Social isolation describes minimal contact with other people, whereas loneliness is a perceived state of isolation, i.e. when a person feels that they lack relationships, closeness and interaction. Although the two are linked and often coexist, it is possible to be socially isolated without feeling lonely and vice versa. Many older people living within nursing homes and large households may report feeling lonely, despite being surrounded by others. As humans we not only desire the presence of others but we also want to be able to form meaningful relationships based on trust, communication, working together and valuing one another (Masi et al., 2011).

WHY ARE PEOPLE LONELY?

Almost 80% of our waking hours are spent with others, be that friends, family, distant relations or co-workers, and generally this time is perceived to be happier and more rewarding than time spent alone (Hawkley & Cacioppo, 2010). Approximately 49% of those aged over 75 years live alone with 6% of older people leaving their house once a week or less (Davidson & Rossall, 2015). Social isolation affects 11%-24% of older people but only 6%-13% of older people report being often or always lonely (Patel et al., 2019). Older people are more often socially isolated due to bereavement, outliving close family and friends and declining health and mobility, which creates difficulties in getting out (see Fig. 71.1). Other risk factors for loneliness include poor self-reported health, household size, housing ownership, dependence for activities of daily living (ADLs), having multiple eye conditions and marital status (Campaign to End Loneliness, 2016).

Loneliness is typically a transient feeling and has been likened to hunger or thirst as a prompt to alter our behaviour. In this case it encourages us to maintain and repair relationships, to enable us to lead a happier and more fulfilling life. Importantly, from a biological point of view, these social connections may result in gene transmission and survival of the human species. If the opportunity to form such associations is lost, the state of loneliness becomes chronic with detrimental effects (Masi et al., 2011).

WHY DOES IT MATTER?

The consequences of loneliness are of concern (see Fig. 71.2), and it can be considered a disease state (Tiwari, 2013). Predictably there are effects on mental health with higher rates of depression and cognitive impairment/dementia. Risk of suicide is increased further in a group of people, who are already considered to be at high risk (Hawkley & Cacioppo, 2010). Physical health effects include increased risk of stroke and cardiovascular disease and subsequent

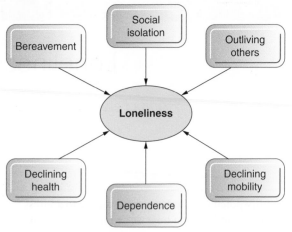

FIG. 71.1 Risk factors for loneliness.

increase in mortality rate. Loneliness is now being compared to the more widely known risk factors of smoking and obesity (Courtin & Knapp, 2017).

There is evidence that loneliness increases progression of frailty with both motor and functional decline (Gale, Westbury, & Cooper, 2018). It is also linked with poor nutrition and sleep disturbance (Choi, Irwin, & Cho, 2015). All of these factors affect the potential for rehabilitation and independent living, with repercussions on both the health and social care systems. People identified as being lonely make more calls to emergency services, request a greater number of GP appointments and are at increased risk of requiring nursing home admission (Hanratty et al., 2018).

When people are lonely they often view themselves in a more negative way and begin to expect rejection. This low self-esteem and resultant anxiety leads them to become more self-conscious in new social situations and less willing to interact with others. This vicious cycle of thoughts and behaviours reinforces the feeling of loneliness and is referred to as maladaptive social cognition (Masi et al., 2011).

MEASURING LONELINESS

Several scales have been developed to measure loneliness, mainly for research purposes, but also useful to service providers. Commonly used in research, but perhaps too long for everyday use, is the "The De-Jong Giervald" 6-Item Loneliness Scale, which was designed specifically for older people and can separate out "social" from "emotional" loneliness. Another widely used instrument is the "UCLA" (University of California, Los Angeles) 3-item scale, although it was originally designed for younger students. Potentially more useful in healthcare settings are single-item scales such as the "English Longitudinal Study of Ageing" (ELSA) single-item question, which simply asks "How often do you feel lonely? Hardly ever, some of the time or often?" This is quick and easy to use, although the reliability has not been extensively tested.

The Campaign to End Loneliness has written guidance on the use of these measurement tools, discussing their advantages, disadvantages and limitations. They have also designed their own loneliness measurement tool which has the advantage of being worded in a more positive language, without mentioning the word "loneliness" (Campaign to End Loneliness, 2015).

WHAT CAN WE DO ABOUT IT?

Preventing loneliness is important in maintaining both physical and psychological well-being. Efforts to reduce loneliness have concentrated on reducing social isolation, which should in part be achievable by increasing independence. Addressing certain health issues increases the likelihood of people getting out and interacting with their local community. Poor mobility is a significant barrier, and simple measures such as foot care, chiropody and addressing pain control can improve this. Other considerations that prevent people from socialising are memory, continence, hearing and visual problems (Cooke, 2018). Such issues should be highlighted as a routine part of a comprehensive geriatric assessment, but health

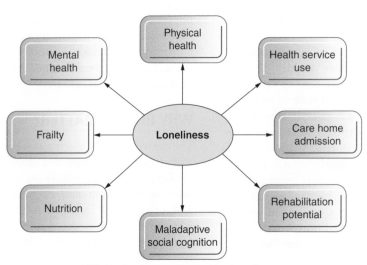

FIG. 71.2 Areas affected by loneliness.

professionals should also enquire about support networks and participation in activities.

Interventions to address loneliness can be delivered either in groups (e.g. support groups, reminiscence therapy) or on a one-to-one basis (e.g. training in computer use, animal companionship, visitor volunteers, befriending schemes) (Landeiro et al., 2017). They can be organised in community settings, supported living facilities or in a patient's own home.

It is suggested that there are four ways to help reduce social isolation and the feeling of loneliness:

1. Training people in social skills by providing education on developing friendships and other social behaviours.
2. Enhancing social support networks. This can include befriending programs and specialist support groups for those with specific health conditions or recent bereavement.
3. Increasing opportunities for social interaction. Provision of transport can allow people to attend events and groups in the community and technology can be used for communication or interactive games and activities.
4. Focusing on maladaptive social cognition, as described above, which can be effectively reversed by using social cognitive training (Masi et al., 2011).

ARE INTERVENTIONS SUCCESSFUL?

Reducing social isolation in older people is most effective when tackled using group-based formats and when the individuals are required to actively participate (Dickens et al., 2011). Providing social opportunities however will not always solve loneliness as we also need to change the way people approach their social relationships. Addressing maladaptive social cognition through either cognitive behavioural therapy or psychological reframing has shown greater reduction in loneliness compared to those targeting social interactions alone (Masi et al., 2011).

WHO CAN HELP?

Loneliness is recognised as an important issue, and the UK government has demonstrated their commitment to this with the appointment of a Minister for Loneliness. The British Geriatrics Society is welcoming and supporting the development and delivery of the UK government's strategies to reduce social isolation, loneliness and its consequences (Cooke, 2018). Voluntary organisations such as The Red Cross and the UK Royal Voluntary Service offer potential solutions as do other local charity projects. "Social prescribing" is set to become more widespread, with the plan for a network of social prescribing link workers across the UK (Dickens et al., 2011).

This is a service which helps to link people with sources of support and social activities within their community.

"Campaign to End Loneliness" is a charitable organisation in the UK who aim to share approaches to combat loneliness. The three steps to their campaign are:

- Identifying and establishing contact with lonely people
- Understanding the contributory factors in that person's loneliness
- Establishing the best way to address this and then supporting the individual to access appropriate services (Campaign to End Loneliness, 2016).

Age UK has produced loneliness maps to focus attention on the localities likely to benefit from extra support. Health and social care services are being encouraged to create community resource directories detailing services available to older people. They are advised to produce these in a range of electronic and hard copy formats to reach a greater number of people. These could then be distributed to staff and volunteers who come into contact with older people.

Working with registrar departments, hospices, and GP surgeries can help target recently bereaved older people to promote local opportunities for social contact. Engagement with charities, fire and rescue services, housing associations, relevant public services, and businesses such as supermarkets, leisure centres and libraries can also help direct attention where it is required (Campaign to End Loneliness, 2016).

Current research is also focussing on technology, both existing and novel, to promote socialising in order to prevent and treat loneliness. For example, virtual reality, social media, TV-based socialising and near-field communication have been used to try and motivate people to take steps to combat loneliness and such "persuasive technology" could potentially change behaviour. "Socialisation robots" are increasingly being used in some societies such as Japan (Abdi et al., 2018). One particular type of socially assistive robot is the "robotic pet" which has proved useful for some older people.

CONCLUSION

There is a huge amount of work to be done in this area, but there is great potential and desire to tackle the problem. Everyone involved in rehabilitation of older people must be aware of loneliness, understand its impact and look to identify those affected. It is important to be familiar with local services, ensuring opportunities are made available to those would benefit, who are often the more vulnerable members of society. Together we must be at the forefront in developing schemes to combat this important condition.

▌ SUMMARY POINTS

- Loneliness is the perception of feeling isolated and lacking in relationships; it does not necessarily mean minimal contact with people
- There is evidence of significant negative effects on both physical and mental health and of increased use of emergency, primary and social care services

- Addressing loneliness requires recognition of those at risk and knowledge of interventions available. Healthcare staff are often well placed to assist in this
- It is important to ensure that proposed interventions are accessible to patients as it is frequently the more vulnerable and less independent patients who require them

MCQs

Q.1 Which one of the following describes loneliness?
  a. Living a long distance from friends and family
  b. The perception of a lack of meaningful relationships and social interactions
  c. Living alone with no opportunity to meet people
  d. The loss of a spouse, partner or close family member

Q.2 Evidence suggests that the most effective intervention for loneliness is:
  a. Group based intervention to reduce social isolation
  b. One-to-one intervention providing education in social interaction and developing relationships
  c. Group-based intervention enhancing social support networks
  d. Cognitive behavioural therapy focussing on maladaptive social cognition

REFERENCES

Abdi, J., Al-Hindawi, A., Ng, T., & Vizcaychipi, M. P. (2018). Scoping review on the use of socially assistive robot technology in elderly care. *BMJ Open, 8*, e018815.

Campaign to End Loneliness. (2016). *The missing million: in search of the loneliest in our communities*. Retrieved from: https://www.campaigntoendloneliness.org/wp-content/uploads/The-Missing-Million-report-FINAL.pdf.

Campaign to End Loneliness. (2015). *Measuring your impact on loneliness in later life*. Retrieved from: https://www.campaigntoendloneliness.org/wp-content/uploads/Loneliness-Measurement-Guidance1.pdf.

Choi, H., Irwin, M. R., & Cho, H. J. (2015). Impact of social isolation on behavioural health in elderly: systematic review. *World Journal of Psychiatry, 5*(4), 432–438.

Cooke, C. (2018). BGS response to call for evidence on tackling loneliness. 27 July 2018. Retrieved from: https://www.bgs.org.uk/policy-and-media/bgs-response-to-call-for-evidence-on-tackling-loneliness.

Courtin, E., & Knapp, M. (2017). Social isolation, loneliness and health in old age: a scoping review. *Health and Social Care in the Community, 25*(3), 799–812.

Davidson, S., & Rossall, P. (2015). Age UK Loneliness Evidence Review July 2015. Retrieved from: https://www.ageuk.org.uk/globalassets/age-uk/documents/reports-and-publications/reports-and-briefings/health--wellbeing/rb_june15_lonelines_in_later_life_evidence_review.pdf.

Dickens, A. P., Richards, S. H., Greaves, C. J., & Campbell, J. L. (2011). Interventions targeting social isolation in older people: a systematic review. *BMC Public Health, 11*(1), 647.

Gale, C. R., Westbury, L., & Cooper, C. (2018). Social isolation and loneliness as risk factors for the progression of frailty: the English Longitudinal Study of Ageing. *Age and Ageing, 47*(3), 392–397.

Hanratty, B., Stow, D., Moore, D. C., Valtorta, N. K., & Matthews, F. (2018). Loneliness as a risk factor for care home admission in the English Longitudinal Study of Ageing. *Age and Ageing, 47*(6), 896–900.

Hawkley, L. C., & Cacioppo, J. T. (2010). Loneliness matters: a theoretical and empirical review of consequences and mechanisms. *Annals of Behavioral Medicine, 40*(2), 218–227.

Landeiro, F., Barrows, P., Nuttall Musson, E., Gray, A. M., & Leal, J. (2017). Reducing social isolation and loneliness in older people: a systematic review protocol. *BMJ Open, 7*, e013778.

Masi, C. M., Chen, H. Y., Hawkley, L. C., & Cacioppo, J. T. (2011). A meta-analysis of interventions to reduce loneliness. *Personality and Social Psychology Review, 15*(3), 219–266.

Patel, R. S., Wardle, K., & Parikh, R. J. (2019). Loneliness: the present and the future. *Age and Ageing, 48*(4), 476–477.

Perlman, D., & Peplau, L. A. (1981). Towards a social psychology of loneliness. In R. Gilmour, & S. Duck (Eds.), *Personal relationships 3: relationships in disorder* (pp. 31–56). London: Academic Press.

Tiwari, S. C. (2013). Loneliness: a disease? *Indian Journal of Psychiatry, 55*(4), 320–322.

72

Continuing Rehabilitation at Home

Vanda Cummins & Elissa Burton

LEARNING OBJECTIVES

- Identify key components of community-based care plans
- Categorise older adults based on their function and activity levels, not their age
- Discuss recommended strength, balance and physical activity levels
- Describe key enablers and barriers to staying fit for life

INTRODUCTION

There are three sections to this chapter. Section 1 explores re-adjusting to the home environment, changes in health and social supports, expectations and care plans.

Section 2 categorises older adults by functional ability and looks at maximising independence through modifiable influences of physical activity and exercise. Section 3 looks at enablers and barriers to staying fit for life.

SECTION 1: TRANSITIONING FROM HOSPITAL TO HOME

On returning home after a stay in hospital, the rehabilitation focus changes from "what do I need to do to get home?" to "what do I need to do to keep myself at home?" Emotions can range from relief at being home to worry about coping without 24-hour hospital support. A support team may include family, friends, healthcare and social care providers. The rehabilitation environment changes, and community-based occupational therapists and physiotherapists may be needed to advise and assist with mobility issues and additional equipment in the home, garden and community surrounds. Opportunities to adapt and safely use these environments to meet rehabilitation needs should be sought. For example balance activity supports could include kitchen counter tops, tables or narrow hallways.

Person-Centred Care Plans

To help the transition home, the hospital team should develop a patient-centred discharge care plan. Community-based rehabilitation services and teams should be involved in this process. Good communication is crucial to manage roles and responsibilities while keeping the needs, preferences and expectations of the older person and their family at the centre of care. A study of 1000 people readmitted to hospital after a recent discharge found that whilst the majority reported no difficulties understanding their care plan, most reported difficulties carrying it out (Greysen et al., 2017). Knowledge

was not enough; planning skills and a willingness to implement their plan were also needed to successfully self-manage (Greysen et al., 2017). For example, not only do you need to know to take your medications (knowledge), you also need to fill your pill box with the right tablets in the right time slots (planning) and take your pills at the right time as prescribed (willingness to carry out the plan) (Greysen et al., 2017). Care providers both in hospital and community services should consider all these skills along with social influences and motivational and behaviour change strategies. The British Geriatrics Society (2017) recommends that community-based care plans consider the following:

- Person designated to coordinate care and reviews
- Health and social care summary
- Well-being maintenance plan including goals and actions
- Escalation plan if issues arise
- Urgent care or advanced care plan (if necessary).

This planning should support the physical and emotional needs of the older person and their carer along their rehabilitation journey and across their changing spectrum of need.

Case 1: 80-Year-Old Bert (See Fig. 72.1)

"Coming home from hospital after my second hip replacement was much tougher. It took a long time for me to accept I wasn't able to do what I used to. My children have busy lives and I didn't want to bother them. People don't want to hear you moaning. I went into myself and I'd say I got depressed. What helped me most was those who gave me hope. Hope is a great thing. I needed to feel listened to and supported. I needed encouragement to start group exercises and meet others and I'm very grateful to the primary care team who motivated me to start. There's strength in numbers. My advice looking back on where I was is don't be hard on yourself. Adjust your expectations to help yourself feel less 'stuck'. Feeling better won't just happen, you have to make an effort to do more for yourself. Express how you feel to people. Find things to make you hopeful. Don't depend on tablets. Try new things like meditation, group exercises and health and wellbeing advice. Start by doing

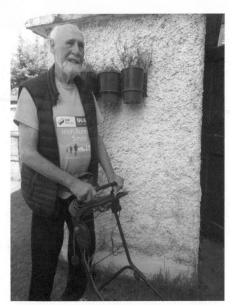

FIG. 72.1 Bert who keeps busy by helping his daughter in her garden.

what you can. Do a little bit, then a little bit more. Get involved in something you love so you can give back a bit to others even if that means having to change how you do it."

SECTION 2: CATEGORISING OLDER PEOPLE ACCORDING TO FUNCTION AND PHYSICAL ACTIVITY LEVELS AND NOT AGE

Older people have a wide range of functional needs that services need to support. The UK National Service Framework for Older People (Department of Health United Kingdom, 2001) describes three broad groups with different health and social care policy goals:

1. **Entering old age:** Independent and regularly active, so goals should promote and extend healthy life.
2. **Transitional phase:** Functional ability declining towards frailty, so goals should identify emerging problems ahead of crisis and ways to effectively respond.
3. **Frail older adults:** Independence and quality of life are compromised, so goals should anticipate and respond to problems recognising the complex interaction of physical, mental and social care factors.

The Rockwood Clinical Frailty Scale (Rockwood et al., 2005) is a clinical measure of fitness and frailty that has nine categories of function ranging from very fit to completely dependent.

Why Is Physical Activity and Exercise Important for Older People?

Maintaining independence is a key priority for older people. As we age, there is a normal decline in function; however, this can be reduced by staying physically active, building muscle and bone strength, improving balance and avoiding long periods of sedentary behaviour (Skelton & Mavroeidi, 2018).

Sedentary lifestyles (sitting or lying for long periods) lead to loss of muscle and bone strength. Loss of muscle mass is known as sarcopenia or 'flesh poverty' and can be concomitant with an increase in fat mass, so total body weight may not change (Kim & Choi, 2013). Sarcopenia is not inevitable and can potentially be reversible with strength training (Skelton & Mavroeidi, 2018). If functional decline continues below the 'disability threshold', the consequences can be life changing as the older person is now unable to stand up off a chair or toilet on their own. This leads to loss of autonomy and a greater dependence on carers.

A study with 90+ year old nursing home residents showed that when they took part in a 12-week strengthening programme, their leg strength almost doubled (Fiatarone et al., 1990). This study also supports a "dosage-response" curve showing the frailer a person is before starting exercise, the greater their potential gains, in other words they have the most to gain. Also, Harvey, Chastin, & Skelton (2018) showed that if older people broke up sedentary behaviours by adding extra 'sit to stands' throughout the day for 10 weeks both their speed in getting out of a chair and ability to walk and turn were improved.

Guidelines for Physical Activity and Strength and Balance Activities

Exercise at the right dosage and duration is called "The miracle cure" (Livingston et al., 2017). However, there is no ideal exercise or physical activity to suit everybody, and participation levels vary depending on abilities, needs and preferences. Igniting motivation and self-efficacy skills can enhance participation levels (see Fig. 72.2).

Exercise guidelines (World Health Organization, 2011) for adults over 65 years recommend at least 150 minutes of moderate activity a week, with daily activity preferable. Extended periods of sedentary behaviour should be broken up, and strength and balance activities should be undertaken at least twice a week. However, research shows that fewer than 20% of older populations around the world participate in strength and balance training, and these figures decrease with age (Bennie et al., 2016, Humphries, Duncan, & Mummery, 2011, Mayer et al., 2011, Merom et al., 2012, National Center for Health Statistics, 2015).

In the latest Cochrane Review of effectiveness of exercise on reducing falls for older people living in the community, balance and functional exercises showed the greatest effect in reducing both the rate of falls and the number of people experiencing falls (Sherrington et al., 2019). Multiple types of exercise such as balance, functional and strength training combined also showed a positive effect as did Tai Chi although the quality of evidence was not as high for Tai Chi (Sherrington et al., 2019). Sherrington et al. (2017) suggest that to be effective in the prevention of falls, exercise programmes should be undertaken for at least 3 hours a week (this can be a combination of group and home-based exercise). Programmes should involve challenging and progressive balance and resistance training and exercise in a standing position. The 3 hours a week exercise should continue for

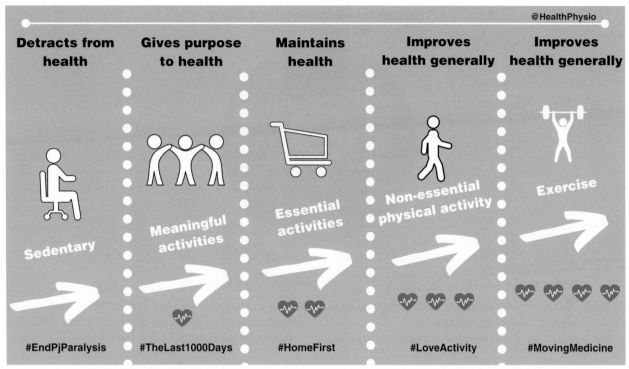

FIG. 72.2 Continuum of meaningful activities. (Reproduced with kind permission from Chris Tuckett 2019 @ HealthPhysio.)

a minimum of 50 hours (dosage) over a period of at least 6 months (duration).

Interventions that integrate functional exercise into daily life are a promising alternative or complement to structured exercise (Weber et al., 2018. These programmes were preferred by older people who disliked the concept of exercise or who felt they did not have the time to do exercises (Burton et al., 2014). See Resources section of book for further details of these and other evidence-based falls prevention exercise programmes such as "Otago" and "Falls Management Exercise Programmes" and links to movement campaigns like "Make Every Contact Count" and "Movement is Medicine".

Case 2 (See Figs 72.3 and 72.4)

To reduce feelings of unsteadiness and her fear of falling, Marlene was taught how to embed Lifestyle integrated functional exercises (LiFE) into everyday activities so they become

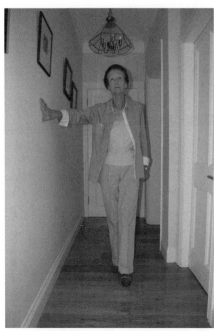

FIG. 72.3 Marlene in hallway.

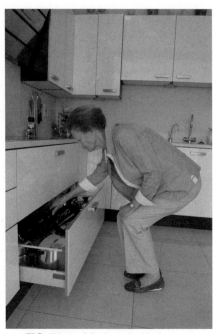

FIG. 72.4 Marlene in kitchen.

**Focus on the exercise donut (the whole)
and not just the hole**

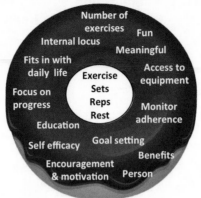

FIG. 72.5   The exercise donut. (Reproduced with kind permission from Ben McCormack 2019 @CorKinetic.)

a daily habit. Now every time she masters a challenge, she sets herself a new slightly harder one. For example,

Picture 1. Every time she walks down her hallway, she challenges her balance reactions by narrowing the width of her steps as if walking on a line (she can progress this further by not touching the wall or closing her eyes).

Picture 2. Every time she reaches into her saucepan drawer or empties the dishwasher, she focuses on using her legs as much as possible during the squat. As this becomes easier, she tries squatting further.

SECTION 3: ENABLERS AND BARRIERS TO STAYING FIT FOR LIFE

In a study of older adults wanting to live independently in their own homes, the main motivations to be physically active were maintaining or improving health and well-being, followed by enjoyment, and to be socially active particularly with family and friends (Burton, Lewin, & Boldy, 2013). Walking as their means of transport to the shops or medical appointments also motivated some people (Burton et al., 2013).

Barriers to being physically active included lack of time, cost and having no one to be active with. Having a pet, or combining a walk with a family member perhaps to the local café helped (Burton et al., 2013). Integrating exercise into activities such as watching television helped removing the barrier of no time.

Ongoing injury or illness can be a major barrier (Burton et al., 2013). Many believe that when they experience pain, such as with osteoarthritis, the best thing to do is restrict activity and hope the pain subsides. Studies show for osteoarthritis, strength training can reduce pain as well as improve functional aspects if completed correctly ((Li et al., 2016)). If pain is reduced, they may be more likely to stay physically active over the longer term.

Another barrier reported is that they are "too old" (Burton et al., 2013). However, a 90-year-old who has been physically active all their life may be healthier and living independently more easily than a 75-year-old who has never been active, is now experiencing health issues and refuses to be active.

CONCLUSION

Embedding routine physical activity into daily life helps maximise independence. Physical, mental, social and emotional health can influence physical activity levels. Fig. 72.5 "The Exercise donut" considers meaningful 'hooks' or personal values and shows it is not a one-size-fits-all approach.

SUMMARY POINTS

- Care plans should support the physical and emotional needs of older people and their carers and be responsive to changing needs along their rehabilitation journey

- To prevent falls, strength and balance exercises should be progressively challenging and undertaken for at least 3 hours a week for a minimum of 6 months
- No one-size-fits-all and exercise programmes should suit abilities, needs and preferences

MCQs

Q.1 In general, healthy older people should participate in the following amount of physical activity every week to gain health benefits:
  a. 150 minutes of walking only

  b. 150 minutes of moderate-intensity aerobic activity, plus strength and balance training twice a week
  c. Strength and balance training four times a week
  d. None of the above; as people age they should not be active

Q.2 Which one of the following strategies has the greatest effect on preventing falls for older people living in the community?

a. Participate in a strength, balance and functional training programme on a regular basis

b. Stay seated and do not move around in case the person falls

c. Walk every day

d. Start swimming regularly

REFERENCES

Bennie, J., Pedisic, Z., van Uffelen, J., Charity, M., Harvey, J., Banting, L., Vergeer, I., Biddle, S., & Eime, R. (2016). Pumping iron in Australia: prevalence, trends and sociodemographic correlates of muscle strengthening activity participation from a national sample of 195,926 adults. *PlOS One, 11*, e0153225.

British Geriatrics Society. (2017). *Fit for frailty Part 1 and Part 2. Consensus best practice guidance for older people living in community and outpatient settings*. London: British Geriatrics Society.

Burton, E., Lewin, G., & Boldy, D. (2013). Barriers and motivators to being physically active for older home care clients. *Physical & Occupational Therapy in Geriatrics, 31*, 21–36.

Burton, E., Lewin, G., Clemson, L., & Boldy, D. (2014). Long term benefits of a lifestyle exercise program for older people receiving a restorative home care service: a pragmatic randomized controlled trial. *Healthy Aging & Clinical Care in the Elderly, 6*, 1–9.

Department of Health United Kingdom. (2001). *National service framework for older people*. London: Department of Health United Kingdom.

Fiatarone, M., Marks, E., Ryan, N., Meredith, C., Lipsitz, L., & Evans, W. (1990). High-intensity strength training in nonagenarians. Effects on skeletal muscle. *JAMA, 263*, 3029–3034.

Greysen, S., Harrison, J., Kripalani, S., Vasilevskis, E., Robinson, E., Metlay, J., & Auerbach, A. (2017). Understanding patient-centred readmission factors: a multi-site, mixed-methods study. *BMJ Quality & Safety, 26*, 33–41.

Harvey, J., Chastin, S., & Skelton, D. (2018). Breaking sedentary behaviour has the potential to increase/maintain function in frail older adults. *Journal of Frailty, Sarcopenia and Falls, 3*, 26–34.

Humphries, B., Duncan, M., & Mummery, W. (2011). Prevalence and correlates of resistance training in a regional Australian population. *British Journal of Sports Medicine, 44*, 653–656.

Kim, T., & Choi, K. (2013). Sarcopenia: definition, epidemiology, and pathophysiology. *Journal of Bone Metabolism, 20*, 1–10.

Li, Y., Su, X., Chen, S., Zhang, Y., Zhang, Z., Liu, C., …, & Zheng, N. (2016). The effects of resistance exercise in patients with knee osteoarthritis: a systematic review and meta-analysis. *Clinical Rehabilitation, 30*(10), 947–959.

Livingston, G., Sommerlad, A., Orgeta, V., Costafreda, S., Huntley, J., Ames, D., …, & Mukadam, N. (2017). Dementia prevention, intervention, and care. *The Lancet, 390*, 2673–2734.

Mayer, F., Scharhag-Rosenberger, F., Carlsohn, A., Cassel, M., Müller, S., & Scharhag, J. (2011). The intensity and effects of strength training in the elderly. *Deutsches Ärzteblatt International, 108*, 359–364.

Merom, D., Pye, V., Macniven, R., van der Ploeg, H., Milat, A., Sherrington, C., Lord, S., & Bauman, A. (2012). Prevalence and correlates of participation in fall prevention exercise/physical activity by older adults. *Preventive Medicine, 55*, 613–617.

National Center for Health Statistics. (2015). *Health, United States, 2014: with special feature on adults aged 55–64*. Hyattsville, MD: National Center for Health Statistics.

Rockwood, K., Song, X., Macknight, C., Bergman, H., Hogan, D., McDowell, I., & Mitnitski, A. (2005). A global clinical measure of fitness and frailty in elderly people. *Canadian Medical Association Journal, 173*, 489–495.

Sherrington, C., Fairhall, N., Wallbank, G., Tiedemann, A., Michaleff, Z., Howard, K., …, & Lamb, S. (2019). Exercise for preventing falls in older people living in the community. *Cochrane Database of Systematic Reviews, 1*, CD012424.

Sherrington, C., Michaleff, Z., Fairhall, N., Paul, S., Tiedemann, A., Whitney, J., …, & Lord, S. (2017). Exercise to prevent falls in older adults: an updated systematic review and meta-analysis. *British Journal of Sports Medicine, 51*, 1749–1757.

Skelton, D., & Mavroeidi, A. (2018). How do muscle and bone strengthening and balance activities (MBSBA) vary across the life course, and are there particular ages where MBSBA are most important? *Journal of Frailty, Sarcopenia and Falls, 3*, 74–81.

Weber, M., Belala, N., Clemson, L., et al. (2018). Feasibility and effectiveness of intervention programmes integrating functional exercise into daily life of older adults: a systematic review. *Gerontology, 64*(2), 172–187.

World Health Organization. (2011). *Global recommendations on physical activity for health 65 years and above* [Online]. Geneva, Switzerland. Retrieved from: http://www.who.int/dietphysicalactivity/physical-activity-recommendations-65years.pdf (Accessed 26 July 2017).

73

Driving Assessment and Rehabilitation

Desmond O'Neill

LEARNING OBJECTIVES

- Explain why assessment and management of driving and transport has become an important element of rehabilitation for older people
- Describe the importance of a due balance between mobility and safety
- List the principles and resources required for assessment of fitness to drive
- Discuss the ethical and legal implications of medical fitness to drive for older people

Driving is an instrumental activity of daily life of huge consequence at all ages and in particular in later life (O'Neill, 2015) but the empirical literature is modest, and a number of background issues contribute to the gaps in our knowledge.

These include failure of the public health community to recognise transport mobility as a vector of well-being and social inclusion. The chapter on transport in one of the key (and otherwise excellent) texts of public health (Marmot & Wilkinson, 1999) makes for unhappy reading: accidents, pollution and the impact of cars on exercise, and no mention of the association of lack of access to transport with impaired health and social inclusion (Hjorthol, 2013).

Gerontologists have also failed to appreciate the importance of driving: there is little or no coverage of driving in most longitudinal studies of ageing, with disproportionate emphasis on public transport (Bartley & O'Neill, 2010). This neglect has extended into clinical services, with doctors not enquiring about driving and transport status of patients in a range of relevant conditions, and poor awareness of guidelines on medical fitness to drive.

Although there has been progress on developing methodologies for assessment and rehabilitation of driving for individual conditions such as stroke, Parkinson's disease and arthritis, there has been almost no attention paid to driver rehabilitation for multimorbidity. Transport is an issue of great importance to older people and also provides a pragmatic illustration of the positive attributes of ageing, that of an exemplary safety record for older drivers despite high levels of multimorbidity (Cicchino & McCartt, 2014).

A KEY ELEMENT OF SOCIAL INCLUSION AND WELL-BEING

The most major change in the literature of transport and health in the last decade has been the recognition that the focus on medical fitness to drive must maintain a due equilibrium between mobility and safety (OECD, 2001). The literature for the first 100 years has been almost obsessively concerned with safety (Oxley & Whelan, 2008).

Private cars and walking are the predominant forms of transport for the general public and older people in the developed world: even if usage of public transport is increasing among older US citizens, it remains below 3% of trips (Lynott & Figueiredo, 2011). Driving cessation is associated with a range of negative health outcomes, including depression (Marottoli et al., 1997), nursing home placement (Freeman et al., 2006) and death (Edwards et al., 2009). Negative social outcomes and impaired quality of life (Banister & Bowling, 2004) are causes of concern (Davey, 2007) affecting spouses and partners (Curl et al., 2015), and reducing spending in the wider economy (Kim & Richardson, 2006).

THEORETICAL BASIS OF MOBILITY

The theoretical framework for aligning transport with health and well-being has advanced in recent years. A useful concept is that of the life space, concentric areas of expanding distance within and outside the home with increasing requirements for independent mobility (May, Nayak, & Isaacs, 1985). Higher scores on life space are correlated with increased quality of life in older people (Rantakokko et al., 2013), and lower scores with impaired physical performance and lower sense of autonomy (Portegijs et al., 2014).

CLINICAL ASPECTS OF DRIVING AND AGEING

Given that medical factors have a relatively small role to play in accident causation (Marshall, 2008), including dementia and stroke (Chee et al., 2017; Rapoport et al., 2019), that older drivers strategically adapt to their age-related disability (De Raedt & Ponjaert-Kristoffersen, 2000), and that transport

TABLE 73.1 **Sample diseases and conditions for which appropriate assessment and remediation may be of benefit.**

FRAILTY AND DECONDITIONING REHABILITATION (Marottoli et al., 2007)	
Neuropsychiatric	
Stroke	Driving-specific rehabilitation (Akinwuntan et al., 2005)
Parkinson's disease	Maximising motor function, treatment of depression, assessment of cognitive function (O'Neill, 2008)
Delirium	Treatment and resolution
Depression	Treatment: if antidepressant, choose one with least potential of cognitive/motor effects (Rubinsztein & Lawton, 1995)
Mild dementia	Assess, treat depression, reduce/eliminate psychoactive drugs, advice not to drive alone (Breen et al., 2007)
Cardiovascular	
Syncope	Advice pending investigation: treat cause (Sorajja et al., 2009)
Respiratory	
Sleep apnoea	Treatment of underlying disease (Alvarez et al., 2008)
Vision	
Cataract	Surgery, appropriate corrective lens and advice about glare (Monestam & Wachtmeister, 1997)
Metabolic	
Diabetes	Direct therapy to avoid hypoglycaemia (Stork, van Haeften, & Veneman, 2007)
Musculoskeletal	
All arthritides	Driving-specific rehabilitation programme (Jones, McCann, & Lassere, 1991)
Iatrogenic	
Polypharmacy	Rationalise medications (Ray, Thapa, & Shorr, 1993)
Psychoactive medication	Rationalise, minimise (Ray et al., 1992)

is so important in optimal ageing, the healthcare team need to move from the traditional position of arbiter of who should not drive to that of enabler of safe transport.

There is an impressive range of evidence for interventions that improve comfort and safety for older drivers (Table 73.1). In addition, licence restriction is associated with lower crash risk (O'Byrne, Naughton, & O'Neill, 2015), holding out promise that graduated driving reduction may be a viable alternative to driving cessation. While patients require advice for many medical conditions to protect them and other road users from harm (Redelmeier, Yarnell, & Tibshirani, 2013), they also need access to these enabling and rehabilitative strategies which facilitate continued and more comfortable driving.

The philosophy and practice of geriatric medicine provide a good basis for assessment of medical fitness to drive in older people. This is not a charter for dilettantism: rather, it is a challenge to develop the extra resources required to ensure that we have adequate support when making decisions about safe mobility of older people. This parallels the task of assessing safety at home or capacity to manage financial affairs: in these cases, it is good practice to liaise with an occupational therapist or a neuropsychologist. Further support can be gained from a range of guidelines on medical fitness to drive (American Geriatrics Society and Pomidor, 2016; Rapoport et al., 2015).

ELEMENTS OF THE DRIVING ASSESSMENT

Physicians assessing older people for transport/driving capability in rehabilitation need to know:
1. How does the older adult meet their transportation needs?
2. What intrinsic factors contribute to driving ability and how can we assess them?
3. What interventions should clinicians pursue?
4. What is the physician's responsibility in regard to driver licencing and insurance authorities?

TAKING A DRIVING/TRANSPORTATION HISTORY

Although it may seem obvious that transportation should figure in a comprehensive assessment, this is not necessarily the case: for example, many patients do not receive formal advice or assessment about driving after stroke (McNamara et al., 2014) or syncope (MacMahon, O'Neill, & Kenny, 1996). The patient's own assessment of driving should be assessed: a promising approach in this regard is the Adelaide Self-Efficacy Scale (George et al., 2007). A collateral (witness) history of driving abilities is important if the patient has cognitive impairment, cognisant of a potential conflict of interest of a spouse who does not drive (Adler et al., 2000): a proxy rating of self-efficacy may be helpful

BOX 73.1   Altered Driving Behaviours Which Should Arouse Concern

- Becoming lost in familiar areas
- Driving too fast
- Reacting too slowly
- Consistently making poor judgements
- Failure to notice street signs
- Having more accidents
- Receiving indecent gestures from other drivers
- Miscalculating speed and distances
- New dents on the car
- Knocking off rear view mirrors
- Showing poor judgement when making turns
- Impaired ability to recognise or understand road or traffic signs.

(Stapleton, Connolly, & O'Neill, 2012) and a new proxy instrument, the Fitness-to-Drive Screening Measure, shows potential (Winter, Classen, & Shanahan, 2014).

For patients with cognitive impairment, physicians should enquire about new unsafe driving behaviours. These behaviours present in a range of brain pathology, from head injury to dementia, and raise concerns about continuing driving privileges. It is important to recognise behaviours that represent a *change* from baseline (Box 73.1).

WHAT FACTORS ARE IMPORTANT IN DRIVING ASSESSMENT?

There are three main categories of medical conditions relevant to driving. The most important are those which affect *self-regulation*: at younger ages this mostly relates to immaturity, risky personality, alcohol dependence and psychiatric illness, but for older drivers is predominantly related to dementia. The second category is that of *physical impairments* relevant to driving, including those of vision, strength and coordination. Finally, some conditions can *suddenly disable* a driver, most commonly syncope, seizure and hypoglycaemia.

An older person can present with a combination of all three – for example Parkinson's disease with associated Lewy body disease and a tendency to fall asleep, further complicated by fluctuations – but in general it is the ability to self-regulate and behave in a prudent manner relative to the current clinical condition that is the key determinant of fitness to drive. This is consistent with risk homeostasis, the concept that best explains the complex and hierarchical processes of driving (Fuller, 2005).

Traditional neuropsychological test batteries do not reflect this model: unsurprisingly, psychometric approaches to assessing self-regulation have been disappointing (Ranney, 1994). All such batteries should be seen as an aid to an overall assessment of the functional status of the patient rather than as an indicator of whether or not the patient is fit to drive (Molnar et al., 2006).

The most effective clinical approach to the risk homeostasis model is the hierarchy of Michon of strategic, tactical and operational factors (Michon, 1985). The strategic level is the choice of whether or not to travel, the tactical decision is whether or not to overtake and the operational level is what to do when overtaking and faced with an oncoming car. The strategic and tactical levels are generally more important in terms of driving safety than the operational level, and experienced clinicians will be alert to this.

The most common personnel for driver assessment involves a combination of physician, occupational therapist and/or neuropsychologist, specialist driving assessor and/or social worker. Not all disciplines will be needed by all patients, as a trichotomy is usually the result of preliminary assessments (Molnar et al., 2006): should not drive (i.e. severe cognitive deficits) with referral to the social worker to plan alternative transportation as appropriate; no problem with driving (i.e. mild cognitive impairment); and those who require further evaluation, off- and/or on-road.

The overall interdisciplinary assessment should attempt to provide solutions to both maintaining activities and exploring transport needs. However, even in a skilled rehabilitation setting, the predictive value of team assessments may be low for diseases such as stroke (Akinwuntan et al., 2002): it is increasingly clear that early recourse to an on-road assessment is the optimal approach for those with cognitive impairment who need further assessment (Breen et al., 2007). Simulators may represent opportunities for both driver rehabilitation (Akinwuntan et al., 2005) (analogous to training aeroplane pilots) and assessment, albeit limited by increased simulator sickness with advancing age (Brooks et al., 2010).

On-road driver assessment is the near-optimal standard and should be offered to all patients who are not clearly dangerous when driving (Fig. 73.1). The assessor will require a full clinical report, and may choose to use one of the recently developed scoring systems for on-road assessment of

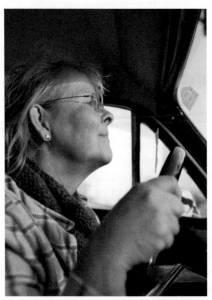

FIG. 73.1   On-road assessment should be offered to all patients who are not clearly dangerous when driving. (From Mik Lav/Shutterstock.com)

patients with dementia (Kowalski, Tuokko, & Tallman, 2010). This should ideally involve some degree of cognitive loading, which will tend to bring out the degree and extent to which the older driver can manage complex situations safely (Uc et al., 2004). Clarification of the skill set and training of on-road driving assessors remains an unresolved issue in most countries around the world (Di Stefano & Macdonald, 2010): relative to need in the USA, for example, there are very few trained on-road assessors (Betz et al., 2014).

There are certain limitations with road assessments. Occasionally a patient may perform well on an assessment but the proxy history and clinical examination may suggest a background pattern of driving and capabilities which seem unduly hazardous: in such cases, the clinical decision should outweigh the on-road assessment. Expenses for driving evaluations vary from USD $200 to $500, and health insurance or government health providers may not cover the cost. However, it is also argued that such a cost is not unreasonable in view of the other maintenance costs associated with the upkeep of a car.

WHAT INTERVENTIONS CAN WE MAKE?

Depending on the illnesses present, there is potentially a wide range of interventions that we can undertake (Table 73.1). Car adaptation on advice from an occupational therapist, physiotherapist or specialist driving assessor can improve driving comfort and safety as demonstrated in the CarFit programme (Stav, 2010). Follow-up review should be organised for those with progressive illness such as dementia and parkinsonism. A review period of 6–12 months is reasonable with a progressive neurodegenerative dementia (Duchek et al., 2003). However, patients and carers should be advised to seek an earlier review if they perceive a significant decline in the status of the dementia or in driving abilities.

For progressive neurological conditions, the physician needs to help the patient and their family prepare for eventual driving cessation. Early and appropriate diagnosis disclosure is likely to be important (Bahro et al., 1995) in conjunction with a modified Ulysses contract outlining that driving cessation needs to be planned for (Howe, 2000). This is named after the hero who made his crew tie him to the mast on the condition that they did not heed his entreaties to be released when seduced by the song of the sirens. It forms the basis of a useful patient and carer brochure (Hartford, 2000).

The act of highlighting the potential of compromised driving ability may have a therapeutic benefit, promoting increased vigilance among patient and carers that their social contract for driving privileges is not the same as that of the general public. Support is given to this concept by the success of restricted licencing for people with medical illnesses (O'Byrne et al., 2015). While the effect might arise from the restrictions (avoidance of motorways, night-time driving), it is also possible that the labelling of these drivers may heighten self-awareness.

A clear recommendation should be made to the patient and recorded in the medical record: this should include advice to inform their insurance company of relevant illnesses, as well as any statutory requirement to inform their driver licencing authority.

WHEN DRIVING IS NO LONGER POSSIBLE

At this stage, alternative options should be discussed with the patient, and friends and family as appropriate, as well as drawing on locally available resources. Training to use public transport and engaging with providers of public transport to adapt to the needs of those with acquired age-related disability is an underdeveloped rehabilitation practice with older people (Risser et al., 2015). State or local sponsored services may provide door-to-door transport for older adults in large vans, many of which are lift-equipped. Local communities, societies, retirement centres or local church groups may use funds or volunteers to provide services to physician offices, grocery stores and meetings. The place of mobility scooters in meeting this need is controversial: while not suitable for those with moderate-to-severe dementia, their role for those with physical disabilities is unclear (Auger et al., 2008) but they are increasingly popular (May, Garrett, & Ballantyne, 2010), and neither road nor pavements are currently configured for their safe use.

WHEN PATIENTS CONTINUE TO DRIVE DESPITE ADVICE TO CEASE

Previous medical fitness to drive guidelines may have laid too much emphasis on the role and responsibility of the doctor, and not enough on the responsibilities of drivers and other citizens, overmedicalising the response paradigm. When concerns arise over continued driving by a person with dementia and their driving habits are dangerous, it is misguided kindness to consider dangerous driving in terms of diagnosis and treatment of the underlying cause. Dangerous driving is not only a hazard to the driver and other road users, but also a statutory offence and should be reported to the police in the first instance.

This approach can lift a weight off doctors' shoulders, as not uncommonly a relative will ask the doctor to 'do something' about dangerous driving the relative has witnessed. As second-hand information, the doctor should remind the relative that they have a citizen's duty to report the dangerous driving to the police: the medical aspects can be dealt with subsequently.

It is also inappropriate and unfair to expect doctors to be the sole conduit for reporting driving that poses hazard to the general public: this responsibility, in the absence of a family member or carer witness, should lie with any healthcare professional witnessing the behaviour.

Breaking physician confidentiality faced with likelihood of hazard to other members of the public is almost universally supported by most codes of medical practice. It is expected that the clinician will have tried persuading patient and family in the first instance: breaking confidentiality should only occur if both of these approaches have failed and the patient is deemed to represent a significant risk to other road users.

A grey area is determination of what represents a significant risk to other road users. A relatively low threshold is indicated for a progressive neurodegenerative illness where insight is impaired: if a patient refuses assessment and is reported by a third party to be driving erratically or in an unsafe manner, then it is probably appropriate to consider breaking patient confidentiality.

To whom this should be reported poses a practical ethical challenge. The traditional route of reporting to driver licencing authorities may have relatively little benefit: removal of a licence is likely to have little impact on a driver with reduced insight into deteriorating driving skills. It is important that this disclosure has some likelihood of impact and results in the least traumatic removal of the compromised older driver from the road. In such instances, the family may be able to intervene in terms of disabling the car and providing alternative modes of transport. In my own experience, I rarely have had to invoke official intervention, but find that a personal communication with a senior police officer in the patient's locality may result in a sensitive visit to the patient and cessation of driving.

SUMMARY POINTS

- Transportation and driving represents an important if relatively neglected aspect of rehabilitation of older people, and health professionals need to provide due attention to incorporating outdoors mobility into research and practice

- Assessment of driving has become an integral part of the clinical assessment of older people
- Multidisciplinary teams in geriatric medicine, appropriately supported by specialist on-road assessment, can help to support safe mobility and social inclusion in later life

MCQs

Q.1 Which of the following is true?
  a. Older drivers are more likely to be in a road accident
  b. Public transport should be recommended for all older people
  c. Older drivers strategically adapt to their disability
  d. All drivers over 70 years of age should have an on-road assessment
  e. Removal of a driving licence is a completely effective way to stop dangerous driving

Q.2 Which of the following is true regarding fitness to drive?
  a. All patients should be assessed by a psychologist and occupational therapist

  b. Several instruments exist which can be relied upon to accurately predict fitness to drive
  c. It is the sole responsibility of the doctor to refer a patient for driving assessment
  d. The ability to self-regulate and behave in a prudent manner relative to the current clinical condition is the key determinant
  e. Simulators are more accurate for assessing fitness to drive in older people

REFERENCES

Adler, G., Rottunda, S., Rasmussen, K., & Kuskowski, M. (2000). Caregivers dependent upon drivers with dementia. *Journal of Clinical Geropsychology, 6*, 83–90.

Akinwuntan, A. E., de Weerdt, W., Feys, H., Pauwels, J., Baten, G., Arno, P., & Kiekens, C. (2005). Effect of simulator training on driving after stroke: a randomized controlled trial. *Neurology, 65*, 843–850.

Akinwuntan, A. E., Feys, H., Deweerdt, W., Pauwels, J., Baten, G., & Strypstein, E. (2002). Determinants of driving after stroke. *Archives of Physical Medicine and Rehabilitation, 83*, 334–341.

Alvarez, F. J., Fierro, I., Gomez-Talegon, M. T., Vicondoa, A., & Ozcoidi, M. (2008). Patients treated with obstructive sleep apnea syndrome and fitness to drive assessment in clinical practice in Spain at the medical traffic centers. *Traffic Injury Prevention, 9*, 168–172.

American Geriatrics Society & Pomidor, A. (Eds.) (2016). *Clinician's guide to assessing and counseling older drivers*, 3rd edition. Washington, DC: National Highway Traffic Safety Administration.

Auger, C., Demers, L., Gélinas, I., Jutai, J., Fuhrer, M. J., & DeRuyter, F. (2008). Powered mobility for middle-aged and older adults: systematic review of outcomes and appraisal of published evidence. *American Journal of Physical Medicine & Rehabilitation, 87*, 666–680.

Bahro, M., Silber, E., Box, P., & Sunderland, T. (1995). Giving up driving in Alzheimer's disease: an integrative therapeutic approach. *International Journal of Geriatric Psychiatry, 10*, 871–874.

Banister, D., & Bowling, A. (2004). Quality of life for the elderly: the transport dimension. *Transport Policy, 11*, 105–115.

Bartley, M., & O'Neill, D. (2010). Transportation and driving in longitudinal studies on ageing. *Age Ageing, 39*, 631–636.

Betz, M. E., Dickerson, A., Coolman, T., Schold Davis, E., Jones, J., & Schwartz, R. (2014). Driving rehabilitation programs for older drivers in the United States. *Occupational Therapy in Health Care, 28*, 306–317.

Breen, D. A., Breen, D. P., Moore, J. W., Breen, P. A., & O'Neill, D. (2007). Driving and dementia. *BMJ, 334*, 1365–1369.

Brooks, J. O., Goodenough, R. R., Crisler, M. C., Klein, N. D., Alley, R. L., Koon, B. L., …, & Wills, R. F. (2010). Simulator sickness during driving simulation studies. *Accident Analysis & Prevention, 42*, 788–796.

Chee, J. N., Rapoport, M. J., Molnar, F., Herrmann, N., O'Neill, D., Marottoli, R., …, & Carr, D. B. (2017). Update on the risk of motor vehicle collision or driving impairment with dementia: a collaborative international systematic review and meta-analysis. *The American Journal of Geriatric Psychiatry, 25*(12), 1376–1390.

Cicchino, J. B., & McCartt, A. T. (2014). Trends in older driver crash involvement rates and survivability in the United States: an update. *Accident Analysis and Prevention, 72*, 44–54.

Curl, A. L., Proulx, C. M., Stowe, J. D., & Cooney, T. M. (2015). Productive and social engagement following driving cessation: a couple-based analysis. *Research on Aging, 37*, 171–199.

Davey, J. (2007). Older people and transport: coping without a car. *Ageing & Society, 27*, 49–65.

Di Stefano, M., & Macdonald, W. (2010). Australian occupational therapy driver assessors' opinions on improving on-road driver assessment procedures. *American Journal of Occupational Therapy, 64*, 325–335.

Edwards, J. D., Lunsman, M., Perkins, M., Rebok, G. W., & Roth, D. L. (2009). Driving cessation and health trajectories in older adults. *The Journals of Gerontology Series A Biological Sciences and Medical Sciences, 64*, 1290–1295.

Freeman, E. E., Gange, S. J., Munoz, B., & West, S. K. (2006). Driving status and risk of entry into long-term care in older adults. *American Journal of Public Health, 96*, 1254–1259.

Fuller, R. (2005). Towards a general theory of driver behaviour. *Accident Analysis and Prevention, 37*, 461–472.

George, S., Clark, M., & Crotty, M. (2007). Development of the Adelaide driving self-efficacy scale. *Clinical Rehabilitation, 21*(1), 56–61.

Hartford, F. (2000). *At the crossroads: a guide to Alzheimer's disease, dementia and driving*. Hartford, CT: Hartford Foundation.

Hjorthol, R. (2013). Transport resources, mobility and unmet transport needs in old age. *Ageing and Society, 33*, 1190–1211.

Howe, E. (2000). Improving treatments for patients who are elderly and have dementia. *Journal of Clinical Ethics, 11*, 291–303.

Jones, J. G., McCann, J., & Lassere, M. N. (1991). Driving and arthritis. *British Journal of Rheumatology, 30*, 361–364.

Kim, H., & Richardson, V. E. (2006). Driving cessation and consumption expenses in the later years. *The Journals of Gerontology Series B Psychological Sciences and Social Sciences, 61*, S347–S353.

Kowalski, K., Tuokko, H., & Tallman, K. (2010). On-road evaluation: its use for the identification of impairment and remediation of older drivers. *Physical & Occupational Therapy in Geriatrics, 28*, 75–85.

Lynott, J., & Figueiredo, C. (2011). *How the travel patterns of older adults are changing: highlights from the 2009 National Household Travel Survey*. Washington DC: AARP Public Policy Institute.

MacMahon, M., O'Neill, D., & Kenny, R. A. (1996). Syncope: driving advice is frequently overlooked. *Postgraduate Medical Journal, 72*, 561–563.

Marmot, M. G., & Wilkinson, R. G. (1999). *Social determinants of health*. Oxford; New York: Oxford University Press.

Marottoli, R. A., Allore, H., Araujo, K. L., Iannone, L. P., Acampora, D., Gottschalk, M., Charpentier, P., Kasl, S., & Peduzzi, P. (2007). A randomized trial of a physical conditioning program to enhance the driving performance of older persons. *Journal of General Internal Medicine, 22*, 590–597.

Marottoli, R. A., Mendes de Leon, C. F., Glass, T. A., Williams, C. S., Cooney, L. M., Jr., Berkman, L. F., & Tinetti, M. E. (1997). Driving cessation and increased depressive symptoms: prospective evidence from the New Haven EPESE. Established Populations for Epidemiologic Studies of the Elderly. *Journal of the American Geriatrics Society, 45*, 202—206.

Marshall, S. C. (2008). The role of reduced fitness to drive due to medical impairments in explaining crashes involving older drivers. *Traffic Injury Prevention, 9*, 291–298.

May, D., Nayak, U. S., & Isaacs, B. (1985). The life-space diary: a measure of mobility in old people at home. *International Rehabilitation Medicine, 7*, 182–186.

May, E., Garrett, R., & Ballantyne, A. (2010). Being mobile: electric mobility-scooters and their use by older people. *Ageing and Society, 30*, 1219–1237.

McNamara, A., McCluskey, A., White, J., & George, S. (2014). The need for consistency and equity in driver education and assessment post-stroke. *Journal of Transport & Health, 1*, 95—99.

Michon, J. A. (1985). A critical view of driver behaviour models: what do we know, what should we do? In L. Evans, & R. C. Schwing (Eds.), *Human behavior and traffic safety* (pp. 485–520). New York: Plenum.

Molnar, F. J., Patel, A., Marshall, S. C., Man-Son-Hing, M., & Wilson, K. G. (2006). Clinical utility of office-based cognitive predictors of fitness to drive in persons with dementia: a systematic review. *Journal of the American Geriatrics Society, 54*, 1809–1824.

Monestam, E., & Wachtmeister, L. (1997). Impact of cataract surgery on car driving: a population based study in Sweden. *British Journal of Ophthalmology, 81*, 16–22.

O'Byrne, C., Naughton, A., & O'Neill, D. (2015). Is driver licensing restriction for age-related medical conditions an effective mechanism to improve driver safety without unduly impairing mobility? *European Geriatric Medicine, 6*, 541–544.

O'Neill, D. (2008). Driving and safe mobility in Parkinson's disease. In J. Playfer, & J. Hindle (Eds.), *Parkinson's disease in the older patient*. Oxford: Radcliffe Publishing.

O'Neill, D. (2015). Transport, driving and ageing. *Reviews in Clinical Gerontology, 25*, 147–158.

OECD. (2001). *Ageing and transport: mobility needs and safety issues*. Paris: OECD.

Oxley, J., & Whelan, M. (2008). It cannot be all about safety: the benefits of prolonged mobility. *Traffic Injury Prevention, 9*, 367–378.

Portegijs, E., Rantakokko, M., Mikkola, T. M., Viljanen, A., & Rantanen, T. (2014). Association between physical performance and sense of autonomy in outdoor activities and life-space mobility in community-dwelling older people. *Journal of American Geriatrics Society, 62*, 615–621.

Ranney, T. A. (1994). Models of driving behaviour: a review of their evolution. *Accident & Analysis and Prevention, 26*, 733–750.

Rantakokko, M., Portegijs, E., Viljanen, A., Iwarsson, S., & Rantanen, T. (2013). Life-space mobility and quality of life in community-dwelling older people. *J Am Geriatr Soc, 61*, 1830–1832.

Rapoport, M. J., Plonka, S. C., Finestone, H., Bayley, M., Chee, J. N., Vrkljan, B., …, & O'Neill, D. (2019). A systematic review of the risk of motor vehicle collision after stroke or transient ischemic attack. *Topics in Stroke Rehabilitation, 26*, 1–10.

Rapoport, M. J., Weegar, K., Kadulina, Y., Bédard, M., Carr, D., Charlton, J., …, & Marshall, S. (2015). An international study of the quality of national-level guidelines on driving with medical illness. *QJM, 108*, 859–869.

Ray, W. A., Gurwitz, J., Decker, M. D., & Kennedy, D. L. (1992). Medications and the safety of the older driver: is there a basis for concern? *Human Factors, 34*, 33–47. discussion 49-51.

Ray, W. A., Thapa, P. B., & Shorr, R. I. (1993). Medications and the older driver. *Clinics in Geriatric Medicine, 9*, 413–438.

Redelmeier, D. A., Yarnell, C. J., & Tibshirani, R. J. (2013). Physicians' warnings for unfit drivers and risk of road crashes. *New England Journal of Medicine, 368*, 87–88.

Risser, R., Lexell, E., Bell, D., Iwarsson, S., & Ståhl, A. (2015). Use of local public transport among people with cognitive impairments–a literature review. *Transportation Research Part F: Traffic Psychology and Behaviour, 29*, 83–97.

Rubinsztein, J., & Lawton, C. A. (1995). Depression and driving in the elderly. *International Journal of Geriatric Psychiatry, 10*, 15–17.

Sorajja, D., Nesbitt, G. C., Hodge, D. O., Low, P. A., Hammill, S. C., Gersh, B. J., & Shen, W. K. (2009). Syncope while driving: clinical characteristics, causes, and prognosis. *Circulation, 120*, 928–934.

Stapleton, T., Connolly, D., & O'Neill, D. (2012). Exploring the relationship between self-awareness of driving efficacy and that of a proxy when determining fitness to drive after stroke. *Australian Occupational Therapy Journal, 59*, 63–70.

Stav, W. (2010). CarFit: an evaluation of behaviour change and impact. *The British Journal of Occupational Therapy, 73*, 589–597.

Stork, A. D., van Haeften, T. W., & Veneman, T. F. (2007). The decision not to drive during hypoglycemia in patients with type 1 and type 2 diabetes according to hypoglycemia awareness. *Diabetes Care, 30*, 2822–2826.

Uc, E. Y., Rizzo, M., Anderson, S. W., Shi, Q., & Dawson, J. D. (2004). Driver route-following and safety errors in early Alzheimer disease. *Neurology, 63*, 832–837.

Winter, S. M., Classen, S., & Shanahan, M. (2014). User evaluation of the Fitness-to-Drive Screening Measure. *Physical & Occupational Therapy in Geriatrics, 33*, 64–71.

74

Advance Care Planning

Rónán O'Caoimh & Marie Condon

LEARNING OBJECTIVES

- Describe the core principles of advance care planning and how these can be applied in a rehabilitation setting
- Explain the importance, risks and benefits of advance care planning for older adults
- Describe the different and complimentary roles of each member of the multidisciplinary team in advance care planning

WHAT IS ADVANCE CARE PLANNING?

The ageing of society, while something to be celebrated, is also associated with an increased incidence of frailty, disability and functional decline. These impact negatively upon quality of life, often resulting in a mismatch between the number of years of life lived and healthy life years. Compounding this, many older people may lack mental capacity to be fully involved in decision-making in relation to their financial and healthcare matters (Silveira, Kim, & Langa, 2010). Capacity in the context of healthcare refers to the extent to which someone is able to understand the information provided to them, appreciate it as it applies to them, reason and consider their options and express their preference in a clear and consistent way (Palmer & Harmell, 2016). This includes the ability to make a will, select a course of treatment and accept or decline medical investigations. These become particularly difficult at the end of life (EOL) when many people will require support to make decisions (Silveira et al., 2010).

Advance care planning (ACP) is a preparatory activity, a series of steps and behaviours, leading to the documentation of a person's preferences for their care at a future time point. In this way it allows an individual to retain a voice after they are no longer able to make informed choices for themselves. It is a voluntary, structured and formal process whereby an individual, their family and healthcare professionals come together to understand, plan, document and communicate future decisions for if or when they cannot make these for themselves (Detering et al., 2010).

The process results in the creation of an advance care plan, a written record of people's personal choices and preferences for their health, financial and personal care for use at a future time. This is also called an advance directive, advance decision or anticipatory care plan, depending on the country. In the past, ACP would have been synonymous with the term "living will" and this can be a helpful and concrete way to explain the concept before beginning the discussion. ACP is usually initiated at an early stage of a chronic and progressive disease such as dementia or heart failure, where there is an anticipated and often predictable decline (Mullick, Martin, & Sallnow, 2013). Without an advance care plan, sudden events can lead to challenging family discussions and medicolegal situations (see Box 74.1).

CASE STUDY OF ADVANCE CARE PLANNING IN REHABILITATION

The following case study provides a typical example of an older adult who could benefit from initiation of ACP in rehabilitation, exploring the steps and roles of the healthcare professionals involved.

Fiona is a 79-year-old woman who has many medical problems including heart disease, hypertension and diabetes mellitus. She had a stroke resulting in word-finding difficulty (expressive aphasia) and right-sided weakness. She is currently receiving inpatient rehabilitation. The rehabilitation team discussed during the multidisciplinary team (MDT) meeting that Fiona would benefit from completing an ACP. Her family are devout and believe God will decide Fiona's fate.

Professional Roles:

1. **Determining Fiona's decision-making capacity:** In the presence of a communication deficit, occupational therapy (OT) and speech and language therapy (SLT) worked together to assess if Fiona has sufficient cognitive abilities to partake in the discussions and to explore how they could help promote her autonomy.
2. **Engage with Fiona and her family:** Medical social work (MSW) facilitated discussions between Mrs Williams and her family to help encourage and support them to engage in ACP while taking into account their spiritual beliefs. She also involved the chaplain to help engage with the family.
3. **Provide information:** Fiona's consultant provided clear information regarding her current medical status, her comorbidities and the risk of future events and the implications they may have on her decision-making capacity. Individual interdisciplinary team members delivered the

BOX 74.1   The Case of Nancy Cruzan

Historical Case: Nancy Cruzan

Nancy Cruzan suffered irreversible brain damage and went into a persistent vegetative state in 1983. She was tube fed to avoid dying from dehydration or starvation. Nancy's family wanted the tube removed as they believed Nancy would not have wanted to live in a persistent vegetative state. No advance care plan was in place. The case went to the Supreme Court after a battle between her family and the Missouri Department of Health. The Supreme Court ruled there was a right to die and Nancy's feeding tube was removed eight years after she entered a persistent vegetative state. This was the first such case and lead to the development of advance care directives (ACD). Following from this, the US Congress passed the Right to Die act and received more than 300,000 requests for ACD forms (Orentlicher, 1990).

relevant information required to help Fiona identify her goals, values and priorities for her future care. This informative conversation was facilitated by the SLT who helped break down information into an aphasia-friendly format. The OT and older person clinical nurse specialist used the recommended communication aids when they were discussing ACP with Fiona.

4. **Documentation:** The MSW and SLT helped Fiona document an advance care plan (resources section) in the presence of her family. She signed it and it was witnessed by one of the MSWs. A date for review was documented. The MSW shared a copy with Fiona, her family including her nominated spokesperson, and sent it to her general practitioner, her geriatrician and a copy was kept in her medical chart.

THE IMPORTANCE OF ADVANCE CARE PLANNING

Preparation and forward planning are especially important when thinking about your future healthcare needs. Prompt initiation of ACP is important for everyone involved in the process from the person themselves and their friends and family to healthcare professionals (see Fig. 74.1). It benefits the person making the plan by protecting their personal beliefs and preferences, allowing them to retain their voice and control over their care. In this way, ACP not only enhances autonomy, it can also increase satisfaction and quality of life (Detering et al., 2010). ACP makes it more likely that people will receive treatment that is broadly in keeping with their previously stated wishes (Silveira et al., 2010). This reduces stress and anxiety as well as the potential for conflict for all those involved. It also fosters an environment of openness amongst those participating. This in turn can help patients and their families understand the condition, pharmacological and non-pharmacological treatment options, and potential complications.

ACP is acceptable and achievable for most people including those living at home and nursing home residents (Weathers et al., 2016) and should be considered for all individuals with chronic diseases, especially where people are at risk of losing their ability to make decisions, e.g. those with early dementia. While robust data from randomised controlled trials on the direct benefits are as yet lacking, several programmes show ACP minimises unwanted and often unnecessary hospital admissions (Graverholt, Forsetlund, & Jamtvedt, 2014; Molloy et al., 2000). Similarly, although there is insufficient evidence to support the economic benefits of ACP (Weathers et al., 2016), they may lower costs to healthcare systems by reducing use of acute care services (O'Sullivan et al., 2016).

BARRIERS AND FACILITATORS

ACP discussions can be difficult, and many people feel uncomfortable with the idea of exploring their mortality. In addition, few older adults even at EOL are recognised by healthcare professionals to have a limited life expectancy, meaning that these discussions are often put off until it is inappropriate or even impossible to start (Glare et al., 2003). Reflecting this, awareness of the ACP process remains suboptimal and uptake is variable, ranging from as low as 4% in Norway to as high as 70% in the United States of America (Osborn et al., 2014; Teno et al., 2007). Common barriers are insufficient time,

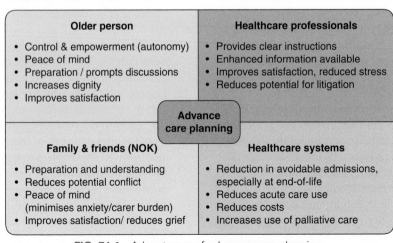

FIG. 74.1   Advantages of advance care planning.

Emma is a 62-year-old woman with chronic obstructive pulmonary disease (COPD). Her husband passed away 3 years ago and her daughter lives in Australia. She has had three hospital admissions last year due to recurrent chest infections. She is now attending pulmonary rehabilitation classes in her local health centre.

Seamus is a 79-year-old man with ischaemic heart disease, osteoarthritis and a history of falls. His wife has noticed he has become more forgetful recently and has some short-term memory loss. His general practitioner is concerned he may have dementia and has referred him to a geriatrician to assess his memory loss.

poorly developed IT systems to facilitate electronic transmission of advance care plans and poor understanding, education and awareness of ACP amongst the general public and healthcare providers (Howard et al., 2018).

What can be done to improve uptake? Healthcare professionals should offer scheduled meetings to discuss goals of care, involve families and systems should have policies in place to educate staff and access past information (Simon et al., 2015). ACP should be considered at transitions of care and after the diagnosis of or recovery from life-threatening illness, e.g. within survivorship care planning, especially older adults with chronic disease where it is often overlooked (O'Caoimh et al., 2017). See Box 74.2 for some examples. It is also helpful if positive and open conversations take place regularly and that relationships between patients, families and healthcare professionals are strong. Where they are not, ACP is less likely to take place.

Unlike planning a will or power of attorney, a lawyer or solicitor is not required for completion of an advance care plan. Reminding families of this is helpful as legal costs can be prohibitive. While the legal status of advance directives varies internationally, where they are completed correctly, they carry weight and should also be taken into account when planning treatments. They are not legally binding in all cases, and patients, relatives and healthcare professionals should consult locally when preparing or acting upon one (Thompson, 2015). Considering the sensitive nature of the topic, healthcare professionals are advised to prepare for ACP discussions. Ensuring the correct facts regarding all recent and relevant test results and liaising with other healthcare professionals involved in the person's care to ensure consistency of information provided is vital. Understanding an individual's cultural and religious beliefs is beneficial as these may also influence the discussion (Balboni et al., 2007).

MAKING AN ADVANCE CARE PLAN – KEY COMPONENTS

Lots of people can and should be involved in making an advance care plan. This includes older people themselves, their healthcare providers and if appropriate, family and friends. The process is dynamic and can continue to be updated over time. It is flexible and should be bespoke, tailored to the individual and their readiness and ability to participate. Reflecting this, ACP falls under a number of different approaches based on the stage of the disease: general (broadly considering goals of care, often at the early stage of a condition or when a person becomes frail) and disease-specific (clearly establishing treatment and other options when life-limiting conditions are present, active and progressive). ACP should involve a number of steps including initiation, exploration and documentation that may happen over several discussions (Kononovas & McGee, 2017) (Fig. 74.2).

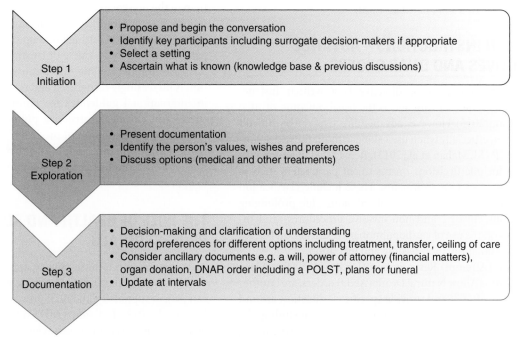

FIG. 74.2   Key steps in general advance care planning.

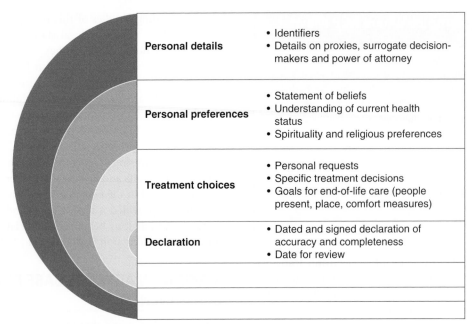

Personal details	• Identifiers • Details on proxies, surrogate decision-makers and power of attorney
Personal preferences	• Statement of beliefs • Understanding of current health status • Spirituality and religious preferences
Treatment choices	• Personal requests • Specific treatment decisions • Goals for end-of-life care (people present, place, comfort measures)
Declaration	• Dated and signed declaration of accuracy and completeness • Date for review

FIG. 74.3   Core elements included in an advanced care plan.

While advance care plans differ in their approach and structure, there are common elements that should be included. Basic personal information should be included such as the family and relevant proxies. Preferences including an expression of someone's personal beliefs (what that person wants, what matters to them, expressions of spirituality) as well as their healthcare choices at EOL should then be included. The next section should establish clear personal preferences regarding future options including the documentation of discussions about palliative care and medical treatments including expectations for EOL care. Other common elements include a date for review, and a declaration by the person themselves and relevant healthcare professionals supporting the completion of the plan (Fig. 74.3).

WRITTEN INSTRUCTIONS – ADVANCE DIRECTIVES AND DNAR ORDERS

An advance care plan or directive is a written instruction to guide medical care and is the usual outcome of ACP (Thompson, 2015). However, advance directives can be difficult to interpret, especially when used alone without the wider context of ACP (McMahan et al., 2013). Items listed in an advance directive include decisions on treatment parameters such as the refusal of certain treatments. These include clarification on the ceiling of treatment (use of antibiotics, life-prolonging medications, invasive and non-invasive procedures) and instructions on the use of cardiopulmonary resuscitation (CPR), artificial ventilation, tube-feeding and hydration.

Do Not (Attempt) Resuscitation (DNR or DNAR) orders, also known as Allow Natural Death (AND) orders, are another component of ACP and provide specific clarification around a patient's preferences relating to resuscitation including the use of CPR (cardiac massage) and ventilation (breathing tube) in the event of cardiopulmonary arrest. As with ACP,

these orders promote autonomy by making the wishes of patients expressly clear. Physicians may implement such orders when CPR will be futile or harmful. Documenting a DNAR in the medical records provides clear instructions to the team as to the course of action to be taken if a patient stops breathing or their heart stops beating (Breault, 2011). Communication around such orders is critical in order to prevent misunderstandings, particularly with families.

CARE PLANNING IN REHABILITATION

Rehabilitation is an important setting to begin ACP as it affords patients time to identify their values and priorities rather than in the presence of an acute illness where decisions are required quickly. Health and social care professionals (HSCPs) in the rehabilitation setting build up strong relationships with patients during their course of treatment putting them in an ideal position to facilitate ACP discussions. ACP in rehabilitation is increasingly recognised and is currently recommended in international guidelines for chronic conditions such as stroke and chronic obstructive pulmonary disease (Hebert et al., 2016). Presentation of prognostic information is essential to ensure the older adult and their families understand that while the emphasis of rehabilitation is recovery, it is vital to appropriately plan for the future.

THE ROLE OF HEALTH AND SOCIAL CARE PROFESSIONALS

ACP requires a multidisciplinary approach (Cornally et al., 2015). HSCPs are becoming increasingly aware of the role they can play in supporting the ACP process (Detering et al., 2010; Korn et al., 2019). Individual MDT members can provide their own expertise, breaking down relevant information over time to formulate both a broad and disease-specific ACP. HSCPs should provide objective information on the risks, benefit and potential harm of treatments and the consequences of refusal of treatment. Some examples of the role of HSCPs in ACP discussions include:

- SLTs can help those with communication difficulties to understand information, and support the decision-making process.
- Dieticians and SLTs can explain the concept of feeding despite an unsafe swallow and artificial nutrition and hydration.
- Physiotherapists can approach topics including non-pharmacological treatments for symptoms including pain management and respiratory care while pharmacists can detail pharmacological management options towards EOL.
- Physiotherapists and OTs can initiate conversations regarding environmental and functional considerations in relation to place of care.
- MSWs interface with patients, families and other healthcare professionals during the ACP process due to their interpersonal skills in support, mediation and advocacy.

They can facilitate discussions between and provide emotional support during this time.

HSCPs should understand ACP and appreciate the appropriate times to engage in discussions. UK guidelines recommend ACP is initiated in primary care (Royal College of Physicians, 2009), and indeed many HSCPs work with patients in the community with chronic disease and life-limiting conditions building strong relationships, which is vital for starting ACP discussions (Wenrich et al., 2001). ACP has, in recent years, been introduced to HSCP-led programmes such as pulmonary rehabilitation (Korn et al., 2019). Education on the topic helps create an awareness and early initiation of ACP discussions. While ACP is generally well received by HSCPs, concerns are raised regarding the need for specific training on the topic (Korn et al., 2019; Weathers et al., 2016). HSCPs should have a broad understanding of the patient's condition including the physical, psychological, social and spiritual issues as well as the legal and ethical considerations around ACP. Online training, ACP workshops and user-friendly resources will help HSCPs to facilitate more ACP discussions (Cornally et al., 2015).

SUMMARY POINTS

- Advance care planning promotes autonomy for older people with chronic disease and frailty allowing them to retain a voice in their care decisions, even when no longer able to do so because of ill health and should be considered by all those with life-limiting conditions
- Rehabilitation is an ideal setting to consider beginning advance care planning discussions and health and social care professionals should be actively engaged in the process
- More education is required for all participants in advance care planning to increase uptake, which at present is suboptimal

MCQs

Q.1 Which one of the following is true about advance care planning (ACP)?
- a. ACP allows an individual to retain a voice after they are no longer able to make informed choices for themselves
- b. ACP should be completed as close to death as possible
- c. The primary reason for completing an ACP is to avoid medicolegal problems
- d. ACP should not be considered in the rehabilitation setting

- e. Patients should be obliged to have an ACP after acute illness

Q.2 Which of the following should be included in an advance directive?
- a. Basic personal information
- b. Preferences including an expression of someone's personal beliefs
- c. Healthcare choices at EOL
- d. A declaration by the person themselves
- e. All of the above

REFERENCES

Balboni, T.A., Vanderwerker, L.C., Block, S.D., Paulk, M.E., Lathan, C.S., Peteet, J.R., & Prigerson, H.G. (2007). Religiousness and spiritual support among advanced cancer patients and associations with end-of-life treatment preferences and quality of life. Journal of Clinical Oncology: *Official Journal of the American Society of Clinical Oncology, 25*(5), 555.

Breault, J. L. (2011). DNR, DNAR, or AND? Is language important? *Ochsner Journal, 11*(4), 302–306.

Cornally, N., McGlade, C., Weathers, E., Daly, E., Fitzgerald, C., O'Caoimh, R., Coffey, A., & Molloy, D. W. (2015). Evaluating the systematic implementation of the 'Let Me Decide' advance care

planning programme in long term care through focus groups: staff perspectives. *BMC Palliative Care, 14*, 55.

Detering, K. M., Hancock, A. D., Reade, M. C., & Silvester, W. (2010). The impact of advance care planning on end of life care in elderly patients: randomized controlled trial. *BMJ, 340*, 1345–1353.

Glare, P., Virik, K., Jones, M., Hudson, M., Eychmuller, S., Simes, J., & Christakis, N. (2003). A systematic review of physicians' survival predictions in terminally ill cancer patients. *BMJ, 327*, 195–198.

Graverholt, B., Forsetlund, L., & Jamtvedt, G. (2014). Reducing hospital admissions from nursing homes: a systematic review. *BMC Health Services Research, 14*, 36–43.

Hebert, D., Lindsay, M. P., McIntyre, A., Kirton, A., Rumney, P. G., Bagg, S., …, & Teasell, R. (2016). Canadian Stroke Best Practice Recommendations: Stroke Rehabilitation Practice Guidelines, update 2015. *International Journal of Stroke*, *11*(4), 459–484.

Howard, M., Bernard, C., Klein, D., Elston, D., Tan, A., Slaven, M., Barwich, D., You, J. J., & Heyland, D. K. (2018). Barriers to and enablers of advance care planning with patients in primary care: survey of health care providers. *Canadian Family Physician*, *64*(4), e190–e198.

Kononovas, K., & McGee, A. (2017). The benefits and barriers of ensuring patients have advance care planning. *Nursing Times*, *113*, 1, 41–44.

Korn, B., Bailey-Scanlan, M., Ribeiro, L. H., & Broderick, J. (2019). Advance care planning education sessions during pulmonary rehabilitation in Ireland. *Journal of Cardiopulmonary Rehabilitation and Prevention*, *39*, 8–10.

McMahan, R.D., Knight, S.J., Fried, T.R., & Sudore, R.L., (2013). Advance care planning beyond advance directives: perspectives from patients and surrogates. *Journal of Pain and Symptom Management*, *46*(3), 355–365.

Molloy, D. W., Guyatt, G. H., Russo, R., Goeree, R., O'Brien, B. J., Bédard, M., & Dubois, S. (2000). Systematic implementation of an advance directive program in nursing homes: a randomized controlled trial. *JAMA*, *283*, 1437–1444.

Mullick, A., Martin, J., & Sallnow, L. (2013). An introduction to advance care planning in practice. *BMJ*, *347*, f6064.

O'Caoimh, R., Cornally, N., O'Sullivan, R., Hally, R., Weathers, E., Lavan, A. H., & Molloy, D. W. (2017). Advance care planning within survivorship care plans for older cancer survivors: a systematic review. *Maturitas*, *105*, 52–57.

Orentlicher, D. (1990). The right to die after Cruzan. *JAMA*, *264*(18), 2444–2446.

Osborn, R., Moulds, D., Squires, D., Doty, M. M., & Anderson, C. (2014). International survey of older adults finds shortcomings in access, coordination, and patient-centered care. *Health Affairs*, *33*, 2247–2255.

O'Sullivan, R., Murphy, A., O'Caoimh, R., Cornally, N., Svendrovski, A., Daly, B., …, & Molloy, D. W. (2016). Economic (gross cost) analysis of systematically implementing a programme of advance care planning in three Irish nursing homes. *BMC Research Notes*, *9*(1), 237.

Palmer, B. W., & Harmell, A. L. (2016). Assessment of healthcare decision-making capacity. *Archives of Clinical Neuropsychology*, *31*(6), 530–540.

Royal College of Physicians. (2009). *Advance care planning – national guidelines. Concise guidance to good practice. A series of evidence-based guidelines for good clinical management.* London: RCP.

Silveira, M. J., Kim, S. Y., & Langa, K. M. (2010). Advance directives and outcomes of surrogate decision making before death. *New England Journal of Medicine*, *362*, 1211–1218.

Simon, J., Porterfield, P., Bouchal, S. R., & Heyland, D. (2015). 'Not yet' and 'Just ask': barriers and facilitators to advance care planning—a qualitative descriptive study of the perspectives of seriously ill, older patients and their families. *BMJ Supportive & Palliative Care*, *5*(1), 54–62.

Teno, J. M., Gruneir, A., Schwartz, Z., Nanda, A., & Wetle, T. (2007). Association between advance directives and quality of end-of-life care: a national study. *Journal of the American Geriatrics Society*, *55*, 189–194.

Thompson, A. E. (2015). Advance directives. *JAMA*, *313*(8), 868–1868.

Weathers, E., O'Caoimh, R., Cornally, N., Fitzgerald, C., Kearns, T., Coffey, A., & Molloy, D. W. (2016). Advance care planning: a systematic review of randomised controlled trials conducted with older adults. *Maturitas*, *91*, 101–109.

Wenrich, M. D., Curtis, J. R., Shannon, S. E., Carline, J. D., Ambrozy, D. M., & Ramsey, P. G. (2001). Communicating with dying patients within the spectrum of medical care from terminal diagnosis to death. *Archives of Internal Medicine*, *161*, 868–874.

75

Health Promotion

Ellen McGough, Rachel Prusynski & Ny-Ying Lam

LEARNING OBJECTIVES

- Describe common secondary conditions associated with disability and age-related health conditions
- Identify modifiable lifestyle factors that affect health in older adults with disability
- Discuss elements of person-centred education and guidance for older adults with disabilities

- Describe health promotion strategies for increasing physical activity and social participation in older adults with disability upon discharge from rehabilitation services

INTRODUCTION

Disability is increasing as the population ages, with more people living with existing or newly acquired disabilities. People with disabilities are more likely than those without disability to report health problems (Kinne, 2008). Health promotion in older adults aims to prevent or delay the onset of disease and disability by identifying risk factors and implementing strategies that promote healthy ageing (Peel, McClure, & Bartlett, 2005). The purpose of this chapter is to provide guidance on how to support older people to lead a healthy lifestyle after rehabilitation.

Health promotion strategies for older adults aim to (1) maintain and increase functional abilities, (2) maintain and improve self-care, and (3) stimulate one's social network (Golinowska et al., 2016). Initiatives to address modifiable lifestyle factors in all older adults include increasing physical activity, reducing smoking and alcohol consumption, and participating in learning and community activities. Health promotion efforts by family and community carers can help people ageing with a disability to mitigate age-related diseases, prevent the loss of functional abilities and maintain meaningful roles in society (Golinowska et al., 2016; Kern et al., 2019; Peel et al., 2005).

HEALTH PROMOTION FOR OLDER ADULTS WITH DISABILITY

Having a disability often increases the risk of developing a secondary health condition. Common disability-related conditions in older adults with stroke, multiple sclerosis and spinal cord injury include pain, fatigue, bowel and bladder dysfunction, sleep difficulties, spasticity, depression and falls (Baylor et al., 2014; Jorgensen, Iwarsson, & Lexell, 2017; Kern et al., 2019). Associated lifestyle factors such as sedentary behaviour or smoking can contribute to additional health problems that are common in older adults, including high blood pressure, heart disease, frailty, pressure ulcers and/or arthritis

(Jensen et al., 2012). A focus on health promotion, by addressing common risk factors, can help to preserve function and reduce the impact of these common health conditions (Fig. 75.1).

POST-REHABILITATION DECLINE

Short-term gains achieved during rehabilitation can rapidly decline after discharge. Over time, older adults with a disability can fall below the minimum threshold for independent function, increasing risk for additional health problems. Forty-seven percent of adults with disability are sedentary compared to 26% of healthy older adults. A sedentary lifestyle in a person with disability leads to deconditioning that negatively impacts health, which in turn creates a cyclic pattern of physical deconditioning (Rimmer, Schiller, & Chen, 2012). The time immediately post-rehabilitation represents a critical window to optimise physical activity and other health promoting activities in order to maintain health and independence. The goal of post-rehabilitation exercise, along with a healthy lifestyle, is to sustain the short-term rehab improvements and continue to make further functional gains (Rimmer et al., 2012; Rimmer & Lai, 2017).

CASE

Jean-Luc is an 81-year-old left-handed man with hypertension, diabetes and heart failure who is completing inpatient rehabilitation after a stroke. He has new right-hand weakness, mild speech difficulty (expressive dysphasia), and difficulties with attention and memory. He is able to walk household distances independently with a walker. He has lived alone in an accessible apartment since his husband died 2 years ago. Jean-Luc will receive home therapies at discharge. His niece will check in on him daily to set up his medications, help with bathing, and take him shopping for groceries and to appointments. Jean-Luc wants to know how best to lead a healthier life to prevent a future stroke and maintain his independence.

> **Common Disability-Related Health Conditions**
> - Pain
> - Fatigue
> - Bowel & Bladder Dysfunction
> - Spasticity
> - Sleep Difficulty
> - Depression
> - Deconditioning
> - Mobility Problems
> - Falls & Injuries

> **Common Age-Related Health Conditions**
> - High Blood Pressure
> - Heart and Lung Disease
> - Dizziness
> - Diabetes
> - Arthritis
> - Peripheral Vascular Disease
> - Vision Impairment
> - Mobility Problems
> - Falls & Injuries

> **Health Promotion Focus for Older Adults with Disability**
> - Healthy Eating
> - Smoking Cessation
> - Minimize Alcohol Consumption
> - Minimize Substance Misuse
> - Medication Management
> - Mental Health & Coping Strategies
> - Fall & Injury Prevention
> - Physical Activity Promotion

FIG. 75.1 Health conditions and health promotion in older adults with disability.

TRANSITIONING FROM REHABILITATION: SCREENING AND PREVENTION INTERVENTIONS

In older adults with disability, interactions between ageing and disability lead to accelerated decline (Jensen et al., 2012; Rimmer & Lai, 2017). Although age and genetics are non-modifiable contributing factors, addressing modifiable lifestyle factors can lead to better health outcomes. Early identification of risk factors and timely intervention are fundamental to preventing, delaying and/or reversing disability in older adults (Jensen et al., 2012). For example, health promotion in older adults with disability includes risk assessments, providing person-centred interventions and education, and evidence-based guidelines for maintaining health (Table 75.1) (Center for Disease Control and Prevention, 2017; Chernoff, 2001; Kuerbis et al., 2014; Thun et al., 2013; World Health Organization, 2010).

BARRIERS TO HEALTHY LIFESTYLE AFTER REHABILITATION

Mobility Limitations

Rehabilitation healthcare professionals focus on restoring physical function and preventing secondary health problems (Rimmer et al., 2012; Rimmer & Lai, 2017). Mobility and self-care are critical targets during this recovery phase. Ongoing exercise, individualised to meet the patient's needs, is important for reducing mobility-related disability. Individualised exercise routines focus on strength, flexibility, balance and locomotion (e.g. walking and wheelchair propulsion). However, due to newly acquired impairments, medical conditions and slower recovery in older patients, many patients may not achieve a high level of physical function even after formal rehabilitation ends (Rimmer & Lai, 2017).

Cognitive Impairment

Patients who undergo rehabilitation for stroke, brain injury or other disorders may have impaired cognition, making it difficult to maintain a healthy lifestyle and participate in social and physical activities. In addition, older adults are at higher risk for cognitive impairment due to ageing and neurodegenerative changes. Barriers caused by cognitive impairment include difficulty planning and scheduling appointments, difficulty keeping up with conversations and exercise groups, and challenges in learning or relearning skills and health information.

Fatigue and Deconditioning

Older adults with certain disabilities, especially multiple sclerosis and stroke, often experience fatigue that limits their participation in exercise, daily activities and community-based activities. Fatigue can also be related to weakness and poor endurance after an illness or prolonged deconditioning (Rimmer et al., 2012). Fatigue can be compounded by depression or a sedentary lifestyle, which is highly prevalent in people with stroke, brain injury and neurodegenerative conditions. Fortunately, there is evidence that physical activity can decrease fatigue in people with disabilities and improve quality of life (Backus, 2016).

Mood and Self-Efficacy

Older adults with a new disability may experience depressive symptoms and reduced self-efficacy, or lack of confidence, in their ability to carry out healthy lifestyle activities. Although formal rehabilitation works towards reducing dependence on others, a poor sense of self-efficacy can negatively affect everyday activities and social participation. Self-efficacy has been shown to be one of the strongest predictors of physical activity in adults (French et al., 2014).

Health Literacy

Health literacy is the degree to which individuals are able to understand health information in order to make informed decisions about their healthcare. In addition to potential

TABLE 75.1 Risk assessment and interventions for older adults transitioning from rehabilitation services.

	ASSESSMENT	PATIENT-CENTRED INTERVENTIONS
Healthy Eating	• Chewing, swallowing, taste and smell difficulties • Ability to cook • Transportation or mobility issues limiting access to food • Signs of malnutrition: unintended weight loss and poor eating habits • Barriers including poverty or social isolation	• Consult a registered dietitian • Connect patient to local food assistance (food bank), home-delivered meals or community senior centre meals programmes
Smoking Cessation	• Tobacco use habits • Behavioural change readiness	• Offer phone Quit-lines • Prescribe tobacco-cessation medications • Promote smoke-free environments • Refer to behavioural intervention programmes (SmokeFree US, EU)
Minimise Alcohol and Substance Misuse	• Screen for substance abuse and addiction • Behavioural change readiness • Social isolation	• Refer to substance use helplines • Screening, brief intervention and referral to treatment (SBIRT) • Refer to addiction or detoxification programmes
Health and Medication Management	• Cognitive or physical changes affecting ability to self-monitor (e.g. check blood sugars, take meds as prescribed) • Review polypharmacy • Sedentary lifestyle • Poor health literacy	• Consider case manager or home nursing • Provide education on health conditions and medications • Create medication management system (e.g. pill box, accurate medication schedule) • Reduce polypharmacy • Refer to Chronic Disease Health Maintenance Programmes to build confidence in self-management
Mental Health and Coping	• Screen for depression • Identify difficulty coping with disability • Assess for suicidal ideation or plan • Difficulty sleeping	• Refer to mental health provider • Teach coping strategies • Promote physical activity and exercise • Promote sleep hygiene • Prescribe medications as needed
Fall and Injury Prevention	• Multicomponent fall risk assessment (e.g. vision, balance, polypharmacy, mobility, cognition) • Home safety check • Ability to get up from a fall • Driving safety	• Refer to outpatient or home rehab services (e.g. physiotherapy, occupational therapy) for balance, mobility and gait training • Refer to fall prevention programme • Recommend community based exercise programmes (e.g. Tai Chi, fitness classes, aquatic exercise) • Educate on home safety and fall risks • Update driving recommendations
Physical Activity	• Assess fall risk • Clarify medical precautions for exercise (e.g. heart conditions, seizures) • Review exercise adaptations needed for disability • Behavioural change readiness	• Design an exercise programme that accommodates for disability-related impairments • Provide an individualised exercise prescription that considers the person's health and precautions • Assist in accessing community-based programmes • Utilise behavioural change techniques

cognitive decline after the onset of an injury or disease, low health literacy may be present in up to 50% of people with chronic diseases. Efforts to identify learning needs and to deliver health information in ways that ensure patient understanding are crucial to enhance adherence to health recommendations and prevent the onset of major health problems (Heijmans et al., 2015).

Family/Carer Support

Many older adults with disabilities experience social isolation or are without family, a carer and community support even prior to a debilitating injury or diagnosis. Combined with physical and/or cognitive impairments, those lacking community support may require more assistance from social services or other networks. For example, in-home carers can help support participation in activities of daily living, increase physical activity and facilitate social engagement.

Financial Resources

Older adults with a disability who struggle financially are at greater risk for functional decline and have access to fewer resources that contribute to health. Fitness centre memberships, nutrition counselling, healthy foods and many over-the-counter products or medications that help people stay healthy can be financially out of reach for older adults with disabilities.

Facilities and Resources

Identifying community programmes for exercise and other activities is essential for maintaining an active lifestyle after rehabilitation. Considerations such as transportation needs, barriers to wheelchairs and/or walkers, and time schedules are important (Backus, 2016). Many people with a new disability lose their ability to drive and must rely on friends, family or community resources for transportation. Community programmes that offer fitness programmes specifically for people with disabilities are more likely to have knowledgeable exercise staff and equipment that is safe and accessible for individuals with disabilities (Rimmer et al., 2012; Rimmer & Lai, 2017). Examples include aquatics programmes, seated exercises and accessible gym equipment for people with physical disabilities.

HEALTH PROMOTION STRATEGIES TO INCREASE PARTICIPATION

Promoting Exercise and Physical Activity

Exercise physiologists, fitness trainers and trained carers can help to overcome barriers when transitioning from healthcare-based exercise to community exercise. A smooth transition can be facilitated by implementing the following strategies to increase opportunities for older adults with disability to stay physically active: (1) identifying and educating healthcare professionals in the community; (2) improving community access; (3) securing safe, affordable and accessible equipment and facilities; and (4) offering socially engaging forms of physical activity that can be maintained across the lifespan (Backus, 2016; French et al., 2014; Motl, Pekmezi, & Wingo, 2018; Rimmer et al., 2012; Rimmer & Lai, 2017).

Older adults with disabilities are unable to participate in the same physical activity programmes and recreational activities as their peers (Campbell, Coulter, & Paul, 2018; Latham et al., 2003). Programmes that facilitate physical activity and incorporate exercise into everyday life may enhance adherence and could be as effective as structured exercise programmes (Pahor et al., 2014). Individuals with cognitive impairment will likely benefit from a cognitively intact exercise partner, step-by-step instructions, high repetition, familiar activities, memory cues and exercise that is enjoyable and tailored to the individual (Teri et al., 2018).

Supporting Behaviour Change Strategies

Commitment, motivation and self-efficacy are critical for anyone to make lifestyle changes that contribute to better health. Behaviour change strategies used with older adults and people with disabilities have been shown to increase attendance at health promotion programmes, improve adherence to exercise recommendations and lead to improved long-term participation in physical activity (Lai et al., 2017). One example of a successful strategy is motivational interviewing, a counselling technique that aims to elicit a person's own motivations for health behaviour change and then connect individual motivation with strategic planning and personal commitment to make changes (Soderlund, 2018).

Additional successful coaching strategies include helping older adults understand and address barriers that affect healthy behaviours and assisting them in setting reachable goals to improve a valued activity. It is important to encourage self-monitoring, motivation and feedback on progress towards their goals (French et al., 2014). To maintain sustained change in a lifestyle behaviour, it is important that participants perceive benefit. Therefore, ensuring that programmes help participants reflect on their personal accomplishments is important in reinforcing healthy behaviours.

Incorporating Technology

Many technological options have been studied to help patients access and adhere to health promotion interventions. Tele-coaching, instructional videos and telephone follow-up calls after educational or exercise interventions can improve long-term adherence and access to health promotion services (Lai et al., 2017). Cell phone applications such as activity trackers or exercise and nutrition apps are effective in helping patients set goals, track their diet and activity status, and provide patients and health professionals with data about challenges and successes. These apps help individuals learn ownership and self-monitoring techniques, which can improve their sense of control over their health (Brickwood et al., 2019).

Overall, sustained health promotion interventions must be holistic in addressing individual barriers for each patient. Rehabilitation and healthcare providers should have a strong understanding of these types of community resources in order to help patients make and sustain healthy behaviours.

CONCLUSION

Health promotion for older adults with a disability includes maintaining health, maximising function and improving participation in meaningful activities. Rehabilitation professionals play a critical role in health promotion through providing guidance for a healthy lifestyle and assisting older adults with a disability in transitioning to community resources. In addition to providing education and guidance to patients and families, rehabilitation professionals can work within their communities to bridge gaps between healthcare and community resources in an effort to provide appropriate and accessible programmes that support physical activity, health resources and social participation for older adults with disability.

SUMMARY POINTS

- Short-term gains achieved during rehabilitation can rapidly decline after discharge
- Identification of risk factors and timely intervention is important for promoting health in older adults as they transition out of rehabilitation
- Older adults with a newly acquired disability face many barriers to a healthy lifestyle
- Rehabilitation professionals can play a key role in increasing sustainable resources, by working within their communities to develop programmes that support physical activity and social interaction for older adults with disability

MCQs

Q.1 Physical activity and exercise programmes for older adults with disability should:
- **a.** Not be recommended for persons with a high fall risk
- **b.** Not include fall prevention and balance exercises
- **c.** Consist of 15 minutes of high intensity exercise 3 days per week
- **d.** Be adapted to each person's medical and physical limitations

Q.2 Health promotion strategies in older adults with disability target factors such as:
- **a.** Substance abuse
- **b.** Stroke
- **c.** Coronary artery disease
- **d.** Bladder incontinence
- **e.** All of the above

Q.3 Recommended strategies to support sustainable healthy lifestyle choices include:
- **a.** Critical analysis of an individual's skill in an activity
- **b.** Immediate feedback techniques to correct errors
- **c.** Interview strategies to elicit a person's own motivations for participation in health promoting activities
- **d.** Coaching techniques to force a person to participate in health promoting activities despite their reluctance

REFERENCES

Backus, D. (2016). Increasing physical activity and participation in people with multiple sclerosis: a review. *Archives of Physical Medicine and Rehabilitation, 97,* S210–S217.

Baylor, C., Yorkston, K. M., Jensen, M. P., Truitt, A. R., & Molton, I. R. (2014). Scoping review of common secondary conditions after stroke and their associations with age and time post stroke. *Topics in Stroke Rehabilitation, 21,* 371–382.

Brickwood, K. J., Watson, G., O'Brien, J., & Williams, A. D. (2019). Consumer-based wearable activity trackers increase physical activity participation: systematic review and meta-analysis. *JMIR Mhealth and Uhealth, 7,* e11819.

Campbell, E., Coulter, E. H., & Paul, L. (2018). High intensity interval training for people with multiple sclerosis: a systematic review. *Multiple Sclerosis and Related Disorders, 24,* 55–63.

Centers for Disease Control and Prevention. (2017). *Important facts about falls.* Retrieved from https://www.cdc.gov/homeandrecreationalsafety/falls/adultfalls.html (Accessed 16 August 2019).

Chernoff, R. (2001). Nutrition and health promotion in older adults. *The Journals of Gerontology Series A Biological Sciences and Medical Sciences, 56,* 47–53.

French, D. P., Olander, E. K., Chisholm, A., & Mc Sharry, J. (2014). Which behaviour change techniques are most effective at increasing older adults' self-efficacy and physical activity behaviour? A systematic review. *Annals of Behavioral Medicine, 48,* 225–234.

Golinowska, S., Groot, W., Baji, P., & Pavlova, M. (2016). Health promotion targeting older people. *BMC Health Services Research, 16 Suppl, 5,* 345.

Heijmans, M., Waverijn, G., Rademakers, J., van der Vaart, R., & Rijken, M. (2015). Functional, communicative and critical health literacy of chronic disease patients and their importance for self-management. *Patient Education and Counseling, 98,* 41–48.

Jensen, M. P., Molton, I. R., Groah, S. L., Campbell, M. L., Charlifue, S., Chiodo, A., Forchheimer, M., Krause, J. S., & Tate, D. (2012). Secondary health conditions in individuals aging with SCI: terminology, concepts and analytic approaches. *Spinal Cord, 50,* 373–378.

Jorgensen, S., Iwarsson, S., & Lexell, J. (2017). Secondary health conditions, activity limitations, and life satisfaction in older adults with long-term spinal cord injury. *PM& R, 9,* 356–366.

Kern, S. B., Hunter, L. N., Sims, A. C., Berzins, D., Riekena, H., Andrews, M. L., Alderfer, J. K., Nelson, K., & Kushner, R. (2019). Understanding the changing health care needs of individuals aging with spinal cord injury. *Topics in Spinal Cord Injury Rehabilitation, 25,* 62–73.

Kinne, S. (2008). Distribution of secondary medical problems, impairments, and participation limitations among adults with disabilities and their relationship to health and other outcomes. *Disability and Health Journal, 1,* 42–50.

Kuerbis, A., Sacco, P., Blazer, D. G., & Moore, A. A. (2014). Substance abuse among older adults. *Clinics in Geriatric Medicine, 30,* 629–654.

Lai, B., Young, H. J., Bickel, C. S., Motl, R. W., & Rimmer, J. H. (2017). Current trends in exercise intervention research, technology, and behavioral change strategies for people with disabilities: a scoping review. *American Journal of Physical Medicine & Rehabilitation, 96,* 748–761.

Latham, N., Anderson, C., Bennett, D., & Stretton, C. (2003). Progressive resistance strength training for physical disability in older people. *Cochrane Database of Systematic Reviews,* CD002759.

Motl, R. W., Pekmezi, D., & Wingo, B. C. (2018). Promotion of physical activity and exercise in multiple sclerosis: importance of behavioral science and theory. *Multiple Sclerosis Journal - Experimental, Translational and Clinical, 4,* 2055217318786745.

Pahor, M., Guralnik, J. M., Ambrosius, W. T., Blair, S., Bonds, D. E., Church, T. S., …, & Williamson, J. D. (2014). Effect of structured physical activity on prevention of major mobility disability in older adults: the LIFE study randomized clinical trial. *JAMA, 311,* 2387–2396.

Peel, N. M., McClure, R. J., & Bartlett, H. P. (2005). Behavioral determinants of healthy aging. *American Journal of Preventive Medicine, 28,* 298–304.

Rimmer, J., & Lai, B. (2017). Framing new pathways in transformative exercise for individuals with existing and newly acquired disability. *Disability and Rehabilitation, 39,* 173–180.

Rimmer, J. H., Schiller, W., & Chen, M. D. (2012). Effects of disability-associated low energy expenditure deconditioning syndrome. *Exercise and Sport Scientific Review, 40,* 22–29.

Soderlund, P. D. (2018). Effectiveness of motivational interviewing for improving physical activity self-management for adults with type 2 diabetes: a review. *Chronic Illness, 14,* 54–68.

Teri, L., Logsdon, R. G., McCurry, S. M., Pike, K. C., & McGough, E. L. (*2018*). Translating an evidence-based multicomponent intervention for older adults with dementia and caregivers. *Gerontologist, 60,* 548–557.

Thun, M. J., Carter, B. D., Feskanich, D., Freedman, N. D., Prentice, R., Lopez, A. D., Hartge, P., & Gapstur, S. M. (2013). 50-year trends in smoking-related mortality in the United States. *New England Journal of Medicine, 368,* 351–364.

World Health Organization. (2010). *Global recommendations on physical activity for health.* Geneva Switzerland: World Health Organization. Retrieved from https://www.who.int/dietphysicalactivity/global-PA-recs-2010.pdf (Accessed 16 August 2019).

Resources for Patients and Families

7 WHAT CAN PATIENTS AND FAMILIES DO TO HELP WITH REHABILITATION?

Practical Ways to Support Rehabilitation and Get the Best Results

Make sure you/your relative has everything needed to take part in rehab – e.g. bring in from home glasses/hearing aids, comfortable clothing/shoes, books, radio, phone, family photos, diary.

Get as much information as possible about the rehab setting – do some research in advance if possible and ask questions (e.g. visiting times, who is in the team, will there be regular meetings to discuss progress?)

Get as much information as you can about you/your relative's current areas of difficulty and the rehabilitation plan – request time to meet with team members if this is not offered routinely. Ask for written summaries of any important discussions.

Make sure the rehab team know you/your relative's personal story – provide key information such as likes/dislikes, background history, and wishes regarding future care. Bring in photographs from home for your relative's room.

Follow the team's recommendations – following the team's advice, engaging fully in sessions, and working on any tasks set between sessions will all help get the most out of rehab. Family members can often be an invaluable source of support with this. If you are unclear about or disagree with advice, then do let the team know of your concerns.

Maintain ongoing/effective communication with the team – honest and open communication with the team is essential. It is important they are aware of your views and wishes. Consider identifying one person within the team to serve as your key contact and to let teams know how you prefer to communicate (e.g. face to face, phone, emails, communication book, through one family member).

And last but not least, it is important that family members also look after their own self-care needs – rehab can be an extremely emotional journey. It is important to take care of yourself and let others know if you are struggling to cope. Formal psychological/counselling support may be available in the rehab unit. If not, talk to your GP about support options.

8 WHAT CAN WE DO TO HELP PATIENTS AND FAMILIES?

Fostering a Family-Focused Environment

- A useful starting point can be the formation of a small multidisciplinary working group who can take a "think family" approach, steer family-focused initiatives and ensure that this ethos is reflected in ward policies and protocols.
- Review all ward policies through a family-focused lens and identify where there might be gaps in thinking about or provision for relatives. For example, do visiting policies accommodate relatives who cannot visit during regular hours, is there provision for virtual visits (e.g. using phones or tablet devices to see each other) for patients whose relatives are infirm and cannot travel or who live too far to visit, can young children and babies visit grandparents who are hospitalised? This is important in supporting existing attachments – and particularly so for any older patients who were providing care for younger family members at the time of their illness. Many units may restrict children visiting and this can cause distress for all involved.
- A "think family" ethos should also guide the development of physical resources; teams can consider whether the layout and amenities on the ward support the family experience of rehabilitation. Are there dedicated, comfortable and private areas for family and patients to meet, are patients and relatives encouraged to eat meals together, is there a safe play area with toys and games for children (such a space can also double as a useful "real-world" therapy space for helping the older person practise role and activity resumption such as changing a grandchild's nappy), are there good quality refreshments available for family, private space where staff can meet with relatives to share news sensitively and away from the unit's main hub areas? Seeking patient and family views on the ward environment and how it could be improved can form the basis of meaningful audit projects.
- Develop a family resource library on the ward: this can provide psycho-educational resources for relatives (materials can be easily accessed free of charge from many of the large third sector disease/condition-specific organisations and can usefully supplement more personalised information relating to their relative's diagnosis). Resource

libraries can also signpost to community-based activities and support options (e.g. local carers groups) that families might access. Monetary grants may be available from hospital fundraising groups and charitable organisations in order to facilitate the development of such resources when none exist and the setting up of a resource library can be a good project for a volunteer or student to undertake. In addition, it can be helpful to coproduce informational materials with previous patients and family members.

- Nominate staff members to be "family champions" who can help orientate relatives to the ward, signpost them to resources and information, serve as a drop-in resource in the evenings and weekends and help to identify family members that might benefit from more formal emotional support. These staff members should be supported to undertake introductory counselling skills training to assist them in effectively helping relatives who are distressed.

- Implement activities and resources that facilitate family orientation, connection and learning such as a Tree of Positivity, where families can leave encouraging messages for other patients and families who are just entering rehabilitation.

- Set rehabilitation goals that focus on and enhance relationships and encourage family activities that are important to the patient (e.g. working on mobility goals that focus on a grandfather being able to kick a football with his grandchildren; helping an older patient and her daughter work on using public transport to allow them to resume attending art galleries together).

Team Checklist for Creating a Family-Friendly Environment

PHYSICAL ENVIRONMENT	WHO IS RESPONSIBLE FOR TAKING THIS FORWARD	DATE COMPLETED	FUTURE WORK IN THIS AREA
• Create comfy areas for families to sit together in			
• Identify a private, quiet space for staff to talk to families in			
• Provide a refreshments station for families			
• Identify a play area with toys and games for younger visitors			
Create a Family Information and Signposting Hub:			
• Search webpages of key organisations to draw up list of key resources (online, paper leaflets)			
• Order information leaflets on range of conditions and create info library			
• Identify information aimed for children and young people to inform about an adult relative's illness			
• Include information on local support agencies			
• Set up a Tree of Positivity (tree graphic on a wall; families write motivational messages on paper leaves and stick them to the tree)			
"Think family" Training and Support for the Team			
• Identify family champions in the team who will lead on family-focused initiatives			
• Identify relevant training, e.g. counselling skills courses, adult and child safeguarding, supporting carers			
• Clinical supervision for staff supporting families			
Audit and Review			
• Review family visiting polices			
• Family suggestions/comments book to receive feedback			
• Regular family satisfaction surveys			

12 PHYSIOTHERAPY: HOW IT WORKS

Physiotherapy Rehabilitation Interventions

ASSESSMENT FINDINGS	INTERVENTIONS	RATIONALE	CONSIDERATIONS
Decreased hip muscle strength	**Progressive resistance exercise** Dose: 80% 1 repetition maximum (1 RM), 8–15 reps, pain free, once/day, alternate days Build to 20 reps for endurance • Active hip abduction, extension • Standing with one hand support • Sit to stand • Step ups on low step • Addition of resistance bands weights	• Early strength training against gravity • When muscles are weak 8–15 reps provides overload to muscles to increase strength • With increasing muscle strength progress to endurance training with greater reps, utilising aerobic pathways	Safety: ensure hand support is stable
Decreased balance	**Balance exercise** Standing at a supportive surface: weight shifts with hips and knees straight leaning forwards and back, increasing ranges Progress to no arm support, feet together, eyes open/closed, single leg support, turning Progress to: walking negotiating obstacles, turning head, carrying objects	Need for high level of challenge, individualised and progressive to be effective Aim to improve the speed and accuracy of the patient's response to unexpected perturbation via use of the ankle, hip, reaching and stepping strategies	Initially, close supervision and safe set up for hand support to build confidence
Repeated falls	• **Education** about risk factors; intrinsic – home hazard: loose rugs, pets; intrinsic risks: check BP sit and standing and educate • **Train in 'backward chaining'** technique – for getting up from floor • Education on use of a pendant alarm	Assist patient to recognise existing and potential hazards in the home Help manage fear of falling by providing skills to reduce falls risk at home Prevent risk of complications associated with a long lie on the floor	Patient may need help with managing heavy household chores such as vacuuming and laundry. Referral for home help support may be necessary
Diminished walking ability	**Task-specific training of gait** Progress from partial weight-bearing with walking frame to full weight-bearing walking on different surfaces Progress to increasing speed for short periods during daily walk. Community mobility training: crossing roads, negotiating public transport	Increase functional and activity levels within home Speed element required to train muscle power for normal function such as crossing the road	Monitor pain, endurance and balance, especially when introducing speed
Decreased endurance	Increase walking distance, while monitoring rating of perceived exertion (RPE). Climbing stairs. Walking outside Build to 20 minutes per day, or 10 minutes x 3 times per day, for 5 days a week	Place demand on aerobic pathways using functional activity	Monitor correct exercise intensity Exercise to point of slight fatigue to reach overload but not to the point of exhaustion
Health promotion: physical activity (PA)	**Physical activity advice** Education about internationally recommended physical activity levels for older adults Use of an activity log and review by therapist	Exercise recommendations for maintaining physical function for older adults: 30 minutes of aerobic activity 3 times/week and static strength and balance exercises	Potential impact of fear of falling on PA levels
Osteopaenia	• Medium impact weight-bearing exercise (post-menopausal) • Moderate intensity muscle-specific resistance training of 70%-80% 1 RM: • Stair climbing, brisk/power walking 30 minutes per day • Postural education	Gradual build-up of exercise that provides increased load and demand on bones during weight-bearing, avoiding joint pain Bone takes several months to adapt to extra use	• Avoid trunk flexion and/or rotation with loading heavy lifting/carrying • Avoid repeated sit-ups • Precautions apply to osteopenia and osteoporosis with/without fracture and corticosteroid induced osteoporosis with normal T-score

17 NUTRITION AND HYDRATION

Eating healthily, combined with regular physical activity, can help a person live a full, active life, preserving independence into older age.

Ten Simple Dietary Guidelines to Help You Stay Well Into Older Age

1. Balance your food intake with physical activity – the more active you are, the more food you need. Keep an eye on your meal portion size; if you are less active choose smaller serving sizes and add plenty of vegetables, salad and fruit.

2. Include a carbohydrate food (bread, rice, pasta, potato or cereal) at each meal. Choose high-fibre options whenever you can (see following section for suggestions).

3. Aim for five servings of fruits and vegetables each day. These are packed with important nutrients to help you stay healthy. Remember these can be fresh, frozen, tinned or dried. Colour is important – have a mixture of different coloured fruits and vegetables each day such as apples, oranges, bananas, spinach, cabbage, carrots, sweet potato, broccoli, cauliflower, peppers and sweet corn.

4. Protein foods help to make new cells and keep your muscles healthy. Stay fit and strong by eating a variety of protein-rich foods each day. Great sources include lean meat, poultry and fish. Salmon, sardines, trout, fresh tuna and kippers are packed with heart-healthy omega 3 fats. Eating beans, eggs and nuts is a simple way of boosting the protein in your diet.

5. Keep your bones healthy by having three servings of low-fat dairy foods (milk, yoghurt or cheese) each day. Dairy foods with added calcium and vitamin D are even better. Look out for these in the supermarket as fortified foods.

6. Choose heart-healthy fats. We all need some fat in the diet but it is a case of choosing the right type:
   ✗ Saturated fat or animal fat can raise your cholesterol level, which can in turn increase the risk of heart disease. Saturated fat is found in butter, hard margarine, lard, cream, cream based sauces, fat on meat, skin on chicken, and processed meats like sausages, burgers, black and white pudding, meat pies and pâté. It is also found in biscuits, cakes, chocolate, toffees, takeaway foods, foods covered in batter and breadcrumbs as well as milk, cheese and yoghurt.
   ✗ Trans fat or hydrogenated vegetable fat also raises cholesterol levels. Trans fat is found in hard margarine, cakes, biscuits and confectionery. It may be listed as hydrogenated fat on food labels and should be avoided.
   ✓ Monounsaturated fat – aim to replace saturated fat with monounsaturated fat to help protect your heart as it helps lower cholesterol level. Monounsaturated fat is found in olive oil, peanut oil and rapeseed oil, unsalted peanuts, cashew nuts and almonds.
   ✓ Polyunsaturated fat can also help to reduce cholesterol levels. Polyunsaturated fat is found in oily fish (omega-3 fat), sunflower oil (omega-6 fat), sesame oil, flax-seed oil, walnuts and hazelnuts.

Remember all types of fats and oils contain the same amount of fat and calories. They can lead to weight gain if used to excess!

7. Use less salt. Too much salt in the diet can contribute to high blood pressure, which in turn can lead to stroke or heart disease. You can reduce the amount of salt in your diet by:
   • Avoiding adding salt to your food at the table and in cooking. Use pepper, lemon juice, herbs and spices to flavour food instead of salt
   • Choosing fresh foods as often as possible, e.g. fresh meat, chicken, fish, vegetables, home-made soups and sauces without salt
   • Limiting intake of processed or canned food
   • Avoiding foods high in salt such as packet and tinned soups and sauces, instant noodles, Bovril, Oxo, Marmite, stock cubes, soy sauce, garlic salt and sea salt
   • Avoiding processed meats such as ham, bacon, corned beef, sausages, burgers, black and white pudding, meat pies, pâté as well as smoked fish
   • Keeping away from snacks such as salted biscuits and salted crisps and nuts
   • Checking food labels to help you choose foods with a low amount of salt. Too much salt is more than 1.5 g (0.6 g sodium) per 100 g of any food item.

8. Limit amount of foods high in 'empty calories' like biscuits, cakes, savoury snacks (crisps, peanuts), sweets and confectionery. These foods are rich in calories, fat, sugar and salt, so remember – not too much and not too often.

9. Stay hydrated. Among other things, dehydration causes tiredness, dizziness and constipation. Get plenty of fluids (water, fruit cordials, juice, milk) on board each day. As a general guide, about 8 glasses a day should be adequate.

10. Alcohol should be enjoyed in moderation. Generally not more than 14 units should be consumed per week on a regular basis. This is equivalent to about 6 pints of beer or 10 small glasses of wine. It is recommended to have several alcohol-free days each week.

Some Important Nutrients to Consider

As we get older, our bodies have different needs, so certain nutrients become especially important for good health:

Fibre: eating fibre-rich foods helps bowels move regularly, lowering the risk of constipation. A high-fibre diet can also lower the risk for many chronic conditions including heart disease, obesity and some cancers. Good sources of fibre include:
   • 100% wholemeal or wholegrain bread
   • Breakfast cereals such as porridge, Weetabix, shredded wheat, bran flakes
   • Other cereals such as brown rice, brown pasta
   • Potatoes eaten in their jackets
   • Fruits and vegetables
   • Pulse vegetables such as beans, peas and lentils.

Breakfast can be a super way to get a high fibre start to the day: add linseed to a wholegrain cereal or to yoghurt or have prune juice instead of orange juice to boost your fibre intake.

Calcium and vitamin D: Older adults need extra calcium and vitamin D to help maintain bone health. Being a healthy weight can help keep bones strong. Take three servings of vitamin D-fortified milk, cheese or yoghurt each day. Other calcium-rich foods include fortified cereals, dark green leafy vegetables and canned fish with soft bones (like sardines).

Iron and vitamin B12: iron is responsible for carrying oxygen around the body, while vitamin B12 keeps your brain and nervous system healthy. Many older adults do not get enough of these important nutrients in their diet. The best sources of iron include red meats such as beef, liver, kidney, lamb, pork, ham, corned beef, and black and white pudding, while fortified cereals, lean meat and some fish and seafood are sources of both iron and vitamin B12. Taking a vitamin C-rich food like orange juice at meal time can help your body to absorb iron. Ask your doctor or dietitian whether you would benefit from an iron or a vitamin B12 supplement.

A word on exercise....

Combining an active lifestyle with a healthy diet is your best recipe for healthy ageing.

Try to be physically active for at least 30 minutes most days.

It is okay to break up your 30 minutes physical activity into 10-minute sessions throughout the day.

If you are currently inactive, start with 5 minutes of exercise, such as walking, gardening, climbing stairs or dancing and gradually increase this time as you become stronger.

Always check with your doctor or nurse before beginning a new physical activity programme.

Irish Nutrition and Dietetics Institute, INDI

https://www.indi.ie/fact-sheets/fact-sheets-on-nutrition-for-older-people/509-good-nutrition-for-the-older-person.html

19 THE PATIENT STORY

Nine Important Things About Me

(Name or sticker)
I like to be called:
My job/role was:
The person who knows me best,
and looks after me, is:
(Please let them come in to support me when I need it)
What I like best is:
What upsets me is:
Foods I like:
Foods I do not like:
Drinks I like (include sugar/milk, etc.):
Drinks I do not like:

BOX 1   The Four BRAN Questions
1. What are the **B**enefits of this proposed treatment?
2. What are the **R**isks of this proposed treatment?
3. What are the **A**lternatives to this proposed treatment?
4. What if we do **N**othing?

BOX 2   Five Questions Worth Asking Your Patient
1. What is your understanding of where you are with your illness at the moment?
2. What are your goals and priorities?
3. What fears or concerns for the future do you have?
4. What outcomes are unacceptable to you? What are you willing to sacrifice (and not)?
5. What would a good day look like?

BOX 3   Five Questions That Every Patient Has, But Never Asks
1. Do you care about me?
2. Are you the best?
3. Can I trust you?
4. Are you treating me differently from others?
5. Will this treatment make my life better?

20 BRAIN HEALTH AND MENTAL CAPACITY

Suggested content of a Mediterranean diet*

FOOD GROUP	LEVEL OF CONSUMPTION	SUGGESTED PORTIONS	EXAMPLES	COMMENT
Meats	Low	2–3 servings per month	Grilled lamb	Use small cuts of lean meats
Poultry and fish	Low-moderate	2–3 servings per week	Skinless chicken or salmon	Oily fish are high in omega-3 fatty acids
Dairy	Low-moderate	1–3 servings per day	Low-fat cheese, Greek style yoghurt	Dairy can be used regularly but in small amounts
Vegetables	High	4 or more servings per day	Non-starchy vegetables, e.g. carrots, broccoli, peppers	Should include a portion of raw vegetables daily
Fruit	High	3 or more servings per day	Dried apricots, plums, clementines	Use as a substitute for desserts
Legumes, nuts and seeds	Moderate	3 or more servings per week	Soybeans, lentils, sunflower or sesame seeds	Rich in fibre, protein, minerals and unsaturated fats. Use as a snack substitute
Olive oil	Moderate	4 tablespoons per day or less	Extra virgin olive oil is highest quality	Used a substitute for butter
Whole wheat grains	High	4 or more servings per day	Whole grain oatmeal or pasta	Whole grains are high in fibre
Herbs and spices	Moderate	As needed	Basil, cinnamon, oregano	Can be used as a substitute for salt
Wine	Moderate	1 glass per day	No specific variety	Potential beneficial antioxidant effect

*The diet also promotes good intake of water, regular physical activity and eating with socially with other people.

28 FALLS, DIZZINESS AND FUNNY TURNS

Main Falls Risk Factors and Specific Intervention Strategies

FALLS RISK FACTORS

Extrinsic Risk Factors

Home hazards
- Insufficient lighting
- Rugs, carpets and tripping obstacles
- Lack of stairs railings or grab bars
- Slippery floor, wet surfaces

INTERVENTION STRATEGIES

Safety assessment and appropriate environmental modifications, e.g.
- Improvements in lighting, particularly at night
- Installation of grab bars next to the toilet and shower
- Use of raised toilet seat
- Use of non-slip bathmats
- Installation of handrails on stairs
- Removal of carpets and tripping hazards
- Painting the edges of the steps

Outdoor hazards, e.g. uneven sidewalks and lack of paved walking areas

Safety assessment and appropriate environmental modifications, e.g. appropriate lighting and paving, installation of railings along walking pathways

Footwear
(poor fitting, laced or buckled, with high heels)

Safe footwear, i.e. shoes of low heel height and high surface contact area

Poor social **support network**

Social support

Intrinsic Risk Factors

Biological risk factors
(advanced age, female gender)

FALLS RISK FACTORS	INTERVENTION STRATEGIES
Medical conditions	Consider specialist referral (neurologist, orthopaedics, …) to optimise treatment
- Neurologic disease (Parkinson, peripheral neuropathies, …)	Foot assessment and referral for appropriate treatment, in case of foot problems
- Vestibular disorders	
- Osteoarthritis	
- Spine disorders and back pain	
- Prior cerebrovascular events	
- Cognitive impairment and mental confusion	
- Diabetes	
- Urinary incontinence	
- Foot problems (deformities, ulcers, …)	
Reduced physical performance	Physiotherapy and rehabilitation
- Impaired balance and posture problems	Use of orthopaedic devices, if indicated
- Gait disorders	
- Sarcopenia	
Visual Impairment	Regular eye examination
(reduced visual field, impaired depth perception, loss of acuity and contrast sensitivity)	Correction of visual problems, when possible (e.g. early cataract surgery)
	Switch from multifocal/progressive to single-lens glasses when walking outdoor
Medications	Medication review (see paragraph 2.4.3)
Vitamin D deficiency	Vitamin D supplements (800 UI/day according to the AGS/BGS guidelines)*
Psychological risk factors	Assessment and treatment
(e.g. depression, fear of falling, …)	
History of falling	Detailed history collection
	Consider Falls and Syncope Service referral**
Alcohol	Suggest avoiding alcohol intake

*Vitamin D deficiency is associated with gait impairment and muscle atrophy, and randomised trials have demonstrated that vitamin D supplementation improves muscle strength, balance and gait speed. The efficacy of supplementation in reducing falls risk is controversial. According to the AGS/BGS guidelines, supplements should be offered to older people with vitamin D deficiency and should be considered for those with suspected deficiency or who are otherwise at high risk for falls.
**Referral to a Falls and Syncope Service should be considered for patients with recurrent unexplained falls or/and falls-related severe injuries to assess potential cardiovascular causes.

Medications Associated with an Increased Risk of Falls, Syncope and Dizziness

DRUG CLASS	MAIN INDICATIONS	MECHANISM
Antihypertensive and vasodilators	Hypertension	Hypotension, vasodilation, reduced heart rate response to standing, reduced cardiac contractility
- Angiotensin-converting enzyme inhibitors		
- Calcium-channel blockers		
- Nitrates		
- Alpha receptors blockers*		
- Clonidine		
- Hydralazine		
Diuretics	Hypertension, heart failure	Dehydration, electrolyte imbalances
Beta-blockers	Hypertension, heart failure, ischemic heart disease	Reduced heart rate, impaired blood pressure and heart rate response to standing
Levodopa	Parkinson disease	Orthostatic hypotension
Opioids	Chronic pain	Central nervous system effects (sedation, confusion)
Psychoactive	Anxiety, depression, sleeping disorders	Sedation, confusion, prolonged reaction times, psychomotor slowing, balance and gait impairment, hypotension, arrhythmias
- Tricyclic antidepressant		
- Benzodiazepine		
- Phenothiazine		
- Haloperidol		
- Benzodiazepine receptors agonists (e.g. zolpidem and zopiclone)		
Hypoglycaemic (sulfonylurea)	Diabetes	Hypoglycaemia

(Continued)

DRUG CLASS	MAIN INDICATIONS	MECHANISM
Vestibular suppressants	Dizziness and vertigo	Balance impairment, hypotension, confusion, psychomotor slowing
Muscle relaxants	Painful musculoskeletal conditions	Muscle tone reduction, sedation and hypotension
Laxatives**	Constipation (over-the-counter medications)	Dehydration and electrolyte unbalances

*In older male adults, alpha receptors blockers might be indicated for obstructive symptoms related to benign prostatic hypertrophy; in that case, selective drugs with a lower incidence of hypotension should be preferred.

**Laxatives should be used occasionally and for short periods of time, and patients should be advised to increase their water intake, which is also helpful to improve constipation.

Lifestyle Measures for Treatment and Prevention of Orthostatic Intolerance

- Hydration

A daily fluid intake of 2–2.5 L is recommended to avoid dehydration and prevent orthostatic susceptibility. Moreover, patients can consider the rapid ingestion of approximately 500 ml of water (bolus), which can raise systolic blood pressure by 30 mmHg within a few minutes. Bolus water drinking has been demonstrated to be one of the most efficacious non-pharmacological therapy for orthostatic hypotension and may be helpful to prevent symptoms in typical predisposing situations (prolonged standing, hot environment, exercise, and so on).

In subjects with low blood pressure, increasing daily diet salt intake can be suggested (2.3–4.6 g of salt per day). This measure should be avoided in patients with congestive heart failure.

- Avoid predisposing situations

Patients should rise slowly from supine/sitting to upright positions and avoid situations favouring venous blood pooling, e.g. prolonged standing (particularly if motionless), hot environments and large meals. Alcohol intake should be avoided due to the associated vasodilation. Patients should be advised to sit on the edge of the bed for some minutes after waking while performing thigh, buttock or calf contractions, since hypotensive symptoms are more likely to occur after nocturnal sleeping.

- Abdominal binders or compression stockings

Compressive waist or thigh-high stockings may be useful to reduce venous blood pooling. Unfortunately, compliance is frequently low, since they are difficult to put on and uncomfortable in hot climates. Abdominal binders offer an effective alternative, are easier to use and equally effective, since most of the pooling occurs in the splanchnic circulation. Although widely used, knee-high stockings are not effective.

- Physical countermanoeuvres

Some physical countermanoeuvres can reduce venous pooling in lower body vessels, activating the muscle pump and translocating blood from the lower body to the heart. These manoeuvres may prevent symptoms occurrence or, if symptoms develop, may delay a possible loss of consciousness allowing the patient to avoid fall-related injuries. Patients should be instructed to perform these manoeuvres in the presence of symptoms or predisposing factors for low blood pressure (e.g. prolonged standing, hot environments). Effective countermanoeuvres include toe raises, thigh, buttock and calf muscle contractions and arm tensing (gripping one hand with the other pulling away the arms). Shifting weight from one leg to the other and marching in place may also be helpful.

- Exercise and physical conditioning

Early mobilisation is crucial to counteract deconditioning and orthostatic susceptibility in bed bound or hospitalised patients; if deconditioning is present, exercise should be recommended. Patients should be cautioned that exercise may temporarily exacerbate symptoms due to increased core body temperature and peripheral vasodilation. Therefore, individuals should be well hydrated prior to exercise and should be careful when standing after an exercise session.

30 COGNITIVE PROBLEMS

Pathway for Assessment of Confusion

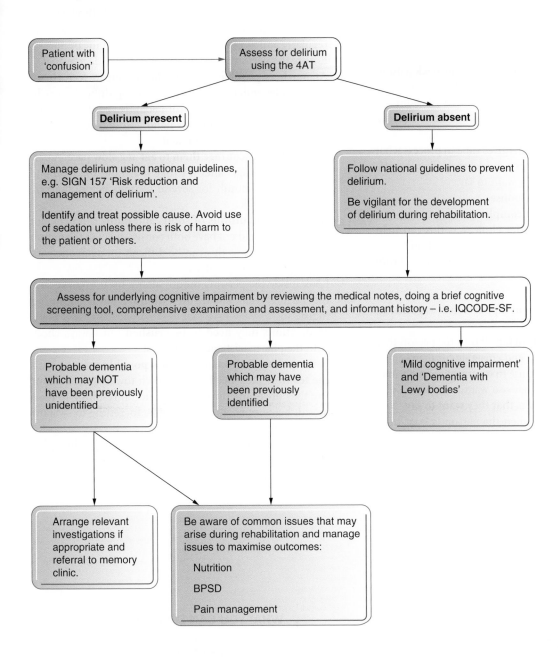

Patient with 'confusion' → Assess for delirium using the 4AT

Delirium present

Manage delirium using national guidelines, e.g. SIGN 157 'Risk reduction and management of delirium'.

Identify and treat possible cause. Avoid use of sedation unless there is risk of harm to the patient or others.

Delirium absent

Follow national guidelines to prevent delirium.

Be vigilant for the development of delirium during rehabilitation.

Assess for underlying cognitive impairment by reviewing the medical notes, doing a brief cognitive screening tool, comprehensive examination and assessment, and informant history – i.e. IQCODE-SF.

Probable dementia which may NOT have been previously unidentified

Probable dementia which may have been previously identified

'Mild cognitive impairment' and 'Dementia with Lewy bodies'

Arrange relevant investigations if appropriate and referral to memory clinic.

Be aware of common issues that may arise during rehabilitation and manage issues to maximise outcomes:

Nutrition

BPSD

Pain management

43 SPEECH AND SWALLOW REHABILITATION AFTER STROKE

How to Support Someone with Communication Difficulties

- Concentrating on communication can be hard for someone after a stroke. **Avoid distractions and background noise** by turning off the radio or TV and making sure you are sitting **face to face** to the person in a **well-lit room.**
- Ensure the person is wearing their **glasses and/or hearing aids** if needed.
- **Speak slowly and clearly** as this gives time to process what you are saying. It also provides a model and helps give the person time to plan what they want to say.
- Allow **plenty of time** for a response.
- Keep **sentences short and uncomplicated.**
- Ask **yes-no questions** and **offer choices** as this can help you and the person identify important information.
- **Repeat important words** and write them down to clarify the meaning.
- Introduce **one idea at a time.**
- Use all types of communication supports such as **gestures, writing** and **pictures.**
- Choose **topics of conversation familiar** to the person that you know will be motivating and engaging for them.
- Acknowledge that you recognise that communication may be hard for the person but that you want to communicate with them and **value what it is that they want to say.**
- Try to **time conversations** when the person is least tired and most able to engage and concentrate.
- Ensure the person has **access to specialised speech and language therapy** and link directly with their SLT to find out what specific goals are being worked on and what strategies help optimise communication.

How to Support Someone with Dysphagia

- **Minimise distractions** within the environment during mealtimes.
- Only give food or drink when the person is **fully alert**. This may mean giving little portions of food and drink more regularly and at times outside of traditional mealtimes.
- Ensure the person is **seated upright** at a 90-degree angle.
- As much as possible, support the person to **feed themselves independently**. If they are having difficulty reaching food, they may benefit from adaptive equipment. You can help by doing 'hand over hand' feeding, i.e. they hold the utensil and you help guide it.
- Feed them or **encourage them to eat at a slow pace.** A person with dysphagia after a stroke may hold the food and drink in their mouth for several seconds before they are able to swallow it.
- **Alternating mouthfuls of solids and fluids** can help, but the person should not have both consistencies in the mouth at the same time as this can be difficult for someone with dysphagia to manage safely.
- Look inside the person's mouth after a meal to make sure that no food is left. **Ensure their mouth is always clean** and moist.
- **Medications may need to be crushed** but always check with the pharmacist and doctor first.
- If the person is drooling, **discuss possible reasons with the team**: Is their head falling down towards their chest? Are they breathing through their mouth resulting in their mouth being open at rest? Are they forgetting to swallow their saliva?
- Always **liaise with the speech and language therapist.** Never give the person something to eat and drink without first checking that it is safe.

44 SWALLOW REHABILITATION IN FRAILTY

Improving Swallowing Outcomes

FACTOR	IMPACT	WHAT YOU CAN DO TO HELP
Poor positioning	• Difficulty reaching, manipulating, controlling and swallowing food or fluid • Reduced ease of swallowing • Increased risk of reflux, heartburn and indigestion, aspiration or choke	• Liaise with the physiotherapist to review sitting and optimise positioning • Encourage sitting out at a table if possible • Sit fully upright with adequate support
Changes to cognition	• Inability to remain sufficiently alert to eat or drink • Reduced appetite • Changes in food and drink preferences • Poor recognition of food, drinks, cutlery or utensils • Reduced ability to self-assess safety of swallowing, resulting in increased risk of aspiration or choking	• Consider the environment and adapt appropriately (levels of light, noise, temperature, etc.) • Monitor levels of alertness and ability to eat and drink safely • Ensure assistance is available from a dysphagia-aware carer for all eating and drinking • Ensure mealtimes coincide with periods of alertness • Eat/drink little and often • Do not offer food or fluid if the person is not sufficiently alert

FACTOR	IMPACT	WHAT YOU CAN DO TO HELP
Reduced vision, dexterity and strength	• Reduced ability to see, manipulate or access food and drink • Limited appetite stimulation and "readiness" to eat or drink • Difficulty cutting, opening, peeling, spreading • Increased risk of aspiration or choking • High reliance on a carer to provide support for eating and drinking	• Liaise with the occupational therapist to promote independence and day-to-day functional abilities • Ensure an appropriate level of assistance is available • Note that adaptive cutlery, plate guards, beakers and straws may increase some swallowing difficulties
Changes to appetite, taste and enjoyment	• Change in food and drink preferences • Reduced appetite and interest in food • Reduced ability to taste sweetness and saltiness • Increased sensitivity to bitter and sour	• Liaise with the dietitian for support and advice on nutrition and hydration • Review and ensure preferred tasting items are available • Review size and frequency of meals • Consider a social dining experience
Poor dentition and oral hygiene	• High potential for pain, ulcers, infection, dry mouth and altered taste • Increased risk of pneumonia from oral bacteria • Difficulties chewing food due to limited dentition, loose dentures or reduced strength and efficiency of chewing action • Reduced saliva production • Loss of appetite	• Liaise with nursing colleagues or dental outreach teams • Encourage regular mouth care and ensure toothbrush, toothpaste and denture care products are available • Secure dentures during the day and remove at night • Consider foods that are easier to chew
Reduced tongue strength	• Difficulty manipulating food in the mouth and reduced delivery to teeth • Poor containment of food or drink in the mouth prior to swallow trigger • Poor initial drive of food or fluid from the mouth when swallowing • Food or drink unintentionally remaining in the mouth after a swallow • Increased risk of aspiration or choking	• Follow your SLT's advice on diet and fluid modification • Ask your SLT before using spouted beakers, sports caps or straws • Encourage and promote and specific compensatory postures, strategies or prompts recommended by your SLT
Reduced hyolaryngeal excursion	• Delayed and incomplete closure of the airway resulting in increased risk of food and fluid entering the airway • Poor opening of the oesophagus resulting in impaired transit, feelings of food 'sticking'	• Encourage regular completion of any targeted rehabilitation exercises • Ask for information, advice or training from your SLT • Encourage physical activity
Reduced pharyngeal strength	• Poor drive of food and fluid through the pharynx resulting in residue post-swallow	

48 REHABILITATION AFTER SURGERY

Risk Factors Associated with Delirium

	THINGS TO CONSIDER
Pain	Is analgesia adequate? Daily review of doses – too high vs too low, remove any unnecessary opioids, ensure simple analgesia prescribed, consider breakthrough analgesia prior to mobilising/activity
Infection	Observe for any signs of surgical site infection/cough/breathlessness or dysuria. Avoid urine dipstick, send MSU (mid stream urine) if any suspicion of UTI (urinary tract infection). Monitor for pyrexia
Nutrition	MUST scoring, food intake charts Good oral care and dentition including dentures Observe for signs of oral thrush and treat as appropriate Refer to dietitian + offer snacks if able to take oral nutrition and intake is poor or weight loss observed Is any assistance needed at mealtimes, is OT involvement required, can relatives/friends be involved at mealtimes? Encourage foods that are enjoyed by the patient, can relatives bring these in? Offer snacks at varying times of day

(Continued)

THINGS TO CONSIDER

Constipation including urinary retention	What is the normal bowel routine for the patient, is this likely to be altered by the surgery, what laxatives do they usually take? Ensure regular opportunity for bowel movements, encourage mobility and good hydration Laxatives may be required if on high-dose opioids Observe for signs of abdominal discomfort, distention and seek medical advice Monitor urinary output, consider bladder scan if urine output poor +/– suprapubic discomfort If acute urinary retention occurs in context of constipation, aim to relieve the constipation and remove catheter as soon as bowels opening well
Hydration	Strict fluid balance monitoring including catheters, drains, vomiting, stoma output Encourage oral intake at every opportunity, consider if any assistance required Supplementary fluids may be necessary if oral intake inadequate Diuretics may not be required in the perioperative period – be aware of what medications are prescribed
Medications	Ensure essential medications can be administered via alternative route if NBM (nil by mouth; not able to take food or drink orally): Parkinson's medications, anti-epileptics, antihyperglycaemics are especially important Avoid blood pressure lowering mediations in hypotensive patients, and ensure clear plans in place for blood thinning medications to be stopped/restarted (aspirin, clopidogrel, anticoagulation) Review of polypharmacy by an older person's specialist wherever possible
Environment and electrolytes	Regular reorientation to time, place, reason for hospital admission Clocks/signage and dates in easy sight Open visiting may be appropriate for those with cognitive impairment, to allow familiar faces and aid reorientation Avoid non-essential ward moves, especially overnight Monitor for electrolyte disturbance (potassium, sodium, calcium) in anyone who develops a delirium, and consider the need to test ferritin/folate/B12 levels + thyroid function

52 VESTIBULAR REHABILITATION

The Components of a Vestibular Rehabilitation Programme

	BALANCE EXERCISES	WALKING	GAZE STABILITY EXERCISES	HABITUATION EXERCISE
Aim	To promote appropriate balance responses in challenging situations (e.g. unsteady surface in the dark)	To improve dynamic balance and gaze stability function, as well as cardiovascular fitness and strength in order to promote participation in daily life	To maintain focus with progressively faster head movement for longer periods, in order to increase gaze stability in dynamic situations in daily life	To increase the tolerance to specific stimuli, positions or situations that provoke symptoms such as dizziness and nausea
Example of programme and progression	Start with wider base of support (e.g. standing with feet at shoulder width apart) and eyes open, performing head movement Progress to an unstable base of support such as a foam mat or a wobble board and eyes closed (crucial for training the vestibular system)	Start at 5 minutes 5 days per week (or current comfortable level) Increase by 5 minutes per week Goal to walk outdoors for 30 minutes, 5 days per week or an alternative realistic goal for the individual	Start with a target of a large letter (e.g. 18 font) Maintain visual fixation on the target for 20 seconds with slow head movement (e.g. 15 turns in 20 seconds) Progress to smaller targets, patterned background with a longer duration (60–90 seconds) at a speed of one turn per second Older people may progress from a seated to a standing position	Identify 2–3 movements or stimuli that provoke mild to moderate symptoms Repeat these for short periods several times per day until symptoms reduce Identify the next most challenging movements or stimuli and repeat

53 REHABILITATION IN DEMENTIA

Facilitating Increased Physical Activity

Recommended for all older adults:

➢ Aerobic activity: 5 days/week for 30 minutes moderate intensity for fitness
➢ Muscle strengthening: 2–3 days/week major muscle group strengthening
➢ Balance activity: 2–3 days/week to reduce risk of falls
➢ Flexibility activity: 2–3 days/week to maintain mobility

Enjoyable	• Exercise activity enjoyed by individual • Fun activities
Environment is positive	• Accepting and normalising • Positive emotional experience
Expectations are realistic	• Meet current level of function • Low frustration
Familiar	• Access implicit memory • Draw on past experiences
Procedural	• Reinforce activities of daily living • Practise basic functional movements
Problem-solving	• Identify reasons for poor participation • Adapt approach
Rest periods	• Recovery periods to sustain exercise • Encourage social interaction during break
Structured routine	• Consistent time and location • Predictable routine
Social support	• Positive interactions • Cognitively intact exercise partner

54 REHABILITATION IN PERIPHERAL VASCULAR DISEASE

Guidance on the Rehabilitation of Older Patients After Surgery

Pain	Pain will undermine any rehabilitation intervention. Pain medication should be used effectively, and timed to allow maximum utilisation of its effects during therapy Different types of pain (e.g. surgical, reperfusion, neuropathic) will require different pain control
Postural hypotension	Characterised by feeling lightheaded on standing. Fluids, early mobility, graded and regular changes to position, and medication review will help
Mobility	Early mobility should be encouraged as soon as feasible after surgery, in order to avoid deconditioning
Communication	Clear expectation-setting, postoperative instructions and goal-setting are essential
Multidisciplinary approach	Necessary to formulate treatment plans, goal attainment, lifestyle management and plan safe discharge
Lifestyle management	Holistic lifestyle management interventions should be addressed, e.g. nutrition, wound care, diabetes control, smoking cessation, promoting increased activity/participation

67 CARE PLANNING MEETINGS

Roles and Responsibilities for Care Planning Meetings

DISCIPLINE	PRE-MEETING PREPARATION	MEETING ROLE(S)
Specialist physician Junior medical staff Advanced nurse practitioner Physician assistant	Get up-to-date information on medical aspects of each patient (e.g. results of investigations, feedback from consults with other specialties) At an early stage, review past use of acute and community health services to gain an idea of problems that are likely to be encountered on discharge and to be addressed by the team as a whole	Often leads the discussion. Provides a resume of long-term and acute medical conditions, the relevant impact of these on care planning and fitness for commencing therapy or discharge Makes a note of instances where early senior clinical liaison with patients/family is required to allay anxieties or differences of opinion over care planning direction and potentially may require referral for second opinions
Ward nurse	Gets relevant ward documentation ready or receives a direct handover from assigned nurses for each patient regarding current levels of mobility and function, identification of any issues with skin integrity, feeding, compliance/tolerance of taking medication, toileting and continence problems, altered mood, impaired cognition and behavioural symptoms Any information gained from conversations with carers/family when visiting and that is relevant to the discharge process may also be noted in advance for the purposes of the meeting	Takes a list of nursing actions that are required for each patient, e.g. insertion/removal of urinary catheters, institution of behaviour diaries, weight charts, referrals to allied disciplines (dietetics, speech and language therapy) and may share responsibilities for ordering of equipment for discharge with the therapists or specialist discharge nurses When patients are close to discharge, they may liaise with the pharmacist to ensure medications are pre-prepared and that the most appropriate formulation of medicines is ordered and/or medicine administration systems (e.g. dosette boxes) to aid adherence
Physiotherapist Occupational therapist	Ensure there are good handovers and up-to-date information on progress with therapy Attempt to gain information on baseline physical functioning for any new patients to the facility	Highlight progress of patients, potential for improvement, need for any equipment to be arranged for eventual discharge and contribute to reviewing and revising as necessary the timescales to achieve goals and estimated discharge date Raise any difficulties with progressing therapy goals, e.g. pain or anxiety that limits progress
Social worker Specialist discharge nurse	Check for any information that might be gained from previous contact with community social workers or from contact with carers/family and which might inform on the potential obstacles to safe discharge	Highlight issues that the medical and/or therapy team might need to tackle in order to allay concerns raised by carers/family. It may also be a case of raising the need for ward nursing staff to undertake a more rigorous and systematic recording of patient behaviours before confirmation of long-term care needs can be made Take an action plan to progress discharge plans (including liaising with patient/family) if it is ascertained from the meeting that there is little scope for further medical or functional improvement
Chaplaincy Meaningful activities coordinator		Take new referrals to their service. Update on conversations with patients/carers that may influence discharge plans and end-of-life care preferences Highlight support that might be needed for carers and contribute to care plans for discharge that might help carers deal with aspects of behaviours (e.g. personal profiles for patients with dementia)
Voluntary sector		Take new referrals to services, e.g. hospital-to-home support

Top Tips for Effective Care Planning Meetings

1. Engage with patients and families at the earliest possible stage so that the multiprofessional team can be appraised of their expectations from the outset and provide some form of benchmark to progress care or discuss alternative options.

2. The various disciplines should try and prepare in advance for the meetings so that discussions can be progressed at a reasonable pace and there are fewer 'unknowns' which can limit the scope of discussions.

3. Physicians should review each patient's past use of acute and community medical services to gain an idea of potential instabilities with their medical status, social/functional status or aberrant health-seeking behaviours. This may highlight problems that are likely to be encountered on discharge and indicate steps that the multiprofessional team could put in place to mitigate anticipated problems.

4. Where it becomes apparent that patient/family preferences for discharge are at variance with the judgements of the multiprofessional team, do not spend too long debating the validity of each side but instead ascertain whether the 'next step' is an allocated member of the team going to discuss these issues one-to-one or whether it will require a wider case conference to be organised.

5. Where differences in opinion exist over the discharge care plans, it needs to be borne in mind that information gathering from the time on the ward may not yet be sufficient to give the complete picture. For example, behaviour charts may not be filled in with enough detail, or there may be factors relevant to the home environment of the individual that might pose hazards to mobility, which can only be gleaned from talking to family/carers. Equally where there are concerns about behavioural symptoms observed on the ward there needs to be an understanding that sometimes it is the unfamiliar and 'distressing' environment of the ward that is responsible for behavioural manifestations and that these may not be as much of a concern in the more familiar environment of their own home.

6. The physician/advanced nurse practitioner/physician associate should expect to be frequently involved in discussions with patients and family, not least to see these as opportunities to discuss advance care plans, patient preferences for future care and treatment escalation plans.

7. All team members should be given some training and empowered to voice opinions on whether an individual patient might be suitable for supportive/palliative discharge planning and have treatment escalation plans/advance care plans put in place. This is formative for the various team members, increases the collaboration of the team and allows for peer review and cross-checking of decision-making.

70 INFORMAL CARE

Ears, Eyes and Mouth

	CARER CONSIDERATIONS	PROFESSIONAL INVOLVEMENT
Dentures	Prioritise wearing at mealtimes, social events, appointments	May need new fitting Examination of gums if painful
Hearing aids	When do they like to have their aids turned on (and off)?	Demonstration of how to turn on, clean and change battery. Ask about use
Glasses	Prompt to wear, offer things of interest to them to read and look at	Up-to-date prescription Inform optician if cognitive impairment; consultation can be adapted

Food and Drink

	CARER CONSIDERATIONS	PROFESSIONAL INVOLVEMENT
Interest in food	Involve in preparation, make an old favourite together When and where did they used to like to eat? Encourage autonomy, give options	Exclude constipation Exclude depression
Small appetite	Do not rush a meal, leave plate on table Offer to reheat if going cold	Large volume of tablets or supplements may be off-putting; review to reduce non-essential medication and timings
Confusion	Try finger foods, simple table setting	

Continence

	CARER CONSIDERATIONS	PROFESSIONAL INVOLVEMENT
Confusion around toileting	Explain what is happening whenever help needed to go to the toilet Prompt to use bathroom regularly, even if wearing pads Change incontinence pads in toilet area Remind them they are on a toilet (may think it is a normal chair)	Medication review: drugs contributing to constipation or incontinence

(Continued)

	CARER CONSIDERATIONS	PROFESSIONAL INVOLVEMENT
Constipation	If no bowel output for more than a day or two, think about using a laxative Exercise Ensure plenty of fluid and fibre in diet	Laxative advice

Skin

	CARER CONSIDERATIONS	PROFESSIONAL INVOLVEMENT
Dry skin	Are they drinking enough? Use a simple moisturiser (and as soap substitute). Do not use bubble bath or shower gel	Community nursing team/ GP to advise on skin regimen
Nutrition	Eating easy-to-eat carbohydrates only? Prioritise protein and fat in meals	Dietician advice Speech and language therapists if swallow changing
Incontinence and moisture	Use barrier sprays and creams twice a day on moisture areas Do not use talcum powder	Skin regime advice
Pressure (on any prominence that takes weight, e.g. heel, bottom, shoulder)	Plan for periods of immobility – are pressure cushions and mattresses needed? If mobility worsening, ask for help Check pressure areas twice a day Change position regularly	Ongoing input, i.e. community nurses and occupational therapists to keep person and caregiver well

Sleep

	CARER CONSIDERATIONS	PROFESSIONAL INVOLVEMENT
Restlessness	Check for pain Check not struggling with toileting	Medical review for physical precipitant
Anxiety	Talk about worries and with reassurance in the day	Mood assessment to exclude depression or anxiety as underlying cause of sleeplessness
Set up for the night during the day	Activity during the day, bedtime routine	
Carer fatigue	Seek help where possible	Assess health needs of the carer, arrange respite

Cognition

	CARER CONSIDERATIONS	PROFESSIONAL INVOLVEMENT
Communication	Everyone should avoid talking about the person as if they are not present – may add to confusion and fear Explain what you are doing even if uncertain they are listening	In new confusion review for physical causes
Orientation	Maintain routines, orientate in activities: "good morning, this is breakfast" Keep clock and calendar in room	
Behaviour that challenges	Avoid argument and taking behaviour personally Seek support Exclude causes of distress that they may be unable to express: pain, hunger, thirst, constipation	Carer support Respite

72 CONTINUING REHABILITATION AT HOME

Falls Prevention

- NHS information on falls section. www.nhsinform.scot/aboutfalls
- Falls Assistant: Use to check your own risk of falls and create a personalised plan. www.fallsassistant.org.uk
- Take the balance challenge and try the 'super six' balance exercises to reduce risk of falls. http://www.knowledge.scot.nhs.uk/fallsandbonehealth/the-national-falls-programme/take-the-balance-challenge.aspx
- Later Life Training UK: Instructor training courses for health professionals and exercise professionals including Otago leader training and postural stability instructor training. www.laterlifetraining.co.uk
- CSP Falls prevention advice and exercises. www.csp.org.uk/public-patient/keeping-active-and-healthy/staying-healthy-you-age

Physical Activity

Make Every Contact count: Training for health professionals to introduce behaviour change techniques during patient interactions. www.makingeverycontactcount.com

- Faculty of Sports & Exercise Medicine UK in partnership with Public Health England and Sport England. Support for health professionals and patients. www.movingmedicine.ac.uk/

- NHS UK: Information on ways to try and achieve recommended physical activity guidelines. https://www.nhs.uk/live-well/exercise/physical-activity-guidelines-older-adults/
- Royal Society of Osteoporosis UK: Information on bone health and osteoporosis, including a series of fact sheets and exercise videos to improve bone health. https://theros.org.uk/

Apps and Games

- **Otago classic app.** Inexpensive app to download. Consists of leg strength and balance exercises designed to reduce falls in older adults who have already had a fall or are at risk of falls. Has videos and audio commentary.
- **Clock Yourself app.** Inexpensive app to download. Consists of progressively challenging balance and cognitive tasks to improve balance reaction times and cognitive function. Can be practised in any safe environment. www.Clockyourself.physio/

74 ADVANCE CARE PLANNING AND REHABILITATION

Example of an advance care plan (derived from the New Zealand ACP Programme. ACP Cooperative 2016. My Advance Care Plan and Guide. Gerontology Nursing Service, Waitemata District Health Board. Available at: https://www.hqsc.govt.nz/assets/ACP/PR/ACP_Plan_print_.pdf)

ADVANCE CARE PLAN

My Details	My Enduring Power of Attorney
Name	Name
Address	Address
Date of birth	Telephone
Telephone	Relationship

Please try to include the following people in decisions about my care

Name	Name
Address	Address
Telephone	Telephone
Relationship	Relationship

What matters to me?

In this section include items like:
- What makes you happy?
- How you like to spend your time?
- Any routines you like

ADVANCE CARE PLAN

My Details	My Enduring Power of Attorney

What worries me?

In this section examples may include:
- How your health might affect your future
- How your heath might affect your family
- Being a burden
- Dying alone

Why am I making an advance care plan?

In this section some things to think about include:
- What illnesses have you had and what could happen to you?
- Does your health stop you from doing some day-to day activities?
- Do you have any health conditions that you are getting treatment for?

As I am dying, my quality of life means:

Consider what quality of life may mean to you at that stage of your life:
- Being aware and thinking for yourself
- Communicating with people who are important to you
- Where is your preferred place of death?

Specific treatment and care preferences:

These expressed preferences should be used to guide clinical decisions in the circumstances I have set out below:

I would/would not want:	In these circumstances:

When I am dying, please consider:

Things to consider
- Let the people who are important to me be with me
- Place of preferred death
- Taking out things, like tubes, that do not add to your comfort
- Stopping medications and treatments that do not add to your comfort
- Religious, cultural and/or spiritual needs

After my death, I would like:

Things to consider include
- Preferences for your death announcement
- Ideas or preferences for your funeral or farewell
- Organ donation
- Last resting place

(Continued)

ADVANCE CARE PLAN
My Details

Signatures
By signing below, I confirm:
- I understand this is a record of my preferences to guide my healthcare team in providing appropriate care for me when I am unable to speak for myself.
- I understand treatments that would not benefit me will not be provided even if I have asked for them.
- I agree that this advance care plan can be made available to all healthcare providers caring for me.

Name
Signature
Date

My Enduring Power of Attorney

By signing below the healthcare professional confirms that:

I am competent at the time I created this advance care plan.

We discussed my health and the care choices I might face.

I have made my advance care plan with adequate information.

I made the choices in my advance care plan voluntarily.

Name
Signature
Date
Title
Telephone

MCQ ANSWERS

CHAPTER 1

1 c
2 e

CHAPTER 2

1 c
2 e
3 d

CHAPTER 3

1 e
2 d

CHAPTER 4

1 d
2 e
3 c and e

CHAPTER 5

1 d
2 b

CHAPTER 6

1 c
2 d
3 c

CHAPTER 8

1 d
2 b

CHAPTER 9

1 d
2 b

CHAPTER 10

1 d
2 b

CHAPTER 11

1 a
2 d
3 d

CHAPTER 12

1 c
2 b
3 c

CHAPTER 13

1 e
2 e

CHAPTER 14

1 e
2 b
3 c

CHAPTER 15

1 d
2 d

CHAPTER 16

1 b
2 d

CHAPTER 17

1 a
2 d
3 c

CHAPTER 18

1 e
2 d

CHAPTER 19

1 e
2 e

CHAPTER 20

1 b
2 d

CHAPTER 21

1 c and d
2 e

CHAPTER 22

1 a
2 c

CHAPTER 23

1 c
2 e

CHAPTER 24

1 a
2 b

CHAPTER 25

1 b
2 b
3 d

CHAPTER 26

1 e
2 c
3 d

CHAPTER 27

1 b
2 d
3 e

CHAPTER 28

1 c
2 b

CHAPTER 29

1 c
2 a

CHAPTER 30

1 d
2 c

CHAPTER 31

1 b
2 d
3 d

CHAPTER 32

1 d
2 d
3 a

CHAPTER 33

1 a
2 d

CHAPTER 34

1 b
2 e

CHAPTER 35

1 c
2 b
3 e

CHAPTER 36

1 d
2 b

CHAPTER 37

1 e
2 b

CHAPTER 38

1 b
2 e
3 d

CHAPTER 39

1 b
2 a
3 c

CHAPTER 40

1 a
2 c

CHAPTER 41

1 c
2 e

CHAPTER 42

1 b
2 d
3 c

CHAPTER 43

1 d
2 e

CHAPTER 44

1 c
2 d

CHAPTER 45

1 b
2 b

CHAPTER 46

1 c
2 d
3 d

CHAPTER 47

1 e
2 c

CHAPTER 48

1 c
2 b

CHAPTER 49

1 a
2 b

CHAPTER 50

1 c
2 b
3 d

CHAPTER 51

1 e
2 b
3 a

CHAPTER 52

1 b
2 b
3 b

CHAPTER 53

1 a
2 c
3 a

CHAPTER 54

1 b
2 e

CHAPTER 55

1 e
2 d
3 e

CHAPTER 56

1 c
2 e

CHAPTER 57

1 d
2 b
3 e

CHAPTER 58

1 b
2 d
3 c

CHAPTER 59

1 c
2 d

CHAPTER 60

1 d
2 d
3 e

CHAPTER 61

1 b
2 c
3 d

CHAPTER 62

1 e
2 c

CHAPTER 63

1 b
2 c

CHAPTER 64

1 d
2 c
3 a

CHAPTER 65

1 e
2 c

CHAPTER 66

1 e
2 a

CHAPTER 67

1 a
2 c

CHAPTER 68

1 b
2 d
3 d

CHAPTER 69

1 e
2 b
3 e

CHAPTER 71

1 b
2 d

CHAPTER 72

1 b
2 a

CHAPTER 73

1 c
2 d

CHAPTER 74

1 a
2 e

CHAPTER 75

1 d
2 e
3 c

INDEX

Note: Page numbers followed by "*b*", "*f*" and "*t*" refer to boxes, figures and tables, respectively.